Microsurgery for Cerebral Ischemia

Microsurgery for Cerebral Ischemia

Edited by

S. J. Peerless and **C. W. McCormick**
University of Western Ontario

With 282 Illustrations

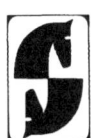

Springer-Verlag
New York   Heidelberg   Berlin

S. J. Peerless, M.D., F.R.C.S.(C)
Professor of Neurosurgery
University of Western Ontario
Chairman, Division of Neurosurgery
Department of Clinical Neurological Sciences
University Hospital
London, Ontario, Canada

C. W. McCormick, M.D., F.R.C.P.(C)
Assistant Professor of Neurology
Department of Clinical Neurological Sciences
University Hospital
London, Ontario, Canada

Library of Congress Cataloging in Publication Data

Main entry under title:
Microsurgery for cerebral ischemia.

   Papers delivered at a symposium held at
University Hospital, London, Ont., Sept. 1978.
   Bibliography: p.
   Includes index.
   1. Cerebral ischemia—Surgery—Congresses.
2. Cerebral arteries—Surgery—Congresses.
3. Microsurgery—Congresses. I. Peerless, Soja
John. II. McCormick, C. W. [DNLM: 1. Cerebral
ischemia—Surgery. 2. Microsurgery. WL355 M6266]
RD594.2.M5   617'.481'059   80-18123

© 1980 by Springer-Verlag New York Inc.

9 8 7 6 5 4 3 2 1

ISBN-13: 978-1-4612-6092-9   e-ISBN-13: 978-1-4612-6090-5
DOI: 10.1007/978-1-4612-6090-5

Contents

Preface

In June 1973, Professor George Austin invited a small group of neuroscientists from Asia, Europe, the United States, and Canada to the Loma Linda University School of Medicine in Loma Linda, California. The fundamental technique of fashioning a small vessel collateral to the brain had been pioneered by Donaghy and Yasargil 5 years before and was now gaining momentum with the increased availability of the operating microscope, fine instruments and sutures, and surgeons trained in microvascular surgery.

The interchange of ideas at this first conference was magic. The handful of participants returned home stimulated with new ideas of technique, patient selection, and postoperative evaluation and resolved to meet again on a regular basis. A Second International Symposium was hosted by Howard Reichman at Loyola University in Chicago, Illinois in June of 1974; a Third Symposium at Rottach-Egern, West Germany in June of 1976 under Professor F. Marguth of the Ludwig-Maximilians-University of Munich.

The Fourth Symposium was hosted by the Department of Clinical Neurological Sciences of the University of Western Ontario, London, Ontario, Canada in September 1978, and this volume is based on the proceedings. More than 200 participants from around the world contributed to this Symposium with many more papers submitted for presentation than could be accommodated in the 2½-day meeting. It was apparent from the sophisticated presentations on brain metabolism, cerebral blood flow, surgical techniques, and patient selection and evaluation that the operation of microvascular anastomosis for cerebral revascularization had come a long way in the 9 years since the first Symposium and was more than simply an elegant technical exercise with an uncertain clinical application.

It was significant, we believe, that this Fourth Symposium was held in conjunction with the first Workshop of the International Cooperative EC–IC Bypass Study. Neurologists and neurosurgeons from more than 50 centers around the world came together in London to discuss the workings of the Bypass Study, a collaborative effort funded by the National Institutes of Health to evaluate the efficacy of cerebral revascularization in a scientific way. This randomized study of matched medically and surgically treated groups was designed to answer the question, "Can microvascular anastomosis reduce the incidence of stroke by 50% or more during the period of follow-up?". Clearly, this is a question of considerable significance during our current epidemic of atherosclerosis. Perhaps the Sixth Conference will be devoted to a spirited discussion of the results of this Study.

The Editors wish to express their appreciation to the Symposium participants for their contributions, as well as, to Mrs. Barbara Valberg who graciously assumed the burden of planning and running the conference and to Heather Carter, Iain Hunter and Michael Peerless for their cheerful secretarial and editorial assistance in assembling this volume.

S.J. Peerless
C.W. McCormick

Contributors

J.M. ALLCOCK, University Hospital, London, Ontario, Canada, *Chapter 23*

A. ANYAI, Nervenklinik der Universitat, Gottingen, West Germany, *Chapter 32*

O. ARENA, Ospedale Maggiore Niguarda, Milan, Italy, *Chapters 13, 24, 25*

K.-E. ARFORS, Department of Experimental Medicine, Pharmacia, Uppsala, Sweden, *Chapter 4*

L.M. AUER, University Clinic for Neurosurgery, Graz, Austria, *Chapter 47*

J.I. AUSMAN, Henry Ford Hospital, Detroit, Michigan, U.S.A., *Chapters 21, 22, 49, 55*

G. AUSTIN, Loma Linda University School of Medicine, Loma Linda, California, U.S.A., *Chapter 7*

W.H. BAKER, Loyola University Medical Center, Maywood, Illinois, U.S.A., *Chapter 16*

C.M. BANNISTER, North Manchester General Hospital, Manchester, England, *Chapter 36*

A. BEDUSCHI, Ospedale Maggiore Niguarda, Milan, Italy, *Chapter 13*

R. BELL, The University of Texas Southwestern Medical School, Dallas, Texas, U.S.A., *Chapter 3*

C.W. BEYER, Jr. The University of Texas Southwestern Medical School, Dallas, Texas, U.S.A., *Chapter 3*

U.W. BLAUENSTEIN, University of Alabama Medical Center, Birmingham, Alabama, U.S.A., *Chapter 9*

S.C. BOONE, North Carolina Memorial Hospital, Chapel Hill, North Carolina, U.S.A., *Chapter 46*

R.M. BORGIA, Ospedale Maggiore Niguarda, Milan, Italy, *Chapter 24*

M.L. BREAM, University Hospital, London, Ontario, Canada, *Chapter 37*

P. BRET, Hôpital Neurologique, Lyon, France, *Chapter 53*

J. CAPDEVILLE, Hôpital Neurologique, Lyon, France, *Chapter 53*

L.P. CARTER, St. Joseph's Hospital and Medical Center, Phoenix, Arizona, U.S.A., *Chapter 8*

S.A. CHAPMAN, North Manchester General Hospital, Manchester, England, *Chapter 36*

N.L. CHATER, Ralph K. Davies Medical Center, San Francisco, California, U.S.A., *Chapters 33, 49, 54*

M. COLLICE, Ospedale Maggiore Niguarda, Milan, Italy, *Chapters 24, 25*

P.W. COOPER, Sunnybrook Medical Centre, Toronto, Ontario, Canada, *Chapter 10*

R.M. CROWELL, Massachusetts General Hospital, Boston, Massachusetts, U.S.A., *Chapter 28*

U. DE GIROLAMI, University of Massachusetts Medical School, Worcester, Massachusetts, U.S.A., *Chapter 28*

R.F. DEL MAESTRO, University Hospitals, Cleveland, Ohio, U.S.A., *Chapter 4*

R. DERUTY, Hôpital Neurologique, Lyon, France, *Chapter 53*

F.G. DIAZ, Henry Ford Hospital, Detroit, Michigan, U.S.A., *Chapters 21, 55*

M. DUJOVNY, Veterans Administration Hospital, Pittsburgh, Pennsylvania, U.S.A., *Chapter 30*

R.J. ERSPAMER, St. Joseph's Hospital and Medical Center, Phoenix, Arizona, U.S.A., *Chapter 8*

F. FAZIO, Hammersmith Hospital, London, England, *Chapters 13, 25*

J.M. FEIN, Albert Einstein College of Medicine, Bronx, New York, U.S.A., *Chapters 6, 38*

W. FEINDEL, Montreal Neurological Institute, Montreal, Quebec, Canada, *Chapters 11, 12*

A. FENSKE, Klinik fur Neurologie, Johannes Gutenberg Universität, Mainz, West Germany, *Chapter 14*

G.G. FERGUSON, University Hospital, London, Ontario, Canada, *Chapter 37*

C. FIESCHI, Clinica Neurologica Universita, Rome, Italy, *Chapter 13*

S. FITZGIBBON, Massachusetts General Hospital, Boston, Massachusetts, U.S.A., *Chapter 28*

A.J. FOX, University Hospital, London, Ontario, Canada, *Chapter 23*

W.A. FRIEDMAN, University of Florida Medical Center, Gainesville, Florida, U.S.A., *Chapter 40*

W. GEE, Allentown and Sacred Heart Hospital Center, Allentown, Pennsylvania, U.S.A., *Chapter 18*

C.W. GOMES, Veterans Administration Hospital, Pittsburgh, Pennsylvania, U.S.A., *Chapter 30*

O. GRATZL, Neurochirurgische Universitätsklinik, Munich, West Germany, *Chapters 26, 41, 45*

V.C. HACHINSKI, Sunnybrook Medical Centre, Toronto, Ontario, Canada, *Chapter 10*

J.H. HALSEY, University of Alabama Medical Center, Birmingham, Alabama, U.S.A., *Chapter 9*

H. HANDA, Kyoto University Hospital, Kyoto, Japan, *Chapters 17, 42*

S. HAYASHI, Massachusetts General Hospital, Boston, Massachusetts, U.S.A., *Chapter 28*

A.C. HAYES, Loyola University Medical Center, Maywood, Illinois, U.S.A., *Chapter 16*

W. HAYWARD, Loma Linda University School of Medicine, Loma Linda, California, U.S.A., *Chapter 7*

M.P. HEILBRUN, University of Utah Medical Center, Salt Lake City, Utah, U.S.A., *Chapter 50*

F. HEPPNER, University Clinic for Neurosurgery, Graz, Austria, *Chapter 47*

R.C. HEROS, Presbyterian University Hospital, Pittsburgh, Pennsylvania, U.S.A., *Chapter 51*

C.P. HODGE, Neurological Institute and McGill University, Montreal, Quebec, Canada, *Chapters 11, 12*

W.F. HOFFMAN, R.K. Davies Medical Center, San Francisco, California, U.S.A.,
Chapter 54

K.-H. HOLBACH, Neurochirurgische Universitätsklinik, Bonn, West Germany,
Chapters 19, 44

P. HOOGLAND, Ursula Clinic, Wassenaar, Holland, *Chapter 29*

Z. ITO, Research Institute of Brain and Blood Vessels, Akita, Japan, *Chapter 20*

M.J. JERVA, Mercy Hospital and Medical Center, Chicago, Illinois, U.S.A.,
Chapter 43

T.H. JONES, Massachusetts General Hospital, Boston, Massachusetts, U.S.A.,
Chapter 28

E. KAZNER, Neurochirurgische Universitätsklinik, Munich, West Germany,
Chapter 26

H.M. KELLER, University Hospital, Zurich, Switzerland, *Chapter 15*

G. KHODADAD, Veterans Administration Hospital, Cincinnati, Ohio, U.S.A.,
Chapter 48

C.F. KIECK, Massachusetts General Hospital, Boston, Massachusetts, U.S.A.,
Chapter 28

A.C. KLASSEN, University of Minnesota Hospitals, Minneapolis, Minnesota,
U.S.A., *Chapter 55*

G. KLETTER, Neurochirurgische Universitätsklinik, Vienna, Austria, *Chapter
32*

N. KOSSOVSKY, Veterans Administration Hospital, Pittsburgh, Pennsylvania,
U.S.A., *Chapter 30*

R.K. LAHA, Veterans Administration Hospital, Pittsburgh, Pennsylvania, U.S.A.,
Chapter 30

R.E. LATCHAW, University of Minnesota Hospitals, Minneapolis, Minnesota,
U.S.A., *Chapters 22, 55*

B.E. LAUX, Washington University School of Medicine, St. Louis, Missouri,
U.S.A., *Chapter 1*

D. LEACHEM, Kantonsspital, Basel, Switzerland, *Chapter 41*

J. LECUIRE, Hôpital Neurologique, Lyon, France, *Chapter 53*

M.C. LEE, University of Minnesota Hospitals, Minneapolis, Minnesota, U.S.A.,
Chapters 22, 55

L. LEFF, Veterans Administration Hospital, Pittsburgh, Pennsylvania, U.S.A.,
Chapter 30

E. LICHTER, Loma Linda University School of Medicine, Loma Linda, California, U.S.A., *Chapter 7*

J.R. LITTLE, Montreal Neurological Hospital, Montreal, Quebec, Canada,
Chapter 11

U. LUETOLF, University Hospital, Zurich, Switzerland, *Chapter 15*

A.E. MADDEN, Allentown and Sacred Heart Hospital Center, Allentown,
Pennsylvania, U.S.A., *Chapter 18*

F. MARGUTH, Neurochirurgische Universitätsklinik, Munich, West Germany,
Chapter 41

I. MATSUDA, Kyoto University Medical School, Kyoto, Japan, *Chapter 17*

M. MAYHOOD, The University of Texas Southwestern Medical School, Dallas,
Texas, U.S.A., *Chapter 3*

H.M. MEHDORN, The University Hospital of San Francisco, San Francisco,
California, U.S.A., *Chapters 5, 33–35, 54*

G. MEINIG, Klinik für Neurologie, Johannes Gutenberg Universität, Mainz,
West Germany, *Chapter 14*

E. MEYER, Montreal Neurological Institute and McGill University, Montreal, Quebec, Canada, *Chapter 11*

R. MEYERMANN, Nervenklinik der Universität, Göttingen, West Germany, *Chapters 31, 32*

A.L. MILLER, Allentown and Sacred Heart Hospital Center, Allentown, Pennsylvania, U.S.A., *Chapter 18*

R.B. MORAWETZ, University of Alabama Medical Center, Birmingham, Alabama, U.S.A., *Chapter 28*

K. MORITAKE, Kyoto University Medical School, Kyoto, Japan, *Chapter 17*

I. NAGATA, Kyoto University Medical School, Kyoto, Japan, *Chapter 17*

M. NARDINI, Department of Neurology, University of Siena, Italy, *Chapter 13*

D. NELSON, Veterans Administration Hospital, Pittsburgh, Pennsylvania, U.S.A., *Chapter 30*

P.N. NELSON, Presbyterian University Hospital, Pittsburgh, Pennsylvania, U.S.A., *Chapter 51*

M. NISHIKAWA, Department of Neurosurgery, University of Zurich, Switzerland, *Chapter 31*

J.W. NORRIS, Sunnybrook Medical Centre, Toronto, Ontario, Canada, *Chapter 10*

A. OKUMURA, Kyoto University Medical School, Kyoto, Japan, *Chapter 17*

V. OLTEANU-NERBE, Neurochirurgische Universitatsklinik, Munich, West Germany, *Chapters 26, 41, 45*

H. ORTEGON, Centro Medico Osler, Monterrey, Mexico, *Chapter 12*

R.B. PHILP, University Hospital, London, Ontario, Canada, *Chapter 37*

C. PINI, Nervenklinik der Universität, Göttingen, West Germany, *Chapter 32*

N. PINTOZZI, Mercy Hospital and Medical Center, Chicago, Illinois, U.S.A., *Chapter 43*

M. POSSA, Department of Neurology, University of Rome, Italy, *Chapter 25*

M.E. RAICHLE, Washington University School of Medicine, St. Louis, Missouri, U.S.A., *Chapters 1, 2*

O.H. REICHMAN, Loyola University Medical Center, Maywood, Illinois, U.S.A., *Chapter 16*

A.L. RHOTON, Jr., University of Florida Medical Center, Gainesville, Florida, U.S.A., *Chapter 40*

D.W. ROWED, Sunnybrook Medical Centre, Toronto, Ontario, Canada, *Chapter 10*

D.S. SAMSON, University of Texas, Dallas, Texas, U.S.A., *Chapter 3*

P. SCHMIEDEK, Neurochirurgische Universitätsklinik, Munich, West Germany, *Chapters 26, 41, 45*

K. SCHÜRMANN, Department of Neurosurgery, University of Mainz, West Germany, *Chapter 14*

G. SCIALFA, Ospedale Maggiore Niguarda, Milan, Italy, *Chapter 24*

W. SELMAN, University Hospitals, Cleveland, Ohio, U.S.A., *Chapter 5*

D. SHAW, Royal Victoria Infirmary, Newcastle-upon-Tyne, England, *Chapter 52*

J. SLOOF, Ursula Clinic, Wassenaar, Holland, *Chapter 29*

R. SPETZLER, University Hospitals, Cleveland, Ohio, U.S.A., *Chapters 5, 35*

F. SPINELLI, Ospedale Maggiore Niguarda, Milan, Italy, *Chapter 13*

H.W. STEPHENS, Allentown and Sacred Heart Hospital Center, Allentown, Pennsylvania, U.S.A., *Chapters 18, 39*

A. SUZUKI, Research Institute of Brain and Blood Vessels, Akita, Japan, *Chapter 20*

D.A. TELLES, University Hospitals, Cleveland, Ohio, U.S.A., *Chapters 5, 34, 35*

M. TERANO, Kyoto University Hospital, Kyoto, Japan, *Chapter 42*

T. TERAURA, Kyoto University Hospital, Kyoto, Japan, *Chapter 42*

J.J. TOWNSEND, University Hospitals, Cleveland, Ohio, U.S.A., *Chapters 5, 33*

C.A.F. TULLEKEN, Ursula Clinic, Wassenaar, Holland, *Chapter 29*

F. VALSECCHI, Ospedale Maggiore Niguarda, Milan, Italy, *Chapter 24*

M.I. VILAGHY, Sunnybrook Medical Centre, Toronto, Ontario, Canada, *Chapter 10*

N. WACKENHUT, Veterans Administration Hospital, Pittsburgh, Pennsylvania, U.S.A., *Chapter 30*

M.M. WADDINGTON, Rutland Hospital, Rutland, Vermont, U.S.A., *Chapter 27*

H. WASSMANN, Neurochirurgische Universitätsklinik, Bonn, West Germany, *Chapter 19*

P.R. WEINSTEIN, University of California Medical Center, San Francisco, California, U.S.A., *Chapters 5, 33–35*

G.E. WHITEHOUSE, Allentown and Sacred Heart Hospital Center, Allentown, Pennsylvania, U.S.A., *Chapter 18*

E.L. WILLS, University of Alabama Medical Center, Birmingham, Alabama, U.S.A., *Chapter 9*

E.M. WILSON, University of Alabama Medical Center, Birmingham, Alabama, U.S.A., *Chapter 9*

Y.L. YAMAMOTO, Neurological Institute and McGill University, Montreal, Quebec, Canada, *Chapters 11, 12*

M.G. YASARGIL, Department of Neurosurgery, University of Zurich, Switzerland, *Chapter 31*

Y. YONEKAWA, Kyoto University Hospital, Kyoto, Japan, *Chapter 42*

D. ZINKE, Loma Linda University School of Medicine, Loma Linda, California, U.S.A., *Chapter 7*

B. ZUMSTEIN, University Hospital, Zurich, Switzerland, *Chapter 15*

I

Lectures by Dr. M. E. Raichle
(Honored Guest of Symposium)

1

Role of Erythrocyte Carbonic Anhydrase in Oxygen Delivery to Brain*

M. E. Raichle and B. E. Laux

The brain is critically dependent for its moment-to-moment function and survival on an adequate supply of oxygen. Because the amount of oxygen stored within the tissue is low, factors concerned with oxygen availability become of paramount importance. These factors include an adequate and responsive blood supply, an adequate oxygen-carrying capacity of the blood, and adequate oxygenation of circulating blood. It is, indeed, the purpose of this conference to focus on the first of these factors, namely, local derangements of cerebral blood flow (CBF) caused by narrowing or occlusion of major cerebral blood vessels.

One aspect of oxygen delivery to the brain which has received little attention in recent years has been the manner in which oxygen is released from hemoglobin on its passage through the cerebral microcirculation. Only recently, through work in other vascular beds,[2] has it become evident that critical time-dependent relationships may exist in the release of oxygen to tissue involving the enzyme carbonic anhydrase (EC 4.2.1.1). It is the purpose of this communication to focus on the role of erythrocyte carbonic anhydrase as it may influence oxygen delivery to the brain.

The enzyme carbonic anhydrase may play an important role in oxygen delivery to brain tissue by facilitating the hydration of metabolically produced carbon dioxide and erythrocytes in brain capillaries, thus permitting the Bohr effect to occur. We have examined the effect of intravenous acetazolamide (30 mg/kg), a potent inhibitor of carbonic anhydrase, upon CBF and oxygen consumption in lightly anesthetized, passively ventilated rhesus monkeys. Details of our experimental setup are presented elsewhere.[4] Cerebral blood flow and oxygen consumption were measured with oxygen-15 labeled water and oxygen-15 labeled hemoglobin,[6] respectively, injected into the internal carotid artery and monitored externally.

The intravenous administration of acetazolamide produced an immediate and significant increase in CBF and an increase in arterial carbon dioxide tension ($PaCO_2$) (Fig. 1-1). The changes in CBF and $PaCO_2$ were accompanied by a significant decrease in cerebral oxygen consumption (Fig. 1-2).

Our study indicates that intravenous acetazolamide in healthy, lightly anesthetized rhesus monkeys produces a significant reduction in cerebral oxygen consumption. This effect occurs within minutes of acetazolamide administration, which is consistent with the 3-minute in-vitro equilibration time between red cell carbonic anhydrase and acetazolamide reported by Maren et al.[3] Furthermore, these data suggest that the effect may in fact be primarily achieved through an effect of acetazolamide on the erythrocyte carbonic anhydrase, since it is unlikely that a significant amount of the drug can cross the blood-brain barrier in this

*This work was supported by U.S. Public Health Service Grants 5 P01 HL 13851 and 5 P50 NS 06833.

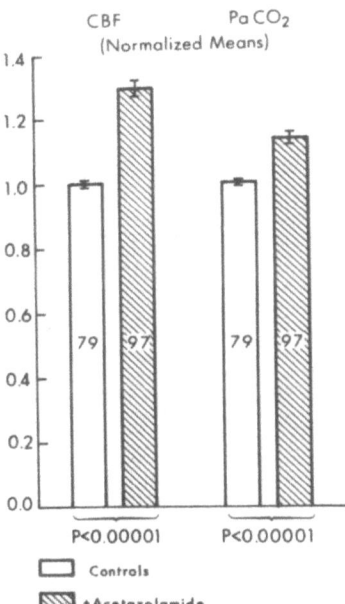

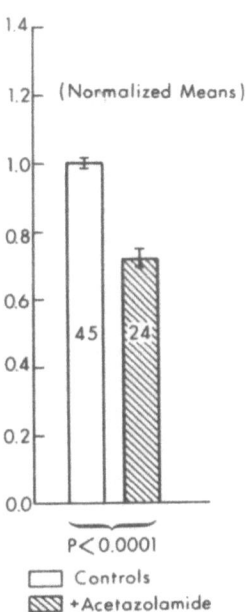

Fig. 1-1. The change in mean cerebral blood flow (CBF) and mean arterial carbon dioxide tension (PaCO$_2$) following IV acetazolamide in rhesus monkeys. The data for these and subsequent histograms have been normalized so that the mean control is 1.0, by dividing the control and experimental data points of each experiment by the mean of the control points for that experiment. The actual mean control CBF was 64.7 ml/100 g/min, and the mean control PaCO$_2$ was 40.7 torr. The number of data points are shown on the bars. The error bars are equal to 2 SEM.

Fig. 1-2. The effect of IV acetazolamide on the cerebral metabolic rate for oxygen (CMRO$_2$). The mean control CMRO$_2$ was 4.16 ml/100 g/min.

time. This is supported by the observation of Roth, Schoolar, and Barlow,[5] who have reported that the entry of ^{35}S-acetazolamide into cat brain has a time course in hours at a dosage level of 150 mg/kg.

If the acetazolamide effect on cerebral oxygen consumption is localized to the blood, what is its mechanism? As has previously been suggested by Cotev et al.,[1] carbonic anhydrase inhibition should interfere with the Bohr shift, the mechanism that augments oxygen release from hemoglobin by an acidic pH shift. Normally, as the oxygen-carrying red cells enter the capillaries, CO$_2$ diffuses in and is virtually instantaneously converted to H$^+$ and HCO$_3$$^-$ by carbonic anhydrase. When the carbonic anhydrase is inhibited by acetazolamide, CO$_2$ cannot convert to H$^+$ and HCO$_3$$^-$ before the blood has left the capillary. Thus the Bohr shift

does not occur and oxygen unloading is inhibited.

The hypothesis that inhibition of erythrocyte carbonic anhydrase with delayed hydration of carbon dioxide and prevention of the Bohr effect poses a significant limitation on oxygen delivery to the brain is supported by two findings in our study. First, the cerebral metabolic rate for oxygen (CMRO$_2$) measured with hemolyzed blood was 11% higher than that measured with normal blood without any carbonic anhydrase inhibition. Second, after acetazolamide was given there was no significant difference between the CMRO$_2$ measured with hemolyzed and normal blood.

We believe these data can be interpreted in the following way. In the hemolyzed blood, carbon dioxide had only to cross the vascular endothelium to achieve immediate access to erythrocyte carbonic anhydrase, which was free in plasma. Thus the time course of the Bohr effect was speeded up and oxygen delivery to the tissue improved. After acetazolamide was given, the presence of carbonic anhydrase and hemoglobin free in the plasma made no difference since the enzyme was inhibited and, thus, once the CO$_2$ crossed the capillary endothelium it still did not have enough time to be hydrated before it left the capillary. It must be emphasized that what is occurring is not caused by a change in arterial hemoglobin saturation (which was always 100%), but by a change in the unloading of oxygen from hemoglobin. This phenomenon could not be reproduced by altering inspired gas O_2 content.

These data support the hypothesis that erythrocyte carbonic anhydrase is important for oxygen delivery to brain tissue. These observations are in accord with the critical nature of the temporal and spatial relationships existing in the microvasculature for erythrocyte carbonic anhydrase as previously emphasized by the work of Forster and Crandall.[2]

It seems reasonable to suggest as a working hypothesis that acetazolamide may induce a critical reduction in tissue oxygen availability which is only partly compensated for by an increase in CBF. Further, the normal response of the cerebrovasculature to hypoxia is attenuated under these circumstances because the PO_2 remains normal in the smooth muscle of a significant portion of the cerebral resistance vasculature. Further work is clearly needed in this area.

Finally, the possibility that acetazolamide may reduce $CMRO_2$ by interfering with the oxygen unloading in the microvasculature must, if substantiated, be taken into considera-

tion in the clinical use of the drug. Thus its use in conditions such as epilepsy where oxygen delivery to the tissue may at times become critical, or in patients with cerebrovascular disease with chronic marginal oxygen delivery to the brain, may need to be reconsidered.

References

1. Cotev, S., Lee, J., Severinghaus, J.W. The effects of acetazolamide on cerebral blood flow and cerebral issue pO_2. Anesthesiology 29:471–477, 1968.
2. Forster, R.E., Crandall, E.D. Time course of exchanges between red cells and extracellular fluid during CO_2 uptake. J Appl Physiol 38:710–718, 1975.
3. Maren, T.H. Use of inhibitors in physiological studies of carbonic anhydrase. Am J Physiol 232(4):F291–F297, 1967.
4. Raichle, M.E., Eichling, J.O., Straatmann, M.G., Welch, M.J., Larson, K.B., Ter-Pogossian, M.M. Blood-brain barrier permeability of ^{11}C-labeled alcohols and ^{15}O-labeled water. Am J Physiol 230:543–552, 1976.
5. Roth, L.J., Schoolar, J.C., Barlow, C.F. Sulfur-35 labeled acetazolamide in cat brain. J Pharmacol Exp Ther 125:128–136, 1959.
6. Welch, M.J., Ter-Pogossian, M.M. Preparation of short half-lived radioactive gases for medical studies. Radiat Res 36:580–587, 1968.

2

Recent Developments in the Measurement of Cerebral Hemodynamics and Metabolism*

M. E. Raichle

Great advances have been made over the past 30 years in the development of techniques for the measurement, in vivo, of the circulation and metabolism of the human brain. The ever-present stimulus for this work has been the general realization that our understanding of disease processes affecting the human brain must ultimately be based upon a direct understanding of regional hemodynamic, biochemical, and metabolic changes. Although many models of human disease have been developed in the laboratory, investigators and clinicians are plagued by the nagging doubt that such models do not faithfully represent the disease as it occurs in humans.

Progress toward the development of a satisfactory means of obtaining biochemical, metabolic, and hemodynamic information on the human brain began with the pioneering work of Kety and Schmidt in 1948. Their introduction of the nitrous oxide technique for the measurement of cerebral blood flow (CBF)[9] when combined with arteriovenous measurements of various substrates and metabolites provided our first clear information on the relationship between substrate delivery and utilization. Although this technique was widely utilized and provided much valuable information, it suffered from the obvious flaw of not providing regional information. Dynamic regional differences in both circulation and me-

tabolism were clearly obscured, if not lost completely, by this approach. The introduction of a method for the measurement of regional CBF based on the external detection of the clearance of a freely diffusible radioactive gas, such as ^{133}Xe, from the brain by Lassen, Ingvar, and their colleagues[6] has provided much additional information on regional hemodynamics in the human brain. However, this technique precluded the measurement of regional metabolism, thus significantly reducing its capacity to provide the type of information necessary. The introduction into the medical environment of cyclotron-produced, positron-emitting radiopharmaceuticals for the measurement of brain hemodynamics and metabolism by Ter-Pogossian and his colleagues[18] partially fulfilled this need for regional metabolic information. Fairly sophisticated techniques were developed for the measurement not only of regional oxygen utilization in the human brain[16] but also of regional cerebral blood volume[5] and regional intracellular pH.[19] These techniques, however, have received only limited application, because they require the intracarotid injection of the radiopharmaceutical, as well as the presence of a cyclotron in the immediate medical environment. Thus until recently we have been unable to obtain more than a quasi-regional assessment of CBF in the human brain and, where circumstances permit, limited metabolic information.

Two significant developments move us closer to the capability of easily and safely acquiring

*This work was supported by U.S. Public Health Service Grants 5 P01 HL 13851 and 5 P50 NS 06833.

truly regional in-vivo biochemical and physiologic information in the human brain. First, the appearance within the medical environment of apparatus for nuclear bombardment such as cyclotrons and linear accelerators, coupled with ingenious techniques for rapid synthesis of radiopharmaceuticals, has provided several radiopharmaceuticals suitable for in-vivo regional hemodynamic and metabolic studies.[20] The parallel development of appropriate mathematical models has provided the basis for practical algorithms that allow parameters of physiologic significance to be estimated from the data.[11] Second, recent major developments in detection systems circumvent most of the disadvantages of conventional detection systems. These systems use the concept of emission tomography, which allows the safe, quantitative, three-dimensional measurement of radioisotope distribution in tissue.

Emission tomography, a nuclear medicine visualization technique that yields an image of the distribution of a previously administered radionuclide in any desired transverse section of the body, is in contrast to transmission tomography, where the image reflects the distribution of x-ray attenuation coefficients. The methods of data acquisition and image reconstruction in emission tomography are similar to those of transmission tomography. Conceptually, it is helpful to view emission tomography as analogous to quantitative tissue autoradiography with the added advantage of allowing in-vivo studies.

Positron Emission Tomography (PET)

Positron-emitting radionuclides are well suited for their imaging by tomography because of one physical property of these particles. This physical characteristic is the generation of annihilation radiation when positrons are annihilated in matter. A number of radionuclides decay by positron emission. These include ^{15}O (2-minute half-life), ^{13}N (10-minute half-life), ^{11}C (20-minute half-life), and ^{18}F (110-minute half-life). Positrons, which are positively charged electrons, are unstable because they include an excess of neutrons with respect to a stable state. Positrons lose their kinetic energy in matter in a manner similar to that of electrons. When positrons are brought to rest, they interact with an electron. The two particles undergo annihilation, and the mass of the two particles is converted into two photons traveling at 180° from each other with an energy of about 511 keV. This is the annihilation radiation.

The annihilation radiation can be uniquely detected by two radiation detectors connected to a coincidence circuit, which records an event only if both detectors sense the annihilation photons simultaneously. This coincidence detection of the annihilation radiation provides a method of "electronic" collimation, since the two detectors can record coincidence events only in a volume of space established by straight lines joining the two detectors. Thus, coincidence detection of the annihilation radiation provides a nearly uniform field of view (or sensitivity) in the region between the two detectors. Coincidence detection of the annihilation radiation also permits an easy, accurate correction for the attenuation of radiation in tissues. Another advantage of annihilation radiation in emission tomography is its high energy (511 keV photons), which gives it greater tissue penetration and thus better detectability than the 140-keV photons of ^{99m}Tc commonly used in gamma-ray emission tomography.

Two disadvantages of PET as compared to gamma-ray emission tomography are: (1) PET is limited to positron-emitting radionuclides, and (2) the dose of radiation delivered to the patient by positron-emitting radionuclides includes contributions from both the annihilation radiation and the kinetic energy of the positrons. These problems are more than offset by the advantages obtained with the use of positron-emitting radionuclides.

A number of PET systems have been designed and constructed and are currently in use. Most of the systems have incorporated scintillation detectors. In its most simple form, a PET system consists of two detectors scanning the imaged object at different angles. However, more detectors can be placed around the imaged object to improve the efficiency of radiation collection. The interested reader is referred to the references for detailed descriptions of the instruments developed to date.[1-4, 7, 10, 17]

Application of PET

Cerebral Metabolism

Cerebral metabolism can be quantified by two different approaches: (1) by using radiolabeled metabolic substrates as tracers, and (2) by using radiolabeled metabolic substrate analogs, which have blocking agents on the molecule to limit the extent of metabolism, as tracers.

The use of a radiolabeled metabolic substrate tracer to study metabolism is illustrated by our method of measuring regional cerebral glucose metabolic rate (CMRGlu) with emission tomography.[12, 13] This approach is based on a modification of a technique previously described and validated.[11] The tomographic measurement of CMRGlu involves a rapid infusion of ^{11}C-glucose intravenously over a 4-minute period. By obtaining the time concentration history of the radioisotope in blood plus emission tomograph images of the brain at the end of the infusion, CMRGlu is calculated with a modification of a previously described mathematical model.[12, 13] In conjunction with the CMRGlu measurement, cerebral blood volume (CBV) is measured using the inhalation of ^{11}CO and PET. This permits the correction of the ^{11}C-glucose scan data for the ^{11}C-glucose present in the brain vascular compartment during the scan. By obtaining the brain image less than 10 minutes from the time of injection, the egress of labeled metabolites from the tissue is insignificant.

This approach to measuring metabolism using radiolabeled metabolic substrates as tracers has several important advantages. First, the tracer is biochemically identical to the compound being traced. Second, the method outlined above is relatively quick, thus permitting repeated measurements should they be required for evaluation of transient phenomena. Third, where only a relative mapping of regional utilization rate is sought with an organ of interest, sampling of peripheral arterial blood is not necessary. Finally and most importantly, this method is not restricted to ^{11}C-glucose nor to the brain. It can be used with a wide variety of available radiopharmaceuticals utilized by the brain, heart, or other organs. A surprising number of positron-emitting radiopharmaceuticals for metabolic studies are currently available.[20]

Another approach to the study of cerebral metabolism is the use of radiolabeled metabolic substrate analogs. An example of this approach is the use of ^{18}F-2-fluoro-2-deoxy-D-glucose (^{18}F-FDG) to measure CMRGlu.[8, 14] ^{18}F-FDG has been administered to man and imaged with emission tomography to determine CMRGlu. This approach has the advantage of trapping the tracer in the tissue so the calculation of metabolic rates is not hampered by the egress of labeled metabolites and free tracer in the tissue. However, these substrate analogs are not biochemically identical to the compound being traced. Therefore, corrections must be made in the tracer model for differences in transport properties and enzyme affinities, which do vary among species.[15] These corrections may present an added difficulty when the organ of interest is diseased, and only a few such compounds are available.

Cerebral Hemodynamics

The quantitative image of a vascular tracer in an equilibrium state is easily performed with emission tomography. Thus, the measurement of CBV tomographically is relatively straightforward. CBV can be quantitated noninvasively by using the inhalation of ^{11}CO to label red blood cells (RBCs). When the labeled RBCs reach equilibrium, emission tomographic images of the ^{11}C-carboxyhemoglobin (^{11}CO-Hgb) activity in the brain are obtained. At the same time venous blood samples are collected to calculate ^{11}CO-Hgb activity in the blood. With appropriate corrections for the density of blood, the brain tissue density, and the ratio of the mean tissue hematocrit of the brain to the large vessel hematocrit, CBV is calculated from the ratio of ^{11}CO-Hgb activity in the brain to the ^{11}CO-Hgb activity of the blood. With this method, in normal humans an average CBV of 4.3 and 3.3 ml/100 g was found in emission tomographic scans obtained 4 and 8 cm above the orbitomeatal line (to be published). Using a similar approach this ^{99m}Tc-labeled RBCs and gamma-ray emission tomography, CBV values of 2 to 4 ml/100 g were found in tomographic sections obtained from various levels of the brain.[21]

The accurate quantitative measure of CBF is not possible with present emission tomographic systems. Current emission tomographic systems do not have the capability to collect statistically adequate data rapidly enough to make a dynamic tracer measurement. This factor precludes the application to emission tomography of various tracer washout techniques currently used to measure CBF with external scintillation detection. Attempts to circumvent this difficulty are currently under way in a number of centers.

With current emission tomographic devices, the accurate quantitative measurement of CBF will require the development of an adequate technique that uses either a steady-state infusion of a radiolabeled tracer or the tissue trapping of a radiolabeled tracer to assure equilibrium during data collection. One positron emission tomographic approach of measuring regional CBF and oxygen metabolism utilizes tomographic imaging of the steady-state distribution of tracer in brain.[21, 22] When ^{15}O-labeled CO_2 is inhaled, the label is rapidly transferred to water. With simple mathematical modeling the equilibrium quantity of ^{15}O-labeled water in a region of the brain can be related to the blood flow of that region. In a companion study the regional steady-state distribution of brain water formed while the subject breathes ^{15}O-labeled oxygen is imaged. The ratio of the two equilibrium images ($^{15}O_2$: $C^{15}O_2$) permits computation of the regional oxygen extraction fraction. The computed CBF and oxygen extraction fraction can be combined with the arterial blood oxygen content to yield the regional cerebral oxygen metabolism. Unfortunately, the computation of CBF with this method is sensitive to uncertainties in the brain tracer concentration due to the nonlinear nature of the blood flow equation. In addition, the ratio approach ($^{15}O_2$:$C^{15}O_2$) of assessing the regional oxygen extraction fraction requires images of good statistical quality because errors in the calculation of either regional value are propagated in the resultant ratio. Also, use of the oxygen extraction fraction as an indicator of cerebral function is unclear because its value reflects both CBF and brain tissue oxygen me-

tabolism. The development of very fast tomographic devices that would circumvent the above-mentioned difficulties in the quantitative measurement of CBF are under study in many centers.

The tomographic imaging of ^{13}N-labeled ammonia ($^{13}NH_3$) at equilibrium has been proposed as an indicator of cerebral perfusion.[23] However, labeled ammonia probably is not a suitable tracer for measuring this aspect of cerebral hemodynamics. The mechanism of ammonia uptake and trapping by the brain is not fully understood, although metabolic factors undoubtedly play a part. The pH of the blood also affects brain ammonia uptake. Furthermore, the uptake of ammonia by the brain seems to be affected by the brain capillary density. For this reason gray-white matter differences in ammonia uptake can be seen on emission tomographic brain images. Brain ammonia uptake also changes with the volume velocity of blood flow, but is not directly proportional to CBF. To compound the problem, with ^{13}N-ammonia the effects of cerebral pathology on ammonia uptake are not known. Thus, the equilibrium emission tomographic imaging of $^{13}NH_3$ is not a measure of CBF and probably is not an accurate measure of cerebral perfusion. The usefulness of $^{13}NH_3$ probably will be limited to that of a qualitative scanning agent capable of demonstrating defects in cerebral perfusion.

Tissue Chemical Composition

Emission tomography provides quantitative measurement in vivo of brain-to-blood partition coefficients for various substrates. This approach is illustrated by our method of quantitatively measuring brain tissue acid-base status using ^{11}C-bicarbonate ($H^{11}CO_3^-$) and ^{11}CO-Hgb.[12] By obtaining equilibrium tomographic images of these two radiopharmaceuticals, one can quantitatively measure the brain-to-blood partition coefficient for CO_2 (λCO_2). This allows the determination of brain CO_2 content on a three-dimensional basis, which can then be used to calculate tissue pH. Values of brain CO_2 content in rhesus monkeys are in accord with previously described measurements of brain CO_2 content.[24] This same approach, using appropriately labeled positron-emitting radiopharmaceuticals, can be used to measure in-vivo parameters such as tissue lipid content, tissue water content, tissue drug concentrations, and the mapping of brain receptors and transmitters.

Blood-Brain Barrier

Gallium-68 in the form of ^{68}Ga-EDTA under normal conditions remains in the vascular space in the brain. However, it accumulates in cerebral lesions in which a breakdown of the blood-brain barrier exists. Thus, this positron-emitting radionuclide is useful in the tomographic demonstration of blood-brain barrier defects to large protein molecules.

Conclusions

PET allows the safe, quantitative, three-dimensional measurement of radioisotope distribution in tissue. This approach, analogous to quantitative tissue autoradiography, offers the opportunity to study tissue metabolism, hemodynamics, and chemical composition with noninvasive methods in humans and animals in both normal and pathologic states. The potential of such a technique is obvious. The requirements for its successful implementation may not be so obvious. It may be clear to most that expensive machinery (cyclotron, imaging device, computers) is a necessary foundation, but not so clear that a critical mass of diverse human talents must be closely coordinated to make the full potential of PET a reality in the biomedical environment. Successful implementation of this technology represents a true collaborative effort among physicists, chemists, mathematicians, and biologists.

References

1. Brownell, G.L., Burnham, C.A., Chesler, D.A., Correia, J.A., Correll, J.E., Hoop, B., Jr., Parker, J.A., Subramanyam, R. Transverse section imaging of radionuclide distributions in heart, lung, and brain. In Reconstruction Tomography in Diagnostic Radiology and Nuclear Medicine, M.M. Ter-Pogossian, et al., editors, University Park Press, Baltimore, 1977, pp. 293–307.

2. Budinger, T.F., Gullberg, G.T. Three-dimensional reconstruction of isotope distributions. Phys Med Biol 19:387–389, 1974.

3. Chesler, D.A. Positron tomography and three-dimensional reconstruction technique. In Tomographic Imaging in Nuclear Medicine, G.S. Freedman, editor, Society of Nuclear Medicine, New York, 1973, pp. 176–183.

4. Cho, Z.H., Eriksson, L., Chan, J. A circular ring transverse axial positron camera. In Reconstruction Tomography in Diagnostic Radiology and Nuclear Medicine, M.M. Ter-Pogossian, et al., editors, University Park Press, Baltimore, 1977, pp. 393–421.

5. Eichling, J.O., Raichle, M.E., Grubb, R.L., Jr., Larson, K.B., Ter-Pogossian, M.M. In vivo determination of cerebral blood volume with radioactive oxygen-15 in the monkey. Circ Res 37:707–714, 1975.

6. Hoedt-Rasmussen, K., Sveinsdottir, E., Lassen, N.A. Regional cerebral blood flow in man determined by intra-arterial injection of radioactive inert gas. Circ Res 18:237–247, 1966.

7. Hoffman, E.J., Phelps, M.E., Mullani, N.A., Higgins, C.S., Ter-Pogossian, M.M. Design and performance characteristics of a whole-body positron transaxial tomograph. J Nucl Med 17:493–502, 1976.

8. Ido, T., Wan, C.N., Fowler, J.S., Wolf, A.P. Fluorination with F_2. A convenient synthesis of 2-deoxy-2-fluoro-D-glucose. J Org Chem 42: 2341–2342, 1977.

9. Kety, S.S., Schmidt, C.F. The nitrous oxide method for the quantitative determination of cerebral blood flow in man. J Clin Invest 27: 476–483, 1948.

10. Phelps, M.E., Hoffman, E.J., Mullani, N.A., Ter-Pogossian, M.M. Application of annihilation coincidence detection to transaxial reconstruction tomography. J Nucl Med 16:210–224, 1975.

11. Raichle, M.E., Larson, K.B., Phelps, M.E., Grubb, R.L., Jr., Welch, M.J., Ter-Pogossian, M.M. In vivo measurement of brain glucose transport and metabolism employing glucose-[11]C. Am J Physiol 228:1936–1948, 1975.

12. Raichle, M.E., Larson, K.B., Higgins, C.S., Grubb, R.L., Jr., Eichling, J.O., Welch, M.J., Ter-Pogossian, M.M. Three-dimensional in vivo mapping of brain metabolism and acid-base status. Acta Neurol Scand (Suppl) 56(64): 188–189, 1977.

13. Raichle, M.E., Welch, M.J., Grubb, R.L., Jr., Higgins, C.S., Ter-Pogossian, M.M., Larson,

K.B. Measurement of regional substrate utilization rates by emission tomography. Science 199:986–987, 1978.

14. Reivich, M., Kuhl, D., Wolf, A., Greenberg, J., Phelps, M., Ido, T., Casella, V., Fowler, J., Gallagher, B., Hoffman, E., Alavi, A., Sokoloff, L. Measurement of local cerebral glucose metabolism in man with ^{18}F-2-fluoro-2-deoxy-D-glucose. Acta Neurol Scand (Suppl) 56(64): 190–191, 1977.

15. Sokoloff, L., Reivich, M., Kennedy, C., Des-Rosiers, M.H., Patlak, C.S., Pettigrew, K.D., Sakurada, O., Shinohara, M. The (^{14}C) deoxyglucose method for the measurement of local cerebral glucose utilization: Theory, procedure, and normal values in the conscious and anesthetized albino rat. J Neurochem 28:897–916, 1977.

16. Ter-Pogossian, M.M., Eichling, J.O., Davis, D.E., Welch, M.J. The measure in vivo of regional cerebral oxygen utilization by means of oxyhemoglobin labeled with radioactive oxygen-15. J Clin Invest 49:381–391, 1970.

17. Ter-Pogossian, M.M., Mullani, N.A., Hood, J., Higgins, C.S., Currie, C.M. A multislice positron emission computed tomograph (PETT IV) yielding transverse and longitudinal images. Radiology 128:477–484, 1978.

18. Welch, M.J., Ter-Pogossian, M.M. Preparation of short half-lived radioactive gases for medical studies. Radiat Res 36:580–587, 1968.

19. Welch, M.J., Eichling, J.O., Straatmann, M.G., Raichle, M.E., Ter-Pogossian, M.M. New short-lived radiopharmaceuticals for CNS studies. In Non-Invasive Brain Imaging, H.J. DeBlanc, and J.A. Sorenson, editors, Society of Nuclear Medicine, New York, 1975, pp. 25–44.

20. Wolf, A.P., Redvanly, C.S. Carbon-11 and radiopharmaceuticals. Int J Appl Radiat Isot 28:29–48, 1977.

21. Jones, T., Chesler, D.A., Ter-Pogossian, M.M. The continuous inhalation of oxygen-15 in assessing regional oxygen extraction in the brain of man. Br J Radiol 49:339–343, 1976.

22. Subramanyam, R., Alpert, N.M., Hoop, B. Jr., Brownell, G.L., Taveras, J.M. A model for regional cerebral oxygen distribution during continuous inhalation of $^{15}O_2$, $C^{15}O$ and $C^{15}O_2$. J Nucl Med 19:48–53, 1978.

23. Phelps, M.E., Hoffman, E.J., Raybaud, C. Factors which affect cerebral uptake and retention of ammonia. Stroke 8:694–702, 1977.

24. Raichle, M.E., Grubb, R.L. Jr., Higgins, C.S. Measurement of brain tissue carbon dioxide content in vivo by emission tomography. Brain Res 166:413–417, 1979.

II

Cerebral Ischemia and Infarction

3

Serum and CSF Brain-Specific Isoenzyme Profiles in Experimental Cerebral Ischemia and Infarction

Duke S. Samson, Chester W. Beyer, Jr., Rodney Bell, and Margaret Mayhood

The goal of our investigative efforts has been to develop an objective means by which ischemic infarction of brain tissue can be promptly and reliably detected and the volume of infarcted tissue can be usefully estimated. The precedent for our investigations stems from the significant role that isoenzyme determination has had in the evaluation of myocardial ischemia and infarction and arises directly from the work of two investigators at our institution[6] who developed the radioimmunoassay technique for the delineation of the brain-specific isoenzyme creatine phosphokinase BB (CK-BB). Utilizing these two investigators' radioimmunoassay technique with their assistance and encouragement, we have attempted to apply this method of quantification to a canine experimental stroke model.

Because of the extensive collateral circulation to the cerebral hemispheres in the dog, the use of this species in the study of cerebral infarction has been somewhat limited. However, we have determined that using a modification of the transorbital approach to the middle cerebral artery in cats[1, 5] we have been reliably able to produce consistent localized infarction in dogs. Adult mongrel dogs of either sex weighing from 18 to 20 kg were selected on the basis of their general health to the extent that could be documented by routine histologic culture and biochemical examination. After an overnight fast, anesthesia was induced with diazepam 0.5 to 1.0 mg/kg given intravenously and was maintained with 70% nitrous oxide inhaled with 30% oxygen. Muscle relaxation was accomplished with pancuronium 0.1 to 0.2 mg/kg initially, with supplemental doses of relaxants as clinically indicated. In each subject, the trachea was intubated and ventilation was controlled with a Harvard animal respirator to maintain the arterial partial pressure of carbon dioxide between 33 and 38 torr. Fluid maintenance consisted of a mixture of one part 5% dextrose in Ringer's lactate to two parts 5% dextrose in water with an additional 20 mEq of potassium chloride per liter of fluid. This was administrated at a rate of 10 to 20 cc/kg/hour with an additional volume of Ringer's lactate to equal surgical blood loss, which was routinely less than 50 cc. This management usually resulted in the near-physiologic maintenance of the dog's cardiovascular respiratory system as indicated by normal blood gases and a constant urine output of 1 to 2 cc/kg/hour as measured by an indwelling catheter in the urinary bladder.

According to the technique described by Redmond,[3] we passed a 20-gauge catheter into the subarachnoid space through a Touhy needle for collection of cerebrospinal fluid samples. The dog was then positioned on his right side for operation, and the blood pressure was recorded as directly measured through a percutaneous catheter in the femoral artery. Control samples of spinal fluid and serum were collected at that time for measurement by radioimmunoassay for brain-specific creatine phosphokinase BB (CK-BB). All assays were performed at our institution in conjunction with Dr. James Willerson, Director of the Center for Ischemic Heart Disease at the University of Texas Health Science Center.

Serum and spinal fluid samples were taken at hourly intervals for 24 hours following occlusion of the middle cerebral artery and thereafter every 4 hours for 72 hours. Observations of changes in the spinal fluid and CSF levels of creatine kinase were correlated with postoperative clinical neurologic examination, infarct size as determined on gross pathologic examination, and computerized volumetric computation, a technique developed by Dr. Joel Kirkpatrick of the Division of Neuropathology at the University of Texas.

The surgical procedure consists of exposure of the left middle cerebral artery by the transorbital approach as outlined previously by Oakes and Kramer.[4] The left orbit is exenterated and the ophthalmic artery is ligated at the level of the orbital fissure. Under microscopic visualization, the orbital strut is drilled away to expose a 2×3 cm area of dura lateral to the intradural portion of the optic nerve. A stellate opening is made in the dura to expose the internal carotid artery at its bifurcation into the anterior and middle cerebral arteries, and the arachnoid cisterns are evacuated of spinal fluid. The internal carotid artery, the proximal middle cerebral artery, and the anterior cerebral artery are then isolated from their pia-arachnoid coverings, coagulated, and divided using the bipolar cautery apparatus and microtechnique. The dura mater is left widely open to allow the orbit to serve as an alternate reservoir for spinal fluid sampling and the eyelid is closed in two layers with nylon sutures.

Very preliminary results indicate that indeed, clinically, these dogs developed lesions which resulted in a consistent degree of neurologic dysfunction; hemiparesis of moderate degree was seen in both right upper and lower extremities with circling to the right and difficulty in maintaining an erect posture for the initial 24 to 48 hours following surgery. However, the dogs were routinely able to feed and care for themselves immediately, awakening from anesthesia promptly following termination of the procedure.

All subjects were observed for 24 hours in a postoperative recovery area and were then returned to their cages for the remainder of the first postoperative week. Seven days following the surgical procedure, the dogs were killed, and the brains were removed at autopsy and immersed in formalin for 21 days. Photographs of the gross hemispheres were made for future reference and for each specimen the volume of infarcted brain was estimated with Dr. Kirkpatrick's technique. Currently the sensitivity of this technique is checked by microscopic examination of H&E preparations at 2-mm coronal intervals. Presently good correlation exists between infarction margins interpreted in computerized volumetric calculations and those demonstrated by microscopic examination of H&E preparation.

In the 15 animals so treated, significant cerebral infarctions that are easily recognizable on gross examination have developed. These range in size from 15% to 35% of the affected hemisphere and are localized to the thalamus and basal ganglia. These results are similar to observations of other models of cerebral infarction based on middle cerebral artery occlusion.

Preliminary results of CSF and serum isoenzyme level determination have been encouraging, but inconclusive. We have noted consistent early peaks in the spinal fluid levels of CK-BB followed by later and less remarkable serum isoenzyme elevations. Unfortunately, it is our feeling and that of Dr. Willerson that the early CSF changes are contaminated by enzyme released from brain tissue traumatized by retraction at the time of middle cerebral artery occlusion, and certainly in several animals we have seen extreme rises in CSF CK-BB levels in CSF removed at the moment of middle cerebral artery occlusion. The radioimmunoassay technique, which is exquisitely sensitive for the presence of the enzyme, being able to detect as little as 0.02 ng/ml of the enzyme in either CSF or blood, is an ideal instrument for use in the evaluation of postischemic enzyme elevations, but the artifact induced into the early measurements by even the minimal brain trauma of microsurgical manipulation invalidates a more in-depth evaluation of our initial enzyme profiles. We have recently begun to examine these same parameters using a modification of Molinari's[2] embolic stroke model and are encouraged that this procedure provides a precise delineation of the temporal and quantitative changes of these potentially important markers in experimental ischemia and infarction.

References

1. Little, D.R. Implanted device for middle cerebral artery occlusion in conscious cats. Stroke 8:258–260, 1977.
2. Molinari, G.S., Laurent, J.P. A classification of experimental models of brain ischemia. Stroke 70:14–17, 1977.
3. Redmond, D.E., Jr., RinderKnecht, H.R., Hudgins, P.J. A technique for repeated access to the subarachnoid space in the dog. J Neurosurg 33: 74, 1970.
4. Oakes, W.J., Kramer, R.S. Unpublished data.
5. Waltz, A.G., Sundt, T.M. The microvasculative and microcirculation of the cerebral cortex after arterial occlusion. Brain 90:681–697, 1967.
6. Willerson, J.T., Stone, M.J., Ting, R., Mukherjee, A., Gomez-Sanchez, C.E., Lewis, P., Hersh, L.P. Radioimmunoassay of CPK-B isoenzyme in human sera: Results in patients with acute myocardial infarction. Proc Nat Acad Sci 74:1711–1715, 1977.

4

Free Radicals and Oxygen During Reperfusion*

R. F. Del Maestro and K.-E. Arfors

A free radical may be defined as any substance which has a lone electron in its outer orbital.[18] These highly reactive compounds may be generated in living tissues by irradiation,[2] homolysis,[18] and during oxidative-reduction reactions.[7, 18] Although free radicals have been implicated in a wide variety of disease states,[1, 9, 13, 20] the precise role played by these substances in normal and pathologic processes remains unclear. The rate of free radical reactions is proportional to the oxygen tension[4, 18] and therefore tissue oxygen availability is an essential factor in the propagation of these reactions. Free radical reactions participate normally in oxidative metabolism and many of the intermediate metabolites involved in the electron transport chain are radical species controlled within the mitochondrial membrane.[5] Cellular membranes, however, may sustain lipid peroxidation damage from free radicals[10] and biomolecules such as hyaluronic acid[13] and DNA[15] undergo depolymerization when exposed to radical species. Free radicals therefore must be carefully controlled within living tissue to prevent damage to cellular components. Cells of aerobic organisms, in contrast to anerobic cells, have evolved a variety of intrinsic enzymatic[6] and scavenging mechanisms[20] to deal with the inevitable free radical by-products of oxidative metabolism and intracellular enzyme function. Enzymes such as catalases, peroxi-

dases, and a variety of superoxide dismutases, along with molecules such as glutathione, cysteine, and vitamin E, may all play a part in controlling free radical reactions.

It has been suggested that cerebral tissue may be particularly susceptible to free radical damage because of its high lipid content[5] and that during cerebral hypoxia and subsequent recirculation[4, 16, 17] membrane peroxidation damage may occur, resulting in cellular disruption and death.

To improve our understanding of the mechanisms of radical control in biological systems we have studied the influence of various enzymes and scavenging molecules on the free radical depolymerization of hyaluronic acid.

Materials and Methods

The in-vitro oxidation of hypoxanthine under aerobic conditions by xanthine oxidase causes formation of free radicals[7] (Fig. 4-1). When purified hyaluronic acid is added to the enzyme mixture its depolymerization as measured by changes in specific viscosity (η sp) is a measure of the free radicals formed. This simple in-vitro system was used to examine the influence of different pharmacologic agents of possible neurosurgical interest.

Each experiment was carried out in duplicate in the same Ostwald viscometer controlled in a temperature bath at $\pm 22.0°C$. The control de-

*This study was supported by the Canadian Medical Research Council.

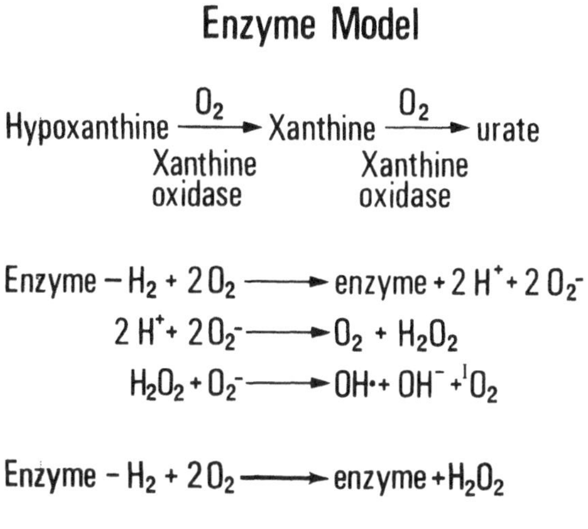

Enzyme Model

$$\text{Hypoxanthine} \xrightarrow[\substack{\text{Xanthine}\\\text{oxidase}}]{O_2} \text{Xanthine} \xrightarrow[\substack{\text{Xanthine}\\\text{oxidase}}]{O_2} \text{urate}$$

$$\text{Enzyme} - H_2 + 2\,O_2 \longrightarrow \text{enzyme} + 2\,H^+ + 2\,O_2^-$$

$$2\,H^+ + 2\,O_2^- \longrightarrow O_2 + H_2O_2$$

$$H_2O_2 + O_2^- \longrightarrow OH\cdot + OH^- + {}^1O_2$$

$$\text{Enzyme} - H_2 + 2\,O_2 \longrightarrow \text{enzyme} + H_2O_2$$

Fig. 4-1. The enzyme model involves the oxidation of hypoxanthine to urate by xanthine oxidase. The enzyme (enzyme-H_2) is oxidized in the presence of oxygen with the subsequent formation of superoxide anion radical (O_2^-) and H_2O_2. These react to form both the hydroxyl radical ($OH\cdot$) and possibly singlet oxygen ($^1O_2$) which may depolymerize hyaluronic acid.

polymerization experiments were carried out in a final volume of 3.3 ml containing 1.6 mg of hyaluronic acid and 2.2×10^{-4} M hypoxanthine in a 0.05 M (pH 7.4) phosphate buffer, with the addition of 0.15 units ml^{-1} of xanthine oxidase initiating the reaction. The influence of the experimental conditions and the individual test compounds on the stability of the hyaluronic acid η sp was studied using denatured enzyme (20 min at 100°C). The amount of scavenging which resulted from the presence of the test compound was determined by comparing the change in hyaluronic acid η sp which occurred in the control depolymerization experiment to that which occurred when the test substance was present. Results were expressed as percentage inhibition of change in hyaluronic acid η sp ($\pm$ SD) after 30 minutes of exposure to active xanthine oxidase. Compounds tested included catalase, superoxide dismutase (SOD), reduced glutathione, L-histidine, dimethyl sulfoxide (DMSO), and dexamethasone.*

*Decadron, Merck, Sharp, and Dohme, Gmbh, Munich.

Results

The addition of active xanthine oxidase to the hyaluronate solutions containing only the substrate hypoxanthine resulted in a 44.4 ± 6.5 (n = 12) percent decrease in hyaluronic acid η sp in 30 minutes. The change in η sp was rapid over the first 10 minutes and then stabilized (Fig. 4-2). Hyaluronic acid η sp remained stable in the presence of denatured xanthine oxidase (Fig. 4-2).

No alterations occurred in hyaluronic acid η sp in the presence of the test substances during experiments using inactive xanthine oxidase.

Catalase and SOD at concentrations of 10 μg ml^{-1} resulted in a 75% inhibition of change in hyaluronic acid η sp (Fig. 4-3) (Table 4-1). This suggests that neither H_2O_2, which would be present when superoxide anion radical (O_2^-) was catalytically scavenged by SOD,[14] nor O_2^-, which would be present when H_2O_2 was removed by catalase, is the active depolymerizing agent, but that both of these substances are

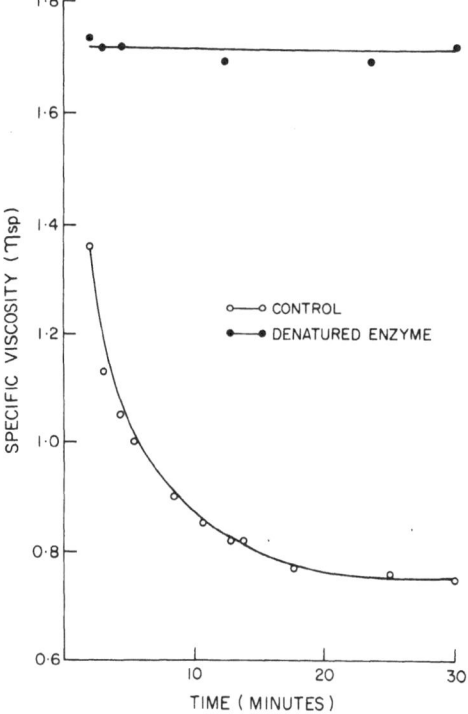

Fig. 4-2. Change in hyaluronic acid η sp following addition of active xanthine oxidase (control) and denatured enzyme with time.

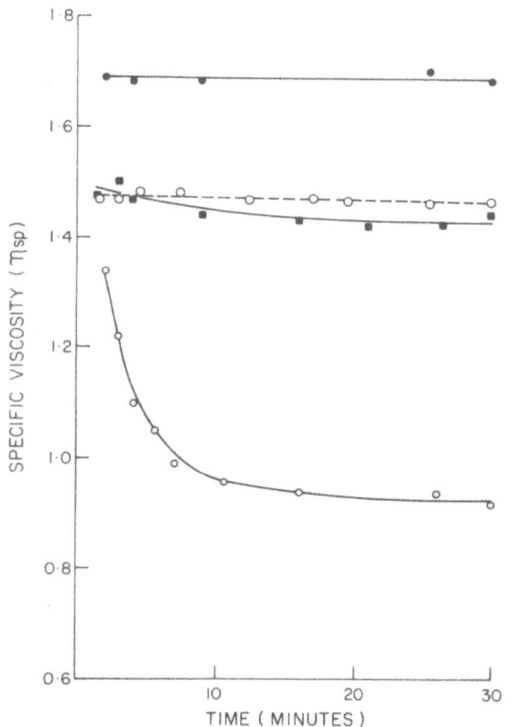

Fig. 4-3. Influence of SOD (■—■) and catalase (o---o) at concentrations of 10 μg ml^{-1} on the change in hyaluronic acid η sp induced by active xanthine oxidase (o—o) with time, hyaluronic acid η sp following addition of inactive enzyme (•—•).

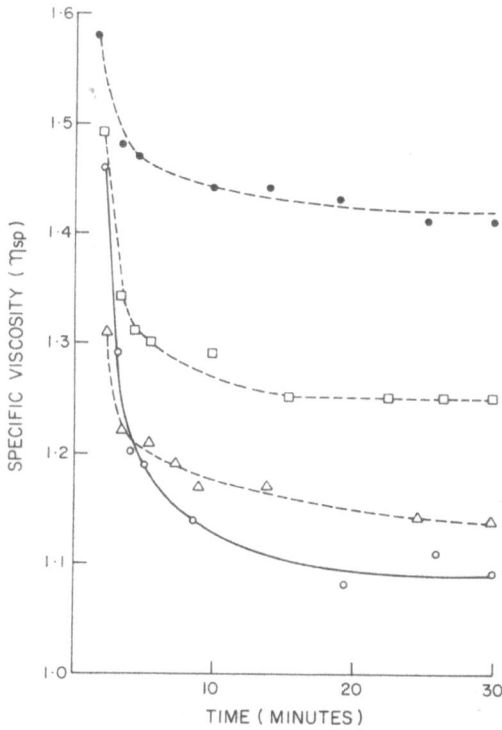

Fig. 4-4. Influence of dexamethasone on change in hyaluronic acid η sp with time. Concentration of dexamethasone used were 0.005 mM ($^{\triangle---\triangle}$), 0.05 mM ($\square$---$\square$), and 0.5 mM ($^{•---•}$). Hyaluronic acid η sp change following active enzyme addition (o—o).

needed to produce the active agent. The most likely mechanism is the Haber-Weiss reaction[8]: $H_2O_2 + O_2^- \rightarrow OH \cdot + OH^- + {}^1O_2$. This would suggest that the hydroxyl radical (OH·), singlet oxygen ($^1O_2$), or both may be responsible for hyaluronic acid depolymerization.

Since L-histidine is an $^1O_2$ scavenger and DMSO an OH· scavenger,[15] this problem could be further clarified by using these agents. Both these substances provided protection at the 5- and 10-mM concentrations (Table 4-1), which further suggests that both $^1O_2$ and OH· may be involved in depolymerization.

The protective influence of reduced glutathione at concentrations tested (Table 4-1) suggests that the intracellular concentrations (1 to 50 $\times 10^{-4}$ M)[11] are sufficient to play a role in the control of free radical reactions.

Dexamethasone at concentrations of 0.005 mM has very limited protective influence, while increasing the concentration to 0.5 mM provides good protection (Fig. 4-4) (Table 4-1).

Table 4-1. Inhibition of hyaluronic acid depolymerization

Substance	Concentration	Inhibition of change in hyaluronic acid η sp (%)	
Catalase	10 μg/ml	76.0	± 6.8
SOD	10 μg/ml	74.2	± 8.3
Glutathione-SH	0.5 mM	24.8	± 16.9
	5.0 mM	47.4	± 8.2
	10.0 mM	72.2	± 3.1
L-Histidine	0.5 mM	25.8	± .02
	5.0 mM	55.5	± 2.5
	10.0 mM	65.4	± 2.8
DMSO	0.5 mM	19.0	± 4.9
	5.0 mM	75.1	± 0.7
	10.0 mM	88.0	± 0.9
Dexamethasone	.005 mM	6.63	± 0.4
	.05 mM	19.4	± 4.1
	.5 mM	58.8	± 4.6

Mean values ± SD of duplicate experiments.

Extrapolation of information obtained from other steroids[21] suggests that attainable intracerebral concentrations of dexamethasone are unlikely to have significant scavenging action.

Discussion

The evolution of life occurred in an oxygen-poor environment and tissue energy requirements were provided by anaerobic processes.[12] Under these conditions very little free radical formation could occur. However, the appearance of plants and their release of O_2 into the atmosphere necessitated the development of adaptive mechanisms to prevent the free radical oxidation of cellular components. The obligatory anaerobes which survive today in environmental conditions free of O_2 have failed to evolve protective scavenging mechanisms. Catalase and SOD along with molecular scavenging molecules are absent or inadequate in anaerobic organisms,[6] while their development in aerobes have allowed their continued evolution in an oxygen-rich environment. Bacteria possess a Mn-based SOD[9] and a member of this species may have been incorporated into primitive organisms which later evolved into the intracellular mitochondria. This MnSOD may have increased the cells' ability to deal with O_2^-.

The mechanisms by which anaerobic organisms succumb to oxygen exposure and the influence of hyperoxia on aerobic organisms may involve an increase in the type or quantity of free radicals produced. The intracellular scavenging mechanisms, decreased or absent in anaerobes and capable of dealing with a limited supply of radicals in aerobes, are overwhelmed with subsequent free radical membrane peroxidation and degradation of biomolecules.

Decreasing oxygen availability to critical levels in cerebral cells results in their adjustment by a switch to anaerobic metabolism. Free radical formation is proportional to oxygen tension,[4, 18] and during complete cerebral ischemia free radicals are unlikely to be involved in cellular damage. In incomplete ischemia free radical formation could continue and result in tissue injury. In the immediate period after the initiation of recirculation cells may be exposed to relatively large amounts of O_2 and must quickly readapt the metabolism to deal with O_2. In the presence of inadequately functioning mitochondria, damaged during the ischemic period (complete or incomplete),[19] and high oxygen tensions the free radical load to the cell may be increased and membrane damage and subsequent cellular death may occur.

This hypothesis (Fig. 4-5) suggests that intrinsic scavenging mechanisms play an essential role not only in the defense against O_2 toxicity but also in free radical control during

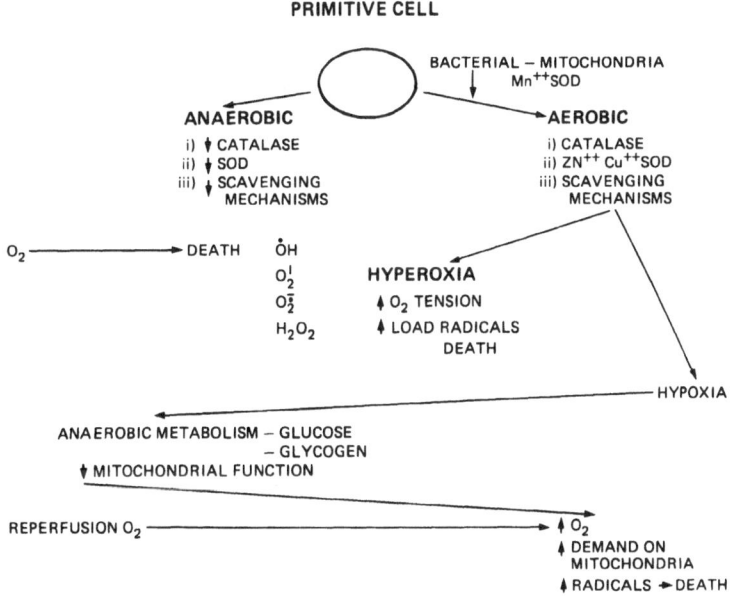

Fig. 4-5. Schematic presentation of the role free radicals and scavenging mechanisms may play in the response of anaerobic and aerobic organisms to oxygen. Exposure of anaerobic organisms to O_2 during recirculation may result in damage due to free radicals.

the recirculation phase of cerebral ischemia. The present in-vitro study suggests that the intrinsic enzymes catalase and SOD, along with reduced glutathione, at in-vivo concentrations can prevent hyaluronic acid depolymerization. Extrinsic scavengers such as DMSO and L-histidine also protect against hyaluronic acid breakdown, and these substances may be useful in cerebral ischemia. De La Torre has shown that DMSO is in fact useful in experimental infarction after middle cerebral artery occlusion,[3] when compared to dexamethasone. This may be related as in the in-vitro model to the ability of DMSO and not dexamethasone to scavenge free radicals at the concentrations achieved. Nordström et al.[17] have suggested that the ameliorating influence of phenobarbital on cerebral ischemia may be related to free radical scavenging.

It appears therefore that more information on the role of free radicals and scavenging mechanisms during ischemia may be useful in developing a new approach to the understanding and treatment of cerebral ischemia.

Acknowledgment

We would like to thank Drs. S.J. Peerless, C.G. Drake, and F.N. McKenzie for their help and advice.

References

1. Babior, B.M. Oxygen-dependent microbial killing by phagocytes. Part 2. N Engl J Med 298: 721–725, 1978.
2. Balazs, E.A., Davies, J.V., Phillips, G.O., Young, M.D. Transient intermediates in the radiolysis of hyaluronic acid. Radiat Res 31: 243–255, 1967.
3. De La Torre, J.C., Surgeon, J.W. Dexamethasone and DMSO in experimental transorbital cerebral infarction. Stroke 7:577–583, 1976.
4. Demopoulos, H.B., Flamm, E., Seligmann, M., Poser, R., Pietronigro, D., Ransohoff, J. Molecular pathology of lipids in CNS membranes. Oxygen and Physiological Function, F.F. Jobsis, editor, Professional Information Library, Dallas, 1977, pp. 491–508.
5. Demopoulos, H.B., Milvy, P., Kakaris, S., Ransohoff, J. Molecular aspects of membrane structure in cerebral edema. In Steroids and Brain Edema, H.J. Reulen and K. Schurmann, editors, Springer-Verlag, New York, 1972, pp. 29–39.
6. Fridovich, I.: Superoxide dismutases. In Annu Rev Biochem 44:147–159, 1975.
7. Fridovich, I. Quantitative aspects of the production of superoxide anion radical by milk xanthine oxidase. J Biol Chem 215:4053–4057, 1970.
8. Haber, F., Weiss, J. The catalytic decomposition of hydrogen peroxide by iron salts. Proc R Soc Ser A 147:332–351, 1934.
9. Hassan, H.M., Fridovich, I. Enzymatic defenses against the toxicity of oxygen and of streptonigrin in Escherichia coli. J Bacteriol 129:1574–1583, 1977.
10. Kellog, E.W., Fridovich, I. Liposome oxidation and erythrocyte lysis by enzymically generated superoxide and hydrogen peroxide. J Biol Chem 252:6721–6728, 1977.
11. Kosower, N.S., Kosower, E.M. The glutathione-glutathione disulfide system. In Free Radicals in Biology, Vol. 2, W.A. Pryor, editor, Academic Press, London, 1976, p. 75.
12. Mains, G. The Oxygen Revolution. New Press, Toronto, 1972.
13. McCord, J.M. Free radicals and inflammation: Protection of synovial fluid by superoxide dismutase. Science 185:529–531, 1974.
14. McCord, J.M., Fridovich, I. Superoxide dismutase. An enzymatic function for erythrocuprein (hemocuprein). J Biol Chem 244:6049–6055, 1969.
15. Morgan, A.R., Cone, R.L., Elgert, T.M. The mechanism of DNA strand breakage by vitamin C and superoxide and the protective roles of catalase and superoxide dismutase. Nucleic Acids Res 3:1139–1149, 1976.
16. Nordström, C-H., Siesjö, B.K. Effect of phenobarbital in cerebral ischemia. Part I: Cerebral energy metabolism during pronounced incomplete ischemia. Stroke 9(4):327–335, 1978.
17. Nordström, C-H., Rehncrona, S., Siesjö, B.K. Effects of phenobarbital in cerebral ischemia. Part II: Restitution of cerebral energy state, as well as of glycolytic metabolites, citric acid cycle intermediates and associated amino acids after pronounced incomplete ischemia. Stroke 9(4):335–343, 1978.
18. Pryor, W.A. Free Radicals. McGraw-Hill, New York, 1966.
19. Rehncrona, S. Personal communication.
20. Slater, T.F. Free radical mechanisms in tissue injury. Pion Ltd., London, 1972.
21. Withrow, C.D., Woodbury, D.M. Some aspects of the pharmacology of adrenal steroids and the central nervous system. In Steroids and Brain Edema, H.J. Reulen and K. Schürmann, editors, Springer-Verlag, New York, 1972, pp. 41–55.

5

A New Model for Chronic Reversible Cerebral Ischemia

R. Spetzler, W. Selman,* P. Weinstein, J. Townsend, H. M. Mehdorn, and D. Telles

Clinically meaningful laboratory investigation of stroke therapy requires a model in which the pathophysiology of cerebral ischemia is similar to events occurring in man. The most effective method for monitoring the course of cerebral ischemia for diagnostic and therapeutic purposes has not yet been established. It would be desirable to employ in the laboratory the same diagnostic tools found in sophisticated clinical medical centers.

We have recently designed a new model for chronic reversible cerebral ischemia which satisfies the above criteria. This report describes our experience with this model and its role in the investigation of cerebral vascular disease.

placed subcutaneously over the skull. Pressure over the reservoir inflates the balloon and occludes the middle cerebral artery. The artery remains occluded until pressure is placed over the valve, decompressing the balloon and allowing flow to resume through the vessel (Figs. 5-1, 5-2).

The occluder has several important features. First, the device is implantable at a time remote from subsequent experimentation. In the interim, the device is not exposed and requires no observation or restraints on the animal. Second, after sealing the skull with cranioplasty, the surgical site is not manipulated through the remainder of the investigation. Third and particularly important, the animal is awake and

Model Description

The model incorporates an implantable vessel occluder designed by Spetzler and co-workers. This device consists of a small Silastic balloon cuff connected by a tiny spring-reinforced catheter to a pressure-sensitive valve and reservoir. Through a standard transorbital approach,[6] the balloon cuff is placed around the middle cerebral artery just distal to its origin. The orbit is filled with cranioplasty and the lid sutured shut. The valve and reservoir are

*Recipient of the Allen Memorial Fellowship, sponsored by the Prentiss Foundation and The University Hospitals of Cleveland.

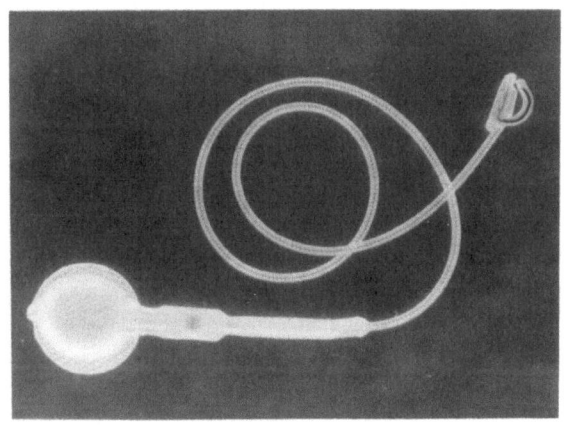

Fig. 5-1. Occluder with balloon deflated.

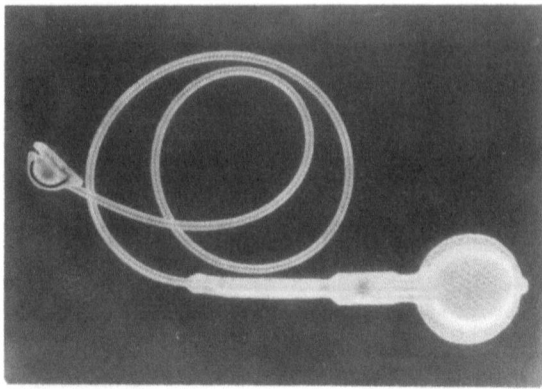

Fig. 5-2. Occluder with balloon inflated.

free from the effect of drugs at the time of occlusion.

Male baboons (sp. Papio anibus) are used as the experimental animals. The choice of these animals is twofold and based on an attempt to design a model relevant to the clinical setting. First, subhuman primates have a cerebrovascular anatomy and potential for collateral blood supply which more closely parallel man's than do those of nonprimate experimental animals. Furthermore, baboons are large enough to allow implantation of our occluder and to permit monitoring of essential clinical parameters, such as detailed neurologic examination, angi-

ography, computerized tomographic scanning, and regional cerebral blood flow studies, with the same methods utilized in humans. We have implanted the occluder in six baboons with the results described below.

Results

Selective cerebral angiography was performed in four animals. A normal pattern of flow was demonstrated in the middle cerebral artery distribution with the balloon deflated. With balloon inflation, absence of middle cerebral artery filling was readily demonstrated. Upon release of occlusion, return of flow was seen in the middle cerebral artery territory. Of particular interest was the dropout of small vessels in those animals undergoing angiography after occlusion (Figs. 5-3, 5-4, 5-5).

All animals were placed in a standard primate restraint chair and observed during various periods of middle cerebral artery occlusion. The animals developed a prompt hemiparesis within 20 seconds of occlusion, which became reversible with reperfusion up to 10 minutes of ischemia. It appeared that there was a "recruitment response" in that the hemiparesis lasted progressively longer each time despite a con-

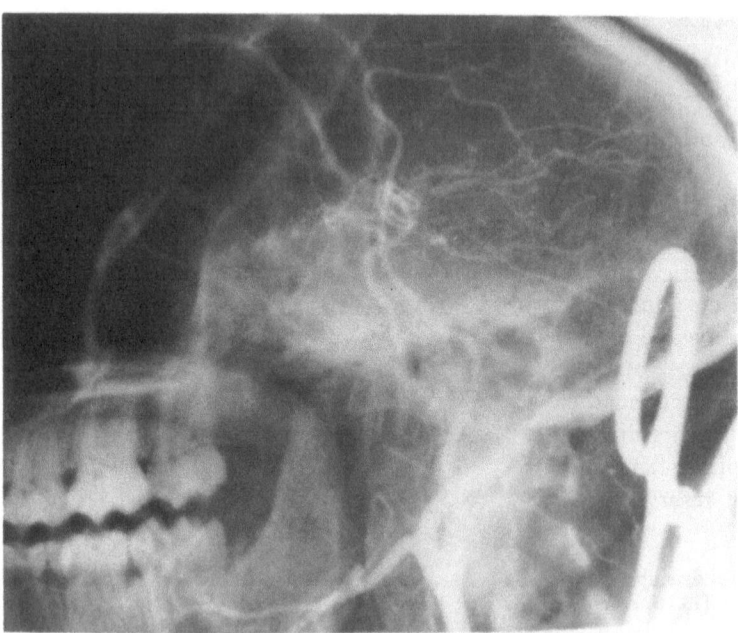

Fig. 5-3. Selective cerebral angiogram, lateral view. Occluder in place. Balloon deflated. Note middle cerebral artery filling.

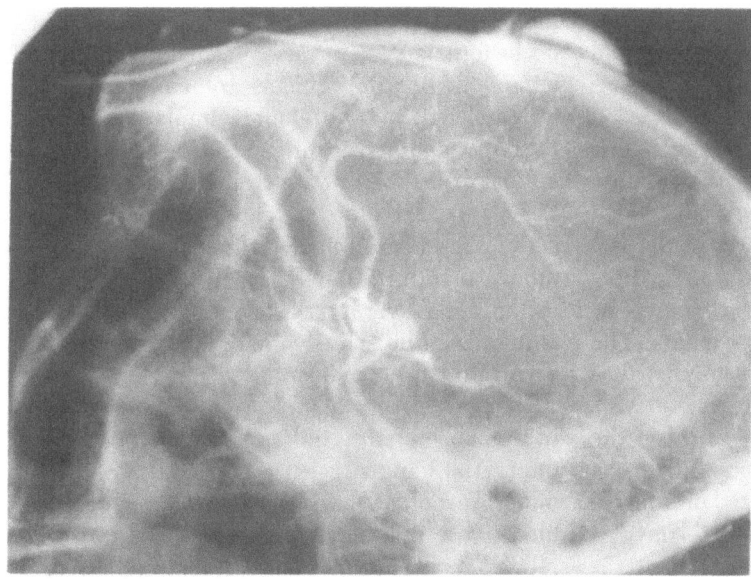

Fig. 5-4. Selective cerebral angiogram, lateral view. Occluder in place. Balloon inflated. Note absence of middle cerebral artery filling.

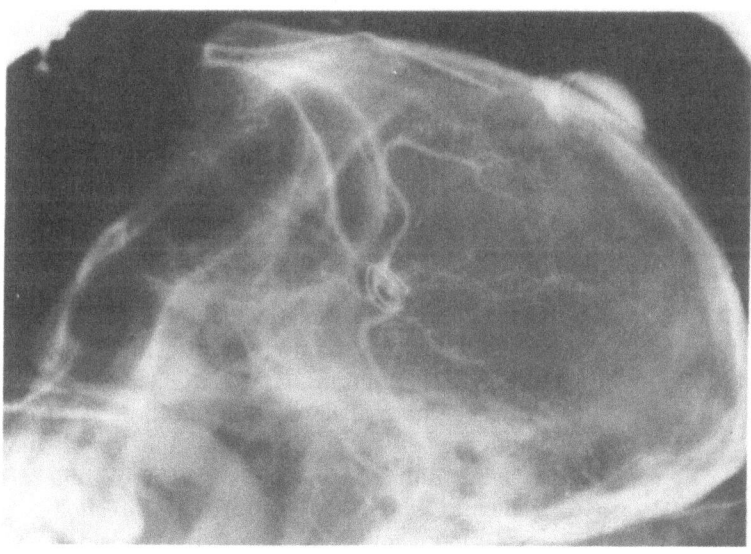

Fig. 5-5. Selective cerebral angiogram, lateral view. Occluder in place. Balloon deflated after previous inflation. Note refilling of middle cerebral artery, with dropout of small vessels.

stant period of occlusion. Moreover, animals studied with angiography after occlusion demonstrated a permanent hemiparesis, whereas those occluded for the same period without angiography had no residual defect.

Computerized tomography was performed in five baboons. Over 500 slices in the coronal plane, with and without contrast, were performed prior to, during, and after occlusion of the middle cerebral artery. Normal scans were seen in control animals while increased enhancement was demonstrated in completed strokes. Low-density changes with peripheral

enhancement were noted during brief (up to 15 minutes) periods of ischemia; these returned to normal within 3 hours.

Regional cerebral blood flow studies were performed in two baboons. Following intracarotid injection of radioactive xenon, decay curves were monitored with 16 collimated scintillation detectors. A prompt decrease in flow in the middle cerebral artery distribution was observed following occlusion of the ipsilateral middle cerebral artery. In one control animal, regional cerebral blood flow was also studied by the xenon inhalation method. Good correlation was observed between the intracarotid and inhalation methods. Autoregulation and CO_2 reactivity were observed to be normal following a 20% elevation of blood pressure and inhalation of 8% CO_2 in room air, respectively.

Gross external neuropathologic examination was unremarkable in all but one brain, which showed mild hemorrhagic softening in the left sylvian fissure. On coronal sections, three brains demonstrated a discrete, pale area of softening in the left putamen and caudate. The area of softening was confined to the distribution of the lateral striate arteries. There were no changes noted in the more distal field of the middle cerebral artery. Microscopically, the area of softening contained sheets of macrophages filled with debris. There was no evidence of hemorrhage. Numerous reactive astrocytes surrounded the ischemic infarct, but only a mild degree of neovascularization was noted. No thrombi were seen in the vessels. These changes were consistent with a subacute infarct. All neuropathologic findings correlated well with clinical examinations. Those animals which had a permanent hemiparesis from occlusion associated with angiography or permanent occlusion demonstrated a stroke at autopsy, whereas the animals with temporary ischemia and complete neurologic recovery revealed no evidence of infarction.

Discussion

Hemodynamically, there are basically two general models with which to study cerebral ischemia: global ischemia, simulating circulatory arrest in humans, and regional ischemia, modeling clinical cerebrovascular occlusive disease. Previous laboratory investigation of regional cerebral ischemia has been hampered by the lack of an adequate clinical model. The effect of both volatile and intravenous anesthetics on cerebral blood flow[10] necessitates that vessel occlusion be performed in an awake animal. To avoid direct trauma and the alterations produced by large craniectomies, a direct approach to the cerebal vasculature, with minimal brain retraction, is required.[6] Since vessel occlusion in man is often temporary,[5] a reliable atrau-

matic method of occlusion which assures post-occlusion patency is also needed. Our model eliminates these problems by employing the inflatable balloon occluder, implanted transorbitally, and performing occlusion in an awake animal at a time remote from implantation.

This model allows us to simulate clinical cerebrovascular occlusive disease, which commonly manifests itself as a neurologic deficit in the middle cerebral artery distribution. This is mimicked by selective middle cerebral artery occlusion in primates.[12, 13] The clinical and pathologic effects of occlusion noted here are in agreement with the results of Astrup, Symon, et al.[1] and suggest the existence of ischemia thresholds varying with degree of local blood flow reduction. These investigators correlated neuronal function with regional cerebral blood flow in baboons. Neurons maintain normal electrophysiologic function as evidenced by normal evoked potentials from flows of 50 ml/100 g/min to 20 ml/100 g/min. This lower level of flow appears critical, since below this level evoked potential diminishes and at 15 ml/100 g/min evoked potential completely disappears. It is not until flow falls below 12 ml/100 g/min that evidence of impending cell death, that is, increased extracellular potassium ion concentration, is seen. The length of time that neurons can remain in the low flow state before cell death occurs is unknown, but return of normal function has been observed with return of normal flow.[1, 2] In addition, Crowell and co-workers suggest that the functional ischemia threshold is independent of time of ischemia, whereas the infarction threshold of local blood flow reduction varies considerably with time.[4] It is important to determine if repetitive occlusion and ischemia alter the functional threshold such that the time independence is lost, as suggested by the "recruitment response" noted in our investigation. Furthermore, it is necessary to determine if these thresholds can be correlated with changes within the resolution of diagnostic studies employed in the clinical setting.

Three major tests are currently employed for cerebral ischemia. Angiography is valuable for defining the vascular anatomy. However, the pathology may not be visualized secondary to clot dissolution or embolic migration. Our results also indicate that angiography in the acute phase of cerebral ischemia may lead to irreversible pathologic changes.

Computerized tomography (CT) has been used to study cerebral ischemia.[3, 11] It is ideal for an initial examination because it can identify fresh blood, ventricular size, and mass effects, but it demonstrates vascular anomalies poorly, and cannot identify a vessel occlusion.

The feasibility of repeated regional cerebral blood flow (rCBF) studies in stroke patients has been shown by several groups.[7, 8] Schmiedek and co-workers argued for the superiority of combined computerized tomography and regional cerebral blood flow studies in the diagnosis of cerebral ischemia because they are complementary.[9] The CT scan may be negative in the early phases of cerebral ischemia, but rCBF will detect early changes in reduced blood flow. It should be noted that our data indicate that CT may be more sensitive to early changes in cerebral ischemia than was previously believed. In old infarcts, rCBF may fail to show the pathology secondary to the "look-through" phenomenon, yet CT will readily demonstrate the defect.

On the basis of these results, we believe that this model will be helpful for future investigation to facilitate both the diagnosis and therapy of cerebral vascular disease.

References

1. Astrup, J., Symon, L., Branston, N., Lassen, N.A. Cortical evoked potential and extracellular K^+ and H^+ at critical levels of brain ischemia. Stroke 8:41, 1977.
2. Branston, N.M., Symon, L., Crockard, H.A. Recovery of cortical evoked response following temporary middle cerebral artery occlusion in baboons: Relation to local blood flow and PO_2. Stroke 7:151, 1976.
3. Constant, C., Renoir, A.M., Caile, J.M., Vernheit, J. Follow-up study of cerebral ischemia with computed tomography (C.T. Acta Scanner). In Cerebral Function Metabolism and Circulation, D.H. Ingvar and N.A. Lassen, editors, Munksgaard, Copenhagen, 1977, pp. 164–165. Acta Neurol Scand Suppl 64, Vol. 56.
4. Crowell, R.M. Personal communication.
5. Fieschi, C., Bozzao, L. Transient embolic occlusion of the middle cerebral and internal carotid arteries in cerebral apoplexy. J Neurol Neurosurg Psychiatry 32:236, 1969.
6. Hudgins, W.R., Garcia, J.H. Transorbital approach to the middle cerebral artery in the squirrel monkey: A technique for experimental cerebral infarction applicable to ultrastructural studies. Stroke 1:107, 1970.
7. Kohlmeyer, K. Relationships between functional cerebral restitution and cerebral circulation in repeated studies of regional cerebral blood flow in stroke patients. In Cerebral Function Metabolism and Circulation, D.H. Ingvar and N.A. Lassen, editors, Munksgaard, Copenhagen, 1977, pp. 532–533. Acta Neurol Scand Suppl 64, Vol. 56.
8. Rao, N.S., Ali, Z.A., Omar, H.M., Halsey, J.H. Regional cerebral blood flow in acute stroke: Preliminary experience with the 133Xenon inhalation method. Stroke 5:8, 1974.
9. Schmiedek, P., Lanksch, W., Olteanu-Nerbe, V., Kazner, E., Gratzl, O., Marguth, F. Combined use of regional cerebral blood flow measurement and computerized tomography for the diagnosis of cerebral ischemia. In Microsurgery for Stroke, P. Schmiedek, O. Gratzl, R. Spetzler, editors, Springer-Verlag, New York, 1977, pp. 67–68.
10. Smith, A.L., Wollman, H. Cerebral blood flow and metabolism; Effects of anesthetic drugs and techniques. Anesthesiology 36:378, 1972.
11. Spetzler, R.F., Wing, S.D., Norman, D. Evaluation of patients with cerebral ischemia using computerized tomography. In Microsurgery for Stroke, P. Schmiedek, O. Gratzl, and R. Spetzler, editors, Springer-Verlag, New York, 1977, pp. 195–200.
12. Symon, L. Studies of leptomeningeal collateral circulation in Macacus rhesus. J Physiol 159:68, 1961.
13. Symon, L., Pasztor, E., Branston, N.M. The distribution and density of reduced cerebral blood flow following acute middle cerebral artery occlusion: an experimental study by the technique of hydrogen clearance in baboons. Stroke 5:355, 1974.

6

Brain Energetics in Patients Undergoing STA–MCA Anastomosis

J. M. Fein

The response of cortical pyridine nucleotide (NADH) fluorescence levels to surface electrical stimulation was evaluated from multiple areas in five patients undergoing STA–MCA bypass. The level of NADH fluorescence as monitored with a reflectofluorometer is a function of the relative amount of reduced NADH in the total NADH–NAD pool within neuronal mitochondria. In the steady state this level is directly related to the severity of ischemia and inversely related to the level of oxidative metabolic activity. Increased electrophysiologic activity produced by direct cortical stimulation, evoked cortical response, seizure activity, or during the initial phase of spreading depression is associated with a rapid change in the NADH level. In this study direct cortical stimulation was chosen to elicit the metabolic response since the topographic and temporal relations of the two facilitate repeated measurement and kinetic analysis of the redox transient.[8, 9, 14]

Intraoperative Studies

Patients with transient ischemic attacks (TIA) were selected for microvascular bypass of the anterior circulation based on clinical and radiographic indications previously described.[10] Five of these patients had complete preoperative and intraoperative studies. Each patient underwent preoperative regional cerebral blood flow studies using the noninvasive technique described by Obrist.[13] This provided weighted measurements of gray matter flow (CBFg) from 16 hemispheric regions. CBFg studies were employed to identify areas of relative focal ischemia (Table 6-1). This was found in two of the five patients. Craniotomy was centered over the area of relative focal ischemia demonstrated in two patients and 3 cm above the tragus in the three other patients. The clinical and CBF data in five patients are summarized in Table 6-1. After exposure of the cortical recipient artery, a flexible fiberoptic instrument was focused on a region of cortex approximately 3.5 mm in diameter. It was divided into three proximal branches, one of which conducted monochromatic light (366 nm) to the cortex. This excites mitochondrial NADH to fluoresce at a wavelength of 450 nm and at an intensity related to the NADH content of the NADH–NAD pool. Some of the excitation light is absorbed by hemoglobin and some is lost by specular reflection from cortical and arachnoidal surfaces. The light signals from the cortex were conducted by the fiberoptic appliance and were filtered through optical filters of 450-nm wavelength, which allowed passage of the fluorescence signal, and 366-nm wavelength, which allowed passage of the reflectance signal to individual photomultiplier tubes. The signals were transduced into analog output using a circuit described by Chance.[1] The corrected fluorescence (F–R) is the difference between fluorescent and reflect-

Table 6-1. Clinical and hemodynamic data on five patients undergoing STA–MCA bypass

Case	Date	Episodic symptoms	Angiogram	CBFg
1	3/21/78	Am. Fug. O.S., R. Hemp.	LICO RICS	nl
2	11/10/77	Am. Fug. O.D.	RICS Cavernous	nl
3	11/16/78	Dysphasia	LICO	RFI–35%
4	1/ 3/78	Dysphasia	LICO	RFI–40%
5	5/11/76	Dysphasia	LMCO	nl

ance signals and is directly related to the level of cortical mitochondrial NADH.

After the steady-state level of corrected fluorescence was recorded, stimulating pulses were delivered to the cortex through a Grass S-88 stimulator and a Grass SIU-5 stimulus isolation unit. The bipolar stimulating electrodes were insulated, except for the tips which were separated by 4.0 mm and straddled the optical recording area on the cortex. These stimulations produced a rapid oxidation slope followed by a rereduction slope. The half-time ($t_{1/2}$ ox) from stimulation to the point at which the maximal amplitude (P_{max}) was achieved and the half-time from the point of maximal amplitude to the initial baseline ($t_{1/2}$ red) were recorded. These kinetic studies were repeated in up to three cortical regions in each patient. The effect of topical phenobarbital application to the cortex and the effect of microanastomosis on these parameters was also studied.

Results

Nonischemic Cortex

Effect of Varying Stimulation Parameters on the Fluorescence Transient. Following an adequate stimulating pulse a linear drop in fluorescence (oxidation) to a point of maximal amplitude change (P_{max}) was followed by a slower return to baseline (rereduction). There was a near-linear increase of P_{max} in response to increasing the stimulating voltage from 2 to 7 volts. Between 7 and 9 volts there were no further changes in P_{max}. Stimulating voltages

greater than 9 volts resulted in fluorescence responses which could not be distinguished from background (Fig. 6-1). There were no significant changes of $t_{1/2}$ ox or $t_{1/2}$ red in response to variations in stimulating voltage between 3 and 10 volts. An increase in train length between 0.6 and 1.6 sec was associated with an increase in P_{max}. Further increases in train length had no significant effect (Fig. 6-1). Varying the train length between 0.6 and 2.2 sec had no effect on $t_{1/2}$ ox or $t_{1/2}$ red. Varying the stimulation rate demonstrated that the maximal deflection of the fluorescent transient (P_{max}) occurred near 16 Hz. Increasing or decreasing the stimulation rate decreased the

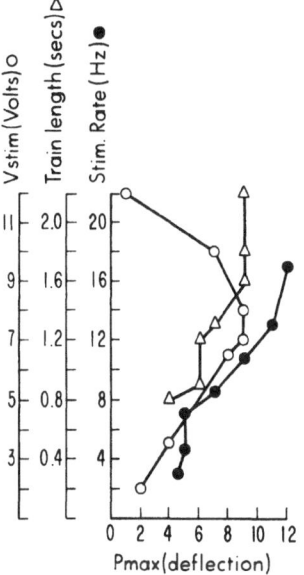

Fig. 6-1. The effect of varying stimulation rate, voltage, and train length on P_{max}.

P_{max} (Fig. 6-1). Variations of stimulation rate between 5 and 20 Hz had no significant effect on $t_{1/2}$ ox and $t_{1/2}$ red. In nonischemic cortex P_{max} is dependent on the stimulus parameters but the kinetic values for the oxidation and reduction responses are independent of stimulus parameters. Further test stimulations were carried out with trains of 7.5 volts at 16 Hz and 1.4 sec train length.

Effects of Varying Metabolism on the Fluorescence Transients.   Phenobarbital was topically applied to the cortex in three patients and measurements of fluorescence transients were carried out in a total of seven areas. There was no effect on $t_{1/2}$ ox or P_{max} but a significant slowing of $t_{1/2}$ red was seen in all areas surveyed (Tables 6-2 and 6-3) within 1 to 8 minutes after topical application. The original rate of rereduction was reestablished 15 to 23 minutes after topical application.

Effect of Anastomosis.   The fluorescence transient response was studied in seven areas in three patients after anastomosis (Table 6-4). This had no consistent effect on $t_{1/2}$ ox, P_{max}, or $t_{1/2}$ red.

Ischemic Cortex

Effect of Varying Stimulating Parameters on the Fluorescence Transient.   Varying stimulating voltage, stimulating rate, and stimulus train length affected P_{max} in a fashion similar to that in the nonischemic cortex. Parameters selected for test stimulation were the same as in the nonischemic cortex. The kinetic values for $t_{1/2}$ ox showed little variation in different areas studied. The $t_{1/2}$ red showed significant variations, depending on the areas studied and the hemodynamic manipulations introduced.

Regional Variations in Rereduction Kinetics. In two areas in Case 3 (Areas a, b) and in one area of Case 4 (Area a), the rereduction kinetics were slower than normal. In one area of Case 3 (Area c) and in two areas of Case 4 (Areas b and c), the reduction kinetics were faster than normal and were associated with an overshoot of the baseline which persisted for an additional 14.5 ± 6.5 sec (Table 6-2).

Table 6-2. $t_{1/2}$ red values in ischemic and nonischemic cortex

Case	Area	$t_{1/2}$ red (sec)
1	a	11.3
	b	11.5
	c	10.7
2	a	10.7
	b	10.5
	c	11.8
3	a	21.6
	b	30.6
	c	6.3
4	a	40.5
	b	5.5
	c	7.6
5	a	11.5
	b	12.5
	c	10.0

Table 6-3. Effects of topical phenobarbital on rereduction kinetics in ischemic and nonischemic cortex

Case	Area	% Δ $t_{1/2}$ red*	Duration of effect (min)
1	a	+ 33	8
	b	+ 20	6
	c	+ 25	19
2	a	+ 60	12
	b	+ 40	11
	c	+ 33	6
3	a	+100	6
	b	–	–
	c	+ 50	10
4	a	+ 25	15
	b	+ 20	10
	c	+ 25	15
5	a	+ 66	18
	b	+ 40	20
	c	+ 50	23

*An increase in $t_{1/2}$ red indicated by + %. Areas not studied indicated by –.

Effect of Topical Phenobarbital.   Five areas were studied after topical application of phenobarbital. In all five areas there was a significant slowing of the rereduction kinetics (Table 6-3). This effect resolved within 15 minutes of the

Table 6-4. Effect of microvascular anastomosis on ischemic and nonischemic cortex

Case	Area	% Δ $t_{1/2}$ red*	Duration to last measurement
1	a	+10%	–
	b	– 8%	–
	c	+10%	–
2	a	+10%	–
	b	0	–
	c	0	–
3	a	+20%	20
	b	+25%	25
	c	+30%	18
4	a	+20%	20
	b	+25%	25
	c	+30%	22
5	a	0	–
	b	+10%	–
	c	– 8%	–

* Increase in $t_{1/2}$ red indicated by + %.

topical application. In each case the kinetics before application were reestablished.

Effect of Anastomosis. Rereduction kinetics were significantly affected by anastomosis in the areas of rapid rereduction associated with an overshoot of the baseline. In Area 3c and in Areas 4b and 4c the mean $t_{1/2}$ red was slowed from 6.6 sec to 11.4 sec and the overshoot of the baseline was eliminated. This effect persisted on studies repeated up to 25 minutes after anastomosis (Table 6-4).

Discussion

The redox level of the mitochondrial coenzyme pyridine nucleotide depends on the rate at which reducing equivalents or electrons are provided to it by citric acid cycle intermediates and the rate at which these are removed by the electron transport chain and the electron acceptor oxygen. The relative level of NADH in the NADH–NAD$^+$ pool in a fixed optical field is directly related to the intensity of the fluorescence signal at 450-nm wavelength. Increases in NADH fluorescence are associated with both anoxic[2] and ischemic[3] insults. Decrease in NADH fluorescence associated with

electrophysiologic and oxidative metabolic activity has also been demonstrated.[11, 12, 14] In animal experiments cortical stimulation produced an evoked metabolic response the kinetic characteristics of which were measurable. Furthermore, the initial oxidation response was slowed by ouabain injection and the secondary rereduction response was slowed by topical application of barbiturate.[15] This indicates that the rate of the oxidation response is a function of the rate of ATP hydrolysis and that the rate of the rereduction response is related to the rate of rephosphorylation of ADP. These results are in general agreement with in-vivo experiments which relate the rate of NADH oxidation to the availability of ADP.[4, 5, 6]

It is recognized that normal energy stores and mitochondrial function are required for recovery of cerebral function after anoxic or ischemic insults. There is disagreement, however, as to the significance of the mitochondrial injury which follows ischemic and anoxic insults which are incomplete and of relatively shorter duration.

Fluorescence transients are related to the flux in local cortical oxidative energy metabolism and can be measured from areas of the cortex exposed during craniotomy for STA–MCA bypass. The characteristic redox transient seen in experimental animals after midcollicular brainstem transection was consistently reproduced despite the presence of anesthetic doses of halothane.

There was little variation in the initial oxidation response between different areas of the craniotomy exposure and between different patients. The presence or absence of low CBFg values was not associated with alterations of the $t_{1/2}$ ox values. The P_{max} achieved within a given cortical field was a function of the stimulating parameters utilized and implies that either a recruitment of more neurons, more mitochondria per neuron, or more complete oxidation of pyridine nucleotides occurs with increased electrophysiologic activity.

The rereduction response showed a significant variation in the ischemic areas compared to normally perfused cortex. Three areas with prolonged $t_{1/2}$ red values were seen. It is tempting to attribute this to a relative prolongation of the oxidation state. This may be related to a state of uncoupled oxidative phosphorylation in which electron transport proceeds relatively uninhibited by available ADP.[7]

The very rapid rereduction kinetics associated with overshoot of the original baseline may be indicative of areas of relative hypoxia. Marginal oxidation may be adequate to maintain a baseline redox level. The sudden burst of activity associated with cortical stimulation may transiently deplete limited oxygen reserves, shifting the redox level until compensatory mechanisms are effective.

The oxybarbiturates are known to slow electron transport processes and the rereduction kinetics. It is unclear at present whether maintenance of a state of relative oxidation during physiologic stress may contribute to protection since the known effects of barbiturates on steady-state NADH fluorescence are in the opposite direction.[15]

A mechanism by which microvascular anastomosis may favorably benefit ischemic areas is tentatively proposed. Augmentation of steady-state tissue oxygen levels by anastomosis was previously demonstrated.[9] The "hypoxic overshoot" seen in some areas of ischemia in patients with TIA may also be eliminated, providing an increased oxygen capacity to the tissue at risk.

References

1. Chance, B., Oshino, N., Sugano, T., Mayevsky, A. Basic principles of tissue oxygen determination from mitochondrial signals. In Oxygen Transport to Tissue Instrumentation, Methods and Physiology, Haim I. Bicher and Duane F. Bruley, editors, Plenum Publishing Corp., New York, 1973.
2. Chance, B., Cohen, P., Jobsis, F., Schoerer, B. Intracellular oxidation reduction states in vivo. Science 137:499–508, 1962.
3. Chance, B. Pyridine nucleotide as an indicator of the oxygen requirements for energy-linked functions of mitochondria. Circ Res 38 (Suppl) 131–138, 1976.
4. Chance, B., Williams, G.R. Respiratory enzymes in oxidative phosphorylation 1. Kinetics of oxygen utilization. J Biol Chem 217:383–393, 1955.
5. Chance, B., Williams, G.P. Respiratory enzymes in oxidative phosphorylation III. The steady state. J Biol Chem 217:409–427, 1955.
6. Chance, B., Williams, G.B., Holmes, W.F., Higgins, J. Respiratory enzymes in oxidative phosphorylation V. A mechanism for oxidative phosphorylation. J Biol Chem 217:439–451, 1955.
7. Chance, B., Williams, G.R. The respiratory chain and oxidative phosphorylation. Arch Enzymol 17:65–143, 1956.
8. Fein, J.M., Moore, C.M. Energy metabolism in experimental middle cerebral occlusion. Proc Research Society of Neurological Surgery, New York, New York, May 1978.
9. Fein, J.M. Intraoperative measurement of cortical energy metabolism in patients undergoing STA–MCA anastomosis. IX International Symposium on CBF and Metabolism. Tokyo, Japan, May 29–June 1, 1979.
10. Fein, J.M. Contemporary techniques of cerebral revascularization. In Microvascular Anastomoses for Cerebral Ischemia, J.M. Fein and O.H. Reichman, editors, Springer-Verlag, New York, 1978.
11. Jobsis, F., O'Connor, M., Vitale, A., Bremar, H. Intracellular redox changes in functioning cerebral cortex. I. Metabolic effects of epileptiform activity. J Neurophysiol 34:735–749, 1971.
12. Lothman, E., LaMama, J., Cordingly, G., Rosenthal, M., Somjen, G. Responses of electrical potential, potassium levels and oxidation metabolic activity of the cerebral neocortex of cats. Brain Res 88:15–35, 1975.
13. Obrist, W.D. Regional cerebral blood flow estimated by ^{133}Xenon inhalation. Stroke 6:245–256, 1975.
14. Rosenthal, M., Jobsis, F. Intracellular redox changes in functioning cerebral cortex. II. Effects of direct cortical stimulation. J Neurophysiol 34:750–762, 1971.
15. Rosenthal, M., LaMama, J.C. Effect of ouabain and phenobarbital on the kinetics of cortical metabolic transients associated with evoked potentials. J Neurochem 24:111–116, 1975.

III

Cerebral Blood Flow

7

Changes in Cerebral Autoregulation in Patients Undergoing Microanastomosis

G. Austin, D. Zinke, E. Lichter, and W. Hayward

Transient ischemic attacks (TIAs), lasting usually seconds or minutes but occasionally up to 24 hours, are thought to have three possible causes: (1) hemodynamic, (2) embolic, or (3) vasospastic.

The hemodynamic type of TIA is thought to arise in patients who have flow-restricting lesions in one of the main arteries in the neck (internal carotid or vertebral), or in the middle cerebral artery, or in one of the main branches of the circle of Willis. These lesions are thought to be subthreshold for TIAs but to attain threshold by transient decreases in cardiac output. An embolic cause for TIAs is thought to arise predominately from platelet emboli or fibrinoplatelet emboli. The origin of these remains unknown. They are believed possibly to arise from atherosclerotic or ulcerative plaques in the internal carotid artery, vertebral artery, middle cerebral artery, or the heart. In addition, activation of platelet emboli is greatly increased by emotional stress. The evidence for a vasospastic origin of TIAs is the least conclusive. Vasospasms of the pial vessels have been seen to occur under the microscope in the human brain during the course of vascular surgery. These spasms usually last up to 5 to 10 minutes in duration and are markedly flow limiting.

All of these potential sources of TIAs exert their effects by limiting blood flow to the brain. Some of them may be focal in flow limitation and some more diffuse. Similarly, TIAs can be of a focal character, such as unilaterally blurred vision, slurred speech, weakness or numbness of an opposite extremity; or nonfocal, as in the case of dizziness, recent-memory loss, confusional episodes, blackout attacks, or emotional instability (frequent unwarranted crying spells). It has been postulated that there is loss of autoregulation in some patients so that the decrease in pressure normally necessary to exceed the balance autoregulation need not occur. If autoregulation were indeed lost, this would make the seriousness of both hemodynamic and, to some extent, fibrinoplatelet emboli and vasospasm more severe.

In the past ten years since the original suggestion by Donaghy and Yasargil,[10] a number of patients have undergone microanastomosis for brain ischemia. This has largely consisted of anastomosis of the superficial temporal artery to the middle cerebral artery on the side of major obstruction. In the course of evaluating potential patients for anastomosis, the usual criteria which have been observed are: (1) a history of TIAs, RINDs, or partial stroke, and (2) a flow-limiting lesion visualized by cerebral angiography which is inaccessible or inoperable.

In addition, over the past six years we have added a further criterion, namely, that cerebral blood flow should be significantly reduced. Although this is mainly reduced in a more or less regional fashion, because of the distributive nature of the circle of Willis, it often occurs over a widespread area and even includes the opposite hemisphere by virtue of a cerebral steal. The authors have previously reported on the technique of measuring rCBF by the non-invasive intravenous injection of ^{133}Xe. This is a 12-minute flow test in which the fast or gray-matter component only has been utilized.[1,2] In over 1,135 patients there has been no morbidity with this technique. In the present paper we present the results of measuring autoregulation in a series of patients undergoing microanastomosis for brain ischemia.

Methods

Measurements were made on a control group of individuals and on patients. The mean flow through the gray matter is approximately 70 ± 6 mm/100 g/min. The reproducibility within a one-week period is ± 14% in controls. Mean blood pressure was increased by an intravenous infusion of 0.004% Neo-Synephrine. The average increase of cerebral blood flow in controls for an increase of 19 mm Hg in mean pressure was 3.37 ± 3.24 ml/100 g/min. A significant increase in CBF (gray) for loss of autoregulation was considered to be the mean plus 2 SD, i.e., 10 ml/100 g/min. Patients who were considered to be adequate candidates for microanastomosis according to the criteria listed above were brought to the cerebral blood flow laboratory and similar studies for autoregulation were done. No sedation was used and the laboratory conditions for controls and patients were the same. The results obtained from patients were then broken down into various groups according to the site of the lesion and whether or not there was a loss of autoregulation (AR).

Results

The mean cerebral blood flow at rest was 74 ± 8 ml/100 g/min. This is close to the average value obtained in all controls previously. There was a mean change in cerebral blood flow of 3.4 ± 3.2 ml/100 g/min when the mean blood pressure change was 19 mm Hg. As mentioned above, the significant change for patients was considered to be 10 ml/100 g/min. The results are shown in Table 7-1. Loss of autoregulation

occurred in 27 of 57 patients who were studied and later underwent microsurgical anastomosis for cerebral ischemia. The highest incidence in loss of autoregulation occurred in 4 out of 6 patients with bilateral internal carotid occlusion or stenosis (66%). The next-highest incidence occurred in those with internal carotid artery stenosis. In those patients with internal carotid artery occlusion, loss of autoregulation occurred in 44% (Table 7-2). There was no difference between the mean blood pressure at rest in those patients who had lost autoregulation and those who had intact autoregulation. Similarly, there was no significant difference in the mean CBF at rest for those who had intact autoregulation and those with lost regulation (Table 7-3). In the 27 of 57 patients who showed loss of autoregulation, there was a change from a control blood flow from 45 ml/100 g/min to 64.4 ml/100 g/min which corresponded to a mean increase in blood pressure of 24 mm Hg (Table 7-4). Follow-up studies of the incidence of transient ischemic attacks were obtained in 22 patients who had

Table 7-1. Controls (AR) N = 9

CBF (resting $\overline{BP}$)	74.03 ± 8.1
CBF (increased $\overline{BP}$)	77.4 ± 10
Mean change in $\overline{BP}$	19 mm Hg
Mean change in CBF	3.37 ± 3.24
Sig. change for patients	3.37 + 2 SD = 10

Table 7-2. Loss of autoregulation 27/57

I.C.O.	12/27	44%
I.C.S.	8/13	62%
M.C.O. & S.	2/9	22%
B.I.C.O. & S.	4/6	66%
V.O. & S.	1/2	50%

Table 7-3. Autoregulation STA–MCA patients (N = 57)

Mean $\overline{BP}$ (intact AR)		100.7
Mean $\overline{BP}$ (lost AR)		98.1
P value	0.44	
Mean CBF (intact AR)		46.2
Mean CBF (lost AR)		45.1
P value	0.67	

Table 7-4. Lost autoregulation patients (N = 27)

Control CBF	45.1 ml/100 g/min
Final CBF	64.4 ml/100 g/min
Change CBF	19.3 ml/100 g/min
Change BP	24 mm Hg

Table 7-8. Postoperative mortality in AR patients

Lost AR	Intact AR	Cause	Postop time
	1 FB.	Septicemia	60 hr
1 KH.		Unknown	23 mo
1 RK.		Stroke—	
		Opp. side	3 days
1 WH.		Same	5 mo
	1 BJ.	Ca lung	7 mo
	1 WF.	Ca colon	7 mo

lost autoregulation. The postoperative incidence of TIAs was decreased markedly in all of those patients and the average decrease in all groups was 82% (Table 7-5). In patients with intact autoregulation, which was present in 26 of 57 patients, the average decrease in TIAs was 92% (Table 7-6). It should be noted that the follow-up in these patients was 15 ± 9.7 months. In patients who had lost AR, minor strokes had occurred preoperatively in 44%, whereas in those with intact AR minor strokes had occurred in only 27% preoperatively (Table 7-7). Postoperatively two deaths occurred within 30 days. One was due to fulminating septicemia thought to have arisen from a very severe tooth abscess which had not been noticed preopera-

tively. This patient had intact autoregulation. The second death occurred three days after operation and was due to occlusion of the opposite internal carotid artery. The patient had lost AR. The opposite internal carotid artery of another patient occluded five months postoperatively. This patient had lost autoregulation. The two other deaths which occurred in patients with intact AR were due to carcinoma of the lung and carcinoma of the colon (Table 7-8).

Table 7-5. TIAs—Lost autoregulation (N = 22)

Lesion	N	Pre	Post	↓ %
I.C.O.	8	19	4	79
I.C.S.	8	27	2	93
M.C.O. & S.	2	8	1	87
B.I.C.O. & S.	4	16	5	69
Follow-up = 15 ± 9.7 mo				

Table 7-6. TIAs—Intact autoregulation (N = 26)

Lesion	N	Pre	Post	↓ %
I.C.O.	13	47	10	79
I.C.S.	5	23	0	100
M.C.O. & S.	6	16	3	89
B.I.C.O. & S.	2	10	0	100
Follow-up = 15 ± 9.7 mo				

Table 7-7. Preoperative strokes in autoregulation patients

Total	20/57 = 35%
In lost autoregulation	12/27 = 44%
In intact autoregulation	8/30 = 27%

Discussion

Autoregulation was first described by Roy and Sherrington in 1890.[18] Essentially it refers to the ability of the brain to maintain a constant perfusion cerebral blood flow over a wide range of mean pressures and down to a level of approximately 70 mm Hg. Below this level blood flow varies linearly with pressure. The main controlling features of cerebral blood flow are thought to be exerted through a myogenic effect by extracellular fluid pH, and possibly by a somewhat more rapidly acting neuronal effect.[11, 13, 16, 20] In addition, cerebral blood flow is responsive to variation in aPO_2. Above 50 mm of aPO_2, the flow remains constant, and below 50 mm the flow increases as the aPO_2 drops. Similarly, with $aPCO_2$ there is a wide and even more sensitive change in CBF.[9, 12, 17, 19] Over a wide range of values (CO_2 30 to 80 mm Hg) CBF varies almost linearly with changes in $aPCO_2$. The best explanation for this is that the intravascular CO_2 diffuses rapidly out of smaller arteries and arterioles into the extracellular space, and by immediate variation of the extracellular fluid pH causes changes in the size of the smaller blood vessels. At present it is known that as the pH of the extracellular spaces decreases there is a marked dilatation of the cerebrovasculature. This has been shown predominately in animals, but also in man, using the Kety-Schmidt inert gas technique[14] and the isotope techniques developed by Harper et al.[12] and by Lassen and Munch,[15] where CBF has been shown to vary widely in proportion to arterial PCO_2.

In the patients and controls in this study, there was no significant change in arterial PCO_2 during the studies. The marked failure of autoregulation in some patients can be explained on the basis of atherosclerotic changes involving the medial walls of small arteries. This makes them less elastic and less able to respond to changes in extracellular fluid pH. To a similar extent, these vessels would be less responsive to neurogenic effects. Finally, there is the possibility that there may be some impairment of brain stem neurogenic effects by virtue of the disease process.

The potential consequences of failure of autoregulation in these patients are marked. In terms of preoperative TIAs or stroke it could accentuate their appearance and severity because the brain PO_2 would vary with the pressure and reach a critical level for the appearance of TIAs quite rapidly. This is based on observations showing changes in cortical oxidative metabolism varying with brain PO_2.[3-5] Other potential dangers of loss of autoregulation are apparent in that there is a significantly higher incidence of preoperative stroke in these patients and a significantly lower decrease in the incidence of TIAs following surgery. The fact that the decrease in TIAs is so high can be partially attributed to the shortness of the follow-up, which averaged 15 months. In the longer follow-up period of 37 months, we have shown an average decrease in all types of TIAs, both focal and nonfocal, of 66%. This was in spite of the fact, however, that 64% of all operated patients were back at full- or part-time work which they could not do before the procedure.

In considering the mortality of autoregulation patients, it appears significant that the only two postoperative strokes occurred in patients who had lost autoregulation. Aside from this, the lessons to be learned from this study are that approximately 50% of all patients undergoing microanastomosis, as judged by the present study, would have lost autoregulation. This suggests the importance of maintaining an adequate perfusion pressure at all times in the hospital, preoperatively, during the period of anesthetic induction, and postoperatively. Undoubtedly some of the problems which arise in the immediate postoperative period might be avoided or ameliorated if a higher level of mean pressure was maintained in these patients.

References

1. Austin, G., Laffin, D., Rouhe, S., Hayward, W. Intravenous isotope injection method of cerebral blood flow measurements: Accuracy and reproducibility. Proceedings of the International Symposium on Cerebral Circulation and Metabolism, Philadelphia, 1973.
2. Austin, G., Laffin, D., Hayward, W. Evaluation of fast component (gray matter) by 12 minute IV method using analog computer analysis. In Blood Flow and Metabolism in the Brain, A.M. Harper, W.B. Jennet, S.D. Miller, and J. Rowan, editors, Churchill Livingston, Edinburgh, 1975, pp. 8.25–8.31.
3. Austin, G.M., Haugen, G., Lichter, E., Hayward, W. Microneurosurgical anastomosis: A biochemical basis for improvement. Acta Med Nagaskiensia 22(1-2):35–49, 1977.
4. Austin, G., Haugen, G., LaManna, J. Cortical oxidative metabolism following microanastomosis for brain ischemia. In Oxygen and Physiological Function, F. Jobsis, editor, Professional Information Library, Dallas, 1976, pp. 531–544.
5. Austin, G.M., Jutzy, R. Noninvasive monitoring of human brain oxidative metabolism. In Frontiers of Biological Energies from Electrons to Tissue. University of Pennsylvania, Philadelphia, 1978.
6. Austin, G.M., Chance, B., Hill, W., Barlow, C. Monitoring of cortical mitochondrial respiration during microanastomosis. Abstract American Association Neurological Surgeons, New Orleans, 1978, pp. 531–544.
7. Austin, G.M., Haugen, G., Brown, D., et al. Cortical mitochondrial respiration following microanastomosis. Abstract American Association Neurological Surgeons, Toronto, 1977.
8. Austin, G.M., Schuler, W., Willey, J. In vivo studies of mitochondrial respiration. In Oxygen Transport to Tissue, I.A. Silver, M. Erecinska,

and H.I. Bicher, editors, Plenum Publishing Corp., New York, 1978, pp. 289–295.

9. Detar, R., Bohr, D.F. Oxygen and vascular smooth muscle contraction. Am J Physiol 214: 245–256, 1968.

10. Donaghy, P., Yasargil, G. Extraintracranial blood flow diversion. Abstract American Association of Neurological Surgeons, Chicago, 1968.

11. Gotoh, F., Ebihara, S.I., Toyota, M., et al. Role of autonomic nervous system in autoregulation of human cerebral evaluation. Eur Neurol 6:203–207, 1972.

12. Harper, A.M., Glass, H.I. Effects of alterations in the arterial carbon dioxide tension on the blood flow through the cerebral cortex and normal and low arterial pressure. J Neurol Neurosurg Psychiat 28:449–452, 1965.

13. James, I.M., Miller, R.A., Purves, M.J. Observations on the extrinsic neurol control of cerebral blood flow in the baboon. Circ Res 75: 77–93, 1969.

14. Kety, S.S., Schmidt, L.F. The effects of altered arterial tensions of carbon dioxide and oxygen on cerebral blood flow and cerebral oxygen consumption on normal young men. J Clin Invest 27:484–492, 1948.

15. Lassen, N.A., Munch, O. The cerebral blood flow in man determined by the use of radioactive krypton. Acta Physiol Scand 33:30–49, 1955.

16. Meyer, J.S., Shimazu, K., Fukuuchi, Y., et al. Cerebral dysautoregulation in cerebral neurogenic orthostatic hypotension (Shy-Drager Syndrome). Neurology 23:262–273, 1973.

17. Reivich, M. Arterial PCO_2 and cerebral neurodynamics. Am J Physiol 206(1):25–35, 1964.

18. Roy, L.S., Sherrington, L.S. Regulation of the blood supply of the brain. J Physiol 11:85–108, 1890.

19. Shinojyo, S., Scheinberg, P., Kogure, K., et al. The effects of graded hypoxia upon transient cerebral blood flow and oxygen consumption. Neurology 18:127–133, 1968.

20. Symon, L., Held, K., Dorsch, N.W.C. On the myogenic nature of autoregulatory mechanism in the cerebral circulation. In Cerebral Blood Flow and Intracranial Pressures. Proceedings 5th International Symposium, Roma-Siena, 1971, Part I. Eur Neurol 6:11–19, 1971/1972.

8

Regional Cortical Blood Flow During Cerebrovascular Surgery

L. Philip Carter and Richard J. Erspamer

The essence of surgery upon the vasculature of the central nervous system is its effect on the blood flow within the tissue. The long-term results can be evaluated by postoperative angiography and radioactive regional blood flow studies; however, acute alterations in tissue perfusion are equally important. These immediate changes can be assessed in the operating room by angiography,[6] electromagnetic flowmeters,[9, 10] measurements of metabolism,[1] observation of the direct cortical response,[5] and radioactive diffusion washout techniques.[11] A thermal diffusion flow probe has some advantages over most methods in that it can give a continuous dynamic quantitative recording of cortical blood flow[4] and the vascular structures need not be disturbed. With the thermal flow probe a thermal gradient is applied directly to the cortex and consequently does not depend upon an adequate concentration of diffusible material arriving at the region in question, as do other diffusion washout techniques.

In 1933 Gibbs[7] described a thermal flow probe which was modified and studied by Grayson[8] who, in 1952, demonstrated the thermal conductivity increment to be a linear function of the rate of blood flow. Brawley[2] constructed a flow probe from a Peltier stack, which Carter et al.[3, 4] have modified and demonstrated to have a relative linear relationship with cortical blood flow. We have monitored regional cortical blood flow in 79 craniotomies; over half have been for vascular problems. The present report describes our experience with aneurysms and superficial temporal artery to middle cerebral artery bypass (STA–MCA).

The previously described probe was constructed from a Peltier stack with gold plates soldered to the hot and cold sides of the stack. Copper constantine thermocouples measure the temperature difference between the gold plates which, during recording, are in contact with the cortex. The difference between the "no flow" probe recording and the probe value for various levels of cortical blood flow as determined by ^{133}Xe in experimental animals was used to calibrate the probe.[3] As expected from Grayson's[8] work, there was a relatively linear relationship between cortical blood flow as determined by the probe (CBF_p) and that determined by ^{133}Xe fast component within the physiologic range.

At craniotomy, after dural opening, the probe was placed on the area of cortex of interest, avoiding surface vessels (Fig. 8-1). The probe was held in place with a suture around the connecting cable secured to the scalp and was covered by the dura or a cotton sponge. Recording was carried out during the operative procedure, frequently moving the probe to assess flow in various regions. In most cases a radial arterial cannula was inserted to record mean blood pressure ($\overline{BP}$) and obtain frequent arterial blood gas studies.

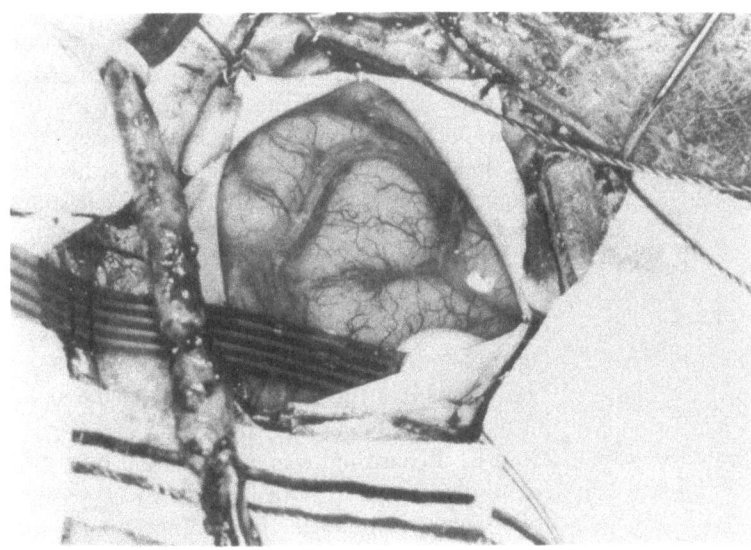

Fig. 8-1. The thermal flow probe rests on the cortex after exposure for STA–MCA. The STA is gently retracted by a rubber band and the recipient cortical vessel is just above the center of the craniotomy. The flow probe is away from the actual site of anastomosis and is tucked beneath a dural edge.

Results

In 33 craniotomies for aneurysm, alterations in regional cortical flow were produced by changes in perfusion pressure, retraction, vascular manipulation, and temporary vessel occlusion.

A typical aneurysm case is illustrated in Fig. 8-2. This recording is from the left frontal lobe during clipping of an aneurysm of the left middle cerebral artery (MCA). When the aneurysm ruptured, an obvious drop in CBF_p occurred while the $\overline{BP}$ was not affected by the hemorrhage. Subsequently as bleeding was controlled, clip applied, aneurysm collapsed, and papaverine applied, a return of CBF_p to prehemorrhage levels occurred. CBF_p always remained

in an acceptable range and the patient made an uneventful recovery. On the other hand, Fig. 8-3 is a tracing from the right frontal lobe of a patient with a right internal carotid aneurysm which demonstrates a significant drop of $\overline{BP}$ with sodium nitroprusside with only a minimal change in CBF_p. Obviously $\overline{BP}$ does not adequately reflect changes in cerebral perfusion.

Manipulation of major vascular channels can produce changes in tissue perfusion (Fig. 8-4). This recording was obtained from the inferior aspect of the left cerebellar hemisphere during an approach to a left vertebral aneurysm. As manipulation of the left posterior inferior cerebellar artery (PICA) occurred a significant drop in CBF_p was observed. CBF_p recovered once

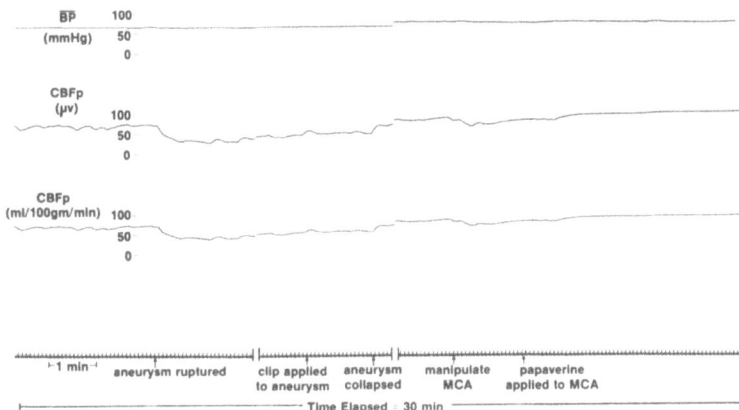

Fig. 8-2. Continuous monitoring of $\overline{BP}$ and CBF_p, as measured by microvolts (μv) and ml/100 g tissue per minute, from posterior inferior left frontal lobe during surgery upon a left MCA aneurysm demonstrates changes in CBF_p without alteration of $\overline{BP}$.

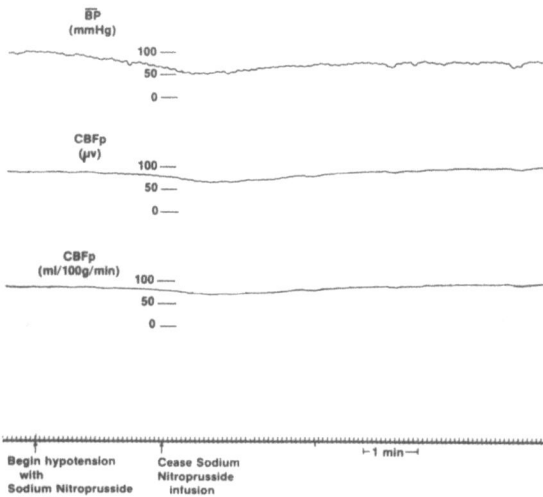

Fig. 8-3. Monitoring from the right frontal lobe during surgery on a large right internal carotid aneurysm shows minimal change in CBF$_p$ with significant drop in $\overline{\text{BP}}$, from 100 to 50 mm Hg.

PICA was released. In contemplating direct surgery on this vessel one must consider the effects of its occlusion upon the blood flow of the cerebellar hemisphere. An example of temporary occlusion of major vascular channels is illustrated in Fig. 8-5, which is a recording from the left temporal lobe during clipping of a left MCA aneurysm. A temporary clip was placed across two branches of the MCA to allow better delineation of the aneurysm. With this maneuver an obvious increase in flow occurred. There was no change with placement of the permanent clip, but the flow returned to the previous level once the temporary clip was removed. This demonstrated excellent collateral circulation, probably through another major branch which was not occluded. The patient had no residual effect from clipping two major MCA branches for five minutes.

Brain retraction at craniotomy is another important factor affecting cerebral blood flow. Fig. 8-6 was recorded before closure from three different regions of the left temporal lobe after clipping of an aneurysm arising in a fenestration of the basilar artery as well as a left MCA aneurysm. During the surgical procedure CBF$_p$ was monitored on the superior temporal lobe and remained in an acceptable range. The self-

retaining brain retractor was on the inferior temporal lobe, providing exposure of the basilar artery. It is apparent that the flow in the inferior portion of the temporal lobe was very low. Postoperatively this patient had a hemorrhagic infarction in the temporal lobe with massive edema.

CBF$_p$ was recorded during six STA–MCA procedures and no changes in CBF$_p$ were observed with occlusion of the cortical vessel. Fig. 8-7 is a recording during left STA–MCA. The PCO$_2$ was the same pre- and postanastomosis, while BP was slightly higher after anastomosis. Recording was made from two different areas, and in both the CBF$_p$ was greater following anastomosis. In addition, once the anastomosis was open and the CBF$_p$ appeared to be stable, the STA was temporarily occluded, demonstrating a drop in CBF$_p$ and recovery with removal of the temporary clip. The CBF$_p$ results were tabulated (Table 8-1). It should be noted that in most cases CBF$_p$ increased following anastomosis; however, in case #69 CBF$_p$ decreased in two recording sites and increased

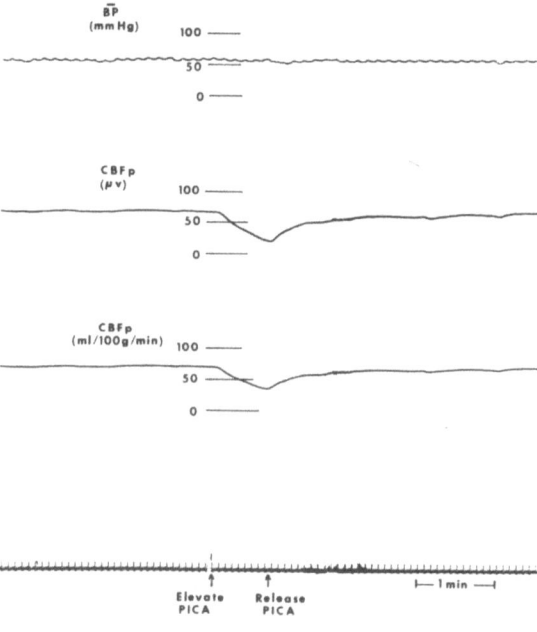

Fig. 8-4. Recording from left inferior cerebellar hemisphere while exposing a fusiform left vertebral aneurysm demonstrates changes in CBF$_p$ with manipulation of left posterior inferior cerebellar artery (PICA).

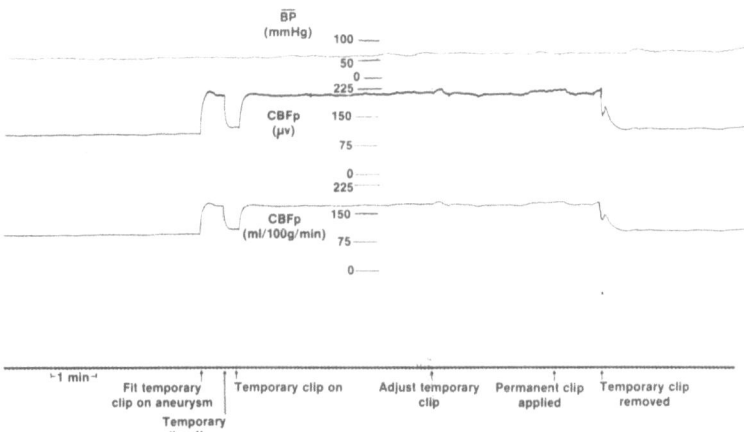

Fig. 8-5. This tracing was obtained from the left temporal lobe during surgery on a left MCA aneurysm. A temporary clip was placed across two branches of the MCA, producing a marked increase in collateral circulation through the cortex being studied.

in a third. This patient had occlusion of the left vertebral artery and stenosis of the other in addition to left MCA occlusion and left internal carotid stenosis. Because the primary symptoms were referable to the left hemisphere

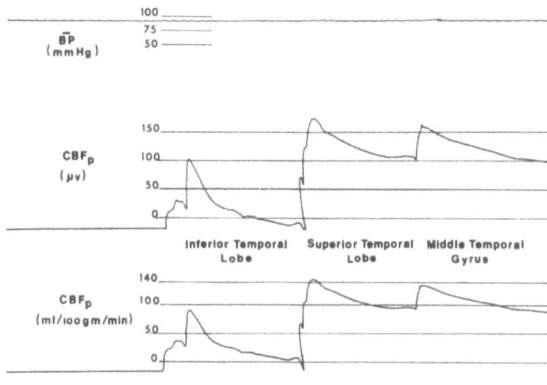

Fig. 8-6. This recording was obtained from three different locations on the temporal lobe following completion of clipping of a difficult basilar aneurysm as well as a small left MCA aneurysm. After the probe is placed at each site approximately one minute is required to reach a steady state which represents the final CBF_p value recorded for each region. The middle and superior temporal gyri had adequate flow in the order of 100 cc/100 g/min but the inferior temporal lobe had markedly diminished blood flow approaching zero.

a left STA–MCA was performed. Postoperatively the patient had some mild dysphasia that was not present preoperatively, but otherwise did well until 38 hours postoperatively when blood pressure abruptly increased and a respiratory arrest occurred. At autopsy it was apparent that the remaining vertebral artery had occluded. Case #59 also had a reduction in CBF_p following anastomosis but showed a good result. This patient had no further TIAs and a patent anastomosis was found on postoperative angiography. The drop in CBF_p demonstrated in case #63 with temporary occlusion of the STA was not demonstrated in two other patients in which temporary occlusion was carried out.

Discussion

The goal of cerebrovascular surgery is to preserve and improve the circulation to the brain. To evaluate changes in cerebral blood flow at the time of surgery we have employed a thermal diffusion flow probe. With this technique abrupt changes in tissue perfusion are readily apparent and reflect changes in blood flow without requiring injection or inhalation of isotopes, perforation of the pial membrane, or manipulation of major vascular channels. Techniques that measure tissue metabolism may indirectly reflect blood flow but may also be affected by other factors, such as anesthetic agents. Obviously changes in tissue metabolism

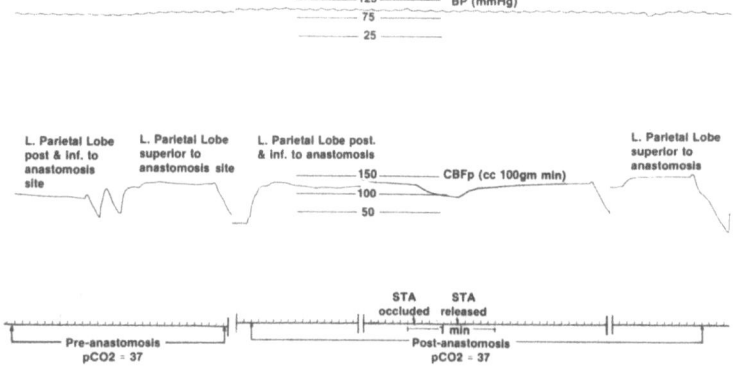

Fig. 8-7. This recording was from two different regions near a STA–MCA. $\overline{BP}$ changed only slightly and the PCO_2 was constant but CBF_p was increased from 95 to 120 and from 135 to 153 cc/100 g/min after anastomosis. In addition, with temporary occlusion of the STA–MCA a significant drop in CBF_p was apparent.

Table 8-1. Results of six STA–MCA patients pre- and postanastomosis

Case #	Patient	Recording site	Preanastomosis			Postanastomosis			Δ		
			PCO_2	CBF_p	$\overline{BP}$	PCO_2	CBF_p	$\overline{BP}$	PCO_2	$\overline{BP}$	CBF_p
33	D.F.	1) 2 cm from anastomosis	38	105	80	−	110	90	−	+ 5	+10
63	H.B.	1) L. parietal lobe, post. & inf. to anastomosis	37	95	83	37	120	98	0	+25	+15
		2) L. parietal lobe, superior to anastomosis	37	135	83	37	153	98	0	+18	+15
69	F.Z.	1) Post. temporo-parietal lobe, posterior to anastomosis	28	52	80	29	40	85	+1	−12	+ 5
		2) Post. temporo-parietal lobe, inferior to anastomosis	28	40	80	29	35	85	+1	− 5	+ 5
		3) Post. temporo-parietal lobe, post. & inf. to anastomosis	28	50	80	29	75	85	+1	+25	+ 5
74	H.W.	1) Post. temporal lobe, posterior to anastomosis	33	70	115	30	85	127	−3	+15	+12
78	A.H.	1) Rt. parietal lobe, posterior to anastomosis	22	60	95	−	70	95	−	+10	0
59	S.L.	1) L. post. temporal lobe	50	110	80	48	80	85	−2	−30	+ 5
		Average:	33.4	79.7	86.2	34.1	102.8	94.2	−0.3	+ 5.6	+ 6.3

Key: PCO_2 = carbon dioxide tension in mm Hg; CBF_p = probe cerebral blood flow in ml/100 g/min; $\overline{BP}$ = mean blood pressure in mm Hg; and Δ = pre- and postoperative differences.

may secondarily alter blood flow in response to the metabolic demand.

Systemic blood pressure is faithfully monitored in aneurysm surgery which, with an open skull without brain retraction, is the same as perfusion pressure. However, as can be seen from Figs. 8-2 and 8-3, CBF_p may change abruptly with no apparent change in $\overline{BP}$ or a significant alteration of $\overline{BP}$ may show only a minimal change in CBF_p. Obviously the cerebral blood flow is affected by many factors in addition to perfusion pressure, such as brain retractor pressure, vascular manipulation, arterial PCO_2, vasospasm, and drugs. The effects on regional flow of vessel occlusion are readily apparent and can give helpful information in some difficult aneurysms when temporary or permanent vessel occlusion is being considered.

We have monitored CBF_p in only six STA–MCA patients and can conclude that some acute changes in tissue perfusion can be detected (Fig. 8-7). This supports Austin's[1] demonstration of acute improvement in tissue metabolism after bypass surgery. The trend seems to be that of increased tissue flow immediately after anastomosis; however, further studies are needed to evaluate different regions in the operative field and compare these areas with pre- and postoperative regional CBF values. Furthermore, while occluding cortical branches we have not found any significant drop in CBF_p, thus supporting the clinical impression that there is such good collateral circulation in the cortex that no tissue ischemia occurs from this maneuver.

Intraoperative evaluation of regional flow may be of help in the future in identifying areas of decreased flow so that augmentation of perfusion can be more accurately directed to these regions. In addition, CBF_p studies may help determine the relative safety of temporary occlusion of major vascular channels so that direct reconstruction or bypass to those vessels can be more safely performed.

Acknowledgment

We thank Hal Pittman, M.D., and William L. White, M.D., for allowing us to include their cases in this study.

References

1. Austin, G., Haugen, G., Schuler, W. Transient ischemic attacks and metabolic aspects of their relief by microsurgical anastomosis. In Microvascular Anastomoses for Cerebral Ischemia, J. Fein and O. Reichman, editors, Springer-Verlag, New York, 1974, pp. 94–102.
2. Brawley, B.W. The pathophysiology of intracerebral steal following carbon dioxide inhalation: An experimental study. Scand J Clin Lab Invest 22 (Suppl 102) XIII:B., 1968.
3. Carter, L.P., Atkinson, J.R. Cortical blood flow in controlled hypotension as measured by thermal diffusion. J Neurol Neurosurg Psychiatry 36:906–913, 1973.
4. Carter, L.P., White, W.L., Atkinson, J.R. Regional cortical blood flow at craniotomy. Neurosurgery 2:223–229, 1978.
5. Eisenberg, H.M., Grossman, R.G., Teasdale, G., et al. The direct cortical response and estimate of cerebral blood flow in man. Proc Am Assoc Neurol Surgeons 44–46, 1978.
6. Feindel, W., Yamamato, Y.L., Hodge, C.P. Intracarotid fluorescein angiography: A new method for examination of the epicerebral circulation in man. Can Med Assoc J 96:1–7, 1967.
7. Gibbs, F.A. A thermoelectric blood flow recorder in the form of a needle. Proc Soc Exp Biol 31:141–146, 1933.
8. Grayson, J. Internal calorimetry in the determination of thermal conductivity and blood flow. J Physiol 118:54–72, 1952.
9. Spetzler, R., Chater, N. Microvascular bypass surgery; Part 2 Physiological studies. J Neurosurg 45:508–513, 1976.
10. Nornes, H., Wikeby, P. Cerebral arterial blood flow and aneurysm surgery. J Neurosurg 47:810–818, 1977.
11. Wilkins, A.G., Cummins, B.H., Griffith, H.B., et al. Repeated measurements of cerebral blood flow during intracranial surgery. Lancet 2:402–403, 1972.

9

The Use of STA–MCA Bypass in the Evaluation of rCBF*

Richard B. Morawetz, James H. Halsey, Jr., Edward L. Wills,
Urs W. Blauenstein, and Edwin M. Wilson

Objective means of evaluating patients who have undergone surgical procedures designed to augment collateral blood supply to the brain are necessary if these patients are to be assessed by means other than ongoing clinical examination and repeated angiography. We have studied seven consecutive patients selected for superficial temporal artery–middle cerebral artery (STA–MCA) bypass by clinical and angiographic criteria using [133]xenon clearance as assessed by the inhalation technique.

Materials and Methods

Seven consecutive patients subjected to STA–MCA bypass are included in this study. Each patient underwent bypass grafting following a preoperative workup which included angiography and at least two [133]xenon inhalation blood flow studies. Graft patency was confirmed by postoperative angiography in every case.

CBF studies were performed using a [133]xenon inhalation blood flow apparatus. Seven regional detectors on each side (Fig. 9-1) allowed simultaneous bilateral blood flow determinations. Data were analyzed using a mathematical model based on the method of Obrist and presented elsewhere.[1, 2] Three parameters were studied in detail:

ISI—This is the initial slope of the recirculation-corrected clearance curve developed in our laboratory by Risberg. It is similar to the widely used gray-matter relative flow rate (f_1) (ml/100 g/min) but has the advantage of being more stable and reproducible in the presence of brain lesions. Like the f_1 it is not very sensitive to nonperfused regions, e.g., infarcts.

Φ—This is an index recently developed in our laboratory which is proportional to the regional total flow (ml/min). Unlike the ISI and f_1 it is sensitive to nonperfused regions.

Q—This is another index developed in our laboratory which attempts to account for the simultaneous behavior of total flow (Φ) and relative flow (f_1, ISI) as their quotient. It appears to behave like regional blood volume (ml), but this interpretation is tentative and the index itself is still under evaluation.

Results presented below include CBF data, blood pressure data, brief clinical summaries and postoperative angiograms of the seven patients in the study. Because of differences in flows obtained in various laboratories, we have calculated mean preoperative values for each region and divided each postoperative value by the mean preoperative value. These data are plotted for right and left sides, the Y axis representing postoperative flow as a percent of preoperative flow, and the X axis showing days following bypass for each postoperative measurement. The same has been done for mean arterial blood pressure (MABP).

*Supported in part by NS 08802.

Discussion

Heilburn et al.[3] have discussed the problems associated with blood flow measurements using the intracarotid injection of [133]xenon in saline in patients who have undergone STA–MCA bypass. The need for a noninvasive technique for regional cerebral blood flow determination which can be carried out in the resting patient free from artifacts associated with anesthesia and the stress of angiography and our belief that serial determinations over time are necessary for the evaluation of these patients have led us to use the inhalation technique for rCBF determination. Many patients subjected to STA–MCA bypass are felt to suffer from ischemia induced by intermittent low-flow states. Areas receiving inadequate blood supply may receive collateral flow from the posterior circulation, from the opposite anterior circulation, and from the ipsilateral external circulation, as well as from bypass grafts. CBF studies carried out using injection techniques cannot take into account multiple sources of blood supply. Inhalation techniques, on the other hand, provide for saturation of all areas with xenon followed by washout by whatever sources of blood supply may be present. Thus it is our opinion that the inhalation technique is better suited to the study of bypass patients than injection techniques.

We have analyzed our data using the mathematical model presented and have presented three indices, ISI, Φ, and Q, which we feel reflect blood flow as expressed in ml/100 g/min and ml/min, and total brain blood volume. Analysis of the data suggests the following overall patterns.

Postoperatively rCBF increased on average by 14% on the operated side and by 8% on the nonoperated side. This interhemispheric difference was significant (p < 0.01). However, flow increases over both hemispheres postoperatively were not significantly greater than those seen preoperatively. A marked improvement in rCBF responses to hypocapnia was seen in patients following bypass grafting, suggesting that the main benefit of STA–MCA bypass in these patients is an increase in the homeostatic cerebrovascular reserve rather than a dramatic increase in the absolute flow to the brain.

In those patients who are neurologically intact following bypass surgery regional flows measured over a hemisphere tend to vary in a similar manner from determination to determination. Those patients with neurologic deficit, either present preoperatively or appearing as a complication of bypass surgery, show hemispheric flows which may vary greatly from region to region (patient TN, Fig. 9-1C).

In patients who are neurologically intact flows over both hemispheres tend to vary in a similar manner. It is our belief that in neurologically intact patients the intact corpus callosum integrates the function of the two hemispheres, and this results in similar blood flows over the two hemispheres in resting patients. Interhemispheric differences appear to be more marked in patients with neurologic deficit (patient TN, Fig. 9-1C).

The following observations were made regarding individual patients. Patient TN (Fig. 9-1C), the only patient to sustain a major neurologic deficit as a result of the surgery, showed a marked reduction in total blood flow (Φ) during the period of his global aphasia. Following clearing of his aphasia, flows (Φ) increased to levels at or above preoperative levels. These changes were not reflected by the ISI values.

Patient WB (Fig. 9-1A) showed an early 30% increase in flow as indicated by ISI and a 40% increase in flow as indicated by Φ. Two weeks after bypass flows had returned to preoperative levels. The patient remained asymp-

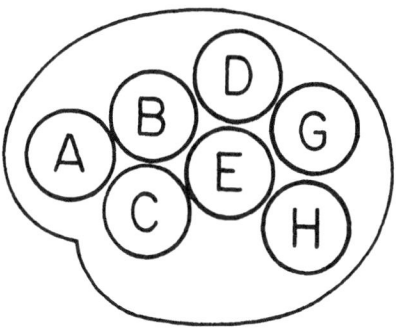

Fig. 9-1. This diagram shows the array of seven detectors and their location over each hemisphere. The letters A, B, C, D, E, G, and H correspond to the flows plotted in Figs. 9-1A through 9-1G.

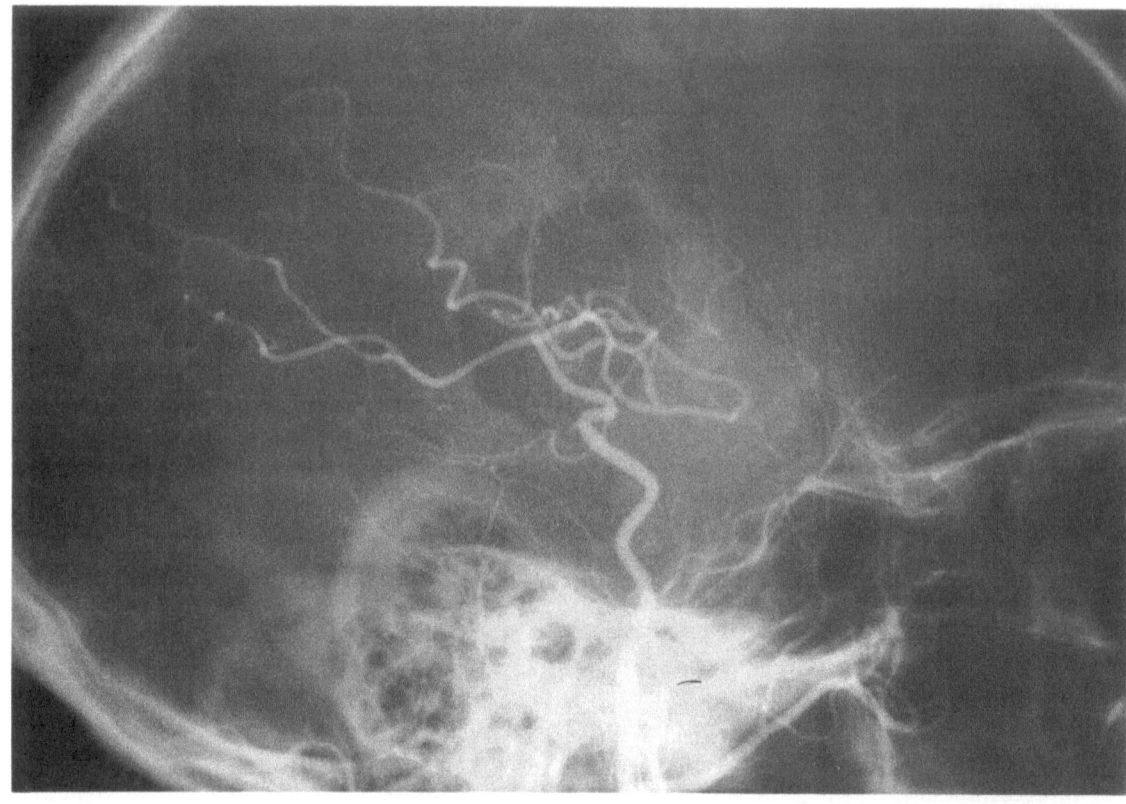

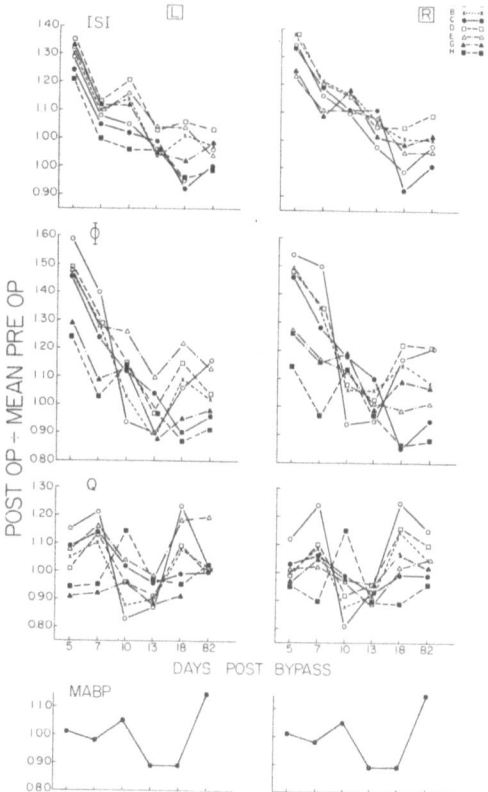

Fig. 9-1A. Patient WB. This 53-year-old man gave a history of left hemiparesis which cleared over several days eight months prior to admission, and the onset of dense right hemiparesis with expressive dysphasia on the day of admission. Angiography showed 80% stenosis of the right internal carotid artery within the cavernous sinus, and complete occlusion of the left internal carotid artery. Left STA–MCA bypass was carried out without complications, and postoperatively the patient had no further ischemic episodes.

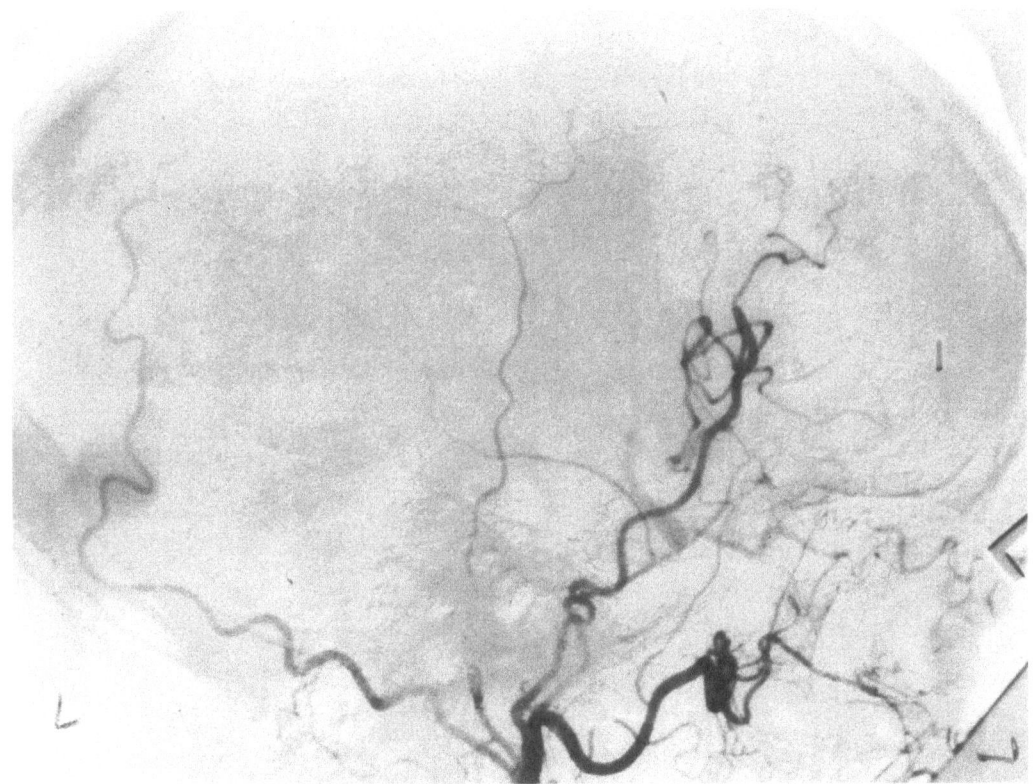

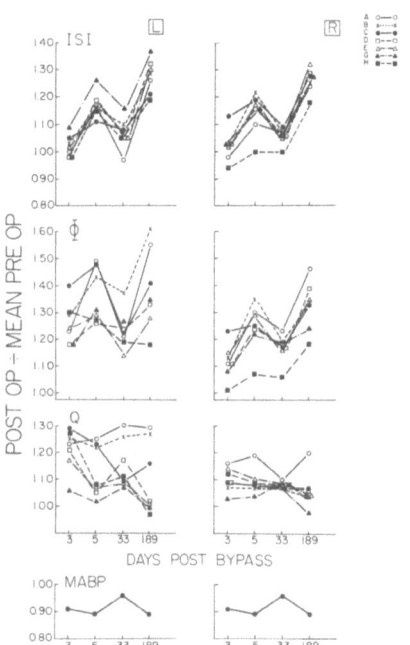

Fig. 9-1B. Patient CE. This 63-year-old man with a history of ischemic heart disease had several episodes of left-sided transient monocular blindness over two months prior to admission. The day before admission the patient suffered two episodes of transient right hemiparesis and aphasia lasting ten minutes. Angiography showed complete occlusion of the left internal carotid artery at its origin. Left STA–MCA bypass was carried out without complications and postoperatively the patient had no further ischemic episodes.

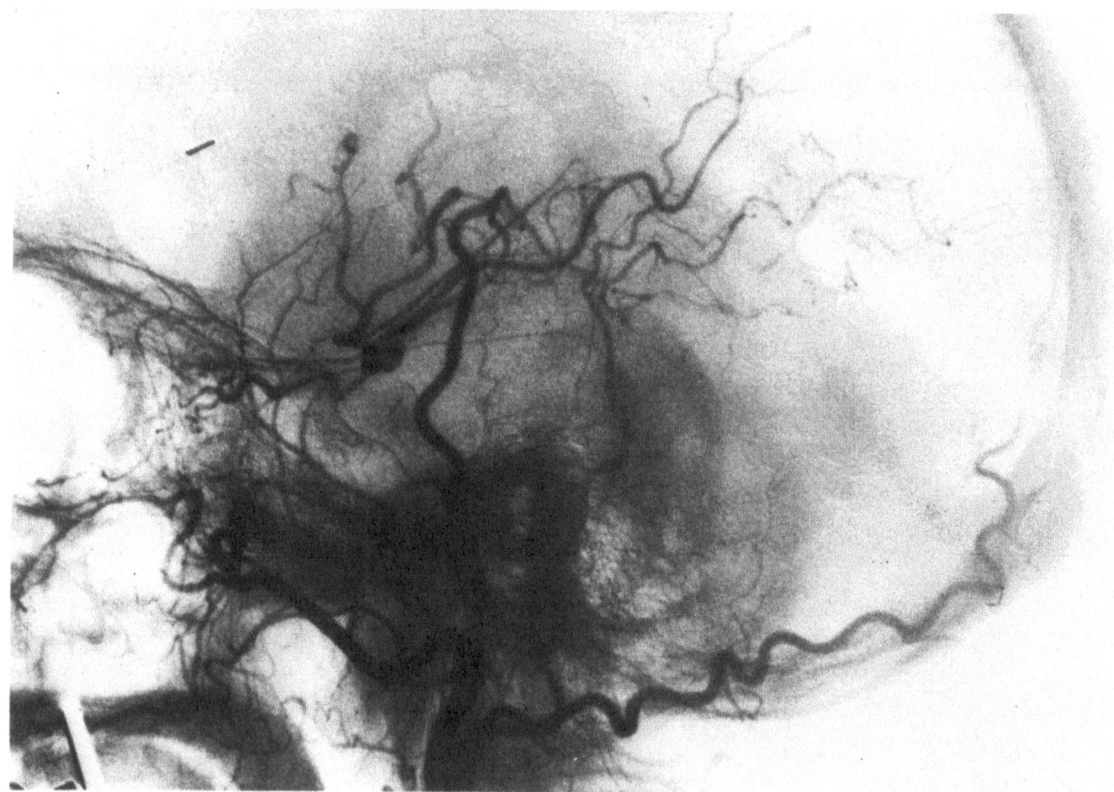

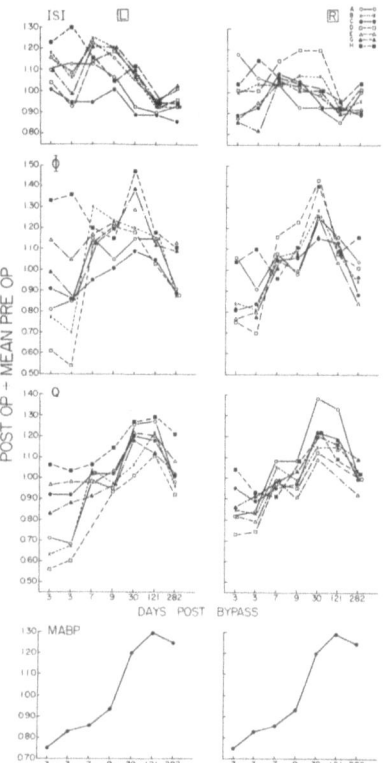

Fig. 9-1C. Patient TN. This 69-year-old man developed left hemiplegia following surgery for an abdominal aortic aneurysm. Angiography at that time showed bilateral internal carotid artery occlusion with intracranial perfusion from both ophthalmic arteries and the posterior circulation. The patient improved over several months and ten months later underwent left STA–MCA bypass. Postoperatively the patient was globally aphasic with no other focal neurologic change. His aphasia cleared over three days and over the next six months improved neurologically relative to his preoperative status. At the time of his last CBF studies, however, the patient had shown worsening of his previously noted left hemiparesis and pseudobulbar palsy.

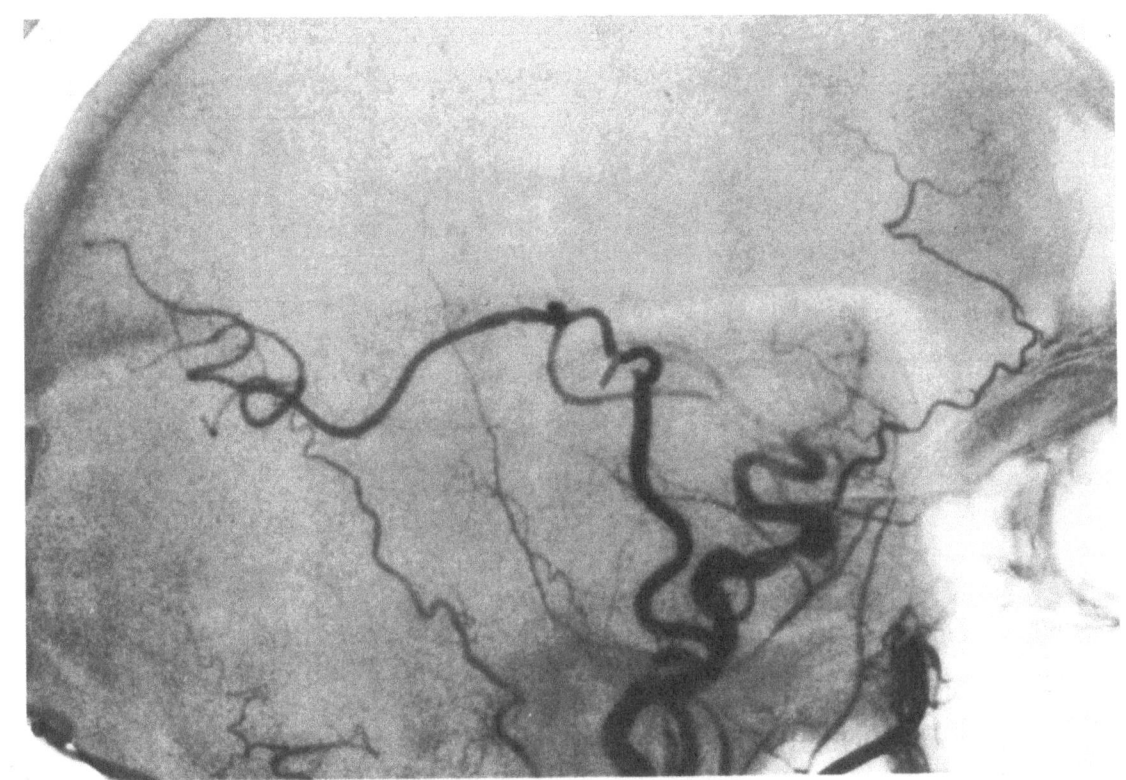

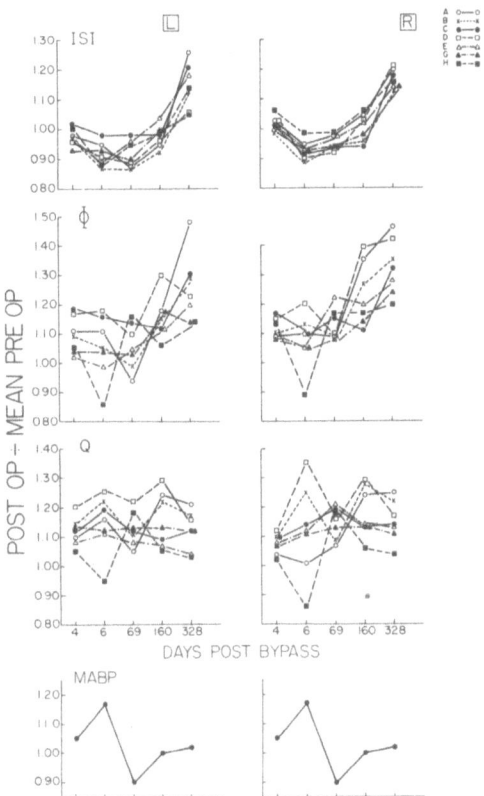

Fig. 9-1D. Patient CB was a 57-year-old man with a one-week history of right transient monocular blindness. Arteriograms showed a 40% stenosis of the right internal carotid artery 1 cm from its origin, and an 85% stenosis of the right intra-cavernous internal carotid artery. Significant supply to the right internal carotid artery distribution from the left internal carotid artery was demonstrated. Following right STA–MCA bypass the patient demonstrated a transient mild left facial weakness which cleared over three days. He remained asymptomatic thereafter.

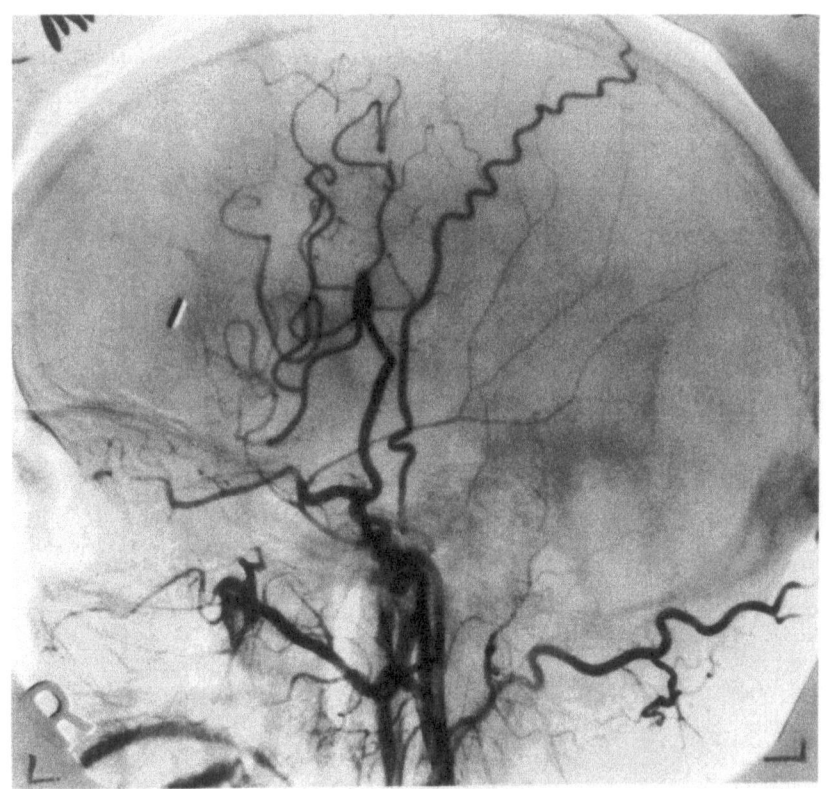

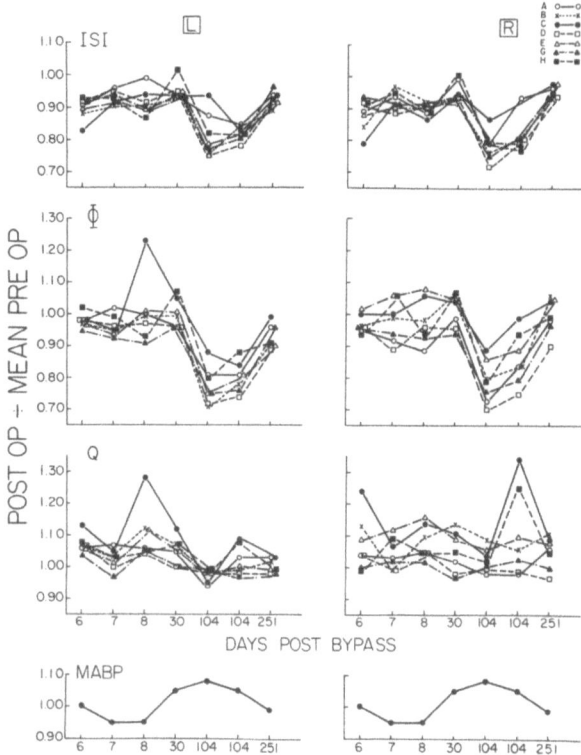

Fig. 9-1E. Patient JM. Several months prior to admission this 53-year-old man experienced an episode of left-sided facial weakness and decreased visual acuity in the left eye. At arteriography both complete occlusion of the left common carotid artery and occlusion of the right internal carotid artery just distal to the ophthalmic artery were demonstrated. Both vertebral arteries were patent. Right STA–MCA bypass was performed without complications. Postoperatively the patient had no further symptoms.

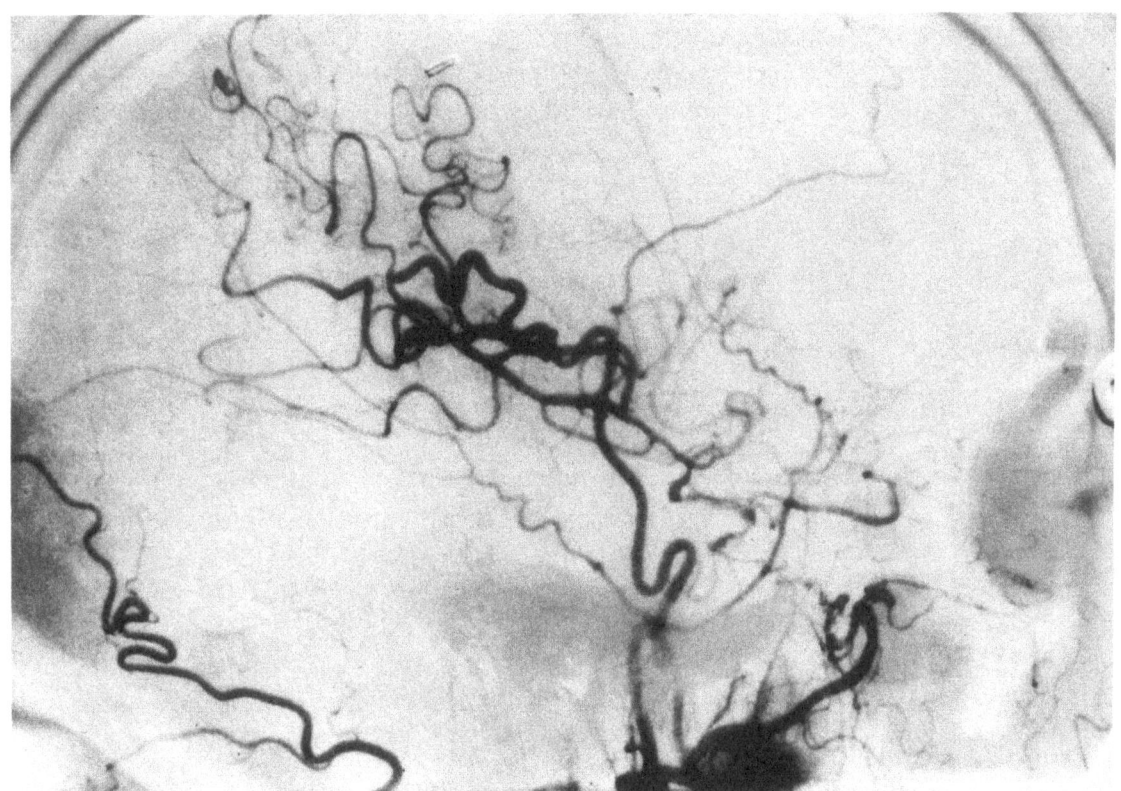

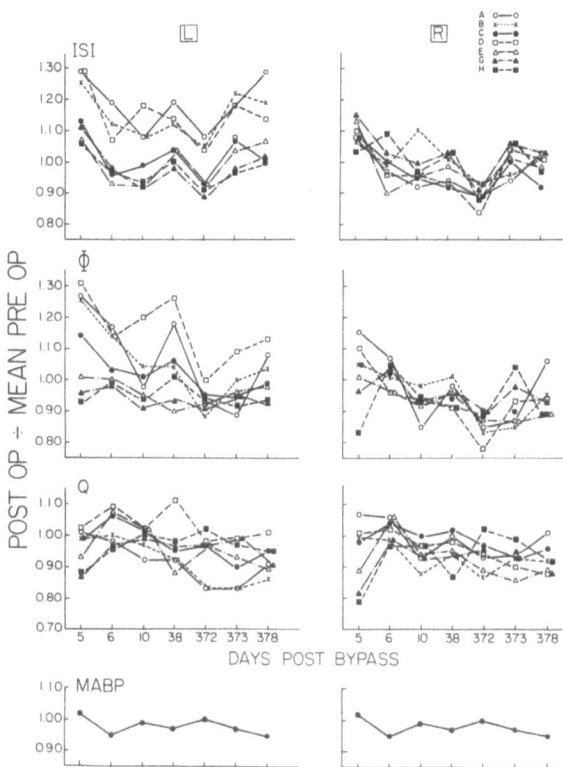

Fig. 9-1F. Patient JG. This 56-year-old man had a three-week history of several episodes of right hemiparesis and dysarthria lasting several hours. Angiography showed occlusion of the left internal carotid artery with left hemisphere perfusion from the right internal carotid artery via the anterior communicating artery. Following left STA–MCA bypass the patient was noted to be neurologically intact and asymptomatic.

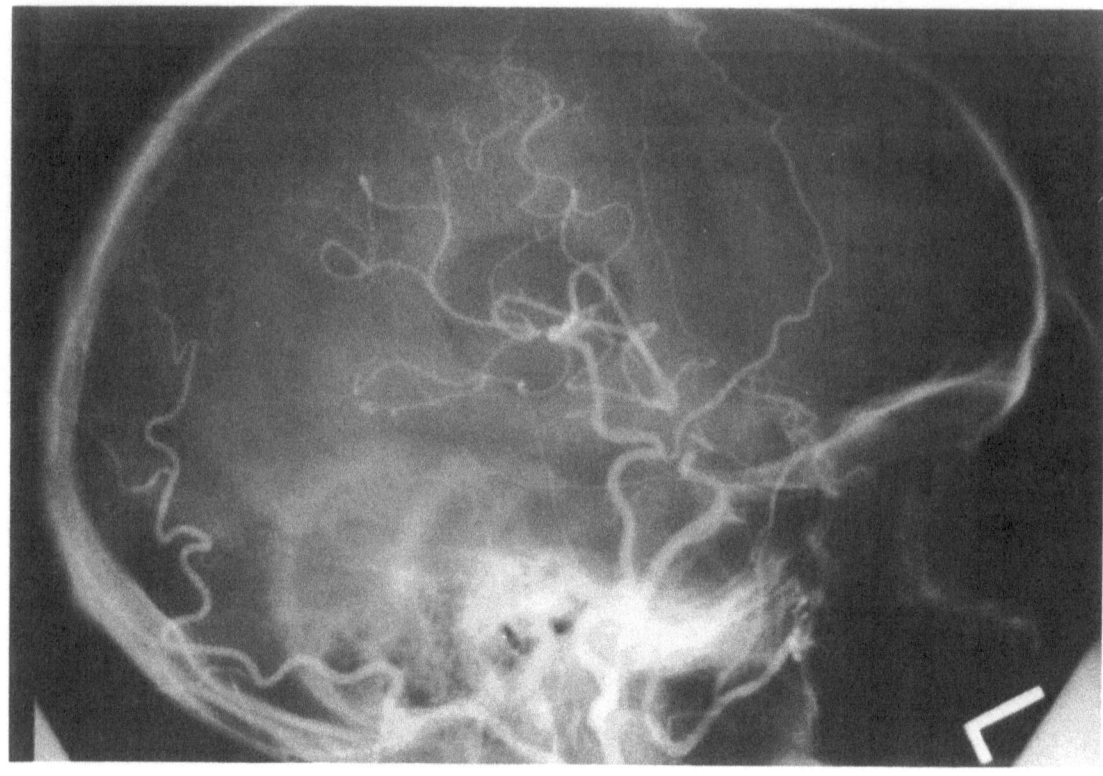

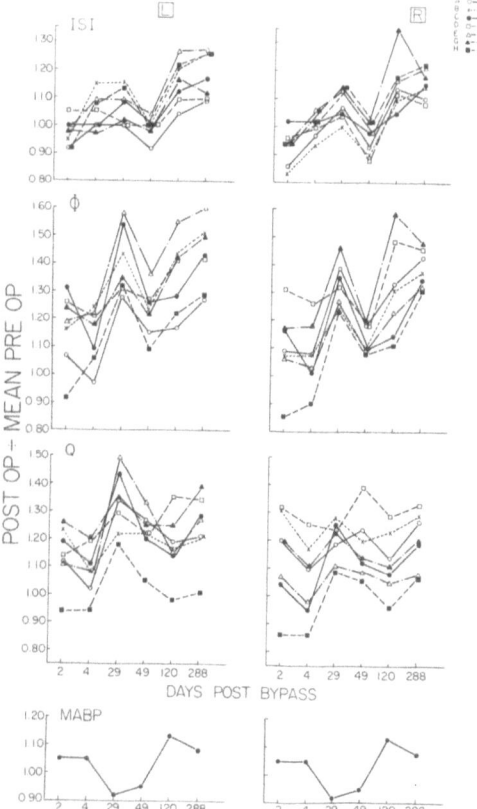

Fig. 9-1G. Patient MH. This 48-year-old man underwent left STA–MCA bypass 18 months after the onset of dense right hemiparesis and motor aphasia and 6 months after open heart surgery for coronary artery bypass and aortic valve replacement. During the 6 months prior to admission the patient had intermittent periods of weakness on the right side and increased inability to express himself and to understand others. Angiography showed a 95% stenosis of the left internal carotid artery at its origin and a 99% stenosis of the left internal carotid artery intracranially at its bifurcation. Following left STA–MCA bypass the patient stated that "my mind cleared" and the patient's family noted that he was much improved in his ability to communicate.

tomatic and neurologically intact and graft patency was documented by angiography.

Patient JM (Fig. 9-1E), the patient with most pronounced decrease in flows postoperatively, remained neurologically intact with graft patency repeatedly confirmed by Doppler examination.

Patient MH (Fig. 9-1G), the patient showing the greatest increase in flow by both ISI (15%) and Φ (40%), was the patient showing the most marked improvement. This patient and his family reported a marked improvement in intellectual function following bypass grafting and improvement in an apparently fixed expressive and receptive dysphasia.

Conclusion

Based on this preliminary study we believe that inhalation [133]xenon blood flow studies may become useful for pre- and postoperative evaluation of patients considered candidates for surgical augmentation of cerebral collateral blood supply. However, it is our opinion that at the present time inhalation blood flow studies are an experimental tool and are not useful in the preoperative selection of patients for STA–MCA bypass grafting. Indeed, our attitude is that patients carefully selected clinically for bypass are useful in the evaluation of our rCBF concepts. Our hope is that with further experience and development the reverse will become true.

References

1. Blauenstein, U.W., Halsey, J.R., Jr., Wilson, E.M., et al. [133]Xenon inhalation method. Analysis of reproducibility: Some of its physiological implications. Stroke 8:92–102, 1977.
2. Blauenstein, U.W., Halsey, J.H., Jr., Wilson, E.M., Wills, E.L. [133]Xenon inhalation method: Significance of indicator maldistribution for distinguishing brain areas with impaired perfusion. An index for total flow. Stroke 9:57–66, 1978.
3. Heilbrun, M.P., Reichman, O.H., Anderson, R.E., Roberts, T.S. Regional cerebral blood flow studies following superficial temporal-middle cerebral artery anastomosis. J Neurosurg 43: 706–716, 1975.

10

rCBF Measurement in Patients with STA–MCA Shunts

M. I. Vilaghy, D. W. Rowed, V. C. Hachinski, J. W. Norris, and P. W. Cooper

Regional cerebral blood flow measurement (rCBF) is one of the best objective methods of selecting patients suitable for the ECA–ICA operation, as well as of assessing the postoperative results of anastomotic surgery.[3] Unfortunately, the resulting changes in skull blood flow sometimes associated with marked increases in caliber of the ECA make the assessment of underlying cerebral circulation difficult when the shunt vessel is injected, since extracranial and intracranial tissues receive the xenon.

Using common carotid injection of radioactive tracer we have found[2] that the contamination of the overlying extracranial tissues reduces estimation of underlying cerebral blood flow by about 17%. However, this effect is not homogeneous.

The present study represents our attempts to overcome the above problems.

Materials and Methods

We have performed 36 rCBF studies on 14 patients at different periods before and after ECA–ICA surgery using the ^{133}Xe method of Ingvar and Lassen.[1]

The injection site was a combination of one or more of the following:
1) The site of the anastomosis
2) The ipsilateral common carotid artery
3) The contralateral internal carotid artery
4) The contralateral common carotid artery
5) Various collaterals such as vertebral arteries or subclavian artery or whenever there is a communication with the intracranial circulation.

Results

1) Fig. 10-1 illustrates the effect of perfusing the ipsilateral brain through the anastomosis as opposed to injecting the contralateral carotid artery allowing perfusion of the ipsilateral hemisphere from the other side.

2) The washout curves recorded by the ipsilateral probes are not "see-through" effects from the contralateral hemisphere. Experiments with cadaver brain (Figs. 10-2, 10-3) show that only 18 to 24% of the radiation recorded is from the contralateral hemisphere. Second, we have studied patients with focal cerebral lesions (angiomas, tumors, epileptic foci) which were not detected by probes placed over the contralateral hemisphere.

3) In cases where the isotope must be introduced through the ipsilateral cerebral circulation, e.g., contralateral carotid occlusion analysis of the curve shape, distribution and behavior may help decide whether the washout curves seen are ECA or ICA in origin.

We have performed comparative studies by injecting the ICA–CCA and ECA in the same

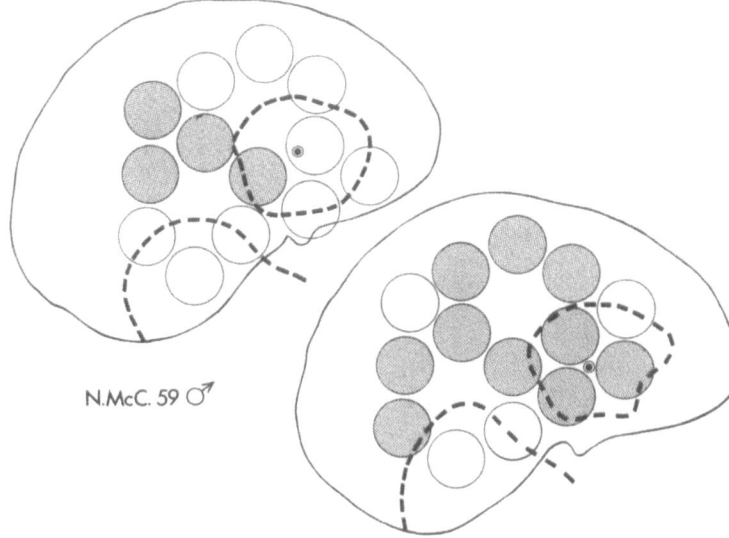

Fig. 10-1. Comparison between injection of ^{133}Xe through the ECA–ICA shunt (left upper) and contralateral internal carotid (right lower). The dotted discs represent areas where rCBF was measured. The empty circles represent areas where the brain was not "seen" because of radiation from extracerebral tissues. Circled dot (⊙) = anastomosis site. Dotted line = craniotomy site and temporal bone mass.

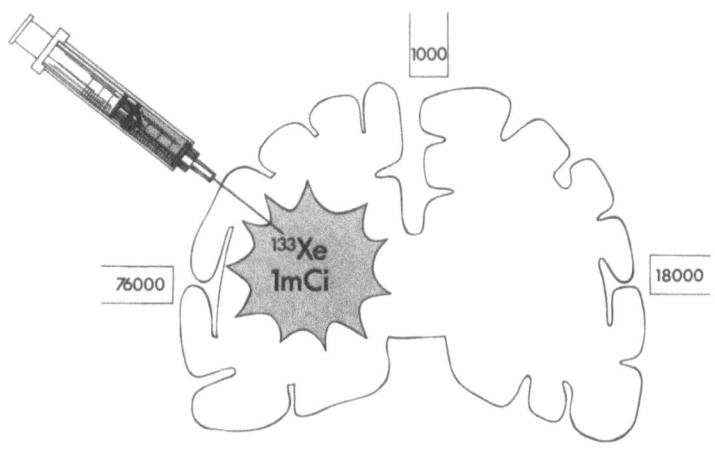

Fig. 10-2. "See through" in cadaver brain. When 1 mCi ^{133}Xe is injected into the centrum semiovale the ipsilateral probe records 76 000 counts, a contralateral symmetrical probe counts 18 000 (of which 1000 is scattered radiation recorded by the contralateral vertical probe). Thus the maximum "see through" (registered counts by a probe looking at the ^{133}Xe pocket) is 17 000/76 000 (=22.4%).

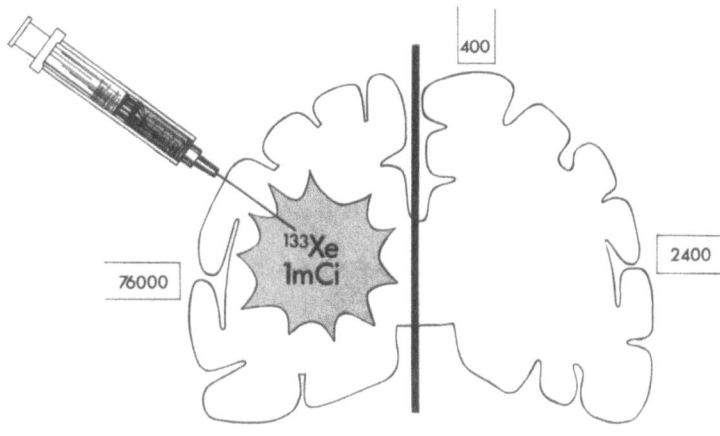

Fig. 10-3. Same experiment as Fig. 10-2 with a lead shield (approx. 0.75 mm thick) between the hemispheres shows that "see through" is reduced to 2000/16 000 (=3.2%).

patients and find that the shape of the curves is a composite of slow-perfusing (scalp) tissue and high-perfusing (brain) tissue (Fig. 10-4).

Further, on hyperventilation when the PCO$_2$

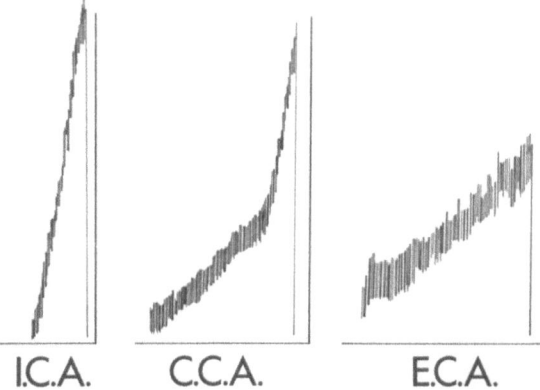

I.C.A.   C.C.A.   E.C.A.

Fig. 10-4. Blood flow curves (logarithmic display). The common carotid (CCA) curve is a composite of internal carotid (ICA) and external carotid (ECA) curves. Since the amount of the increased external carotid circulation is variable, in shunted (ECA–ICA) patients only the ICA type of curves can be accepted as representative of cerebral flow.

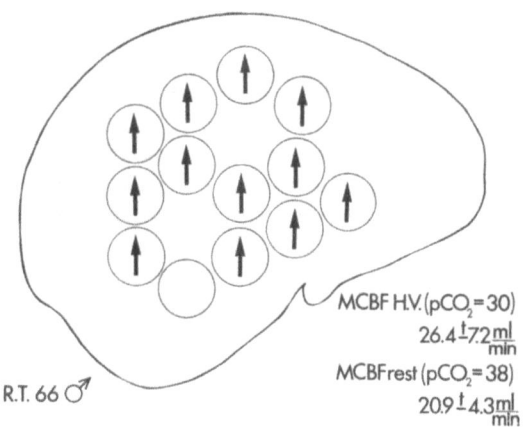

R.T. 66 ♂

MCBF H.V. (pCO₂=30)

$$26.4 \pm 7.2 \frac{ml}{min}$$

MCBF rest (pCO₂=38)

$$20.9 \pm 4.3 \frac{ml}{min}$$

Fig. 10-5. Paradoxical carbon dioxide reaction, i.e., opposite CO_2 reactivity to brain.[2] Regional increases (upward arrows) in blood flow during an 8 mm Hg drop of PCO_2 indicate that all but one of the measured regions represent scalp circulation (and the brain is not "seen") when ^{133}Xe is injected via the anastomosis.

falls, the blood flow becomes slower in brain tissues but faster in the ECA territory (Fig. 10-5).

Third, a biphasic pattern of ECA curves is seen over the distribution of the superficial temporal artery as estimated by angiogram and these curves are sufficiently characteristic to be differentiated from the underlying brain curves (Fig. 10-6).

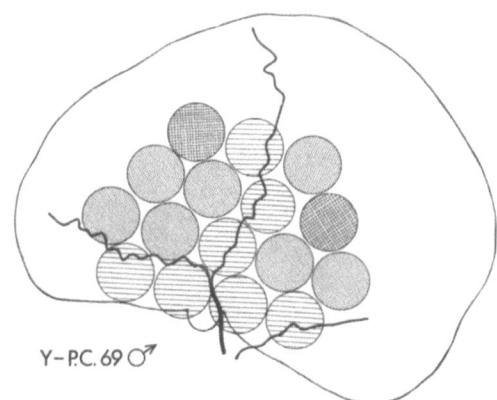

Y–P.C. 69 ♂

Fig. 10-6. Biphasic or "V" pattern. In areas of major ECA branches the underlying rCBF can not be measured because the curves are a composite of brain and external carotid flow. The dotted discs represent areas where ICA type of curves were obtained, thus rCBF readily measured. The stripped circles stand for biphasic rCBF curves that are *not* acceptable in shunted patients. The two checkered regions stand for slightly altered ICA type of display.

Conclusion

Whenever possible isotopes should be injected through the contralateral hemisphere when evaluation of perfusion of underlying ipsilateral brain tissue is desired. "See through" is not a problem since it represents only a fragment of detectable activity. In cases where contamination of overlying ipsilateral scalp tissue occurs these curves can be readily identified.

References

1. Lassen, N., and Ingvar, D. Radioisotopic assessment of regional cerebral blood flow. Prog Nucl Med 1:376–409, 1972.
2. Rudelli, R.D., Hachinski, V.C., Norris, J.W., Cooper, P.W. Regional cerebral blood flow determination by common carotid injection of xenon 133. In Neurology and Neurosurgery, Excerpta Medica, Amsterdam, No. 427, 1977, p. 337.
3. Schmiedek, P., Gratzl, O., Spenzler, R., Steinhoff, H., Enzenbach, R., Brendel, W., Margurth, F. Selection of patients for extracranial–intracranial artery bypass surgery based on rCBF measurements. J Neurosurg 44:303–312, 1976.

11

Cerebral Blood Flow in Superficial Temporal Artery to Middle Cerebral Artery Anastomosis

John R. Little, Y. Lucas Yamamoto, William Feindel, Ernst Meyer, and Charles P. Hodge

Anastomosis of the superficial temporal artery (STA) to a branch of the middle cerebral artery (MCA) has become increasingly popular since its introduction 11 years ago.[3, 20] The efficacy of this procedure in preventing cerebral infarction, however, has yet to be proven despite encouraging clinical results.[2, 6,15, 21] The definition of its role in the treatment of cerebral ischemia will depend partly upon the results of cerebral blood flow (CBF) studies. A few studies[1, 13, 14] demonstrating improvement in regional cerebral blood flow (rCBF) have been reported, but our knowledge of the changes in the cerebral circulation in patients undergoing STA–MCA anastomosis remains limited. The object of this investigation was to provide further information about these changes by studying CBF in a group of patients before, during, and after surgery.

Clinical Material and Methods

CBF studies were performed on 13 consecutive patients undergoing STA to MCA anastomosis. The 11 males and two females ranged in age from 16 to 69 years (mean: 52 years). The clinical presentation in each case was one of cerebral transient ischemic attacks and/or recent, small stroke.

Angiographic studies, with visualization of the aortic arch, carotid arteries, and vertebral arteries, were carried out. There were 11 cases of internal carotid artery (ICA) occlusive disease, including eight with complete obstruction and three with inaccessible, severe stenosis. Two patients had a focal atherosclerotic lesion of the MCA trunk including one complete obstruction and one severe stenosis. The contralateral ICA also was occluded in three patients.

The operative technique used was similar to previous descriptions[12] except: (1) a temporoparietal craniotomy was performed instead of simple trephination, and (2) a continuous suture technique was used for the anastomosis[10] in all but the initial three patients in whom the standard interrupted suture technique was utilized. The largest exposed cortical artery, usually the angular branch, was selected as the receptor vessel. All operative procedures were performed by one surgeon (J.R.L.).

Krypton-77 Positron Emission Tomography ([77]Kr PET)

[77]Kr PET was used to determine rCBF per square centimeter of cerebral tissue in a transverse section of the head. The [77]Kr gas was administered by a simple inhalation technique. The detecting system was remotely connected to a PDP-12 computer for reconstruction of the concentration of [77]Kr every 30 seconds for 8.5 minutes. The clearance rate of [77]Kr in each square centimeter pixel in the cross section of the head was determined. Details of this technique have been published elsewhere.[11, 19]

Examinations were carried out one week before operation and two weeks afterward. Follow-up studies two to six months later were obtained in seven cases.

Intraoperative CBF Studies

The arterial blood pressure was maintained at preoperative levels during these studies. Arterial PCO_2 was kept constant in the 40 ± 3 torr range. The tracers were injected into the ipsilateral common carotid artery (CCA) through a #18 gauge polyethylene catheter which had been inserted percutaneously immediately prior to surgery.

Fluorescein Angiography. Studies were performed before and after anastomosis. Sodium fluorescein (5 ml of a 1% solution) was injected into the ipsilateral CCA through the indwelling catheter and rapid, serial photographs of the cortex were taken. Details of this technique have been described previously.[4, 5, 8]

Xenon-133 (^{133}Xe) rCBF Studies. These were obtained before and after anastomosis. The cortex was covered with a thin plastic film. Four small lithium-drifted semiconductor detectors were placed gently on the plastic film overlying the cortical surface of the inferior frontal gyrus, supramarginal gyrus, angular gyrus, and superior temporal gyrus. ^{133}Xe (10 to 12 mCi) dissolved in 3 ml of isotonic saline was rapidly injected into the ipsilateral CCA through the indwelling catheter. The detecting system was remotely connected through a scaler interface to a PDP-12 computer. The mean rCBF from each cortical area was calculated by a modification of the stochastic analysis.[5, 9, 17]

Results

^{77}Kr PET Studies

Preoperative Findings. Reduced rCBF in the ipsilateral hemisphere was demonstrated in each case. The brain tissue supplied by the MCA was involved predominantly. The reduc-

tion in most cases was heterogeneous with one or more large areas of low flow being identified (Fig. 11-1). These ischemic foci involved cortex, white matter, and basal ganglia. Mean rCBF in ischemic cortex was 19 ± 5 ml/100 g/min (range: 9 to 30 ml/100 g/min) and 30 ± 11 ml/100 g/min (range: 19 to 53 ml/100 g/min) in the subcortical tissue.

Focal rCBF reduction of lesser severity also was observed in the contralateral hemisphere of five patients. In three of them the contralateral ICA was occluded and in two it was patent.

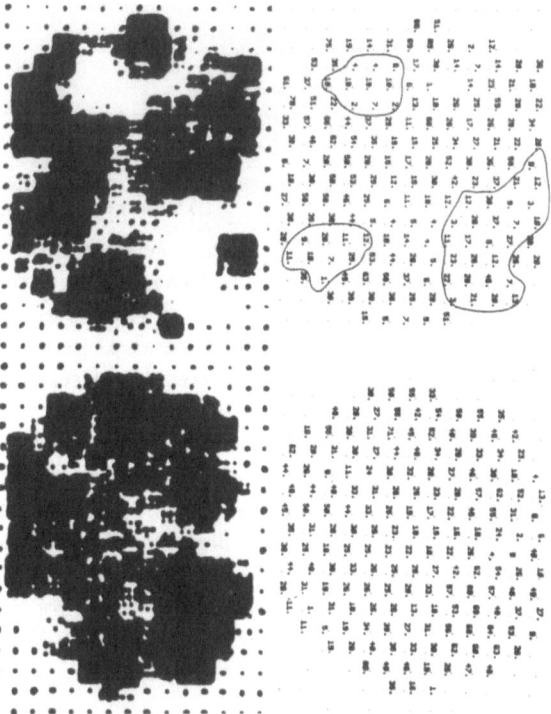

Fig. 11-1. ^{77}Kr PET in a 45-year-old man with occlusive disease of right internal carotid artery. The preoperative gray-scale display of rCBF through a transverse section of the head is shown on the upper left. Black areas indicate normal rCBF and white areas indicate ischemia. A numerical printout of the preoperative study is shown on the upper right. Each number represents rCBF in ml/100 g/min. The postoperative gray-scale display is shown on the lower left and the numerical display on the lower right. Considerable rCBF improvement has taken place in the right frontal and parieto-occipital regions as well as in the deep left frontal lobe.

Postoperative Findings. Substantial improvement of rCBF was observed in all cases. Ischemic foci in the ipsilateral hemisphere either disappeared or were reduced considerably in size. Mean rCBF in previously ischemic cortex was 48 ± 15 ml/100 g/min (range: 27 to 65 ml/100 g/min) and 44 ± 9 ml/100 g/min (range: 34 to 62 ml/100 g/min) in the subcortical tissue. Minimal improvement occurred in one patient with a 70% focal stenosis at the origin of the external carotid artery (ECA). His rCBF values increased considerably following endarterectomy and insertion of a vein graft. Improved rCBF also was demonstrated in the ischemic foci seen preoperatively in the contralateral hemisphere of five patients.

Follow-up Findings. Additional improvement was demonstrated in six of the seven cases studied (mean increase: 13 ± 4 ml/100 g/min). The rCBF values in the other patient decreased slightly.

Intraoperative Findings

Gross Observations. Evidence of previous infarction, consisting of gyral pallor and atrophy, was seen in nine cases. It involved a single gyrus in two cases, two or three gyri in six cases, and more than three gyri in one case. In seven of these nine cases, the cortical infarcts were found to be in the territory of a severely sclerotic, cortical artery. Neovascularization adjacent to these infarcted areas was observed in three cases (Fig. 11-2).

Fluorescein Angiography. Patency of the anastomosis was verified in 12 cases. The other patient was found to have nonfilling of the distal limb of the receptor artery but had improved filling of the other MCA branches. The receptor artery in this case was severely atherosclerotic and had a diameter of less than 1 mm. Improvement in the circulation time (i.e., time between maximal arterial and venous filling) was seen in all cases although focal delays in microcirculatory filling persisted in some cortical regions supplied by severely sclerotic MCA branches.

Two basic patterns of arterial filling follow-ing anastomosis were demonstrated in the 11 patients with ICA occlusive disease. Filling of the cortical MCA branches was generalized in seven (Fig. 11-3) and predominantly in the receptor artery territory in four. In those patients undergoing anastomosis for MCA occlusive disease, the area of cortical microcirculatory filling through the MCA branches was seen to expand.

^{133}Xe rCBF Studies

The results of the preanastomotic and postanastomotic studies are listed in Table 11-1. The preanastomotic rCBF values were similar at the four recording sites in eight cases. In the others, considerable variation from one recording site to the next was observed with areas of very low flow (i.e., $\leqq 25$ ml/100 g/min) interspersed with areas of more normal flow (i.e., $\geqq 40$ ml/100 g/min). The foci with severe rCBF reduction frequently were in the territory of a severely sclerotic cortical artery.

Immediate, substantial increases of rCBF were demonstrated following anastomosis in 10 cases. In two of them, the improvement was predominantly in the receptor artery territory, whereas in the others the improvement was generalized. These findings did not always correlate with results of the fluorescein angiography. Considerable increases of rCBF sometimes occurred in regions where there was relatively little improvement of fluorescein filling (Fig. 11-4).

The patient with postanastomotic occlusion of the distal limb of the receptor artery was found to have reduced rCBF in the region it supplied. The rCBF was not improved in two other patients despite a patent anastomosis. One had a proximal ECA stenosis (i.e., 70%). The other had a narrow (i.e., $<$ 1 mm), diffusely atherosclerotic STA.

The results of the ^{133}Xe clearance studies and ^{77}Kr PET were similar. The lack of spatial resolution of the ^{133}Xe technique,[7] however, did not allow differentiation of cortical and subcortical rCBF. Consequently, the results of the ^{133}Xe studies were found to correspond more closely to the combined cortical and subcortical rCBF values demonstrated by ^{77}Kr PET.

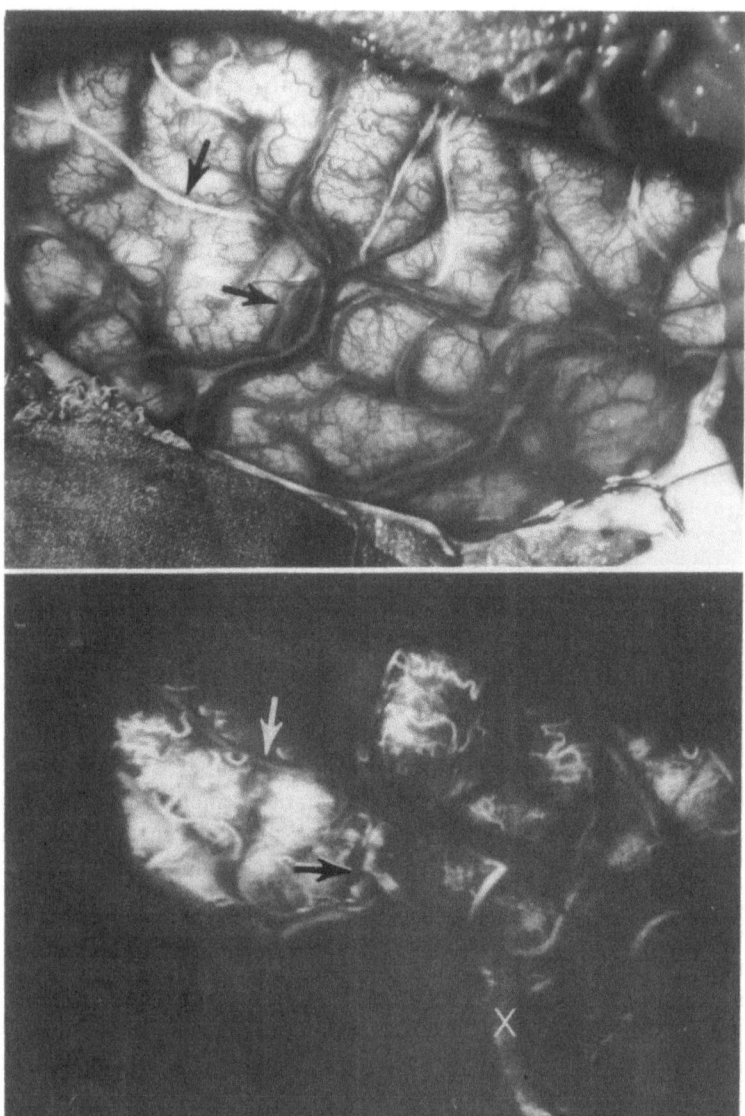

Fig. 11-2. Right parietotemporal craniotomy in a 45-year-old man with right internal carotid artery occlusive disease. Before anastomosis (above), pallor and atrophy of the supramarginal and angular gyri were observed. The main feeding artery (upper arrow) to this region was severely sclerotic. Considerable neovascularization had developed in the vicinity of the sclerotic arteries. The lower arrow indicates the receptor artery. After anastomosis (below), fluorescein angiography (1.5 sec) demonstrated impaired filling of the sclerotic arteries (upper arrow) and adjacent cortical microcirculation. Fluorescein in the STA (X) was obscured by the cuff of connective tissue; however, the anastomotic site was well demonstrated (lower arrow).

Clinical Course

The neurologic status in one patient was slightly worse postoperatively. The anastomosis, using the interrupted suture technique, became partially occluded intraoperatively and attempts to relieve the obstruction were unsuccessful. The cortical receptor artery in this patient was severely atherosclerotic and had a luminal diameter less than 1 mm.

Another patient experienced a single TIA consisting of weakness of the right upper ex-

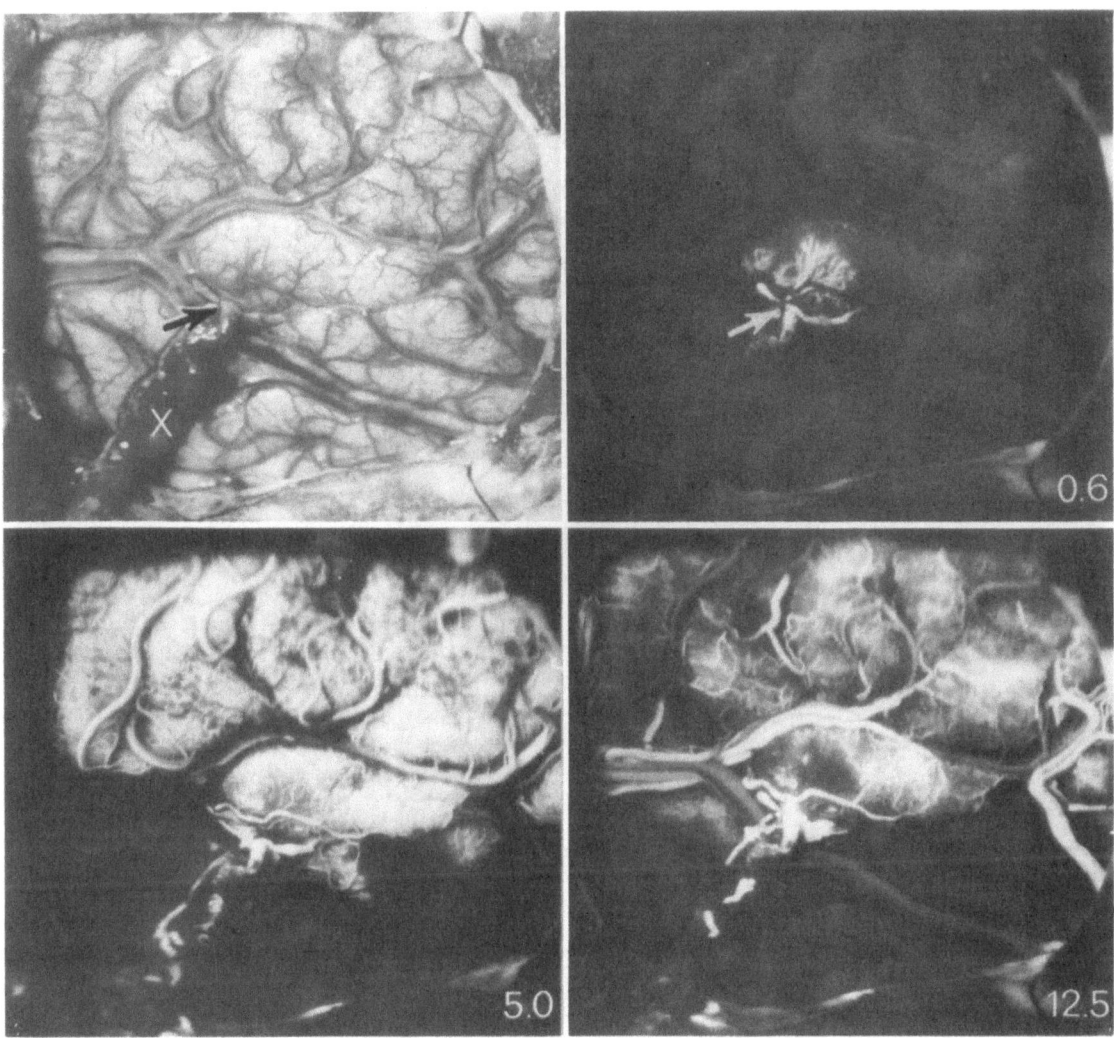

Fig. 11-3. Left parietotemporal craniotomy (upper left) in a 60-year-old woman with left internal carotid occlusive disease showing the STA pedicle (X) and the anastomosis (arrow). Fluorescein angiogram at 0.6 sec showed filling of the STA and cortical receptor artery. Filling of the adjacent microcirculation also was noted. At 5.0 sec, most of the MCA cortical branches had filled. The major cortical veins were well demonstrated at 12.5 sec. Some leakage of fluorescein was seen at the anastomotic site.

Table 11-1. Intraoperative ^{133}Xe rCBF studies

	Mean ^{133}Xe rCBF (ml/100 g/min)			
	Inferior frontal gyrus	Supramarginal gyrus	Angular gyrus	Superior temporal gyrus
Preanastomosis	35 ± 12	32 ± 13	30 ± 10	32 ± 9
Postanastomosis	43 ± 12	37 ± 10	43 ± 14	42 ± 17

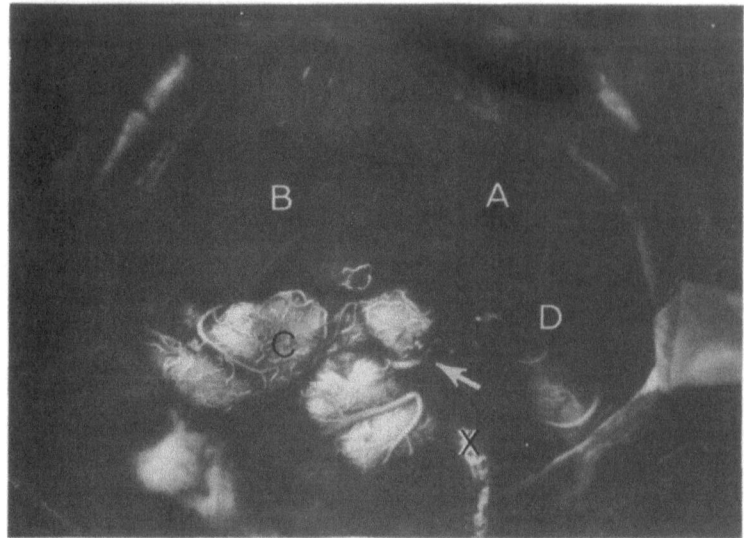

Xe^{-133} Study in O.R.

Detector Position	rCBF (ml/100gm/min)	
	Pre-anastomosis	Post-anastomosis
Inferior Frontal (A)	15	56
Supramarginal (B)	15	33
Angular (C)	17	60
Superior Temporal (D)	20	40

Fig. 11-4. Fluorescein angiogram at 2.4 sec in a 50-year-old man shows filling predominantly in the receptor artery territory. The STA (X) was partly obscured by connective tissue but filling of the receptor artery was well demonstrated (arrow). The letters indicate the sites of the ^{133}Xe detectors. The results of the ^{133}Xe clearance studies are shown below.

tremity and expressive dysphasia during an episode of orthostatic hypotension. Occlusion of a previously stenotic left ICA was demonstrated a few days following a left STA–MCA anastomosis. The remaining 11 patients had no additional TIAs or strokes. Patency of the anastomosis was confirmed in 12 patients undergoing postoperative angiography.

Discussion

^{77}Kr PET was developed for the topographic and quantitative determination of rCBF in every square centimeter of a cross section of the head following inhalation of ^{77}Kr gas.[16, 18, 19] It has proven to be particularly well suited to the assessment of patients undergoing STA–MCA anastomosis. Advantages of the technique include: (1) differentiation of rCBF in cortical and subcortical (i.e., white matter and basal ganglia) tissue, (2) measurement of rCBF in both hemispheres simultaneously, and (3) performance of repeated studies with minimal risk.

The 13 patients selected for anastomosis were shown preoperatively by ^{77}Kr PET to have substantial reduction of rCBF in brain tissue supplied by the ipsilateral MCA. Reduction in flow was more severe in cortex. Mean rCBF in the ischemic cortical tissue was 19 ± 5 ml/100 g/min compared with 30 ± 11 ml/100 g/min in the subcortical tissue. Further slight reduction of flow, particularly in the cortex, would be symptomatic and probably result in infarction. The object of performing the anastomosis in these cases was to improve the flow in the ischemic regions and thereby prevent irreversible injury.

The general pattern of rCBF reduction in the

symptomatic hemisphere was similar in patients with ICA or MCA occlusive disease. The rCBF values were not uniformly low. One or more foci of severe flow reduction invariably were demonstrated. Similar findings have been reported previously by Schmiedek and associates.[13, 14] Unfortunately, their measurement technique did not allow assessment of the subcortical regions or the contralateral hemisphere, which frequently were shown by [77]Kr PET to be ischemic.

The multifocal nature of the rCBF reduction could be explained partly on the basis of occlusive disease of the cortical branches of the MCA. The findings of intraoperative fluorescein angiography and ^{133}Xe clearance studies indicated a relationship between the ischemic foci and the distribution of the sclerotic cortical arteries. In the regions supplied by these diseased vessels, fluorescein filling of the microcirculation invariably was delayed and the rCBF values were low.

Substantial improvement of rCBF was demonstrated immediately following anastomosis by the intraoperative ^{133}Xe clearance studies. The increases in rCBF were not limited to regions adjacent to the anastomotic site but included ischemic foci some distance from it. Some of these regions were shown to receive little or none of the fluorescein supplied by the STA through the anastomosis. This indicated a redistribution of blood flowing through the MCA trunk and the epicerebral collateral channels.

Postoperative [77]Kr PET showed more widespread improvement than indicated by the intraoperative studies. Increased rCBF values were demonstrated in both cortical and subcortical regions. As well, improved rCBF was seen in previously ischemic areas in the contralateral hemisphere of five cases. In two of these patients with a patent contralateral ICA, this was thought to represent reversal of an interhemispheric steal phenomenon.

Follow-up [77]Kr PET studies performed two to six months later demonstrated further increases in rCBF values in six of seven cases studied. Similar improvement was observed in six of fifteen patients examined by Schmiedek and associates.[14] These findings, together with the well-recognized enlargement of the STA during the same period,[6, 10, 15] attest to the physiologic importance of this new collateral channel.

Factors which appeared to limit the success of this procedure included: (1) small (i.e., < 1 mm) size of the STA and/or cortical receptor artery, (2) severe, diffuse atherosclerosis of the STA and/or cortical receptor artery, and (3) severe (i.e., ≧ 70%) stenosis of the proximal ECA. These problems were encountered in three of our cases. Our findings indicate that it is not necessary to use the cortical MCA branch which directly supplies the ischemic zone as the receptor artery. Because of the considerable redistribution of flow following anastomosis a larger, less-diseased branch in another region can be selected. Correction of a proximal, severe ECA stenosis preferably should be performed prior to anastomosis. Poor flow through the donor artery resulting from proximal ECA stenosis undoubtedly limits the effectiveness of the operation and jeopardizes anastomotic patency.

Summary

Cerebral blood flow (CBF) studies were performed before, during, and after surgery on 13 consecutive patients undergoing superficial temporal artery (STA) to middle cerebral artery (MCA) anastomosis. Eleven patients had occlusive disease of the internal carotid artery (ICA) and two had occlusive disease of the proximal MCA. Preoperative krypton-77 positron-emission tomography ([77]Kr PET) demonstrated unifocal or multifocal reduction of regional cerebral blood flow (rCBF), both cortical and subcortical, in the ipsilateral MCA distribution. Mean rCBF in ischemic cortical tissue was 19 ± 5 ml/100 g/min and 30 ± 11 ml/100 g/min in the subcortical tissue. Focal rCBF reduction of lesser severity was observed in the contralateral hemisphere of five cases. Intraoperative fluorescein angiography provided an immediate assessment of anastomotic patency. Fluorescein filling of the MCA cortical branches was generalized in nine cases and predominantly in the receptor artery territory in four. Intraoperative xenon-133 (^{133}Xe) clearance studies demonstrated immediate rCBF improvement following anastomosis. Considerable increases of rCBF sometimes occurred in regions with relatively little fluorescein filling. The multifocal pattern of ischemia appeared to be the result of occlusive disease of the MCA cortical branches. Postoperative [77]Kr PET revealed substantial, widespread increases of rCBF. Mean rCBF in previously ischemic cortex was 48 ± 15 ml/100 g/min and 44 ± 9 ml/100 g/min in subcortical tissue. Improvement in rCBF in the contralateral hemisphere of two patients was thought to represent reversal of an interhemispheric steal phenomenon. The findings of this study indicated that: (1) microvascular anastomosis can substantially improve rCBF in ischemic foci, (2) extensive redistribution of blood flow occurs, and (3) beneficial effects can occur some distance from the anastomotic site.

References

1. Austin, G., Hayward, W., Laffin, D. Use of cerebral blood flow for selection and monitoring of patients. In Microneurosurgical Anastomosis for Cerebral Ischemia, G. Austin, editor, Charles C Thomas, Springfield, 1976, pp. 327–338.
2. Chater, N. Patient selection and results of extra- to intracranial anastomosis in selected cases of cerebrovascular disease. In Clinical Neurosurgery, E.B. Keener, P. Carmel, H. Friedman, et al., editors, Williams and Wilkins Co., Baltimore, 1976, Vol. 23, pp. 287–309.
3. Donaghy, R.M.P. Neurologic surgery. Surg Gynecol Obstet 134:269–271, 1972.
4. Feindel, W., Yamamoto, Y. L., Hodge, C.P. Intracarotid fluorescein angiography. Can Med Assoc J. 96:1–7, 1967.
5. Feindel, W. Yamamoto, Y.L., Hodge, C.P. The cerebral microcirculation in man: analysis by radioisotope microregional flow measurement and fluorescein angiography. In Clinical Neurosurgery, G. Tindall, R.H. Wilkins, and E.B. Keener, editors, Williams and Wilkins Co., Baltimore, 1971, Vol. 18, pp. 225–246.
6. Gratzl, O., Schmiedek, P., Spetzler, R., et al. Clinical experience with extra–intracranial arterial anastomosis in 65 cases. J Neurosurg 44:313–324, 1976.
7. Hanson, E.J., Anderson, R.E., Sundt, T.M. Comparison of krypton-85 and xenon-133 cerebral blood flow measurements before, during, and following focal incomplete ischemia in the squirrel monkey. Circ Res 36:18–26, 1975.
8. Hodge, C.P., Yamamoto, Y.L., Feindel, W. Fluorescein angiography of the brain—the photographic procedure. J Biol Photogr Assoc 46:67–79, 1978.
9. Hohberger, C.P., Yamamoto, Y.L., Thompson, C.J., et al. On-line computer measurement of microregional cerebral blood flow by xenon-133 clearance. Int J Nucl Med Biol 2:153–158, 1975.
10. Little, J.R., Salerno, T.A. Continuous suturing for microvascular anastomosis. J Neurosurg 48:1042–1045, 1978.
11. Meyer, E., Yamamoto, Y.L., Thompson, C.J. Confidence limits for topographical cerebral blood flow values obtained by krypton-77 positron emission tomography. J Comput Assist Tomogr (in press).
12. Peerless, S. J. Techniques of cerebral revascularization. In Clinical Neurosurgery, E.B. Keener, P. Carmel, H. Friedman, et al., editors, Williams and Wilkins Co., Baltimore, 1976, Vol. 23, pp. 258–269.
13. Schmiedek, P., Gratzl, O., Olteanu, V., et al. The contribution of regional cerebral blood flow measurement to the microneurosurgical treatment of cerebral ischemia. In Microneurosurgical Anastomosis for Cerebral Ischemia, G. Austin, editor, Charles C Thomas, Springfield, 1976, pp. 244–255.
14. Schmiedek, P., Gratzl, O., Spetzler, R., et al. Selection of patients for extra–intracranial arterial bypass surgery based on rCBF measurements. J Neurosurg 44:303–312, 1976.
15. Sundt, T.M., Siekert, R.G., Piepgras, D.G., et al. Bypass surgery for vascular disease of the carotid system. Mayo Clin Proc 51:677–692, 1976.
16. Yamamoto, Y.L., Little, J.R., Meyer, E., et al. Changes of topographical regional cerebral blood flow after medical and surgical treatment of stroke evaluated by [77]Kr-positron emission tomography. Stroke 9:107, 1978.
17. Yamamoto, Y.L., Phillips, K.M., Hodge, C.P., et al. Microregional blood flow changes in experimental cerebral ischemia: effects of arterial CO_2 studied by fluorescein angiography and xenon-133 clearance. J Neurosurg 35:155–166, 1971.
18. Yamamoto, Y.L., Thompson, C.J., Little, J.R., et al. Krypton-77 positron emission tomography for measurement of regional cerebral blood flow in a cross section of the head. Acta Neurol Scand 56:48–49, 1977.
19. Yamamoto, Y.L., Thompson, C.J., Meyer, E., et al. Dynamic positron emission tomography for study of cerebral hemodynamics in a cross section of the head using positron-emitting ^{68}Ga-EDTA and [77]Kr. J Comput Assist Tomogr 1:43–56, 1977.
20. Yasargil, M.G., Krayenbuhl, H.A., Jacobson, J.H. Microneurosurgical arterial reconstruction. Surgery 67:221–233, 1970.
21. Yasargil, M.G., Yonekawa, Y. Results of microsurgical extra–intracranial bypass in the treatment of cerebral ischemia. Neurosurgery 1:22–24, 1977.

12

Experimental Cerebral Revascularization Studied by ^{85}Kr Clearance and Fluorescein Angiography After 24 Hours of Permanent Occlusion of the Middle Cerebral Artery in Dogs

Hector Ortegon, William Feindel, Y. Lucas Yamamoto, and Charles P. Hodge

In spite of encouraging clinical results,[1, 17] the definitive role of extra–intracranial bypass in the prevention and treatment of ischemic cerebrovascular disease needs to be further substantiated. Still required are information from clinical cooperative controlled studies and further experimental analysis of the metabolic and hemodynamic changes as well as of the circulatory patterns that follow revascularization in acute and chronic ischemia.

Dogs have been found to be appropriate experimental animals for developing the bypass operations.[7, 10, 11] The hemodynamic effects of cerebral revascularization in these animals has thus far been studied at only short intervals (2 to 3 hours) after vascular occlusion.[3, 9] In a clinical situation it would not be possible to perform an extra–intracranial bypass anastomosis within such a short period after the onset of occlusion.

The aim of the present study was to examine the hemodynamic changes in experimental cerebral revascularization following longer periods of ischemia. We have used a transorbital approach to the middle cerebral artery in dogs, to obviate the need of extensive craniotomy.

Material and Methods

Transorbital Occlusion of the Middle Cerebral Artery

Sixteen mongrel dogs weighing 19 to 24 kg and unselected as to age and sex were used. They were anesthetized with intravenous pentobarbital (25 mg/kg) and supplemental doses were given as needed. Intubation was not required.

The head of the dog was fixed in a holder. After exenteration of the contents of the left orbital cavity and lateral retraction of the temporalis muscle, an 8 × 6 mm craniectomy was made in the portion of the posterior wall of the orbit at the same level and lateral to the orbital fissure. Dural opening was made in a cruciate fashion and, after dissection of the arachnoid, the middle cerebral artery was tied with a 7-0 silk ligature. The point of occlusion verified at postmortem examination has been found to be about 10 mm from the origin of the middle cerebral artery, lateral to the perforating branches and, in 70% of the cases, proximal to its first main cortical bifurcation. The cavity was irrigated with bacitracin solution and a piece of Gelfoam was placed against the craniectomy; although epoxy cement was laid over it, a CSF leak could not always be prevented.

Superficial Temporal–Middle Cerebral Artery Anastomosis

After transorbital occlusion of the left middle cerebral artery, the dogs were allowed to wake up, and 18 to 20 hours later neurologic evaluation was performed. The dogs were then reanesthetized with intravenous pentobarbital. Endotracheal intubation was performed and the dogs were ventilated to control respiratory rate and volume and to maintain a normocapnic state. The femoral artery was catheterized for blood gases and arterial pressure monitoring. The lingual artery was catheterized as well for injection of fluorescein and [85]Kr.

After microsurgical dissection of the superficial temporal artery, a large left hemicraniectomy was performed to expose the cerebral cortex. A transparent polymer film was used to cover the surface of the exposed brain.

Fluorescein angiography of the brain and regional cerebral blood flow studies with [85]Kr were done with the middle cerebral artery occluded.

Following these studies an end-to-side micro-anastomosis was performed between the superficial temporal artery and the main temporal branch of the middle cerebral artery as it entered the sylvian fissure.

When the bypass had been completed, between 26 to 28 hours had elapsed since the proximal middle cerebral artery had been occluded. Fluorescein angiography of the brain was repeated to confirm patency of the anastomosis and to show the change in the pattern of circulation; regional cerebral blood flow as measured by [85]Kr clearance technique quantitated the changes in cortical blood flow for comparison with the preanastomosis values.

Fluorescein Angiography of the Brain

As described previously,[4] 1.6 ml of 1% sodium fluorescein were injected into the common carotid artery through the lingual artery catheter and rapid-sequence fluorescence photographs were taken. This was done approximately 24 hours after transorbital middle cerebral artery occlusion and repeated shortly after STA–MCA anastomosis.

Measurement of Regional Cortical Cerebral Blood Flow

Four semiconductor detectors[5] with a disc of lithium-drifted silicon were placed over the plastic polymer film covering the exposed cortex of the cerebral hemisphere to measure cortical blood flow with [85]Kr before and after STA–MCA anastomosis. Eight to thirteen millicuries (mCi) of beta-emitting [85]Kr dissolved in 3 ml of saline solution were injected into the lingual artery catheter; the isotope clearance curve from each detector was monitored through an on-line computer system (PDP-12),[6] and the flow values were calculated according to Yamamoto's[5, 6] modified form of the original Zierler equation.[18] The depth sensitivity of our semiconductor detector for measurement of 670 keV beta-emitting [85]Kr was found to be within 2.5 mm of brain tissue, indicating that it measures only cortical blood flow in the exposed dog brain.

India Ink Injection

In one of the dogs, 24 hours after middle cerebral artery occlusion both common carotid arteries were cannulated and proximally ligated; the animal was killed with a large dose of intravenous pentobarbital, and 100 ml of india ink were injected immediately afterward through both common carotid arteries simultaneously. The brain was removed and, after fixation in formalin, coronal sections were made; one of them, which passed between the mamillary bodies and the optic chiasm, was stained with H&E for light microscope examination.

The dogs that underwent revascularization were killed at the end of each experiment, and india ink injection, formalin fixation, and coronal sections were performed in the manner described. H&E staining of three different animals, all with patent STA–MCA anastomosis, was done.

Results

One dog had MCA occlusion via transorbital approach and india ink injection only, but no fluorescein angiography brain (FAB) or rCBF measurements were done. Two dogs had technically deficient anastomoses; the other 13, all with patent STA–MCA anastomoses, yielded complete data.

Fluorescein Angiography of the Brain

MCA occlusion was verified and the pattern of collateral circulation was studied. Two types of pattern were observed: (1) either minimum or no filling with dye was seen (Fig. 12-1 A), (2) collateral retrograde flow from the anterior cerebral artery only or intermingled flow from the first cortical bifurcation when the latter had not been occluded via transorbital approach occurred (Fig. 12-1 C, E). In pattern 2, the suprasylvian portion of the hemisphere filled with dye, but the infrasylvian portion showed absence or poor filling with fluorescein at all times. After STA–MCA anastomosis there was a remarkable change in the circulatory pattern in all dogs: the direction of flow went from a retrograde collateral circulation to an antegrade flow, and all areas showed a better filling with fluorescein (Fig. 12-1 B, D, F).

Regional Cerebral Blood Flow (rCBF)

In each of thirteen dogs, four areas of cortex about 1 cm in diameter were examined, usually two above and two below the sylvian fissure. On the basis of the degree of filling with fluorescein and direction of flow, the areas were classified in two divisions: (1) ischemic—minimum or no filling with dye observed during arterial, capillary and venous phases, (2) borderline—filling with fluorescein by retrograde collateral flow from the anterior cerebral artery and/or from the frontal branch of the middle cerebral artery.

A total of 52 areas of cortex were studied, of which 28 were borderline and 24 were ischemic. Most of the borderline areas (18) were located in the suprasylvian region, while most of the ischemic areas were infrasylvian (17), meaning that the latter region has a lesser collateral flow after MCA occlusion.

Since the first rCBF studies in this series were done 24 hours after transorbital occlusion of the MCA, no rCBF values under normal circumstances were obtained. In order to have a control to which these occlusion values were compared, the cerebral blood flow measurements of another series of six dogs[16] with patent middle cerebral artery were used; the methods of analysis were the same. Four areas in each of these six dogs were examined, a total of 24.

After 24 hours of middle cerebral artery occlusion the mean cortical blood flow fell significantly (72%) when compared to dogs with patent middle cerebral artery (Fig. 12-2). This reduction in cortical flow went from a decrease of 59% in borderline areas to 85% in more ischemic areas.

After STA–MCA anastomosis (Fig. 12-3) the mean cortical blood flow increased by 180%, from 135% in the borderline areas to 330% in more ischemic areas.

Neurologic Evaluation

None of the dogs developed a focal neurologic deficit. At the most a few of them exhibited a wide-based gait or appeared moderately apathetic the day following MCA occlusion.

India Ink Injection

Coronal sections of the brain perfused with india ink 24 hours after MCA occlusion show very clearly the area of nonfilling, corresponding to the territory of the occluded artery (Fig. 12-4, top), and involving the frontal and temporal opercula, the upper internal capsule, and the caudate nucleus. There was no macroscopic evidence of edema or shift of the midline structures. Microscopic observation of a section (H&E) passing between the mamillary bodies and the optic chiasm was within normal limits, with good preservation of the cellular architecture of the nonfilling area.

In the dogs that underwent revascularization, both hemispheres showed a uniform epicerebral filling, this being another ratification of patency of the anastomosis. Coronal sections of the brain showed the depth of the revascularized area (Fig. 12-4, bottom). There was no evidence of shift of the midline structures, intracerebral hemorrhage, or any significant amount of swelling. There were no histologic features of infarction when the H&E staining of the coronal sections of the brain of three dogs was observed under the light microscope.

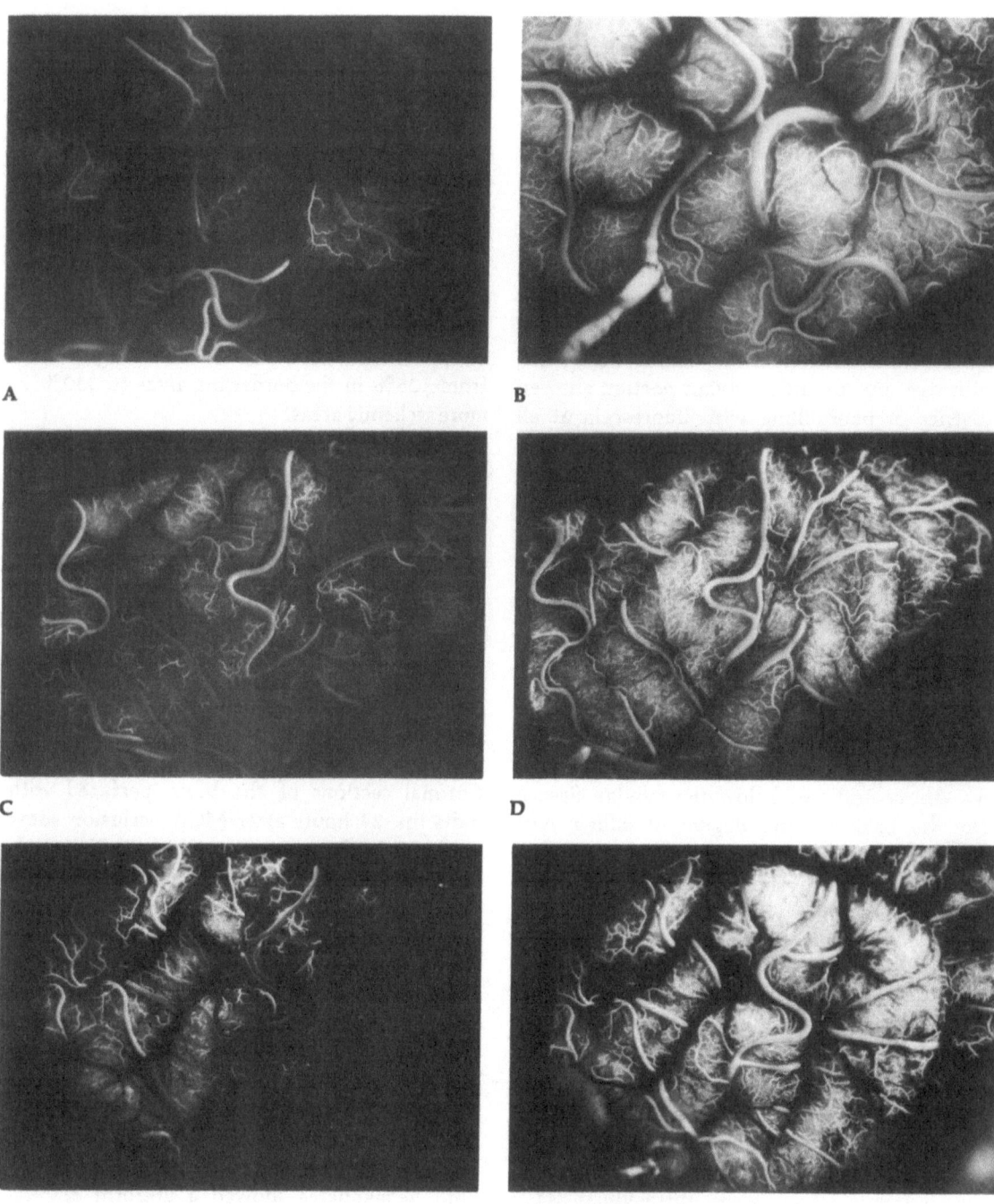

Fig. 12-1. Fluorescein angiography in the dog 24 hours after transorbital occlusion of the left middle cerebral artery and following STA–MCA anastomosis. A. Minimum filling with dye 24 hours after occlusion of the left MCA at 3.08 sec after injection of fluorescein. B. After STA–MCA anastomosis at 3.14 sec after injection of fluorescein. C. Retrograde flow from the anterior cerebral artery, filling the suprasylvian portion of the hemisphere 24 after occlusion of the left MCA, at 3.82 sec after injec-tion of fluorescein. D. After STA–MCA anastomo-sis at 2.57 sec after injection of dye. E. Collateral flow from the anterior cerebral artery intermingled with flow from the first cortical bifurcation of the MCA in a case when the latter was not occluded by the transorbital approach. The infrasylvian (temporal) portion shows no filling with fluorescein 2.62 sec after injection of fluorescein. F. After STA–MCA anastomosis at 2.52 sec after injection of dye.

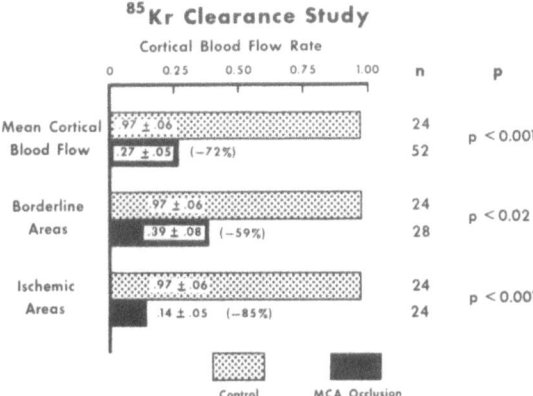

⁸⁵Kr Clearance Study
Cortical Blood Flow Rate

Fig. 12-2. Degree of reduction of cortical blood flow measured with ⁸⁵Kr clearance method 24 hours after occlusion of the middle cerebral artery. n = number of cortical areas examined. Control is based on findings in six dogs of another series with patent middle cerebral artery in which the methods of analysis were the same.

the origin of the MCA, involving the lenticulostriate arteries, a deep infarct of the basal ganglia and internal capsule has always resulted even under normotensive conditions, with a corresponding neurologic deficit.

Molinari[8] was able to embolize the most proximal MCA of dogs with pliable cylinders 1.6 mm in diameter, which assured occlusion of the perforating arteries. A deep infarct involving basal ganglia and internal capsule developed, but consistently throughout his experiments there was sparing of the cortical gray matter of the cerebral hemispheres. This can be accounted for by the extensive network of the leptomeningeal collateral circulation in the dog.[14]

In our experiments a deep infarct would not be expected, since the point of occlusion is distal to the perforating arteries. No neurologic deficit was found in spite of the marked de-

Discussion

It has been reported that occlusion of the middle cerebral artery in dogs does not lead to cerebral infarct unless there is associated hypotension, in which case an infarct of moderate to large extent is consistently present.[13, 15] When the site of MCA occlusion has been precisely verified at postmortem study[8, 12] to be at

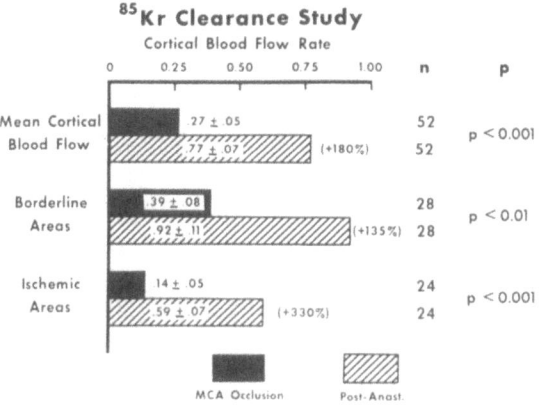

⁸⁵Kr Clearance Study
Cortical Blood Flow Rate

Fig. 12-3. Increase in cortical blood flow measured with ⁸⁵Kr clearance method following STA–MCA anastomosis after 24 hours of MCA occlusion. n = number of cortical areas examined.

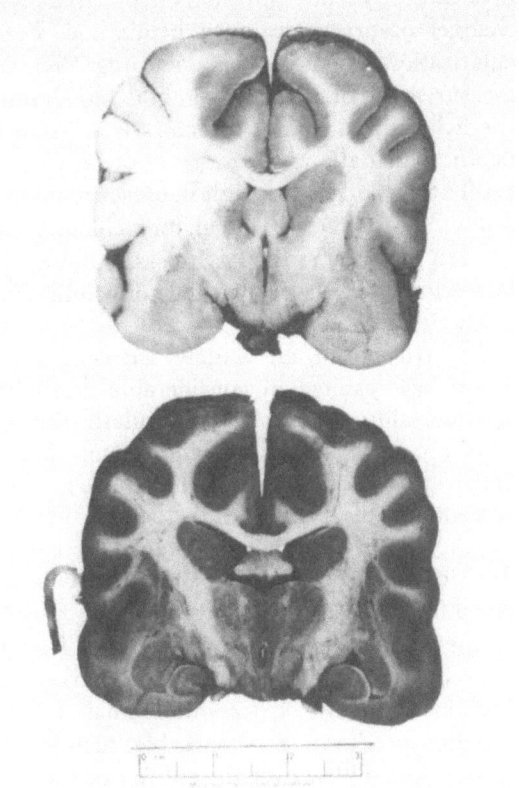

Fig. 12-4. India ink injection. Top: 24 hours after occlusion of the left middle cerebral artery. Bottom: Another specimen following STA–MCA anastomosis after 24 hours of left middle cerebral artery occlusion.

crease in cortical blood flow in the territory of the middle cerebral artery. This could be explained by the sparing of the lenticulostriate arteries, which avoids a deep infarct, and because the integrity of the motor cortex in the dog—which is located not in the sylvian area but in the sigmoid gyrus anteriorly—is maintained by perfusion from the intact anterior cerebral artery.

The canine experimental model has been used extensively in developing the extra–intracranial bypass procedure. The feasibility of these anastomoses remaining patent has been demonstrated experimentally[7, 10, 11] and clinically.[1, 17]

A comparison of graft patency and the presence of an infarct can demonstrate the influence on the ischemic process,[2] but the delineation and extent of an infarct in the fixed brain represents only one end-point in a complex sequence of hemodynamic and metabolic phenomena. Regional cerebral blood flow studies give more dynamic information of circulatory changes occurring during ischemia and revascularization. By using beta-emitting [85]Kr for measurement of regional cerebral blood flow, the field sensed by our detectors is 2.5 mm in depth, which allows for measure of only cortical flow. In correlation with fluorescein angiography, the pattern of circulatory changes can be seen not only in the large vessels but at the microcirculatory level over the convolutions of the brain.

Reperfusion of an acutely ischemic brain lesion has resulted in considerable morbidity and mortality. At present revascularization efforts are aimed mainly at improving chronic impairment of cerebral blood flow. The greatest percentage of patients are helped in this way.[1, 17] Our experimental model resembles this situation of chronic impairment of cerebral blood flow since, although permanent occlusion of the middle cerebral artery did not lead to infarct after 24 hours, it caused a marked reduction of flow. Extra–intracranial bypass grafting produced a remarkable increase in cortical blood flow over the entire middle cerebral artery territory after 24 hours of transorbital occlusion of the middle cerebral artery in dogs.

Summary

The left middle cerebral artery in mongrel dogs was permanently occluded with a 7-0 silk ligature placed through a transorbital microsurgical approach. After 24 hours the left cerebral hemisphere was exposed. The epicerebral circulation was examined by means of fluorescein angiography of the brain and the cortical blood flow was quantitated with [85]Kr clearance technique; after STA–MCA microanastomosis remarkable changes in the circulatory patterns were observed, and increases in cortical blood flow ranging from 135% in borderline areas to 330% in more ischemic areas were documented. At the end of each experiment the brain was perfused with india ink through both common carotid arteries, and after fixation in formalin coronal sections of the brain showed the depth of the revascularized area. Hematoxylin and eosin staining of the coronal sections was done from some of the representative experiments.

References

1. Chater, N., Popp, J. Microsurgical vascular bypass for occlusive cerebrovascular disease. Review of 100 cases. Surg Neurol 6:115–118, 1976.
2. Crowell, R., Olsson, Y. Effects of extracranial–intracranial vascular bypass graft on experimental acute stroke in dogs. J Neurosurg 38:26–31, 1973.
3. Fein, J., Molinari, G. Experimental augmentation of regional cerebral blood flow by microvascular anastomosis. J Neurosurg 41:421–426, 1974.
4. Feindel, W., Yamamoto, Y.L., Hodge, C. Fluorescein angiography of the brain. A new method for examination of the epicerebral circulation in man. Can Med Assoc J 96:1–7, 1967.
5. Feindel, W., Yamamoto, Y.L., Hodge, C. Microregional blood flow changes in experimental cerebral ischemia. J Neurosurg 35:155–161, 1971.
6. Hohberger, C.P., Yamamoto, Y.L., Thompson, C.J., et al. On-line computer measurement of microregional cerebral blood flow by xenon-133 clearance. Int J Nucl Med Biol 2:153–158, 1975.

7. Khodadad, G. Sublingual and lingual-basilar artery anastomosis and carotid–basilar bypass grafts. Surg Neurol 1:175–177, 1973.
8. Molinari, G. Experimental cerebral infarction. II. Clinicopathological model of deep cerebral infarction. Stroke 1:232–244, 1970.
9. Murray, P., Yamamoto, Y.L., Feindel, W. The watershed area following microvascular anastomosis. In Cerebral Function, Metabolism and Circulation, D.H. Ingvar and N.A. Lassen, editors, Munksgaard, Copenhagen, 1977.
10. Nishikawa, M., Yasargil, M.G., Yagi, N., Fish, U. Experimental extra–intracranial anastomosis. Surg Neurol 8:249–253, 1977.
11. Reichman, O.H. Experimenta 1. Lingual–basilar arterial microanastomosis. J Neurosurg 34:500–505, 1973.
12. Rosomoff H.L. Hypothermia and cerebral vascular lesions. J Neurosurg 13:332–343, 1956.
13. Shibata, S., Hodge, C., Pappius, H.M. Effect of experimental ischemia on cerebral water and electrolytes. J Neurosurg 41:146–160, 1974.
14. Symon, L.: Observations on the leptomeningeal collateral circulation in dogs. J Physiol 154:1–14, 1960.
15. Thompson, R.K., Smith, G. Experimental occlusion of the middle cerebral artery during arterial hypotension. Trans Am Neurol Assoc 203, 1951.
16. Yamamoto, Y.L. Personal communication, 1977.
17. Yasargil, M.G., Yonekawa, Y. Results of microsurgical extra–intracranial arterial bypass in the treatment of cerebral ischemia. Neurosurgery 1:22–24, 1977.
18. Zierler, K.L. Equations for measuring blood flow by monitoring of radioisotopes. Circ Res 16:309–321, 1965.

13

Regional Cerebral Perfusion Assessed with [81m]Kr and Emission Computerized Tomography

M. Collice, F. Fazio, C. Fieschi, F. Spinelli, O. Arena, M. Nardini, and A. Beduschi

Functional images of brain perfusion can be obtained by a steady-state method which exploits the peculiar physical characteristics of the radioactive gas [81m]Kr.[2] This is a very short half-lived isotope (13 sec half-life), which can be continuously produced either in the gaseous or the solution phase from its parent [81]Rb (4.6 hours half-life). It emits 190 keV γ rays, an ideal energy for recording with an Anger γ camera. Because of its short half-life, continuous carotid infusion of [81m]Kr in solution will never eventually result in the equilibrium of this diffusible tracer within the brain; during continuous infusion continuous recording of the activity over the brain will therefore reflect at any time regional arrival of tracer, which is a linear function of regional perfusion. Thus, when used in conjunction with an ordinary Anger γ camera, it provides images of cerebral perfusion in two dimensions.

Emission computerized tomography (ECT) is now being developed as a tool for providing more detailed spatial (tridimensional) information in nuclear medicine imaging techniques.[3] A major limitation of ECT is, at the present stage, that very high counting statistics are required to obtain reconstructed images which are reasonably free of noise. This limitation should be, on theoretical grounds, overcome at least in part by the [81m]Kr technique for imaging cerebral perfusion. This is because the short half-life of the isotope enables very high counting statistics to be obtained with a low radiation dose to the patient.

The aim of this paper is to present the preliminary results in a short series of patients in which regional perfusion was assessed using carotid infusion of [81m]Kr and a recently developed ECT system.

Methods

Rubidium-81 generators were produced for us on the M.R.C. Cyclotron Unit at Hammersmith Hospital, London,[1] and shipped to Milan via commercial flights. Krypton-81m solution was continuously recovered from the [81]Rb generator by eluting it with 5% dextrose. This solution was then continuously infused, via a small polyethylene cannula, into the internal or common carotid artery. During the infusion the radioactivity over the head was recorded by means of a commercial device designed for single-photon emission computerized tomography (SELO-GAMMA CAT). This essentially consists of: (1) a large-field γ camera detector, (2) a mechanical gantry suitable to allow a 360° rotation of the detector around the patient's head at a constant adjustable speed, (3) a computer system for collecting data during the detector's rotation and for reconstructing tomographic sections. A run usually consisted of 4 minutes of infusion; over this time approximately 3,000,000 counts were collected. Each run yielded a series of static (two-dimensional) views (right and left laterals, anteroposterior, posteroanterior), axial and coronal sections, the actual thickness of each section being 1.8 cm.

According to the diameters of the skull, 8 to 10 axial sections and 14 to 16 coronal sections were obtained in each study. Coronal and axial sections will, in this paper, be conventionally labeled by a progressive number starting from the front and the base of the skull respectively: the first coronal section (CS 1) will be passing across the frontal regions, approximately 3 cm from the glabella, and the first axial section (AS 1) across the lower part of the hemispheres approximately 3 cm from the external auditory meatus. Coronal and axial sections are respectively perpendicular and parallel to the horizontal plane of the orbitomeatal line.

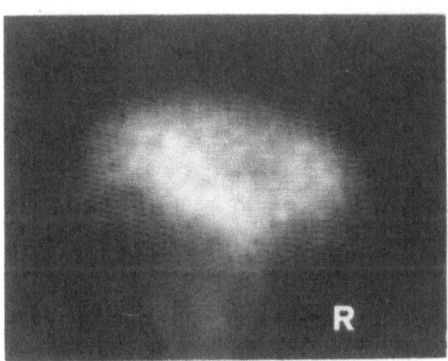

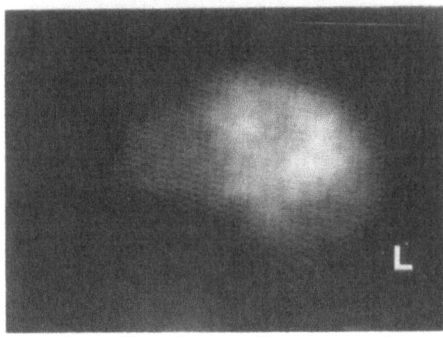

Fig. 13-1. Two-dimensional views of perfusion study from patient with right ICA occlusion obtained by continuous infusion of ^{81m}Kr into the left ICA. Distribution of activity is fairly homogeneous in the right lateral (upper) while in the AP view (lower) beyond the distribution of flow on the left hemisphere a slight activity is present on the right side. In this patient carotid angiography showed both ACAs and only the first segment (1 cm) of right MCA.

Patients

Nine patients with various brain disease were investigated. Diagnoses were established on clinical grounds, by angiographic and transmission computed tomography (TCT) studies, and in some cases by surgical procedure.

Diagnoses were as follows: Patients 1, 2, 3, and 4: complete occlusion of internal carotid artery (ICA); patient 5: right intracerebral frontal hematoma from AVM rupture; patient 6: right frontal glioma; patient 7: postsurgical occlusion of right middle cerebral artery (MCA); patient 8: post-traumatic normal-pressure hydrocephalus (NPH); patient 9: right cerebellar atrophy. Patient 1 was studied both before and after an extra–intracranial arterial bypass (EIAB) procedure, patients 2, 3 and 4 only after such an operation. Patient 5 was studied both before and after operation.

Multiple runs were obtained in each patient (control, hyperventilation, stimuli such as "automatic speech" and "voluntary hand movements"). Only the results of the control runs obtained from patients 1, 5, 6, 7, 8, and 9 are reported in this paper. Results of post-EIAB studies have been reported elsewhere in this volume.

Results

Patient 1

The presenting symptom was reversible ischemic attack from right ICA occlusion. On the left carotid angiograms both the anterior cerebral arteries (ACAs) and only the first segment (1 cm) of the MCA of the right side were visualized. During continuous ^{81m}Kr infusion into the left ICA, the distribution of the activity as recorded from the 2-D left lateral view was nearly uniform (Fig. 13-1 R). On the 2-D anteroposterior (AP) a slight presence of activity could be detected on the right side (Fig. 13-1 L). Coronal and axial sections showed, in addition to the flow distribution to the left hemisphere, a fairly high perfusion corresponding to the territory of distribution of the right ACA and a lesser degree of perfusion to the territory of

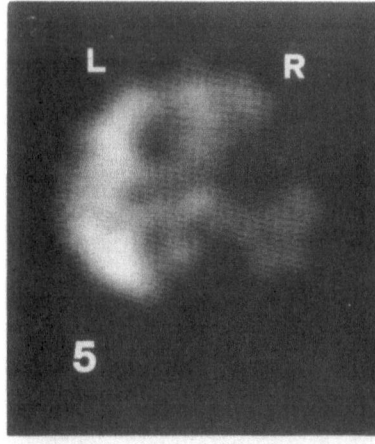

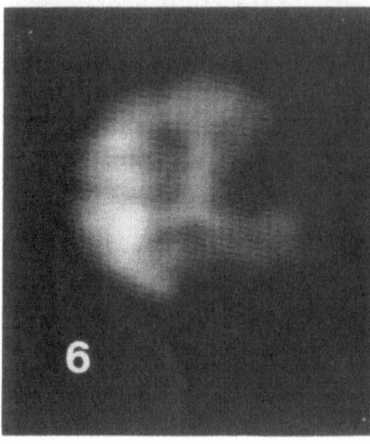

Fig. 13-2. Same patient as in Fig. 13-1 (right ICA occlusion). Tomographic images of perfusion study obtained by continuous infusion of ⁸¹ᵐKr into the left ICA. Two progressive axial sections (5 and 6) passing 7 and 8 cm above OM plane respectively and showing the flow distribution inside the hemispheres. Note the gray-white matter flow distribution and the activity on the right ACA and right MCA regions. In this patient left carotid angiography showed both the ACAs and only the first segment (1 cm) of right MCA.

the right MCA area (Fig. 13-2). These latter appearances were particularly evident in CS 8-10 and in AS 3-5. Moreover, the perfusion in the left hemisphere showed a distribution of activity which was not uniform in the tomographic sections, perfusion to the more central regions (corresponding to the white matter) being lower than perfusion to the more peripheral regions (gray matter).

Patient 5

This patient exhibited moderate intracranial hypertensive signs and slight left hemiparesis. Right carotid angiograms showed frontolateral AVM with indirect signs of space-occupying lesion. TCT scan revealed a high-density lesion of the right frontolateral region. The static 2-D views showed an area of reduced activity (hypoperfusion) corresponding to the frontal region (Fig. 13-3). First to fourth coronal sections, however, showed an area where perfusion was absent corresponding to the white matter of the frontal lobe, surrounded by an area of hypoperfusion (Fig. 13-4). Similar appearances were observed on the axial sections from the third to the seventh section (Fig. 13-5). The largest extension of the "no-perfusion area" was recorded on CS 2 and on AS 4-5. Furthermore, on AS 3-5 an area of hyperperfusion, probably reflecting luxury perfusion, was observed at the periphery of the hematoma in the posterior regions.

Patient 6

(Right frontal glioma.) A small area of hypoperfusion was shown on the right 2-D lateral and AP views. Both coronal and axial sections showed, in addition to this area of hypoperfusion corresponding to the white matter of the frontal lobe, a small area of absent perfusion corresponding to the cortical frontal lateral regions.

Patient 7

(Normal-pressure hydrocephalus.) On the right 2-D lateral view an area of relatively reduced activity was recorded on the frontal region. This was shown by the posteroanterior view to be located at the center of the right hemisphere. On both the coronal and axial sections crossing the ventricular system (CS 6-12, AS 3-6) a dishomogeneous flow distribution (reflecting gray and white matter distribution) was shown around a large area of no perfusion clearly related to the enlarged ventricles.

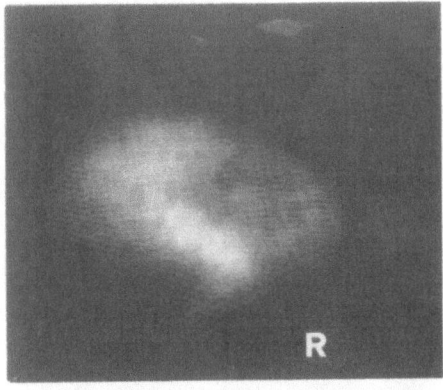

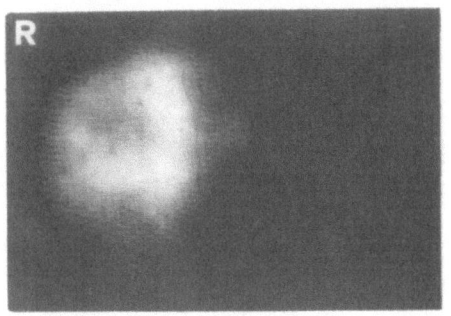

Fig. 13-3. Static two-dimensional views (lateral, upper; AP, lower) of rBP obtained by continuous infusion of [81m]Kr into the right ICA. Note the large area of reduced activity (hypoperfusion on the frontal region).

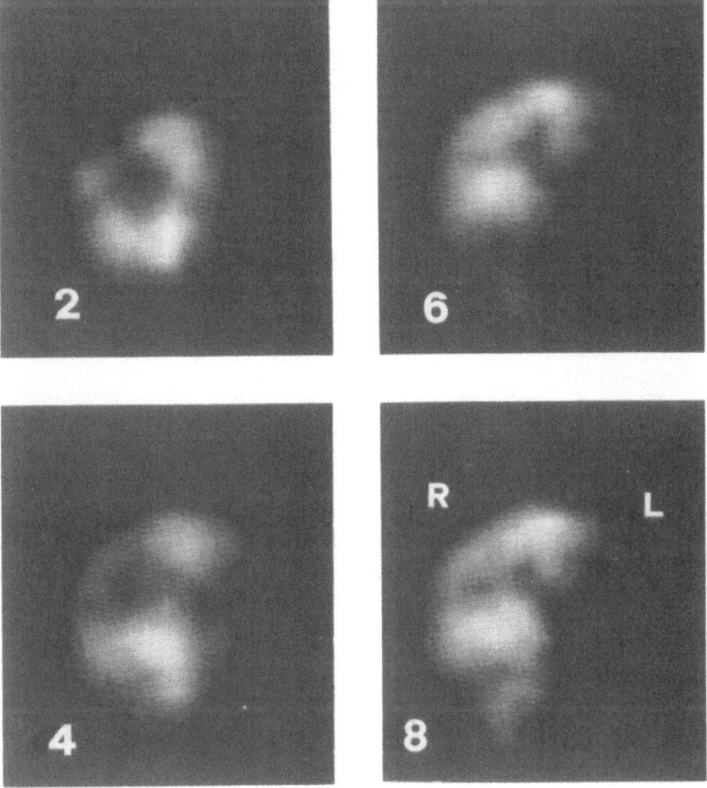

Fig. 13-4. Same case as in Fig. 13-3 (right frontal intracerebral hematoma). Tomographic images of perfusion study obtained by [81m]Kr infusion into the right ICA. Four coronal sections (2, 4, 6, and 8) passing 4, 6, 8, and 10 cm from the glabella, respectively. Note the area of "no perfusion" inside the frontal lobe surrounded by an area of hypoperfusion. The major extent of the no-perfusion area is present on section 2. Also, note the carotid artery image on section 8.

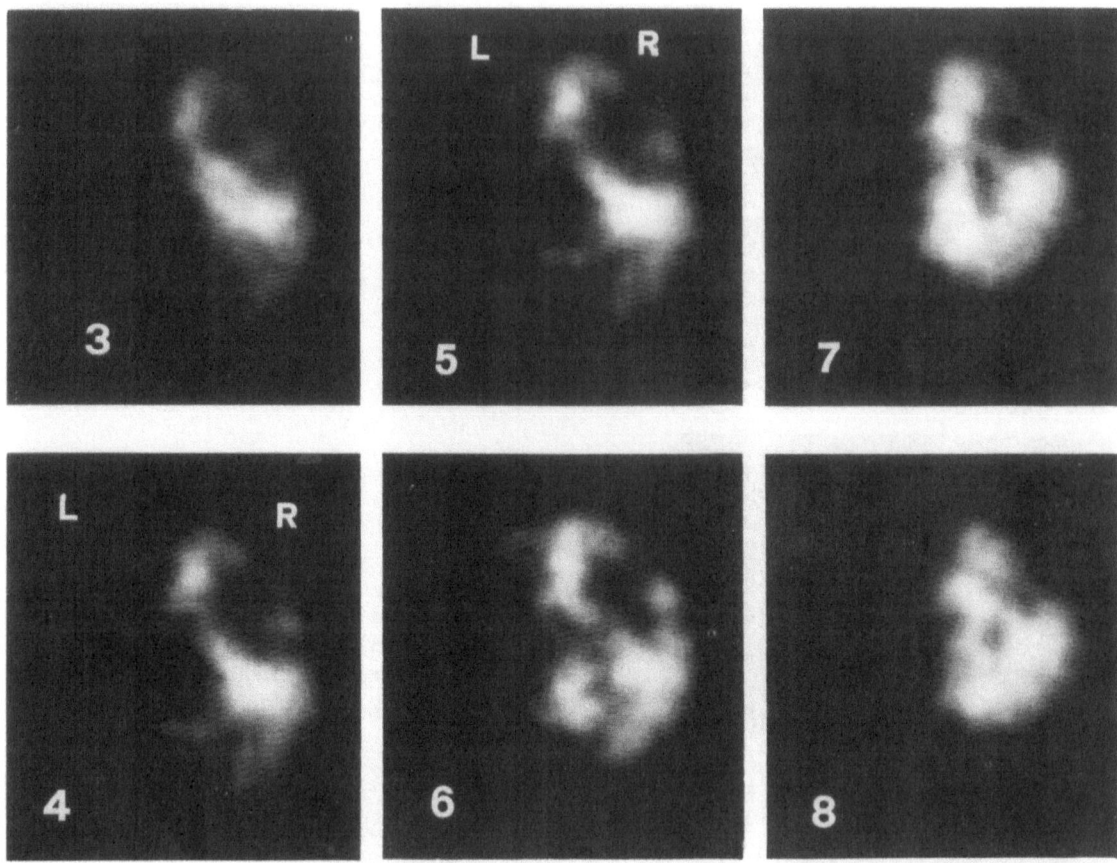

Fig. 13-5. Same case as in Figs. 13-3 and 13-4 (right frontal intracerebral hematoma). Tomographic images of perfusion study obtained by ^{81m}Kr infusion into the right ICA. Six axial sections (3, 4, 5, 6, 7, and 8) passing 5, 6, 7, 8, 9, and 10 cm above OM plane, respectively. Note the area of "no perfusion" inside the frontal lobe (its major extension in sections 4 and 5) and surrounding it an area of hypoperfusion (section 7).

Patient 8

(Post-surgical occlusion of the right MCA.) This patient was studied one month after occlusion of the main trunk of the MCA subsequent to operation for MCA aneurysm. At the study period he exhibited severe hemiparesis; TCT scan demonstrated a large area of low density on the sylvian region and right carotid angiography showed very poor collateral circulation. The right 2-D lateral view showed an area of hypoperfusion on the central area of the hemisphere. The highest axial sections (AS 6-7) showed an area of absent perfusion corresponding to the cortical central area, while on the lower sections (AS 4-5) a smaller area of no perfusion and an area of hypoperfusion were shown. The same appearances were observed on the coronal sections.

Patient 9

This patient with right cerebellar atrophy had a normal TCT scan of the supratentorial regions and normal right and left carotid angiograms. However, both ACAs were better visualized on the left carotid angiogram; on the right angiogram the right ACA was poorly visualized. ECT perfusion study was performed by infusing the tracer into the right ICA. The 2-D right lateral view showed a fairly uniform distribution of perfusion to the whole right hemisphere. The 2-D AP view showed an area of hypoperfusion corresponding to the territory of the right ACA. On both coronal and axial sections the activity was mainly distributed in an area which is anatomically known to be supplied by the right MCA, the perfusion being very poor in the region corresponding to the right ACA. This distribution of cerebral perfusion thus is explained by the angiographic findings of a physiologic variant (underdeveloped first segment of right anterior cerebral artery). Moreover, the perfusion in the territory of the MCA showed dishomogeneous distribution of activity as previously described in patients 1 and 7.

Absorbed Radiation Dose

Absorbed dose to the brain was less than 50 millirads for each run. Absorbed radiation dose to heart and kidney resulting from ^{81}Rb breakthrough was less than 20 millirads.

Discussion and Conclusions

Specific methods for assessing regional cerebral perfusion are particularly useful in reconstructive surgery, as they provide, relative to angiography, detailed information on the presence, extent, and localization of the ischemic areas.

To provide this additional information, these techniques must have high accuracy and spatial resolution. These factors should be significantly improved by the use of emission tomography, which introduces a third dimension for the spatial reconstruction of cerebral perfusion.

This paper shows the feasibility of obtaining, with acceptable absorbed radiation dose to the patients, tomographic images of cerebral perfusion by intracarotid infusion of ^{81m}Kr. These images present definite additional advantages over conventional images in two dimensions, mostly by eliminating the superimposition of activities originating from different regions. These can be summarized as follows: (1) visualization of the perfusion distribution inside the brain including white and gray matter flow distribution, (2) better visualization, localization and evaluation of areas of absent perfusion, hypoperfusion and hyperperfusion as, for example, in the patient with frontal hematoma, (3) detection of cerebral perfusion unpredictable from angiograms alone as shown in the patients with ICA and MCA occlusion, (4) correct interpretation of the areas of apparent hypoperfusion as in the patient with NPH.

Major shortcomings of the technique described in this paper are essentially those previously recognized for ^{81m}Kr carotid infusion and two-dimensional imaging—invasiveness, quantitation, and the fact that one essentially is looking to the flow distribution of the infused vessel rather than to actual cerebral blood flow. In our opinion, however, when the method is used for patient selection for cerebral revascularization the third limitation is the most important, particularly because most of the patients now undergoing reconstruction surgery have a thrombosis of the ICA. This problem could be overcome by infusing ^{81m}Kr in the ascending aorta. This approach, however, still presents significant theoretical and technical problems mainly related to the need, peculiar to emission tomography, of obtaining high counting statistics.

Acknowledgment

We thank the colleagues of the M.R.C. Cyclotron Unit, Hammersmith Hospital, London, U.K., for their cooperation and assistance.

References

1. Clark, J.C., Horlock, P.L., Watson, I.A. Krypton-81m generators. Radiochem Radioanal Lett 25:245–254, 1976.
2. Fazio, F., Nardini, M., Fieschi, C., Forli, C. Assessment of regional blood flow by continuous carotid infusion of krypton-81m. J Nucl Med 18:962–966, 1977.
3. Phelps, M.E. Emission computed tomography. Semin Nucl Med 7:337–365, 1977.

14

The Value of Noninvasive Regional CBF Measurements in Diagnostic and Follow-up Studies in Cerebral Vascular Diseases with Special Regard to EIAB*

G. Meinig, A. Fenske, and K. Schürmann

Assessment of patients with cerebrovascular disease requires precise information on rCBF. In view of the technical improvement of noninvasive rCBF measurement (nrCBF), we have applied noninvasive rCBF equipment in Mainz since 1977. We undertook this study to establish the indication for EIAB and to obtain reliable data for assessment of the results of drug therapy as well as of surgical therapy by follow-up nrCBF measurement.

Methods

Measurement Procedure and Equipment

We use a commercially available 16-channel system with 8-crystal detector $\frac{3}{4} \times \frac{3}{4}$ inches with a 20-mm cylindrical lead collimator on each hemisphere.** The patient was attached to the xenon-administration system by a mouthpiece sealed by surgical self-adhesive drape to avoid loss of radioactivity from the respiration cycle. The end-tidal values of the expired air were measured for xenon activity in a special air detector, and the concentration of CO_2 in a capnograph in the same air sample. Data ac-

cumulation and processing were done by an on-line computer, and the calculations were done by biexponential analysis as described by Obrist et al.[5] and the initial slope index (ISI) as introduced by Risberg et al.[7] Immediately after the study the following parameters were tabulated by the computer: Flow gray (F_g) in ml/100 g/min, the ISI calculated between 2 and 3 min, is independent of the partition coefficient for xenon. Additionally the relative weight of the gray-matter compartment, the fractional flow in percent of the total flow, the decay constant K of the low perfused (white) tissue, and the interhemispheric differences of the corresponding areas were printed out (RIFD = regional interhemispheric flow differences). Using this system a reliable reproducibility could be reached using a xenon concentration of 2.5 to 3 mCi per liter in the inspired air during equilibration of one-minute duration. No spectrum substration for hemispheric x rays was done.

Case Materials

From our patients with cerebrovascular disease in whom nrCBF was performed, we have selected three groups in which all available diagnostic procedures, especially angiography, were performed:

  I. Healthy patients for control (n = 10)

  II. Patients with ICA–MCA obstruction (angiographically proved) (n = 10)

*We wish to express many thanks for the generous financial support by Deutsche Anlagen Leasing GmbH, D-6500 Mainz.

**Cerebrograph available from NOVO-Industrie GmbH Pharmazeutica, Kantstr. 2, D-6500 Mainz.

III. Patients with clinical signs of cerebral ischemia and no significant angiographic correlate (i.e., only minimal arteriosclerotic signs normal for their age) (n = 8).

The nrCBF findings were correlated with the various clinical and diagnostic findings. Moreover, nrCBF was performed following EIAB operation in a limited number of patients.

Results

Fig. 14-1 shows the pattern of flow distribution in normal patients (n = 10). Average hemispheric means of both sides and average flow pattern distribution as well as the distribution in percent of the hemispheric means are given. Our results are similar to those obtained by other groups using nrCBF.[1-7]

In case of ICA–MCA obstruction, we regularly find typical patterns of flow distribution. Fig. 14-2 shows the nrCBF of a 61-year-old female with ICA occlusion for six weeks beyond the bifurcation on the right side. Mean ISI of the affected hemisphere may still be in the normal range (reactive hyperemia in the right frontal and temporal region?). However, comparison of the flow patterns of the affected and nonaffected hemispheres shows a striking reduction of perfusion in the circulation area of MCA on the affected side.

Figure 14-3 shows the pattern of average hemispheric flow distribution of group II. All cases show a regional focal flow decrease on the affected side. The average hemispheric values (n = 10) on the affected hemisphere may be in the lower normal range if each hemisphere is considered on its own. On the other hand, comparison of affected and nonaffected hemispheres (MIFD) reveals a significant difference and evidence for unilateral diminished

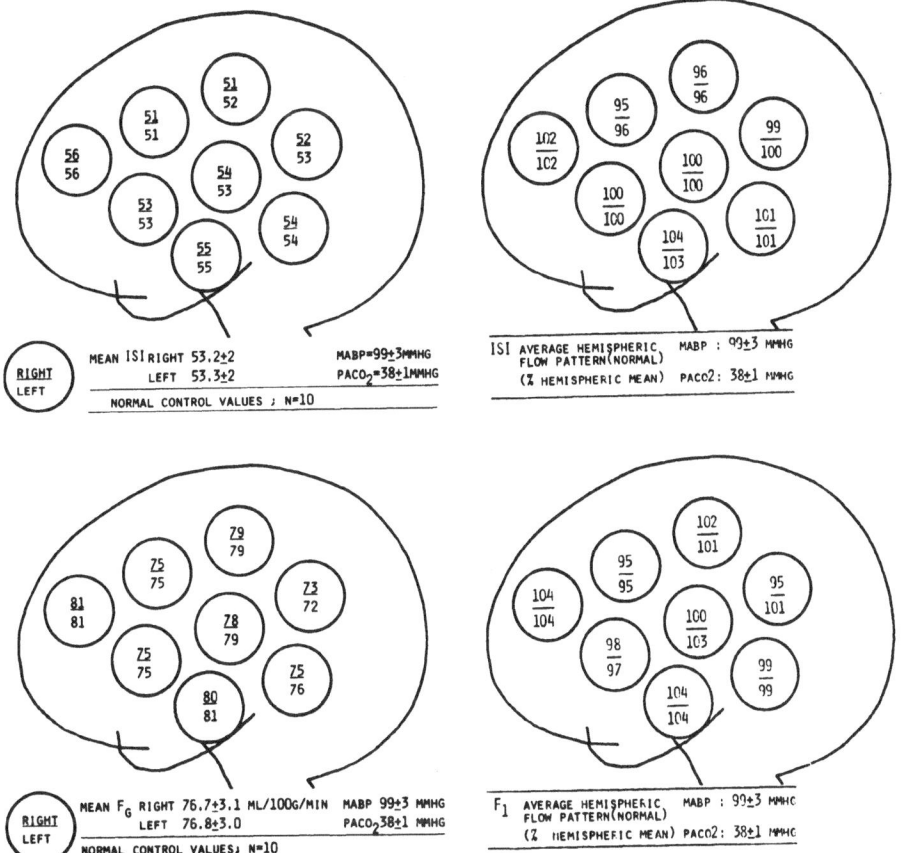

Fig. 14-1. Blood flow in normal subjects.

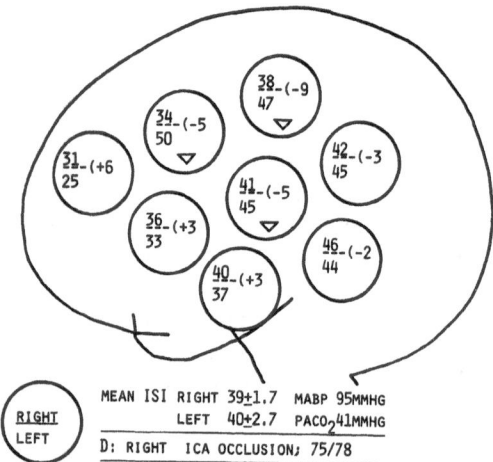

MEAN ISI RIGHT 39±1.7 MABP 95MMHG
            LEFT 40±2.7 PACO₂41MMHG
D: RIGHT ICA OCCLUSION; 75/78

Fig. 14-2. nrCBF pattern of a 61-year-old female with a 6-weeks' ICA occlusion beyond bifurcation.

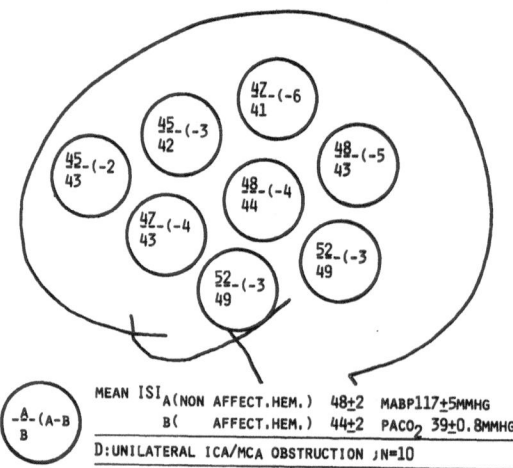

MEAN ISI A(NON AFFECT.HEM.) 48±2 MABP117±5MMHG
          B(AFFECT.HEM.)   44±2 PACO₂ 39±0.8MMHG
D:UNILATERAL ICA/MCA OBSTRUCTION ;N=10

Fig. 14-3. Average nrCBF pattern of 10 patients with ICA–MCA obstruction.

perfusion (Table 14-1). The average regional flow pattern may also still be in the range of lower normal if it is assessed only for the affected side in isolation. The comparison of both sides (RIFD) indicates local pathologic perfusion with accentuation in the region supplied by the MCA. All cases showed a very good correlation between nrCBF and the neurologic and angiographic findings (Table 14-2).

Patient group III seems to be particularly interesting with regard to the sensitivity of the nrCBF method (Fig. 14-4, Table 14-2). Despite normal angiographic findings the nrCBF of patients with symptoms of cerebral ischemia do not seem to be abnormal as compared with the

normal values if the affected hemisphere is considered on its own. Although there is only a slight difference in the mean ISI of both hemispheres, comparison of nrCBF pattern in the affected and non-affected hemispheres indicates local pathologic perfusion.

As Table 14-2 shows, RIFD could be correlated with the neurologic findings in seven of eight cases, while the angiographic finding was negative in all cases.

The number of cases in which we performed nrCBF following EIAB operation is very small. The time interval between EIAB and control of nrCBF was short. Nevertheless, we were able to observe some cases with remarkable im-

Table 14-1. Correlation between rCBF and angiography

Index	Control values, total means	Angiography positive		Angiography negative	
		A.H.	N.A.H.	A.H.	N.A.H.
F_gray	77 ± 3	65 ± 3***	71 ± 3	76 ± 3*	80 ± 3
ISI	53 ± 2	44 ± 2***	48 ± 2	53 ± 3	55 ± 2
Age	44 ± 5	56 ± 2		49 ± 2	
MABP	93 ± 3	117 ± 5		106 ± 3	
PaCO₂	38 ± 1	39 ± 1		38 ± 1	
N	10	10		8	

* = P < 0.05; ** = P < 0.005; *** = P < 0.001, demonstrating significance of interhemispheric differences. Patient with "angiography negative" showed clinically signs of ischemic lesions in the MCA territory of the "affected hemisphere."

A.H. = affected hemisphere.

N.A.H. = nonaffected hemisphere.

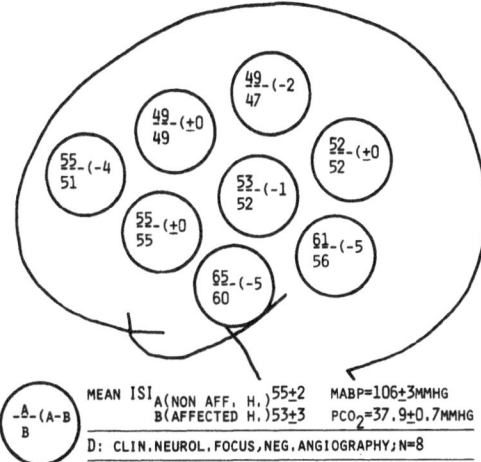

Fig. 14-4. Average nrCBF pattern of 8 patients with clinical signs of cerebral ischemia without angiographic correlates.

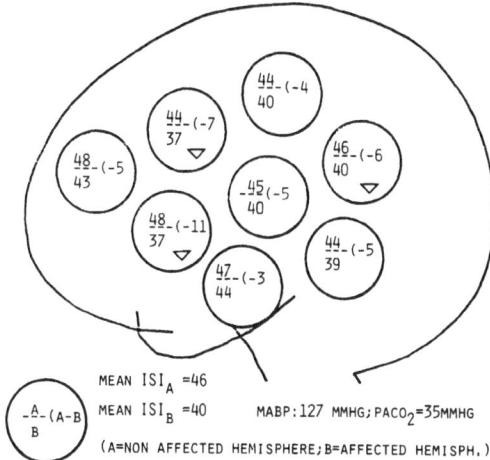

Fig. 14-5. nrCBF pattern of a 61-year-old man with an 8 weeks' ICA occlusion on the right side beyond bifurcation.

prove of nrCBF. For example, Fig. 14-5 shows the nrCBF of a 6-year-old man with a chronic ICA occlusion beyond the bifurcation on the right side. Mean ISI on the affected right side may still be in the normal range. However, it is distinctly reduced as compared to the unaffected side. The flow pattern of the affected side is more or less reduced in all areas which were measured. EIAB was performed on 5 June 1978. Twelve days following the EIAB operation the mean ISI shows an increase of 2 ml/100 g/min (6 ml/100 g/min preoperatively) and the comparison of the nrCBF patterns shows an increase in most areas (Fig. 14-6). Pre- and postoperative regional interhemi-

spheric difference (RIFD) are even more pronounced (Fig. 14-7). Fig. 14-8 shows the postoperative angiogram (from 30 August 1978). Measurement of blood flow in the anastomosis by videodensitometry revealed a value of 73 ml/min.

Discussion

Noninvasive rCBF measurement has advantages for the patient and the on-line equipment is easily handled. Nevertheless, this method is able to provide satisfactory mean and regional

Table 14-2. Relationship between clinically apparent localization of brain vascular lesion and findings using different examination methods

	Angiography		EEG	CT scan	Isotop. A.	Doppler S.	Flow$_{gray}$	ISI	Region (RIFD)
CLIN.	+	(100%)	40(%)	30(%)	50(%)	40(%)	70(%)	65(%)	95(%)
LOC.	(+)	−	10	20	20	20	30	35	5
	−	−	40	40	30	30	−	−	−
II	N.D.	−	10	10	−	10	−	−	−
	+	−	25	12.5	12.5	12.5	62.5	50	87.5
	(+)	12.5	12.5	12.5	−	12.5	12.5	37.5	12.5
	−	87.5	62.5	62.5	87.5	7.5	25	12.5	−
III	N.D.	−	−	12.5	−	−	−	−	−

+ = good correlation to the clinical picture, (+) = poor, (−) = no correlation.
N.D. = not done; group II = 10, III = 8.

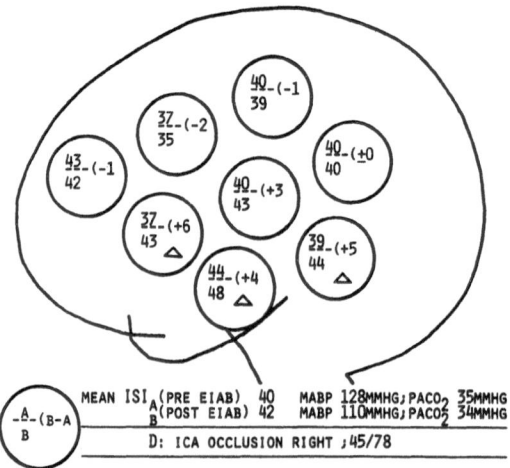

MEAN ISI$_A$(PRE EIAB) 40   MABP 128MMHG; PACO$_2$ 35MMHG
ISI$_B$(POST EIAB) 42   MABP 110MMHG; PACO$_2$ 34MMHG

D: ICA OCCLUSION RIGHT ; 45/78

$\frac{A}{B}$-(B-A)

Fig. 14-6. nrCBF pattern 12 days following EIAB (same patient as in Fig. 14-5).

troversial, it can locate lesions which the unilateral invasive method may not detect. Meanwhile the high diagnostic value of nrCBF in patients with cerebral ischemia and infarction may require that nrCBT measurement is carried out before angiography is performed and in certain cases the nrCBF result may allow the additional invasive methods to be dispensed with. The method permits outpatient preselection before admission to a hospital. To confirm the presented data, which are the result of a few months' measurement of nrCBF, and also to establish the diagnostic value and the reliability of this method, we hope to extend our studies to a larger number of patients very soon.

CBF in patients with cerebrovascular disease. The flow patterns correlate very well with the angiographic and clinical findings. The special advantage of nrCBF is that the perfusion of both hemispheres can be obtained simultaneously. The comparison of mean interhemispheric CBF (MIFD) as well as of regional interhemispheric rCBF (RIFD) patterns thus allows assessment of the cerebrovascular lesion, even in cases which do not show correlation between CT and angiography. Although the accuracy of the nrCBF method has been con-

Summary

The nrCBF findings (Meditronic Cerebrograph) of 10 healthy patients (group I) were compared with the nrCBF measurements of 10 patients with ICA–MCA obstruction (group II) and 8 patients showing cerebral ischemia despite normal angiographic findings (group III). To verify the sensitivity and diagnostic value of the nrCBF method, the results were compared with other diagnostic methods: neurologic correlate, angiography, CT, isotope angiography, Doppler sonography.

In group II the comparison of mean nrCBF of affected and nonaffected hemispheres correlated in more than 60% with the clinical and angiographic findings. It correlated with the interhemispheric regional differences (RIFD) in more than 90%. In group III, mean rCBF correlated in about 50% and RIFD in more than 80% with the clinical findings.

The comparison of the diagnostic reliability of nrCBF with other diagnostic methods (neurologic investigations, angiography, EEG, CT, isotope angiography, Doppler sonography) showed in group III a result which comes near to the reliability of angiography. Of all other methods, nrCBF showed the best correlation with the neurologic finding in group III. Very recent nrCBF measurements following EIAB operation showed great correlation with the clinical findings, angiography, and videodensitometrically measured blood flow.

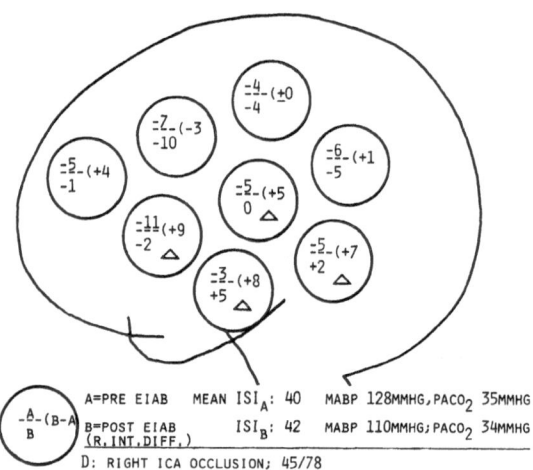

A=PRE EIAB   MEAN ISI$_A$: 40   MABP 128MMHG; PACO$_2$ 35MMHG
B=POST EIAB   ISI$_B$: 42   MABP 110MMHG; PACO$_2$ 34MMHG
(R.INT.DIFF.)

D: RIGHT ICA OCCLUSION; 45/78

$\frac{A}{B}$-(B-A)

Fig. 14-7. RIFD pre- and post-EIAB (same patient as in Figs. 14-5 and 14-6).

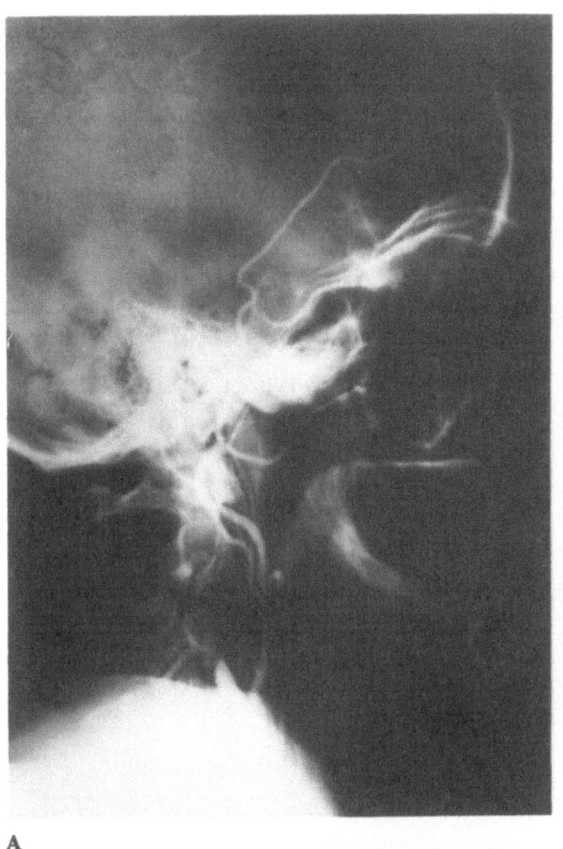

A

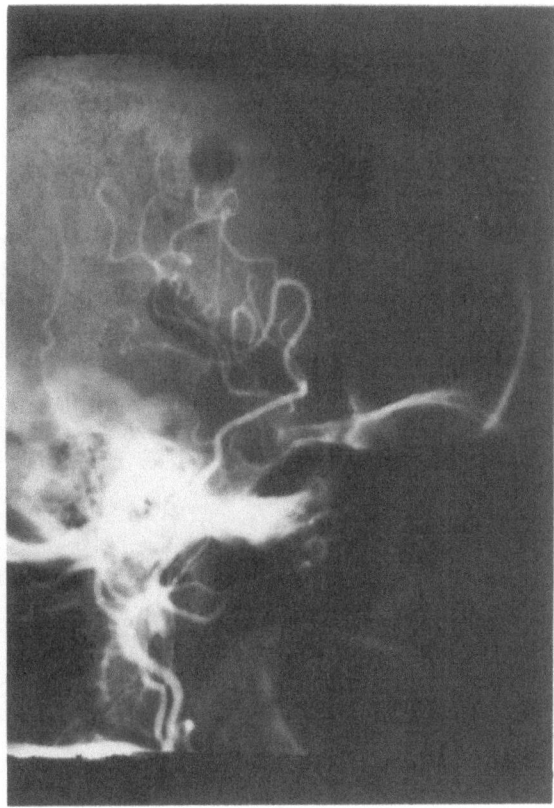

B

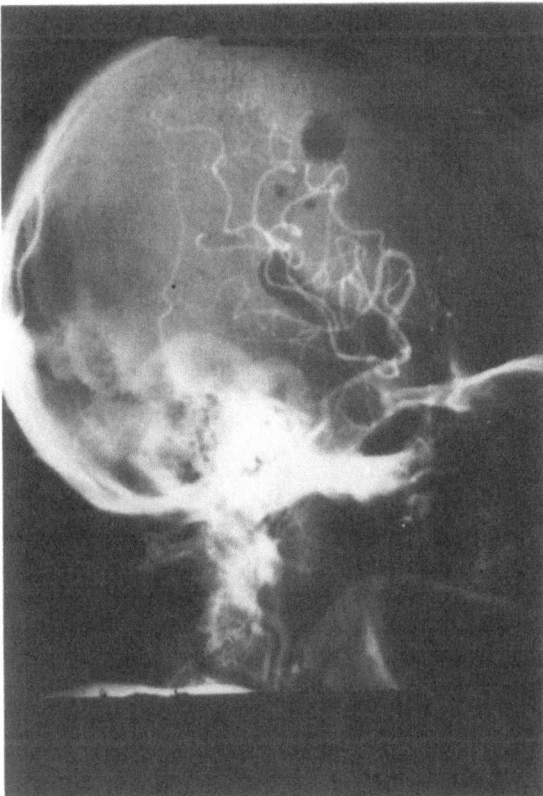

C

Fig. 14-8. A. Preoperative angiogram of patient in Figs. 14-5 through 14-7. B. Postoperative angiogram of same patient. In the bypass the video-densitometric value was 73 ml/min. C. Postoperative angiogram taken 1 sec after B.

References

1. Blauenstein, U.W., Halsey, J.H., Wilson, E.M., et al. [133]Xenon inhalation method: Significance of indicator maldistribution for distinguishing brain areas with impaired perfusion. Stroke 9: 57–66, 1978.
2. Deshmukh, V.D., Meyer, J.S. Noninvasive Measurement of Regional Cerebral Blood Flow in Man. SP Medical and Scientific Books, New York–London, 1977.
3. Meyer, J.S., Ishihara, N., Deshmukh, V.D., et al. Improved method for noninvasive measurement of regional blood flow by [133]xenon inhalation, Part I. Stroke 9:195–205, 1978.
4. Meyer, J.S.: Improved method for noninvasive measurement of regional blood flow by [133]xenon inhalation, Part II. Stroke 9:205–210, 1978.
5. Obrist, W.D., Thompson, H.K., Wang, H.S., et al. Regional cerebral blood flow estimated by [133]xenon inhalation. Stroke 6:245–256, 1975.
6. Reivich, M., Obrist, W., Slater, R., et al. A comparison of the Xe[133] intracarotid injection and inhalation techniques for measuring regional cerebral blood flow. In Blood and Metabolism in the Brain, A.M. Harper, W.B. Jennett, J.D. Müller, J.O. Rowan, editors, Churchill Livingstone, Edinburgh–London–New York, 1975, pp. 8.3–8.6.
7. Risberg, J., Ali, Z., Wilson, E.M., et al. Regional cerebral blood flow by [133]xenon inhalation. Stroke 6:142–148, 1975.

IV

Noninvasive Methods of
Investigation and
EEG Analysis

15

Noninvasive Management of Stroke Patients by Doppler Sonography and Dynamic Radionuclide Brain Scanning

B. Zumstein, H. M. Keller, and U. Luetolf

In recent years cerebrovascular reconstructive surgery has made great progress both technically and in resolving problems of surgical indication. Particularly the STA–MCA anastomosis procedure can be performed with little risk, patency rates above 90%, and good clinical results in preventing further cerebral ischemic events in patients with cerebrovascular occlusive disease.[2, 3, 8, 9, 16, 18, 19] The demonstration of an arterial obstruction by angiography has been a prerequisite for operation. Unfortunately, this procedure is not without risk, especially in patients with generalized atherosclerosis.[11, 15] Another method of investigating such patients is regional cerebral blood flow (rCBF) measurement by radionuclide ^{133}xenon injection.[10] This is again an invasive procedure which requires the cannulation of both carotid arteries.

On the one hand, improved surgical capabilities favor a more intensive investigation of patients suffering from cerebral ischemia, while on the other hand we found by angiography a clearly visible arterial cerebrovascular obstruction requiring surgery in only about 50% of such patients. To evaluate operative results patients must again undergo carotid angiography and/or rCBF measurement.

For these reasons we have evaluated carotid artery Doppler sonography[4, 5, 12] and dynamic ^{99m}Tc brain scanning with qualitative and quantitative analysis of cerebral blood perfusion in this group of patients.[6, 7, 13, 14] These two methods were used as screening procedures rou-

tinely prior to angiography in candidates for EC–IC bypass surgery and in assessing surgical results. It is known that they are capable of detecting significant vascular obstructions.

At the University Hospital of Zurich, the Doppler ultrasound technique was already widely in use as a screening procedure before performing angiography and carotid endarterectomy. The accuracy of predicting a major obstruction of the internal carotid artery (ICA) by this method was found to be 95% compared to angiography in 346 cases.[4, 5] In addition to this diagnostic purpose, we have also used the method for assessing the patency of STA–MCA bypass anastomoses.

Dynamic brain scanning has been used only occasionally for the evaluation of stroke patients. In this study we used it routinely both preoperatively and for assessing the effect of cerebral revascularization.

Our experience with the routine use of these two procedures in the noninvasive management of stroke or stroke-prone patients will form the basis of this report.

Materials and Method

The study consists of three different parts: (1) screening of patients with cerebrovascular occlusive disease by Doppler sonography and qualitative radionuclide brain scanning (35 cases), (2) pre- and postoperative evaluation of patients with STA–MCA bypass anastomoses by Doppler sonography (64 cases), and (3) quantitative ^{99m}Tc brain scanning (in the 10 most recent cases of the 64).

Thirty-five consecutive patients suffering from cerebral ischemia (TIA or little stroke) were investigated by carotid artery Doppler sonography and dynamic brain scanning prior to angiography. Over a 15-month period all patients underwent carotid angiography regardless of the results of the two previous tests. The results of the three procedures were compared. The details of the Doppler technique will not be elaborated here. We used a bidirectional ultrasound Doppler device (Parks 806) with stereo earphones and a 2-channel recorder. For the radionuclide dynamic brain scanning the most common technique with rapid ^{99m}Tc–DTPA intravenous bolus injection was used, the patient in a position for an anterior Towne view under a ON 110 Gamma camera (Ohio Nuclear). The screening and preoperative evaluation were purely qualitative, inspecting the sequential frames for differences in cerebral perfusion. The count rates were stored in a computer for quantitative analysis postoperatively (PDP-11 computer, Digital Equipment Corp.).

Since 1975 the above-mentioned Doppler equipment has been employed to examine 64

patients before and after STA–MCA bypass surgery to assess the patency of the artificial anastomosis. In addition to the usual sonographic criteria of flow signals, bypass patency was determined by the ability to follow the STA up to the site of craniotomy with the Doppler probe and by increased diastolic flow signals compared to the preoperative findings and/or contralateral side (Fig. 15-1). All patients underwent follow-up angiography and the results were compared.

In the 10 most recent cases of 64 who underwent bypass surgery, the dynamic brain scanning procedure was repeated two weeks after surgery and in 3 cases to date three months later, to investigate flow changes on the operated side. The method of postoperative flow evaluation by numerical computer analysis is shown in Fig. 15-2. The flow data were collected by the computer in 2 frames/sec for 30 sec after injection. On dynamic playback images on a color video screen, four regions of interest (ROI) were designated bilaterally: a representative area of the cerebral hemisphere, the middle cerebral artery (MCA), the superficial temporal artery (STA), and the cervical carotid artery (Fig. 15-3). Quantitative activity data were displayed in the form of computer-generated graphs of count rates versus time for each ROI. The activity flow curves of the L-

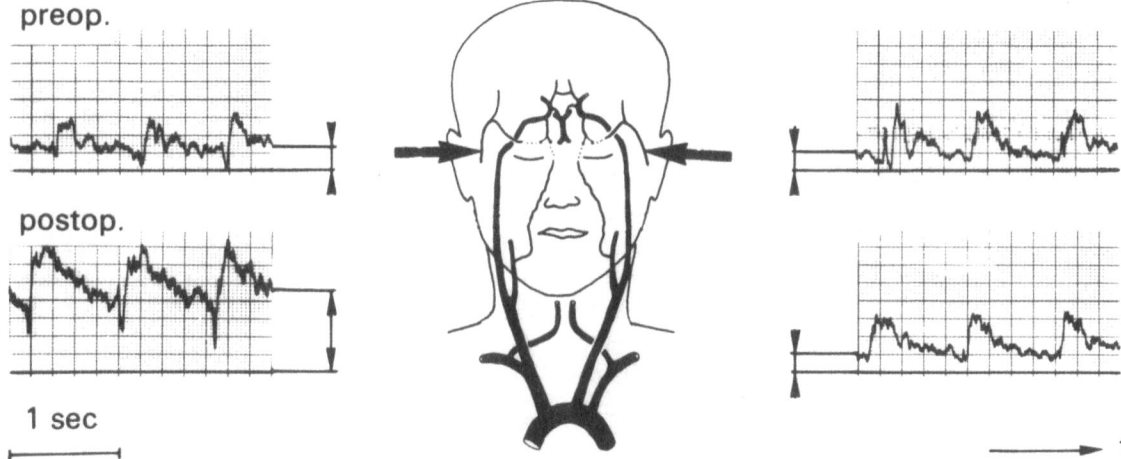

Fig. 15-1. Results of direct Doppler measurements over the STA on the side of anastomosis and contralaterally in a 56-year-old patient with occlusion of the right ICA and minor neurologic deficit. *Before surgery* Doppler signals of the STAs were symmetrical in amplitude and diastolic flow. *After surgery* diastolic flow on the operated side is increased approximately 3 times compared to preoperative and contralateral findings.

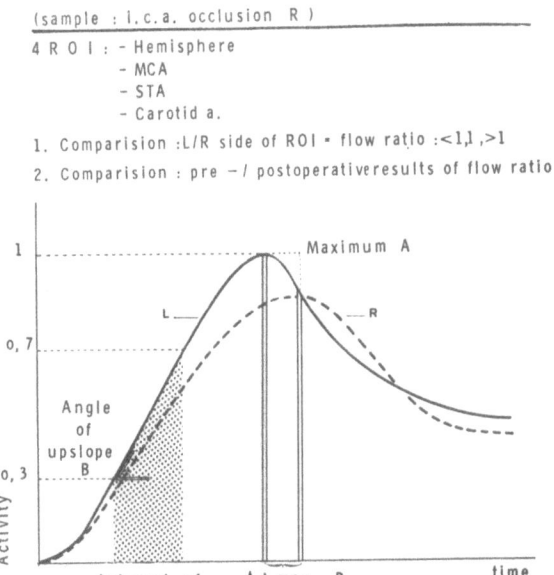

Time / activity curves L and R side.
(sample : i.c.a. occlusion R)

4 R O I : - Hemisphere
          - MCA
          - STA
          - Carotid a.

1. Comparision :L/R side of ROI = flow ratio :<1,1 ,>1

2. Comparision : pre −/ postoperative results of flow ratio

Fig. 15-2. *Above:* Method of cerebral flow evaluation by numerical computer analysis comparing (1) flow curves of L and R side and (2) pre- and postoperative flow ratios in 4 different ROI (see Fig. 15-3). *Below:* Illustration of 2 symmetrical MCA–ROI curves, in a case of right ICA occlusion. Flow curves are described by 4 parameters: A = maximum activity, B = angle of upslope, C = integral of upslope, D = time difference of maximum activity.

sided ROI were compared to the R-sided ones to obtain a perfusion ratio for each ROI pair. Finally, the pre- and postoperative ratios of each ROI pair were compared. Improvement or normalization of flow in a region of previously altered perfusion led to a L:R vascular flow ratio close to 1:1 or even to an inversion of the ratio (Fig. 15-4 A, B).

All of these 10 consecutive cases had well-functioning anastomoses documented by conventional carotid angiography.

Results

Screening and Preoperative Evaluation

Of the 35 patients admitted for evaluation of cerebral ischemia since April 1976, 20 (57%) demonstrated a clear vascular obstruction by angiography: 12 complete occlusions and 4 70% stenoses of the proximal internal carotid artery (ICA), 2 occlusions and 2 stenoses of the middle cerebral artery (MCA). All proximal obstructions of the ICA were diagnosed correctly by Doppler sonography. Four complete occlusions and 2 stenoses of the proximal ICA were missed by the qualitative brain scanning, but the 4 obstructions of the MCA were clearly visualized. The 15 cases with negative Doppler and negative brain scanning results revealed no significant vascular obstruction in the carotid angiograms.

Postoperative Evaluation by Doppler Sonography

In 64 cases having EC–IC bypass surgery the assessment of functioning (62 cases) or non-

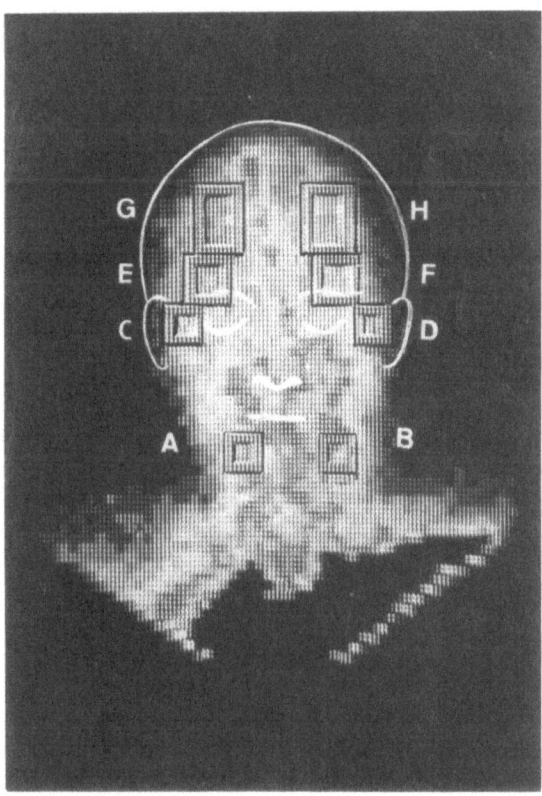

Fig. 15-3. Dynamic brain scan image on the video screen with superimposed drawing of facial outline. Four ROI have been designated bilaterally: a representative area of the cervical carotid artery (A, B), the STA (C, D), the MCA (E, F), and the cerebral hemisphere (G, H).

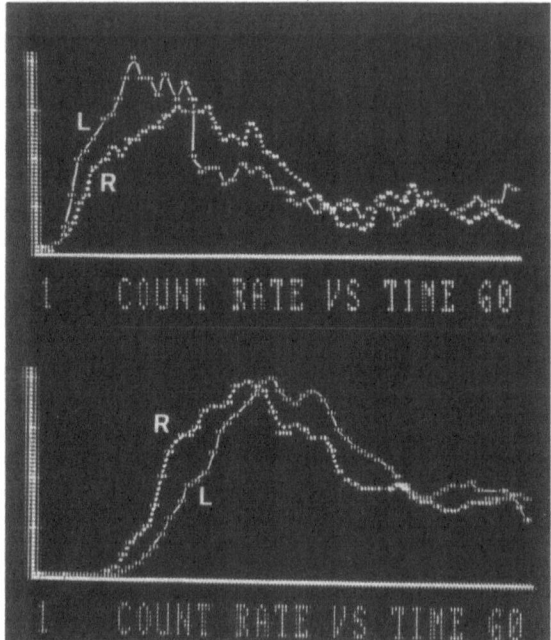

Fig. 15-4. Computer-generated flow curves (count rate vs time) of the L and R MCA–ROI in a case of R ICA occlusion as seen on the video screen. Preoperative (above): maximum activity on the R side is decreased and flow is slower. Postoperative (below): maximum activity is equal on L and R side, flow is faster on R side. On the color video screen L is red and R is yellow. For better black and white visualization the dots forming the curves have been connected by additional lines (L) and dots (R).

functioning (2 cases) was correct in accordance with angiography. In all cases of patent anastomosis, the diastolic flow was definitely increased in the STA of the operated side compared to the other side and to the preoperative findings. Good flow signals of the STA were present up to the site of craniotomy. In only 12 cases was it possible to find a change of the flow direction in the ophthalmic artery despite good intracerebral filling of the MCA by the anastomosis.

Postoperative Evaluation by Dynamic Brain Scanning with Numerical Computer Analysis

In 6 of the 10 patients with angiographically proven patency of the anastomosis who underwent a second an a third brain scanning after surgery, it was possible to demonstrate an improvement of cerebral blood perfusion either by increase of maximum activity or faster circulation. In 4 of these cases the ratios of L:R MCA or hemisphere perfusion approximated 1:1. In 2 cases a slight inversion of the ratios was seen; this means that the perfusion rate of the operated side was superior to that of the unoperated side. In 4 cases the results were indeterminate because of an incorrect bolus injection in 2 cases and unexplained perfusion changes of the nonoperated side in the other 2 cases.

The results of the flow patterns over the ROI of the STA and carotid artery were inconsistent. In 3 cases flow was increased, in 4 there was no change, and in 3 cases flow was actually decreased.

Discussion

The fact that only 57% of the randomly admitted patients with signs and symptoms of cerebral ischemia had significant vascular obstruction proves the importance of noninvasive screening methods. For this purpose the ultrasonic Doppler method appears to be valuable. A positive result in the standard procedure gives a clear indication for carotid angiography. In addition, direct measurements at the site of an anastomosis proved able to demonstrate patency of the EC–IC bypasses. However, the method was not capable of revealing the degree of intracranial filling by an anastomosis. Despite complete filling of the entire MCA territory by a patent anastomosis and no angiographic visualization of the ophthalmic artery, even in 2 cases with improved vision, Doppler sonography still showed unchanged results in the standard examination used to diagnose carotid artery obstructions. A further important point is that the reliability of the method depends on the experience of the person performing this test. In an active cerebrovascular center one full-time person with experience in angiology and neurology should have responsibility for the procedure.

In addition to the Doppler method, qualitative dynamic brain scanning proved valuable. MCA obstructions would be missed by using

Doppler sonography alone as a screening procedure. In the 4 cases with MCA obstruction, dynamic brain scanning was able to detect these lesions accurately. On the other hand, in 4 complete occlusions and 2 stenoses of the ICA, brain scans demonstrated symmetrical extra- and intracranial flow patterns. The failure to visualize an intracranial flow difference in these cases can be explained by adequate collateral circulation. It may be that in the future this point should be considered more carefully in establishing surgical indications. As a diagnostic procedure dynamic scanning is more accurate for detecting MCA than ICA obstructions.

The two screening procedures together were capable of excluding significant vascular lesions in 15 consecutive cases controlled by angiography. We therefore feel that carotid angiography may be withheld in patients with negative results in both tests, especially in patients with increased risk for any reason.

The ability to investigate the effect of an EC–IC anastomosis on cerebral blood flow by a noninvasive method such as quantitative radionuclide brain scanning seems to be promising and was successful in 6 of 10 cases. In a recent publication[1] intracerebral steal phenomena were successfully demonstrated by this method in a case of carotid cavernous fistula. Difficulties arise in cases with similar perfusion rates of both hemispheres in the preoperative examination. In 3 such cases this may be the reason for the failure to demonstrate only a minor increase of blood flow 2 weeks after surgery. A further problem is found in the bolus injection of the dye, which has to be the same in the pre- and postoperative study. We tried to overcome this variable by measuring the integral and the angle of the ascending portion of the curve. This was successful in 2 cases. The parameters of the ROI must be as equal as possible for each procedure, a requirement which necessitates considerable experience. The variable of flow measurement over the STA and cervical carotid artery is probably due to incorrect location of the ROI. The perfusion changes of the unoperated side in 2 cases would have needed further angiographic evaluation for explanation; this was not done because of the uneventful postoperative course in these patients.

This report concerning postoperative evaluation of STA–MCA bypasses by brain scanning has to be considered as preliminary. Our aim is to call attention to this method because it can be performed safely and the equipment required for these studies is already widely used in most departments of nuclear medicine.

Conclusion

In patients suffering from cerebral ischemia with a normal carotid artery Doppler test and a normal dynamic brain scan, it is rare to find a major obstruction of a vessel needing operation. Direct Doppler measurement over the STA of an EC–IC anastomosis is an accurate method to prove a patent bypass and may replace follow-up angiography. Quantitative dynamic brain scanning can be used to prove increased intracranial blood flow in cases with functioning bypass, but more experience and further results are needed to establish its definite value.

References

1. Barnes, B.D., Rosenblum, M.L., Pitts, L.H., et al. Carotid-cavernous fistula. Demonstration of asymptomatic vascular "steal." J Neurosurg 49:49–55, 1978.
2. Chater, N.L., Weinstein, Ph., Spetzler, R. Microvascular bypass for cerebral ischemia—an overview 1966–1976. In Microsurgery for Stroke, P. Schmiedek, editor, Springer-Verlag, New York, 1977, pp. 79–90.
3. Gratzl, O., Schmiedek, P., Spetzler, R., et al. Clinical experience with extra–intracranial arterial anastomosis in 65 cases. J Neurosurg 44: 313–324, 1976.
4. Keller, H.M., Meier, W.E., Yonekawa, Y., Kumpe, D.A. Noninvasive angiograph for the diagnosis of carotid artery disease using Doppler ultrasound (carotid artery Doppler). Stroke 7:354–363, 1976.
5. Keller, H.M., Meier, W.E., Zumstein, B. Nichtinvasive Doppler-Ultraschall Abklärung cerebrovasculärer Patienten: Carotis- und Vertebralis-Doppler-Untersuchung. In Ultraschall-Doppler-Diagnostik in der Angiologie, A. Kriessmann and A. Bollinger, editors, Thieme, Stuttgart, 1978.
6. Messert, B., Tyson, I.B., Barron, S.A. Limita-

94 B. Zumstein, et al.

tions of radionuclide flow studies in bilateral carotid thrombosis. Stroke 6:67–71, 1975.

7. Moses, D.C., Natarajan, T.K., Previosi, T.J., et al. Quantitative cerebral circulation studies with sodium pertechnetate. J Nucl Med 14:142–148, 1973.

8. Peerless, S.J., Chater, N.L., Ferguson, G.F. Multiple-vessel occlusions in cerebrovascular disease—a further follow up of the effects of microvascular bypass on the quality of life and the incidence of stroke. In Microsurgery for Stroke, P. Schmiedek, editor, Springer-Verlag, New York, 1977, pp. 251–259.

9. Reichmann, O.H., Anderson, R.E., Roberts, T.S., et al. Treatment of intracranial occlusive cerebrovascular disease by STA–cortical MCA anastomosis. In Microneurosurgery, H. Handa, editor, Igaku Shoin, Tokyo, 1975, pp. 31–46.

10. Schmiedeck, P., Gratzl, O. Selection of patients for extra–intracranial bypass surgery based on rCBF measurement. J Neurosurg 44:303–312, 1976.

11. Taveras, J.M., Wood, E.H. Cerebral angiography, morbidity and complications. In Diagnostic Neuroradiology, Section 1, Part III, Vol. 2. The Williams and Wilkins Company, Baltimore, 1976, pp. 567–575.

12. Von Reutern, G.M., Buedingen, H.J., Hennerici, M., Freund, H.J. The diagnosis of stenoses and occlusions of the carotid arteries by means of directional Doppler sonography. Arch Psychiatr Nervenkr 222:191–198, 1976.

13. Wagner, H.N., Jr. Nuclear tracer studies of the cerebral circulation. Hosp Pract 7:94–101, 1975.

14. Witherspoon, L.R., Preissig, R.S., Mahaley, M.S., et al. Characterization of malignant gliomas and cerebrovascular disease by cerebral dynamic studies. Stroke 6:199–205, 1975.

15. Wylie, E.J., Ehrenfeld, W.K. In Extracranial Occlusive Cerebrovascular Disease. Diagnosis and Management. W.B. Saunders Co., Philadelphia, 1970, p. 231.

16. Yasargil, M.G., Yonekawa, Y. Results of microsurgical extra–intracranial arterial bypass in the treatment of cerebral ischemia. Neurosurgery 1:22–24, 1977.

17. Yonekawa, Y., Yasargil, M.G. Extra–intracranial anastomosis. Clinical and technical aspects. Results. In Advances and Technical Standards in Neurosurgery, Vol. 3, H. Krayenbühl, editor, Springer-Verlag, New York, 1976, pp. 47–78.

18. Zumstein, B., Probst, Ch. Microneurosurgical contribution to cerebral ischemic apoplexy treatment (Ger, Engl. Abstr.). Schweiz Rundschau Med (Praxis) 66:781–786, 1977.

19. Zumstein, B., Yonekawa, Y., Yasargil, MG. Extra–intracranial arterial anastomosis for cerebral ischemia. Technique and results. In International Conference on Atherosclerosis, R. Paoletti, editor, Raven Press, New York, 1978, pp. 257–263.

16

Noninvasive Evaluation of Superficial Temporal to Middle Cerebral Artery Anastomosis

Andrew C. Hayes, William H. Baker, and O. Howard Reichman

Noninvasive assessment of the patient with carotid occlusive disease has reached a degree of accuracy greater than 90%.[1, 2, 5] Noninvasive techniques include bruit analysis by carotid phonoangiography, comparison of timed ocular pulse volume changes by oculoplethysmography, and assessment of collateral flow patterns using a Doppler flowmeter. These tests are used not only to diagnose carotid lesions in patients with carotid bruits or complaints of cerebrovascular disease but also to assess the postoperative status of carotid endarterectomy.

Extracranial–intracranial bypass is an established method of restoring flow to the cerebral hemisphere in patients with an occluded internal carotid artery or other intracranial stenosis. Whereas subjectively these patients have had excellent postoperative clinical courses, to date objective assessment is dependent upon contrast angiography with its attendant risks and expense. We wondered whether our noninvasive laboratory tests would be affected by a successful intracranial bypass, and thus this report details our experience with noninvasive testing in 15 patients who have undergone 16 superficial temporal to middle cerebral artery anastomoses.

Noninvasive Testing

A battery of noninvasive tests, the Doppler ultrasound cerebrovascular evaluation, carotid phonoangiography, and oculoplethysmography, was done in each patient.

The Doppler cerebrovascular examination[2] demonstrates functioning collaterals to the ophthalmic artery. Normally blood courses up the internal carotid artery, out the ophthalmic artery and its branches, the supraorbital and frontal arteries, to supply the scalp over the eye. In patients with severe proximal internal carotid artery stenosis, blood courses via branches of the external carotid artery, retrograde through the frontal and ophthalmic arteries to supply the distal internal carotid artery. The Doppler cerebrovascular examination is designed to detect this collateral flow pattern.

With the patient in the supine position, a directional Doppler pencil probe is placed over the supraorbital or frontal artery. Flow is noted to be either out of the eye or reversed in toward the orbit. While the flow is continuously monitored, digital compression of the superficial temporal artery in front of the ear, the infraorbital artery under the eye, and the facial artery as it crosses the mandible is performed sequentially. Normally the flow will not be diminished by these compressive maneuvers, although it may be increased. Digital compression of the common carotid artery low in the neck is next performed to prove dependence on the ipsilateral common carotid artery. Therefore, this should diminish flow in the ipsilateral frontal artery.

If pressure over any of the branches of the external carotid artery reduces audible flow, the examination demonstrates collateral flow. When compression over the common carotid artery does not diminish flow, collateral flow via the contralateral carotid or vertebral system exists. This may be distinguished by compression of contralateral external carotid branches and common carotid artery.

Bruit analysis by phonoangiography[5] is next performed. A hand-held microphone is placed over the high, mid, and low positions of the neck. The bruit is displayed on an oscilloscope and photographed on Polaroid film. A bruit which does not extend to the second heart sound is called a short bruit, and we have found that this has no significance.[1] A bruit which extends through the second heart sound is a long bruit and represents at least a 50% steno-sis. In patients who have a total or near-total occlusion, no bruit may be heard, as is the case with minimal bifurcation lesions.

Oculoplethysmography[5] examines the timed ocular pulse volume changes. After the cornea is anesthetized, fluid-filled eye cups are placed on each eye and light sensing clips on each ear. Tracings are obtained from the above sources and compared. A mechanically produced differential tracing comparing the orbit volume changes is simultaneously generated. Normally the ocular volume changes synchronously right and left, as does the ear pulse. Therefore, the differential line is flat. In our experience, a slight differential shift is present with a 50 to 75% stenosis. A visible delay in the beginning of an eye pulse compared to the other eye pulse or an ear trace is diagnostic of stenosis greater than 75%.

Table 16-1. Patient summary

Patient #	Preop angio	Preop lab	Operations	Postop lab	Postop angio
1	Rt ICA occ	R > 75%	Rt STA–MCA	Rt > 75%	—
2	Rt ICA occ	R > 75%	Rt STA–MCA	Rt > 75%	Patent anastomosis
3	Rt ICA occ	R > 75%	Rt STA–MCA	Rt > 75%	—
4	Lt ICA occ	L > 75%	Lt STA–MCA	Lt > 75%	—
5	Lt ICA occ	L > 75%	Lt STA–MCA	Lt > 75%	—
6	Lt ICA occ	L > 75%	Lt STA–MCA	Lt > 75%	Patent anastomosis
7	Lt CCA occ	L > 75%	1) Lt CCA–TEA	Lt > 75%	
	Lt ICA occ		2) Lt STA–MCA	Lt > 75%	Patent anastomosis
8	Lt ICA occ	Bilat > 75%	1) Lt STA–MCA	Bilat > 75%	Patent anastomosis, lt
	Rt ICA FMD		2) Rt ICA dilatation	Bilat > 75%	(No postdilatation angio)
9	Rt ICA occ				
	Lt siphon stenosis	Normal	Rt STA–MCA	Normal	—
10	Lt MCA stenosis	Normal	Lt STA–MCA	Normal	Patent anastomosis
11	Lt ICA occ	—	Lt STA–MCA	Lt > 75%	—
12	Lt ICA occ	—	Lt STA–MCA	Lt > 75%	Patent anastomosis
13*	Lt ICA occ	—	1) Lt STA–MCA	Normal	—
	Rt ICA	—	2) Rt carotid TEA	Normal	
14	Rt MCA stenosis	—	Rt STA–MCA	Normal	Patent anastomosis
15	Rt siphon stenosis	—	1) Lt STA–MCA	Bilat > 75%	Patent anastomosis, lt
	Lt siphon stenosis	—	2) Rt ECA–TEA		(No postrt STA– MCA angio)
			3) Rt STA–MCA		

STA–MCA = Superficial temporal artery to middle cerebral artery bypass.
ICA = Internal carotid artery.
CCA = Common carotid artery.
ECA = External carotid artery.
Occ = Occlusion.
TEA = Thromboendarterectomy.
FMD = Fibromuscular hyperplasia.
*See text: patient had normal results post STA–MCA bypass both before and after the contralateral carotid TEA.

Clinical Study

Fifteen patients who had 16 superficial temporal to middle cerebral artery (STA–MCA) bypasses were examined (Table 16-1). Two patients had middle cerebral artery stenoses, 12 had total internal carotid artery occlusion, and one bilaterally had stenoses of the internal carotid artery at the siphon. In addition to STA–MCA bypass, one patient had an ipsilateral common carotid endarterectomy reestablishing flow into the external carotid artery, one had an ipsilateral external carotid endarterectomy, one had a contralateral dilatation of fibromuscular dysplasia of the internal carotid artery, and one had a contralateral carotid bifurcation endarterectomy. Ten patients were studied using the described noninvasive tests both pre- and postoperatively but five patients were examined only postoperatively.

Results

Nine patients with total occlusion were examined preoperatively. In eight the lesion was correctly demonstrated. The one lesion not demonstrated by any test (false negative) was contralateral to a severe carotid siphon stenosis. The tenth patient had a middle cerebral artery stenosis with a normal carotid system and had normal noninvasive testing. Postoperative testing was unchanged in each of the ten patients.

Five patients were examined only after the operation. One patient with a middle cerebral artery stenosis had normal noninvasive testing. One patient with bilateral carotid siphon stenoses and bilateral STA–MCA bypass was abnormal on each side. Two patients with total occlusion had abnormal tests after extracranial–intracranial bypass. One patient with an internal carotid occlusion had normal testing (false negative) that did not change with superficial temporal artery compression. In addition, this patient had a contralateral stenosis at the origin of the internal carotid artery that tested normal. Repeated testing after the contralateral carotid endarterectomy remained unchanged.

Follow-up contrast angiography was obtained in eight of the fifteen patients with patency of the anastomoses demonstrated in all patients studied (Fig. 16-1). Although not all of the patients had postoperative angiography demonstrating patency, all patients so tested did indeed have patent anastomoses and in our total STA–MCA bypass experience the overall angiographic patency is 100%.

Discussion

It is somewhat disappointing but not totally surprising that conventional noninvasive tests do not revert to normal after STA–MCA bypass operations. First, there would be no expected change in carotid phonoangiography. This test evaluates only bruit analysis, and in patients with intracranial stenosis or total occlusion bruit analysis in the neck is unfruitful. Postoperatively one should expect no change.

The OPG detects disparate timed volume changes of the orbit. Kartchner et al.,[5] using an electromagnetic flowmeter, found that a visible eye pulse delay correlated with a greater than 40% reduction in internal carotid artery flow. If flow via a normal internal carotid artery is approximately 250 ml/min, the oculo-

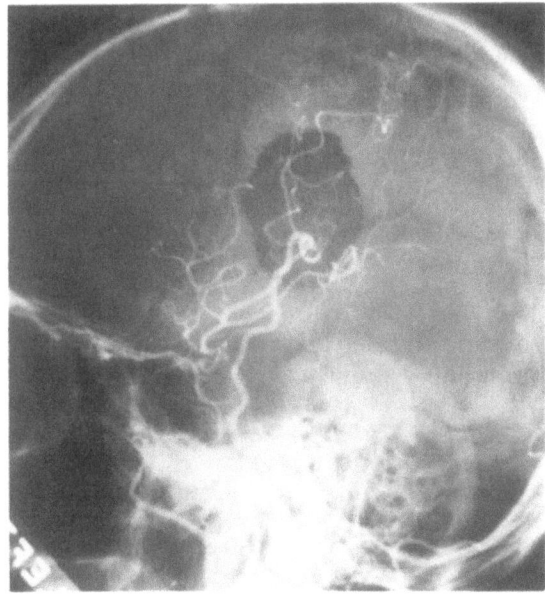

Fig. 16-1. Postoperative arteriogram of patient 15 demonstrating patency of extracranial–intracranial anastomoses on the left side.

plethysmograph should detect a change when blood flow is reduced to approximately 150 ml/min.

Obviously blood flow via the STA–MCA bypass must not be sufficiently increased to cause equalization of the timed ocular volumes. Blood flow through an STA–MCA bypass has been estimated using timed angiography.[6] Although the values varied, the average flow of 86 ml/min was well below Kartchner's 150 ml/min. Furthermore, this flow does not go directly into the internal carotid artery but is routed distally into the middle cerebral artery. Whereas the quantity of flow is enough that patients with MCA symptoms improve clinically, it does not change the oculoplethysmograph back to normal.

The Doppler cerebrovascular examination detects collateral flow patterns via the supraorbital artery. The increased blood flow via the STA–MCA bypass is not enough to alter these patterns.

The oculoplethysmograph used in our laboratory does not measure pressures as does the Gee-OPG. Gee[4] and Carney[3] have each reported an increase in the ipsilateral ophthalmic artery pressure measured by a Gee-OPG. Furthermore, these pressures decreased with digital compression of the superficial temporal artery, further demonstrating that the anastomosis was patent. Additional experience with this mode of testing will be necessary to document postoperative technical success routinely and to determine whether it is sensitive enough to detect stenosis of the bypass.

Summary

Noninvasive cerebrovascular testing was performed in 15 patients who underwent 16 STA–MCA bypasses. Carotid phonoangiography, oculoplethysmography, and Doppler cerebrovascular examinations were performed. Nine of ten patients examined preoperatively were properly diagnosed but these tests did not change after a successful bypass graft. Whereas the amount of blood flow delivered by a successful STA–MCA bypass is sufficient for clinical improvement, it is not sufficient to change noninvasive cerebrovascular testing results.

References

1. Baker, W.H., Hayes, A.C. Non Invasive Laboratory Evaluation, the Loyola Experience, in Diagnosis and Treatment of Carotid Artery Disease, W.H. Baker, editor, Futura Publishing Co., Mt. Kisco, N.Y., 1979, pp. 82–89.
2. Barnes, R.W., Russell, H.E., Wilson, M. Doppler Ultrasonic Evaluation of Cerebrovascular Disease, University of Iowa Press, Iowa City, 1975.
3. Carney, A.L. Ocular plethysmography and suction ophthalmodynammometry in the diagnosis of carotid occlusive diseases. In Microvascular Anastomoses for Cerebral Ischemia, J.M. Fein and O.H. Reichman, editors, Springer-Verlag, New York, 1978.
4. Chater, N.L., Weinstein, P.R., Gee, W. Augmentation of collateral hemispheric blood pressure following superficial temporal to middle cerebral artery anastomosis: Documentation by ocular plethysmography. In Microvascular Anastomoses for Cerebral Ischemia, J.M. Fein and O.H. Reichman, editors, Springer-Verlag, New York, 1978.
5. Kartchner, M.M., McRae, L.P., Morrison, F.D. Noninvasive detection and evaluation of carotid occlusive disease. Arch Surg 16:528, 1973.
6. Reichman, O.H. Estimation of flow through STA bypass grafts. In Microvascular Anastomoses for Cerebral Ischemia, J.M. Fein and O.H. Reichman, editors, Springer-Verlag, New York, 1978.

17

Intraoperative Hemodynamic Study by Doppler Ultrasonic Flowmeter in the Extracranial–Intracranial Arterial Bypass

Hajime Handa, Kouzo Moritake, Izumi Nagata, Yasuhiro Yonekawa, Atsushi Okumura, and Isao Matsuda

With recent advances in technology of Doppler flowmeters, it is now possible to detect the direction of blood flow and visualize the flow patterns in vessels in spectrographic display.[3, 4, 7, 8] In the present study, the flow patterns were analyzed intraoperatively in the donor and recipient arteries just before and just after the extracranial–intracranial bypass in 9 cases.

The flowmeter used in this study is a Model EUD-4 ultrasonic Doppler flowmeter made by the Hitachi Medical Corporation (Fig. 17-1). This apparatus consists of 6 different parts: (1) a Doppler flowmeter in the narrow sense, (2) a frequency analyzer of Doppler sound, (3) an electric integrator which computes the relative blood flow volume and the relative mean blood flow velocity from the Doppler sound spectrogram, (4) an analog computer which integrates the relative blood flow volume and the relative mean flow velocity per one cardiac cycle, (5) a monitoring television, and (6) an ultraviolet line-scan recorder.

The technique is fundamentally based on the Doppler shift principle, whereby the sound scattered by moving corpuscles is shifted in frequency from the incident sound waves by an amount proportional to the blood flow velocity.

A standard transducer used for transcutaneous measurement and a microtransducer for intraoperative use are shown in Fig. 17-2. These transducers are placed on the skin or the vessel through the medium of ultrasonic sol or saline

with an incident angle of 60°, and the transmitted frequency is 5 MHz.

The transcutaneously recorded pattern, which is the sound spectrogram of the flow

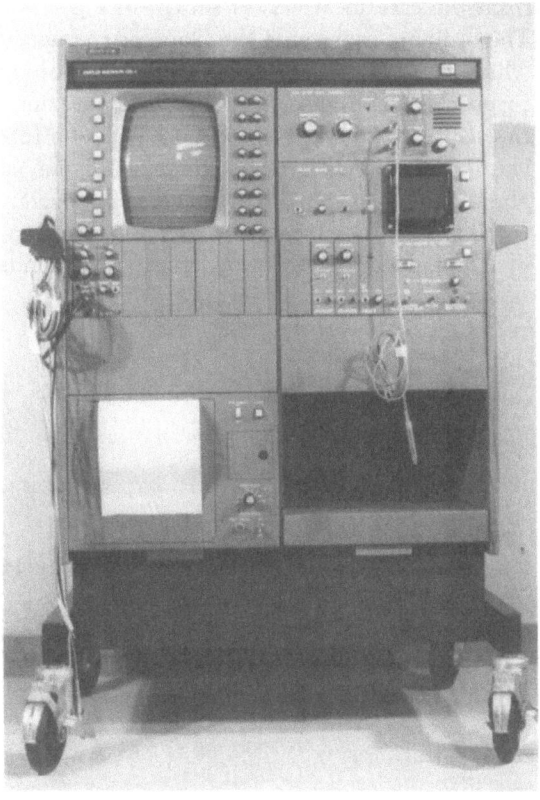

Fig. 17-1. Model EUD-4 ultrasonic Doppler flowmeter made by the Hitachi Medical Corporation.

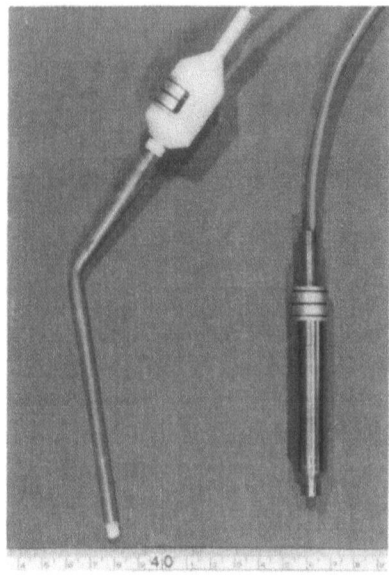

Fig. 17-2. A standard transducer used for transcutaneous measurement and a microtransducer for intraoperative use.

signal (hereafter called the flow pattern) taken from the carotid artery, is shown in Fig. 17-3. The ordinate represents the Doppler frequency which is proportional to the velocity of blood corpuscles. The abscissa represents the time; the scale on page is 1 cm per 0.1 sec. The forward flow, which is normograde, is displayed above the baseline, while the reverse flow below the baseline. The frequency of 1 kHz of Doppler sound shown on each figure corresponds

to the corpuscular speed of about 30 cm/sec on the assumption of incident angle of 60°. The darkness of the pattern correlates with the output voltage, which is proportional to the square root of the number of blood corpuscles per unit volume of the blood. The relative blood flow volume, relative mean flow velocity, and their integrated values per one cardiac cycle are displayed together with the sonagram and electrocardiogram.

Case Presentation

Nine patients, 6 males and 3 females with an age range of 27 to 58 years, examined during the operation are listed in Table 17-1. Middle cerebral artery stenosis accompanied by ipsilateral intracranial internal carotid artery occlusion is found in one case (case 1), intracranial internal carotid artery stenosis in one case (case 2), middle cerebral artery occlusion in 2 cases (cases 3 and 4) one of which (case 3) had also contralateral middle cerebral artery stenosis, internal carotid artery occlusion at its origin in two cases (cases 5 and 6) one of which (case 6) was accompanied by contralateral internal carotid artery stenosis, cerebrovascular "moyamoya" disease in two cases (cases 7 and 8), and a giant aneurysm of the intracavernous portion of the internal carotid artery in one case (case 9). In the case of giant aneurysm, STA–

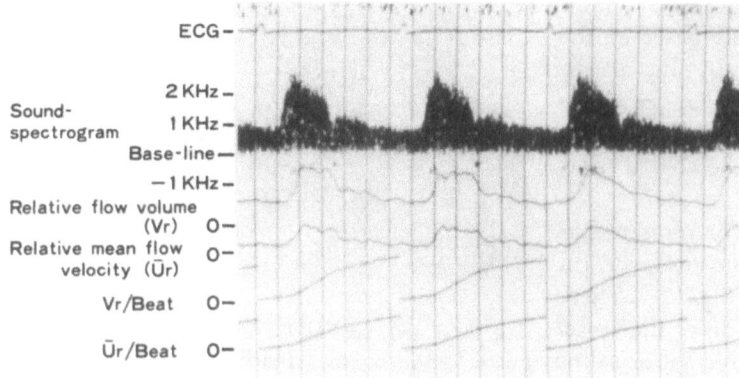

Fig. 17-3. Case 2.

Table 17-1. Results of nine cases measured intraoperatively

Case no.	Age (yr)	Sex	Clinical diagnosis	Angiographic diagnosis	CT finding	Op. side	Intraoperative Doppler study			
							MCA flow	Graft patency	Flow change after anastomosis	
									Distal	Proximal
1. T.S.	50	M	CS	Rt MCS Rt ICO	Low density	Rt	++	++	↑	↓
2. H.Z.	53	M	CS	Lt ICS	Low density	Lt	++	++	↑	Reversed
3. W.M.	58	M	CS	Lt MCS Rt MCO	Atrophy	Lt	+	++	↑	↓
4. W.S.	51	M	PRIND	Rt MCO	WNL	Rt	+	++	↑	Reversed
5. T.T.	53	M	CS	Rt ICO	Low density	Rt	+	++	↑	↓
6. K.T.	44	M	PRIND	Lt ICO Rt ICS	WNL	Lt	++	++	↑	Reversed
7. F.M.	27	F	PRIND	Moyamoya Bil ICO	Low density	Lt	+	−	−	−
8. A.M.	34	F	CS	Moyamoya Lt ICO Rt ICS	Low density	Lt	+	−	↓	↓
9. T.T.	27	F		Giant aneurysm of internal carotid artery	WNL	Lt	++	++	↑	↓

Bil = bilateral.
CS = completed stroke.
ICO = internal carotid artery occlusion.
ICS = internal carotid artery stenosis.
Lt = left.
MCO = middle cerebral artery occlusion.
MCS = middle cerebral artery stenosis.
PRIND = persistent reversible ischemic neurologic deficit.
Rt = right.
WNL = within normal limits.

MCA anastomosis was indicated not for the preexisting ischemic state but for the prevention of cerebral ischemia following the therapeutic carotid ligation. The remaining 8 cases had been suffering from cerebral ischemic attacks and in 6 cases some neurologic deficits remained at the operation.

Method and Results

After a small craniectomy, unilateral anastomosis was performed between a branch of the superficial temporal artery and a cortical branch of the middle cerebral artery.

During the operation direct flow measurement of the donor and recipient arteries of the anastomosis was performed just before and just after the anastomotic procedure. Flow of the cortical branch of the middle cerebral artery was normograde in all cases. In cases with MCA occlusion or bilateral internal carotid occlusion, the flow of a cortical branch of the middle cerebral artery was small, while in cases with only stenotic lesion or well-developed collateral circulation from the contralateral circulation, the flow was large. These findings on

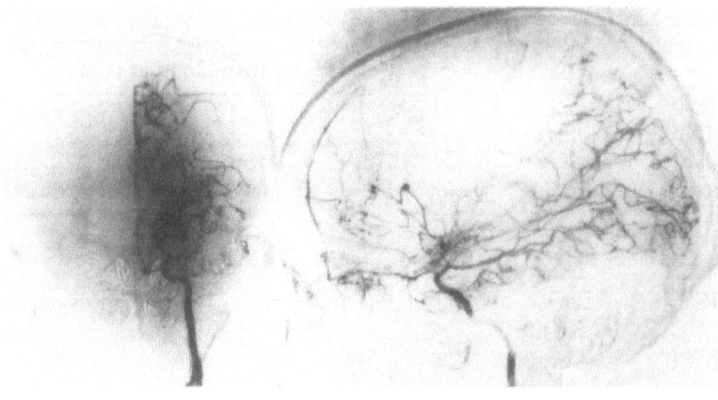

Fig. 17-4. Angiograms of case 7.

the volume and direction of the cortical flow of the middle cerebral arteries correlated with the findings of preoperative angiography in all cases.

After the anastomotic procedure, the bypass flow was examined by direct Doppler measurement. In two cases with so-called moyamoya disease, for one of which angiography is shown in Fig. 17-4, the flow-through bypass was not detectable. However, in all other cases, the graft patency was excellent. The flow in a cortical branch of the middle cerebral artery distal to the anastomosis increased when the clip on the donor artery was removed, and decreased when the clip was reapplied. The flow in the branch of the middle cerebral artery proximal to the anastomosis decreased in five cases and reversed in two cases.

Fig. 17-5 shows the angiogram of case 4 with Rt MCO. Fig. 17-6 shows the results of intraoperative measurement in this case. The flow of the middle cerebral artery distal to the anastomosis increased just after the clip was released from the donor superficial temporal artery. The flow in the branch proximal to the anastomosis reversed from normograde to retrograde, but when the clip was applied its flow again became normograde. Fig. 17-7 shows the result of a transcutaneous flow measurement of the superficial temporal artery ten months after the operation. Good function of the STA–MCA anastomosis was estimated.

Fig. 17-8 shows the angiogram of case 1 with Rt MCS and Rt ICO. Fig. 17-9 shows the results of intraoperative measurement in this case. The flow in the branch proximal to the

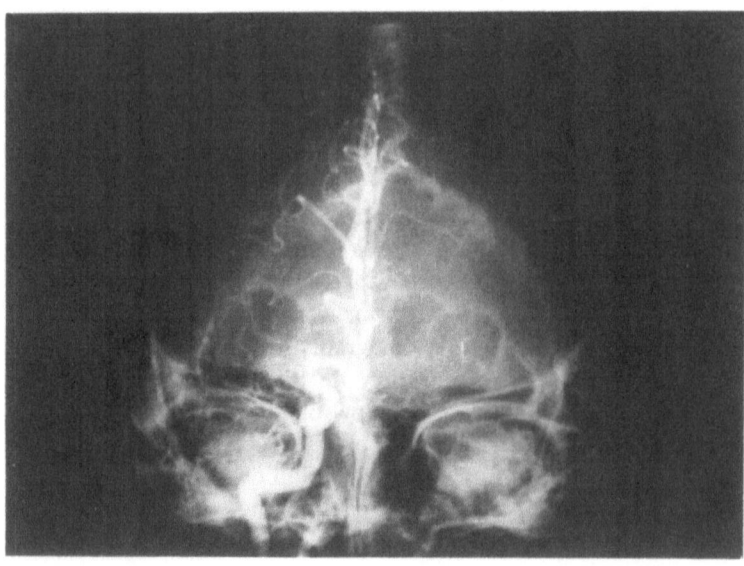

Fig. 17-5. Angiogram of case 4.

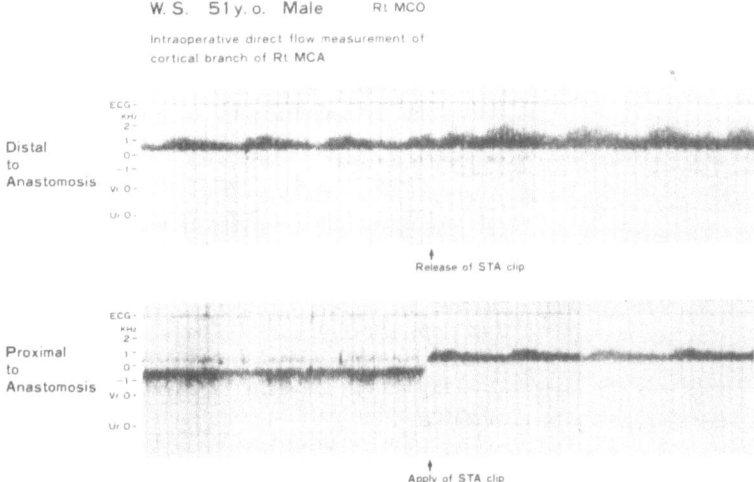

W. S. 51 y. o. Male   Rt MCO

Intraoperative direct flow measurement of
cortical branch of Rt MCA

Distal
to
Anastomosis

Release of STA clip

Proximal
to
Anastomosis

Apply of STA clip

Fig. 17-6. Case 4.

anastomosis decreased with release of the clip on the donor artery, but in the branch distal to the anastomosis the flow increased remarkably.

In cases with so-called moyamoya disease, the graft patency was questionable by the intraoperative direct flow measurement, but excellent graft patency was confirmed postoperatively by the Doppler flowmeter and angiography.

Discussion and Summary

Superficial temporal artery–middle cerebral artery (STA–MCA) anastomosis has been accepted as a relatively safe and effective proce-

dure for relieving cerebrovascular insufficiency and preventing the recurrence of cerebral ischemic attacks. For selection of appropriate candidates or evaluation of the effectiveness of bypass surgery, several methods have been widely used: 4-vessel angiography,[1, 2] rCBF study by ^{133}Xe intracarotid injection,[10] intraoperative pressure measurement,[9] Doppler ultrasonic flowmeter, and computed tomography. Among them, hemodynamic study by Doppler ultrasonic flowmeter is an excellent noninvasive method.

Our results demonstrate that useful information is obtained by Doppler flowmeter on the flow condition of the recipient artery before and after the anastomosis, except in cases with moyamoya disease, in which the results of

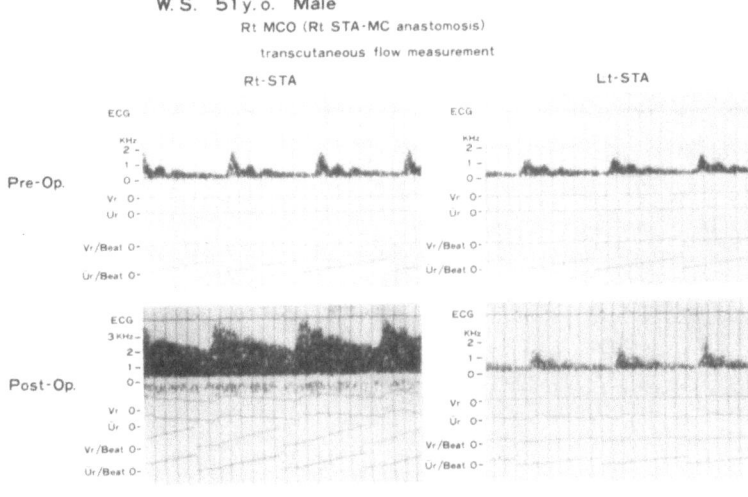

W. S. 51 y. o. Male
Rt MCO (Rt STA-MC anastomosis)
transcutaneous flow measurement

Rt-STA   Lt-STA

Pre-Op.

Post-Op.

Fig. 17-7. Effect of STA–MCA anastomosis. Postoperative measurement taken one week after anastomosis shows good function.

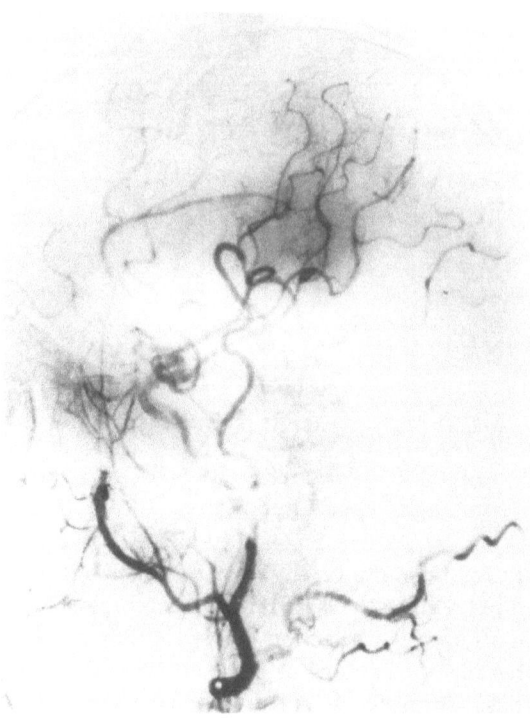

Fig. 17-8. Angiogram of case 1.

intraoperative direct measurement could not be decisive regarding graft patency after anastomosis. This is probably due to widespread narrow recipient arteries and also to arterial spasm of the donor in moyamoya disease.[5, 6]

References

1. Anderson, R.E., Reichman, O.H., Davis, D.O. Radiological evaluation of temporal artery—middle cerebral artery anastomosis. Radiology 113:73–79, 1974.
2. Ausman, J.I., Latchaw, R.E., Lee, M.C., Ramirez–Lassepas, M. Results of multiple angiographic studies on cerebral revascularization patients. In Microsurgery for Stroke, P. Schmiedek, editor, Springer-Verlag, New York, 1977, pp. 222–229.
3. Handa, H., Niimi, H., Moritake, K., Okumura, A., Matsuda, I., Hayashi, K. Analysis of sound spectrographic pattern for assessment of vascular occlusive disorders by continuous wave ultrasonic Doppler flowmeter. Arch Jpn Chirurg 46:214–225, 1977.
4. Hopman, H., Gratzl, O., Schmiedek, P., Schneider, I. Doppler-Sonographie bei mikrovaskulärem Bypass. Neurochirurgia 19:190–196, 1976.
5. Khodadad, G. Transient postoperative occlusion of the superficial temporal–middle cerebral artery branch anastomosis: spasm, swelling, or thrombosis. Surg Neurol 3:341–345, 1975.
6. Kikuchi, H., Karasawa, J. Extra–intracranial arterial anastomosis in ten patients with moyamoya syndrome (occlusion of the circle of Willis). In Microsurgery for Stroke, P. Schmiedek, editor, Springer-Verlag, New York, 1977, pp. 260–263.
7. Matsuo, H., Nimura, Y., Kitabatake, A., Hayashi, T. Analysis of flow patterns in blood vessels with the directional ultrasonic Doppler technique through a transcutaneous approach. Jpn Circ J 37:735–745, 1973.

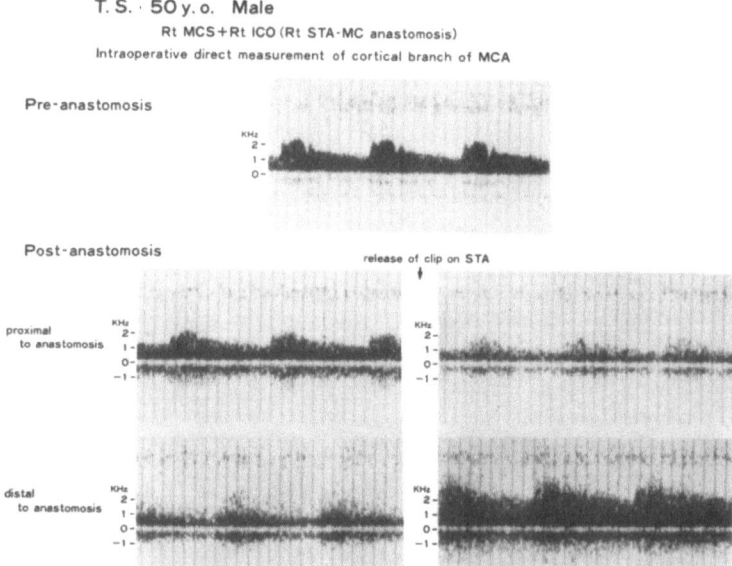

Fig. 17-9. Case 1.

8. Matjasko, M.J., Williams, J.P., Fontanilla, M. Intraoperative use of Doppler to detect successful obliteration of carotid-cavernous fistulas. Technical note. J Neurosurg 43:634–636, 1975.

9. Mizukami, M., Kin, H., Sakuta, Y., Nishijima, M., Araki, G. Cortical arterial pressure in occlusive cerebrovascular disease and results of bypass surgery. In Microsurgery for Stroke, P. Schmiedek, editor, Springer-Verlag, New York, 1977, pp. 233–239.

10. Schmiedek, P., Lanksch, W., Olteanu-Nerbe, V., Kazner, E., Gratzl, O., Marguth, F. Combined use of regional cerebral blood flow measurement and computerized tomography for the diagnosis of cerebral ischemia. In Microsurgery for Stroke, P. Schmiedek, editor, Springer-Verlag, New York, 1977, pp. 67–78.

18

Ocular Pneumoplethysmography in Carotid Occlusive Disease

William Gee, Ann L. Miller, Alice E. Madden, Harry W. Stephens, and Gary E. Whitehouse

The noninvasive assessment of arterial stenosis or occlusion has been the subject of intensive study over the past three decades. A broad review of this work has been assembled by Bernstein.[1] In this review, the role of pressure measurements in vascular disease has been extensively surveyed by Carter,[2] who states, "Studies in humans indicate that systolic pressure . . . is a far more sensitive index of the occlusive or stenotic process than a measurement of blood flow." Winsor[7] was one of the pioneers in the documentation of the significance of the systolic pressure index, relating central systolic pressure to the most distal systolic pressure in an extremity. We have applied this concept to the supreme extremity, the head. Unique to this extremity is a triad arterial supply (carotids, basilar) with triad communications in the circle of Willis (anterior and two posterior communicating arteries). However, two vessels, the ophthalmic arteries, are available for the accurate measurement of distal systolic pressures. The bilateral simultaneous measurements of these two systolic pressures with the ocular pneumoplethysmograph (OPG-Gee), and the correlation of these pressures with the brachial systolic pressure as determined by arm cuff and auscultation, are the subject of this report.

Reports by three independent groups of investigators[4-6] have documented an accuracy of 97% in detecting unilateral or bilateral pressure-significant (50% diameter, 75% cross-sectional area, or greater) carotid stenoses, with the OPG-Gee. A recent report[8] describes a modification of the basic instrument, which allows for the precise measurement of the ophthalmic systolic pressures up to a level of 140 mm Hg. It is uncommon (less than 1%) for a patient to have ophthalmic systolic pressures in excess of this figure. The actual test, which requires about 30 seconds, is simple to perform. The instrument is available commercially, and the details of its application and interpretation have been described.[3-6]

The modified OPG-Gee was used in the present study. In 171 patients who underwent carotid angiography for various reasons (brain tumor, intracranial aneurysms, transient ischemic attacks, etc.), OPG-Gee studies and brachial systolic pressures were obtained. In none of these patients was a significant carotid stenosis found on angiography. Figure 18-1 is a graphic representation of the data derived from the noninvasive testing. Each dot represents the equal ophthalmic systolic pressures of one patient. The three lines represent the mean and the two standard deviations (positive and negative) of this mean index of the ophthalmic systolic pressure as measured by the OPG-Gee, and the systemic (brachial) systolic pressure as determined by arm cuff and auscultation. Where Y represents the ophthalmic systolic pressure and X represents the systemic systolic pressure, the mean index is represented by the following formula:

$$Y = 53.74 + 0.4216\,X$$

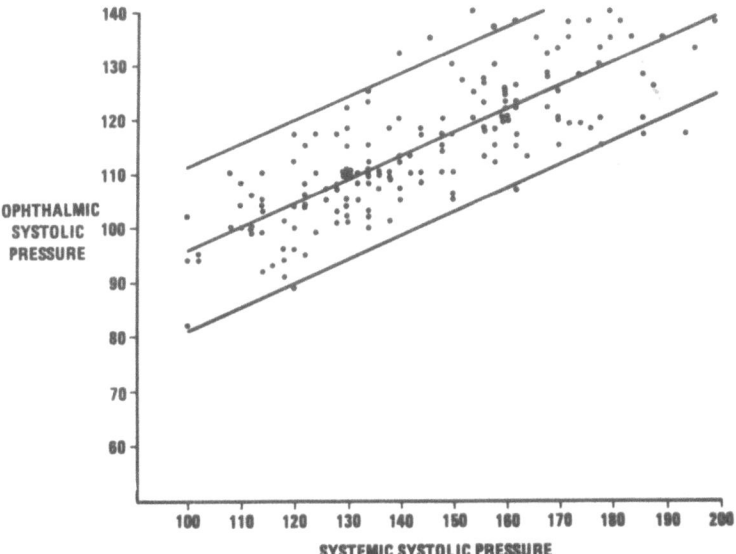

Fig. 18-1. Correlation of systemic (brachial) and ophthalmic systolic pressures in 171 patients.

One standard deviation (SD) equals 7.4. Theoretically, 97.5% of individuals without significant carotid stenosis should fall above the — 2SD line, represented by the following formula:

$$Y = 38.94 + 0.4216\,X$$

The graph indicates that 97.7% of the 171 patients fell above this line.

Previous reports emphasize that a difference in the respective ophthalmic systolic pressures of 5 mm Hg or more in a patient is diagnostic, with 97% accuracy, of a pressure-significant (75% cross-sectional area or greater) carotid stenosis on the side of the lower ophthalmic systolic pressure. However, if both ophthalmic systolic pressures, no matter what the difference between them, fall below the — 2SD line, bilateral pressure-significant carotid stenoses are strongly suspect. Figure 18-2 is a graph representing the data derived from 16 patients with bilateral internal carotid occlusions documented by angiography. Each pair of dots represents one patient. Note that 7 of the 16

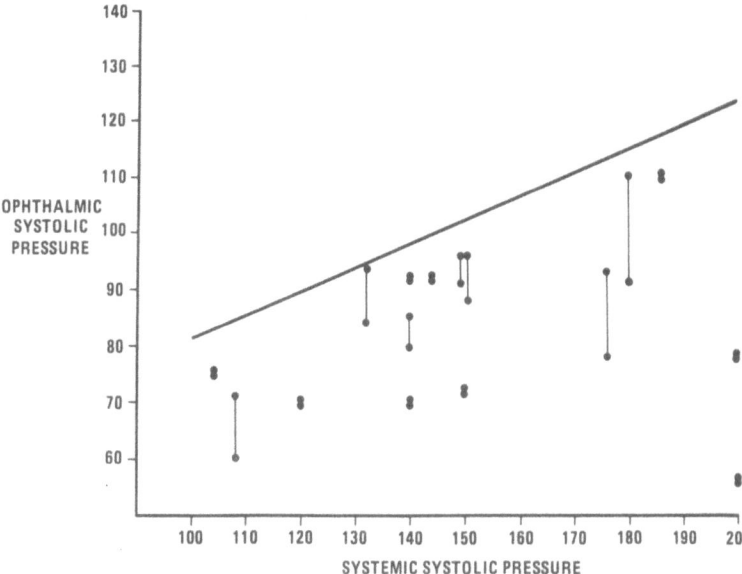

Fig. 18-2. Correlation of systemic (brachial) and ophthalmic systolic pressures in 16 patients with bilateral carotid occlusions.

patients had unequal ophthalmic systolic pressures, and the respective data in each of these patients is connected by a vertical line. These data indicate that at least 40% of such patients have significant variation in the respective collateral hemispheric blood pressures. An additional observation in these 16 patients is that the 2 patients represented by the two pairs of dots at a systemic systolic pressure of 200 mm Hg both died as an immediate result of the second carotid occlusion. It takes little imagination to exclude these 2 patients from the remaining 14 patients by an oblique line which closely parallels the — 2SD line on the graph. This latter, imaginary line would theoretically represent an OSP/SSP index below which would be found carotid occlusions that would progress to fatality.

In a previous report[8] a comparison was made between 17 patients who underwent carotid endarterectomy and 19 patients who underwent external carotid to internal carotid (EC–IC) shunts. The 17 patients who underwent endarterectomy all had angiographically documented unilateral internal carotid artery occlusions and contralateral pressure-significant internal carotid artery stenosis. A comparison of the preoperative and postoperative OPG-Gee studies of these 17 patients revealed that all improved on the side of the endarterectomy, and that 13 of the 17 (76%) improved on the side of the internal carotid occlusion. Of the

19 patients who underwent EC–IC shunt, the procedure was bilateral in 6, for a total 25 procedures. However, one of these procedures connected an occipital artery to a posterior cerebral artery. In this latter circumstance, the OPG-Gee is felt to have no validity. Of the 24 EC–IC shunts evaluated preoperatively and postoperatively by the OPG-Gee, 17 of the 24 (71%) demonstrated improvement. The improvement was unilateral in 4 of the 17 (25%). The improvement was definitely bilateral in 8 of the 17, and possibly bilateral in 5 of the 17 (75%). Figure 18-3 is a graph of the data from two of the EC–IC shunt patients. The patient data labeled *A* is on the left side of the graph. This patient underwent bilateral EC–IC shunts. Prior to the first procedure, at a systemic systolic pressure of 104 mm Hg the ophthalmic systolic pressures were equal, at a level of 5 mm Hg. After the second procedure, at a systemic systolic pressure of 130 mm Hg, the ophthalmic systolic pressures remained equal, at a level of 91 mm Hg. Clinically, the patient was much improved. However, the increase in the ophthalmic systolic pressures is probably principally the result of the increase in the systemic systolic pressure. It is our feeling that, at best, the shunts have only slightly improved the physiologic status of the patient, and may have contributed in no way to his clinical improvement. In contrast, the data labeled *B*, on the right side of the graph, is from a patient

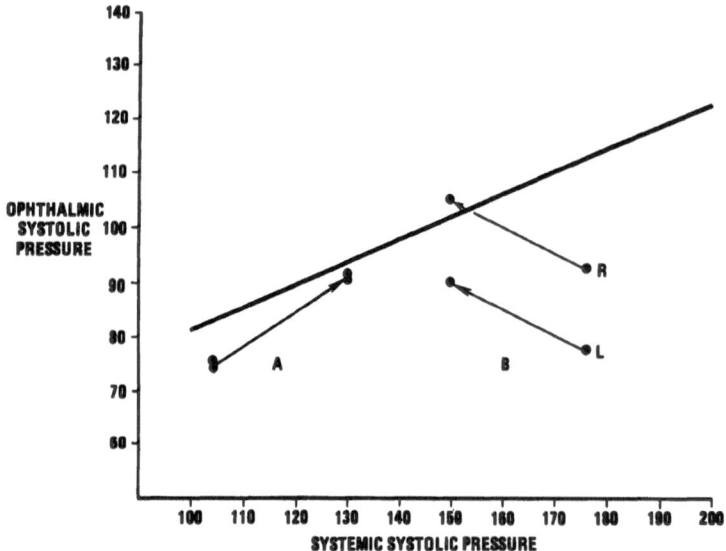

Fig. 18-3. Correlation of systemic (brachial) and ophthalmic systolic pressures in two patients (A on the left, B on the right), before and after the construction of EC–IC shunts. The respective arrows point from the preoperative to the postoperative data.

who underwent only one EC–IC shunt, on the right side. The patient became symptomatic only when his antihypertensive regimen resulted in orthostatic hypotension. Angiography confirmed bilateral internal carotid occlusions and a significant left external carotid stenosis. Preoperatively, at a systemic systolic pressure of 176 mm Hg, the right and left ophthalmic systolic pressures were 93 and 78 mm Hg, respectively. After his right EC–IC shunt, at a systemic systolic pressure of 150 mm Hg, the right and left ophthalmic systolic pressures were 105 and 90 mm Hg, respectively. Thus, in spite of a 26 mm Hg fall in the systemic systolic pressure, there has been an elevation of the ophthalmic systolic pressures of 12 mm Hg. Note that the postoperative right ophthalmic systolic pressure is within normal limits. The patient remained asymptomatic, although his antihypertensive regimen was continued.

The data presented in this report confirm the conclusion of many investigators that accurate measurement of central and distal systolic pressures, and a correlation of these measurements, is the most precise way to characterize significant arterial stenosis or occlusion. Serial determinations in the same patient, especially before and after operations to remove stenoses or to bypass occlusions, is particularly valuable in the objective assessment of operative results. The technique and instrumentation described provide the best method by which the physiology of significant carotid arterial stenoses or occlusions can be monitored.

References

1. Bernststein, E.F. (ed.) Noninvasive Diagnostic Techniques in Vascular Disease. C.V. Mosby, St. Louis, 1978.
2. Carter, S.A. Role of pressure measurements in vascular disease. In Bernstein, E.F. (ed.) Noninvasive Diagnostic Techniques in Vascular Disease. C.V. Mosby, St. Louis, 1978, pp. 261–287.
3. Gee, W., Miller, A.L., Madden, A.E., Stephens, H.W., Whitehouse, G.E. Ocular pneumoplethysmography in the evaluation of patients with brain ischemia. Submitted for publication.
4. McDonald, K.M., Gee, W., Kaupp, H.A. Screening for significant carotid stenosis by ocular pneumoplethysmography. Am J Surg 137:244–249, 1979.
5. McDonald, P.T., Rich, N.M., Collins, G.J., Anderson, C.A., Kozloff, L. Doppler cerebrovascular examination, oculoplethysmography, and ocular pneumoplethysmography. Use in detection of carotid disease: A prospective clinical study. Arch Surg 113:1341–1349, 1978.
6. Machleder, H.I., Barker, W.G. Noninvasive methods for evaluation of extracranial cerebrovascular disease. Arch Surg 112:944–946, 1977.
7. Winsor, T. Influence of arterial disease on the systolic blood pressure gradients of the extremity. Am J Med Sci 220:117–126, 1950.

19

Changes in Collateral Circulation and EEG Analysis Following Extra–Intracranial Anastomosis

K.-H. Holbach and H. Wassmann

Angiography and rCBF measurement by the various isotope clearance methods do not give information whether or to what extent changes in cerebral circulation are related to changes in neuronal functions. The latter, however, can be revealed by EEG and particularly by EEG analysis.

In patients with cerebral ischemia caused by occlusive vascular lesions we studied the changes in CBF and in EEG following EIAB surgery and in particular assessed the relationship between both parameters.

Methods

An extra–intracranial anastomosis operation was carried out in 80 patients to bypass an occlusion or severe stenosis in the internal carotid or middle cerebral artery. Angiographic, neurologic, and electroencephalographic follow-up examinations were performed in some patients up to 3½ years postoperatively. For the assessment of the electroencephalographic changes we used an EEG interval-amplitude-analysis system.[4] This system and the typical findings in normal persons have been described previously.[3] The system enabled us to obtain values for local electrical brain activity in the form of electrical power equivalent (EPE).

Results

A 54-year-old patient suffered from transient weakness in his left arm. Sometimes several of these episodes occurred during the day. Angiography revealed a right internal carotid occlusion and a well-developed frontal branch of the superficial temporal artery (STA), which was used for extra–intracranial arterial bypass (EIAB) surgery. Six days after operation angiography showed a patent anastomosis. The STA irrigated mainly the central sulcus arteries. There was also retrograde filling of the enlarged ophthalmic artery (Fig. 19-1A). Repeated angiography done up to two years postoperatively showed that the STA was filling not only the central sulcus artery but also newly developed small tortuous collateral vessels in the site of the craniotomy (encephalo-myosynangiosis described by Henschen[2]) (Fig. 19-1B). This convolution of vessels also received blood from an enlarged branch of the meningeal artery. Via these vessels mainly the STA filled also the parietal and the operculofrontal arteries. The diameter of the STA and of the cerebral arteries which were filled by the STA appeared to be enlarged while the diameter of the ophthalmic artery appeared to be reduced.

In relation to the preoperative EEG analyses,

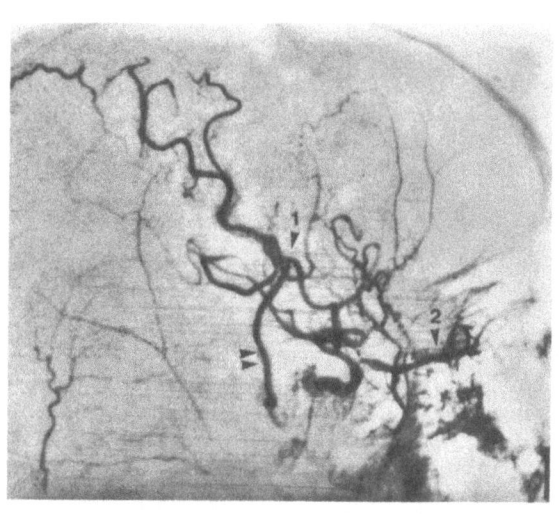 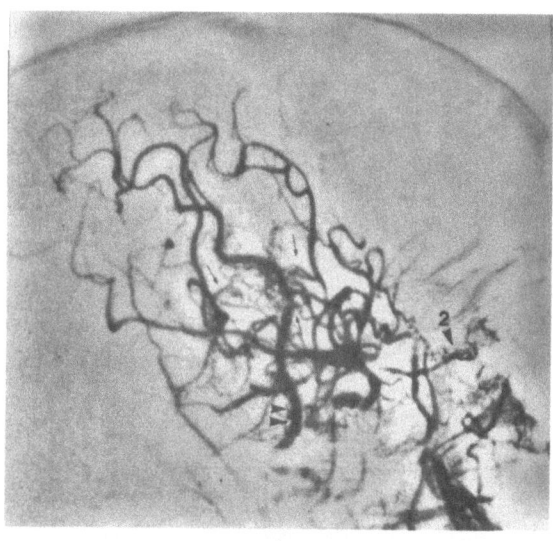

A   B

Fig. 19-1. Right carotid angiography done 6 days following surgery (A): ► = superficial temporal artery (STA), ▼¹ = anastomosis between STA and cortical branch of middle cerebral artery, ▼² = ophthalmic artery. Follow-up angiography 9 months later (B): = convolution of small tortuous collateral vessels.

the postoperative analyses showed an increase of alpha- and beta-wave activity over the affected hemisphere and over the contralateral side (Fig. 19-2). This improvement was found to be maintained at the last EEG analyses done two years following operation. At this time digital compression of the right STA was performed for 2 minutes. This resulted in a distinct temporary reduction of the alpha- and beta-wave activity over both sides. Since operation, the patient has not noted any signs of cerebral ischemia.

A 56-year-old patient suffered from a moderate left hemiparesis caused by an occlusion of the right internal carotid artery in the neck. The patient underwent right EIAB surgery

4½ months following the completed stroke. Eight days postoperatively angiography revealed a patent bypass. The STA irrigated the angular artery and the temporal arteries (Fig. 19-3). There was retrograde filling of the well-developed ophthalmic artery. Follow-up angiography done to date showed an enlargement of the STA and particularly of the cerebral arteries close to the shunt. During the follow-up the STA had taken over the filling of the total territory of the middle cerebral artery and the retrograde flow in the ophthalmic artery had ceased (Fig. 19-4).

In relation to the preoperative EEG alterations, there was considerable improvement of the electrical brain activity during the post-

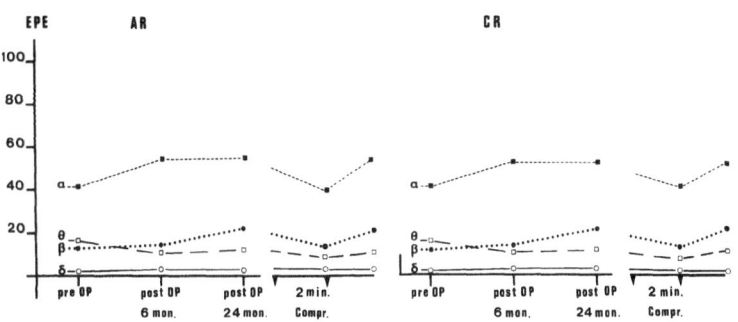

Fig. 19-2. Follow-up EEG analyses and effect of digital STA compression 2 years after EIAB surgery. (EPE = electrical power equivalent value, AR = affected region, CR = contralateral region.)

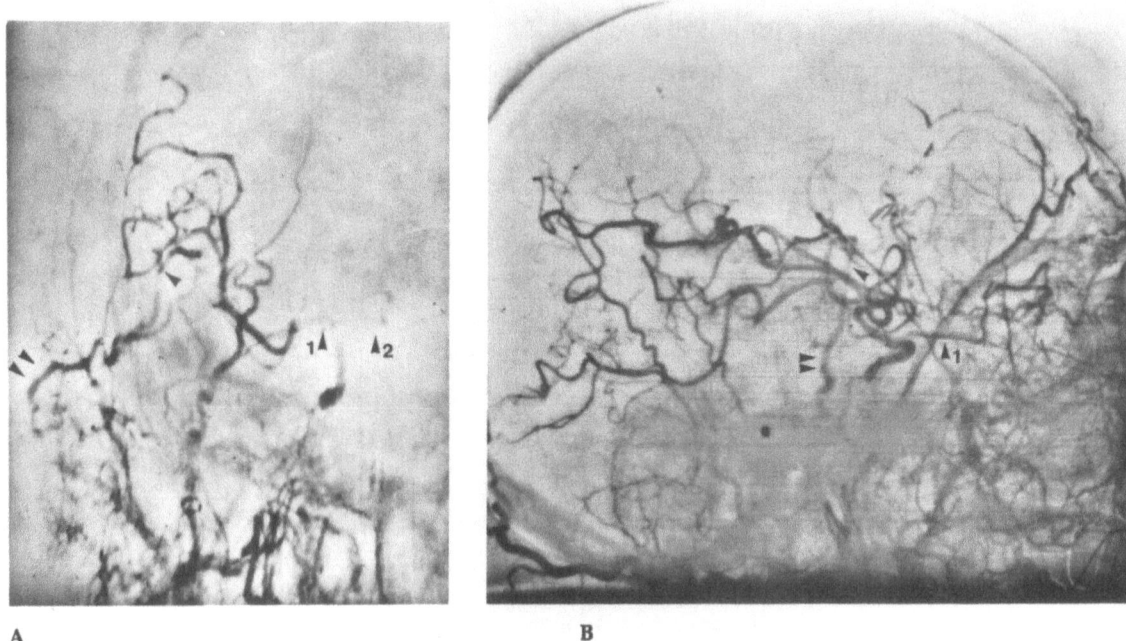

Fig. 19-3. Right carotid angiography done 8 days following surgery. ► = superficial temporal artery (STA), ► = anastomosis between STA and cortical branch of the middle cerebral artery. A: ▲₁ = middle cerebral artery, ▲₂ = anterior cerebral artery. B: ▲₁ = ophthalmic artery.

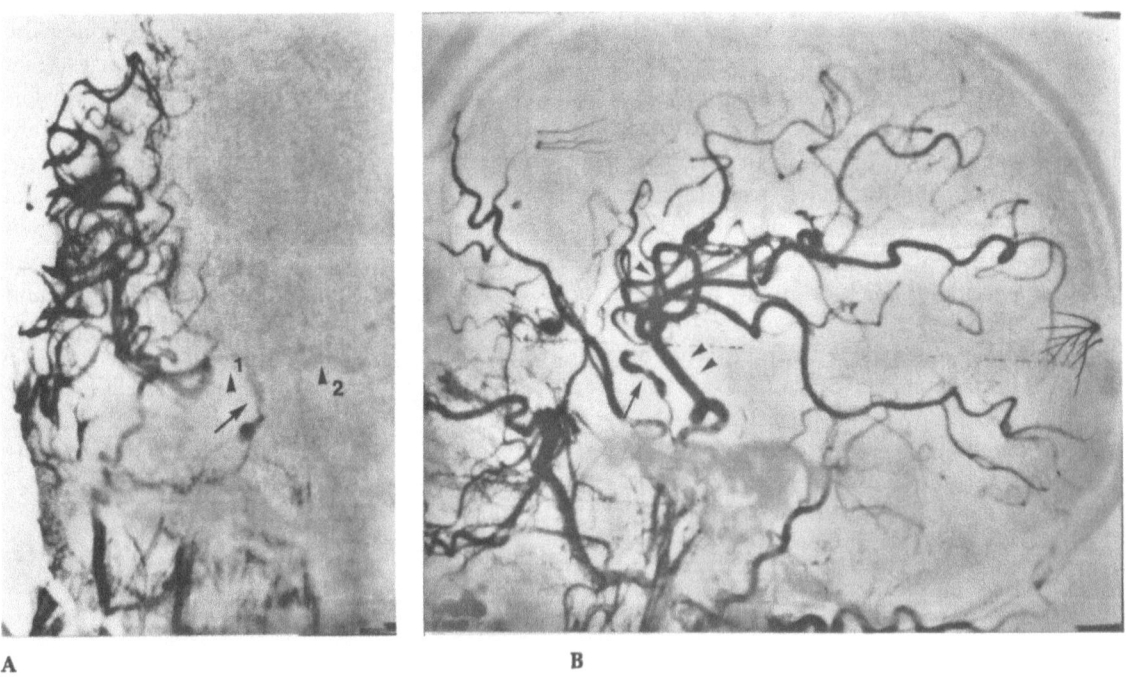

Fig. 19-4. Follow-up angiography done 18 months following surgery. A: Retrograde filling of middle cerebral artery = ▲₁, internal carotid artery = →, and right and left anterior cerebral arteries = ▲₂. B: ► = enlarged STA, ► = site of anastomosis, → = internal carotid artery.

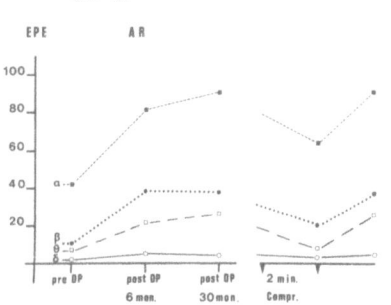
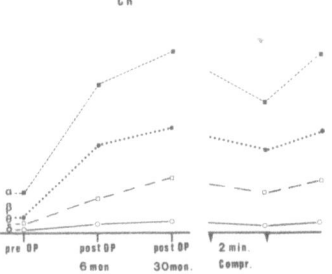

Fig. 19-5. Follow-up EEG analyses and effect of STA compression 30 months postoperatively. (EPE = electrical power equivalent, AR = affected region, CR = contralateral region.)

operative follow-up (Fig. 19-5). The last EEG analytical examinations were performed 2½ years postoperatively and the effect of digital STA compression on the EEG was tested. The interruption of cerebral blood supply from the STA resulted in a considerable bilateral reduction of the electrical brain activity. After compression the electrical brain activity immediately returned to its previous level.

Following EIAB surgery the neurologic deficit of this patient was almost completely reversed and has been maintained at the improved level for nearly 3 years.

A 56-year-old patient had considerable left hemiparesis caused by occlusion of the right middle cerebral artery. The anterior cerebral artery filled most of the middle cerebral territory via leptomeningeal collaterals (Fig. 19-6). Eight weeks following stroke EIAB surgery was carried out. Postoperative angiography re-

vealed a patent anastomosis. The STA filled the angular, the posterior temporal, the middle temporal, and the parietal opercular arteries. The branch of the angular artery that was retrogradely filled from the anterior cerebral artery before operation was anterogradely perfused from the STA after operation (Fig. 19-7).

The postoperative follow-up EEG analyses showed an improvement of the EEG. A reduction of the electrical brain activity occurred during the compression of the STA. Thereafter the electrical brain activity immediately returned to the previous level (Fig. 19-8).

Following surgery the left hemiparesis improved slightly. There was, however, some improvement of reduced mental function.

A 41-year-old patient was suffering from increasingly severe temporary speech disorders, right hemiparesis, various psychological alterations, and seizures. Angiography revealed a

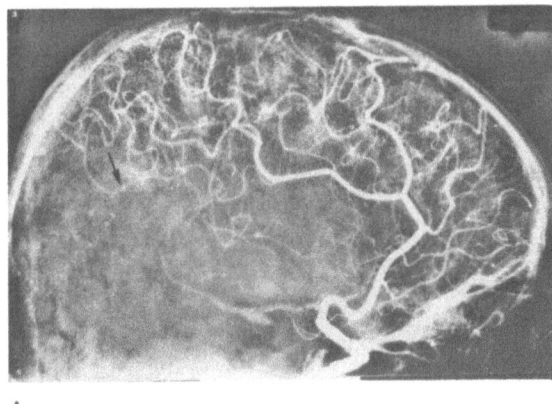
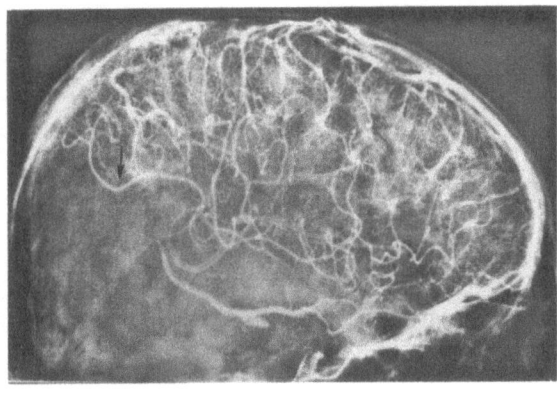

A

B

Fig. 19-6. Right carotid angiography revealing occlusion of middle cerebral artery and leptomeningeal anastomoses. → = retrograde filling of the angular artery.

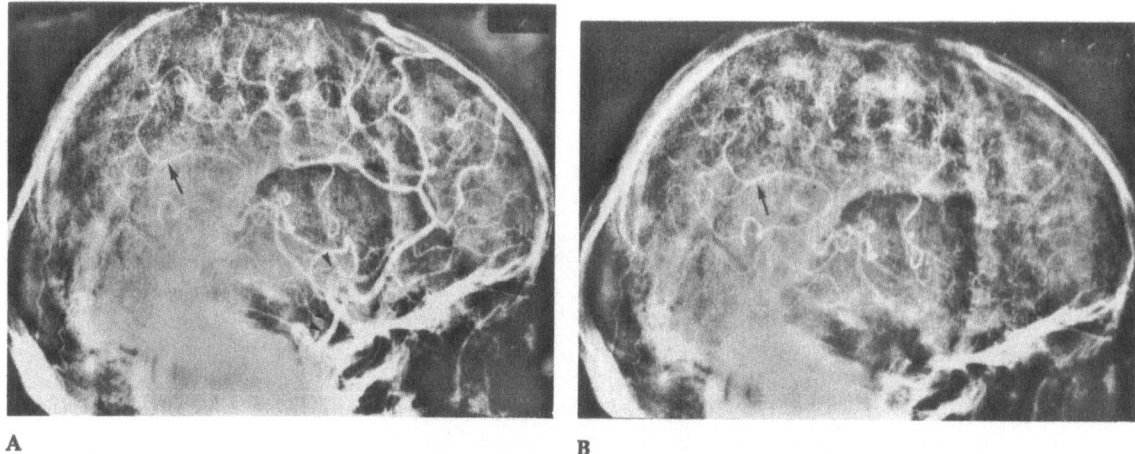

A   B

Fig. 19-7. Postoperative angiography. ▶ = STA, ▶ = anastomosis between STA and cortical branch of middle cerebral artery, → = anterograde filling of the angular artery.

severe stenosis of the right internal carotid artery and an occlusion of the middle cerebral artery. There was only partial filling of the anterior cerebral artery and of the anterior choroidal arteries. The latter perfused retrogradely the pericallosal artery via a rete of fine collateral vessels, causing the typical opacification found in moyamoya disease. The enlarged meningeal arteries filled via fine transdural collaterals to the angular artery. The vascular pathology on the left side was similar. There was also a severe stenosis of the left internal carotid artery. The anterior cerebral artery was occluded and from the nearly occluded middle cerebral artery only a temporal branch was poorly irrigated. The enlarged left meningeal arteries irrigated retrogradely, via fine transdural anastomoses, the anterior cerebral artery,

a part of the middle cerebral territory, and in particular the angular artery (Fig. 19-9).

Five days following EIAB surgery on the left side, angiography showed that the STA was filling nearly the complete territory of the middle cerebral artery, including those regions which were retrogradely perfused via a rete of fine transdural collaterals before surgery. Only the temporal branch of the middle cerebral artery was still filled by the internal carotid artery and a branch of the angular artery was still irrigated via the fine rete of transdural collaterals (Fig. 19-10).

At this time EEG analyses revealed a considerable bilateral increase of the electrical brain activity, particularly of alpha-wave activity (Fig. 19-11). This EEG improvement almost completely receded during the 2-min compres-

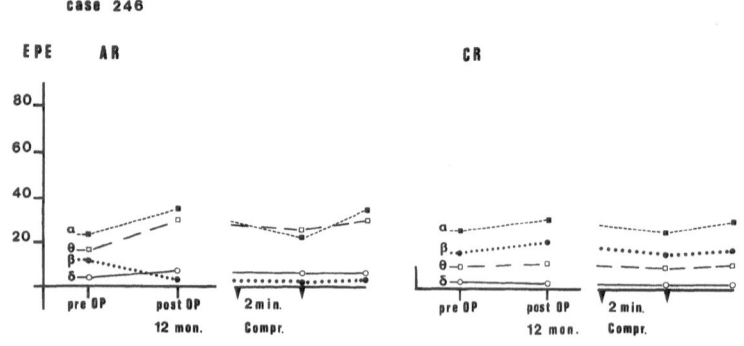

Fig. 19-8. Follow-up EEG analyses and effect of digital STA compression 1 year after surgery. (EPE = electrical power equivalent, AR = affected region, CR = contralateral region.)

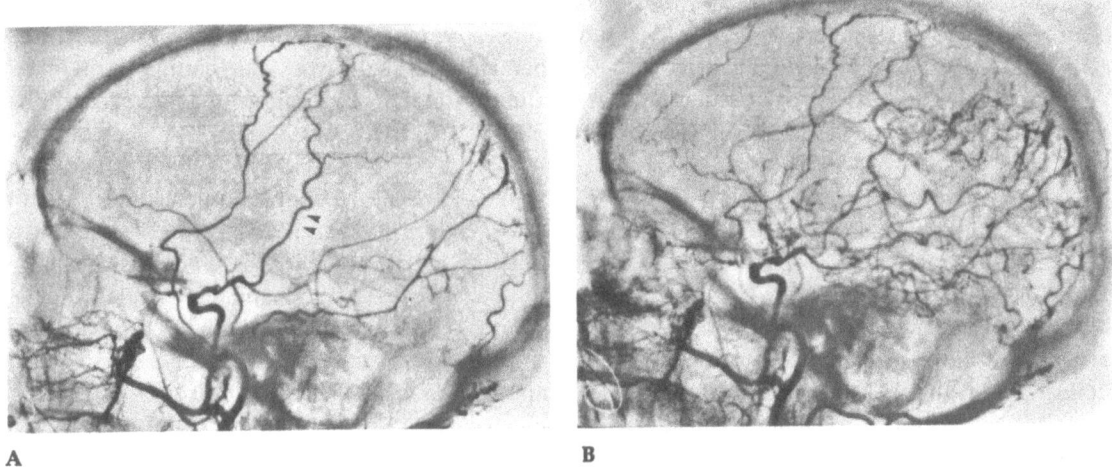

Fig. 19-9. Angiography of the left common carotid artery. ► = superficial temporal artery (STA).

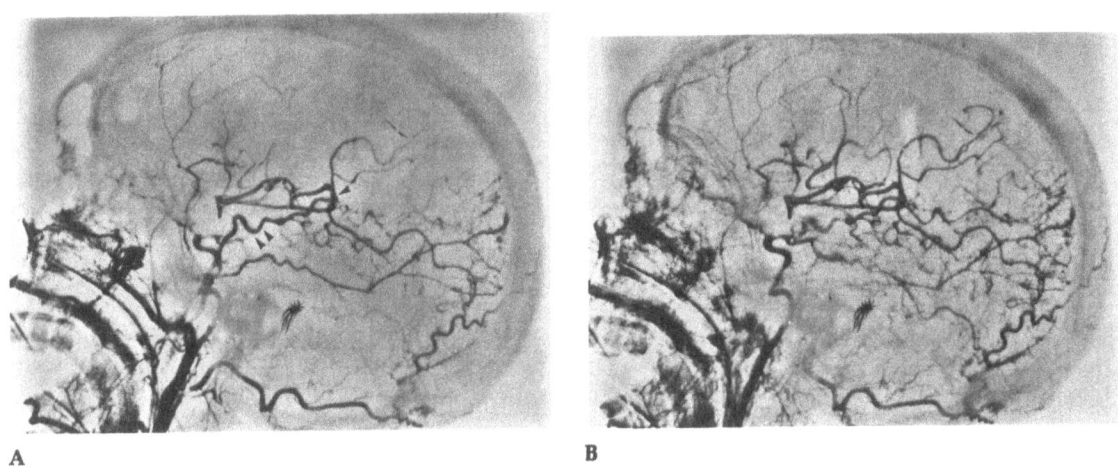

Fig. 19-10. Postoperative angiography. ► = STA, ► = site of anastomosis.

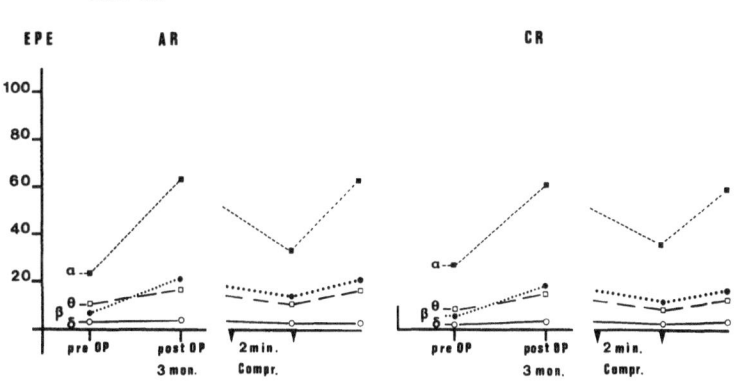

Fig. 19-11. Follow-up EEG analyses and effect of digital STA compression 3 months following surgery. (EPE = electrical power equivalent, AR = affected region, CR = contralateral region.)

sion of the STA. Immediately following digital compression of the STA the electrical brain activity returned to its previous level.

The patient has not experienced any postoperative signs of renewed cerebral ischemia.

Conclusions

On the basis of these results we may summarize as follows: The follow-up angiography indicated that the STA and the cerebral arteries close to the shunt can enlarge considerably, that new collateral vessels can develop in the site of the craniotomy—a phenomenon described as encephalomyosynangiosis—that the new collateral channel is able to take over a steadily increasing part of the cerebral circulation and also to irrigate territories of the brain that were previously well perfused by leptomeningeal or transdural collaterals or from the ophthalmic artery. In some cases this was associated with a reversal of the direction of blood flow in such collaterals.

The follow-up EEG analyses and those done during postoperative digital STA compression indicated that the blood supply from the new collateral channel was usually associated with an increase in electrical brain activity, and that the persistence of the level of EEG improvement was dependent on the cerebral blood supply from the STA. The postoperative bilateral increases in electrical brain activity, which were generally more pronounced over the affected hemisphere than over the contralateral side, allow for the assumption that not only the mainly affected operated side but also the contralateral hemisphere benefit from the blood supply. This is strongly supported by Austin et al.,[1] who found significant increases in mean rCBF on the side of the anastomosis and usually to a lesser extent on the contralateral side. Consequently, redistribution in the cerebral circulation or reversal of intracerebral steal appears to play an important role following EIAB surgery.

References

1. Austin, G., Haugen, G., Lichter, E., Hayward, W. Microneurosurgical anastomosis: A biochemical basis for improvement. Presented at 4th Conference on Occlusive Cerebrovascular Disease, Nagasaki, Japan, March 1977, in press.
2. Henschen, C. Operative Revascularisation des zirkulatorisch geschädigten Gehirns durch das Anlegen gestielter Muskellappen. (Encephalo-Myo-Synangiose). Langenbecks Arch Klin Chir 264:392–401, 1950.
3. Holbach, K.H., Wassmann, H., Hohelüchter, K.L. Reversibility of the chronic post-stroke state. Stroke 7:296–300, 1976.
4. Reetz, H. EEG-Analyse mit digitaler Intervall- und Amplituden-Klassierung. Z EEG-EMG 2: 32–36, 1971.

20

The Emergency STA–MCA Bypass Evaluated by the Induced-Functional EEG Analysis in Acute Ischemic Stroke

Zentaro Ito and Akifumi Suzuki

The extra–intracranial arterial bypass (EIAB) has been performed widely for ischemic stroke patients with transient ischemic attacks (TIA), reversible ischemic neurologic deficits (RIND), and complete strokes.

It has been generally accepted that the EIAB is not always beneficial for severe ischemic stroke in the acute stage, because revascularization can bring severe brain swelling and hemorrhagic infarction.

However, it has been often experienced that the development of cerebral infarctions can be brought on by gradual progress and extension of cerebral ischemia, but that early spontaneous recanalization brings good results under some conditions in cases with middle cerebral artery (MCA) occlusions.[5]

From these experiences, it is considered that emergency bypass surgery may prevent the development of cerebral infarction in acute ischemic stroke, and the results of the bypass would be closely correlated with the pathophysiologic conditions of ischemic brain damage in each case.

Ito[4] has already developed a new method to select suitable candidates for the bypass in the chronic stage, where functional reversibility of ischemic brains could be directly evaluated by changes of somatosensory evoked potentials (SEP) under induced hypertension.

The purpose of this paper is to describe whether or not the changes of percent power spectrum in EEGs and SEPs under induced hyper- or hypotension and administration of glycerol can determine the postreflowed functional reversibility in 15 cases with acute ischemic strokes.

Materials and Methods

We studied 8 surgically and 7 conservatively treated patients, ranging from 43 to 78 years, with a mean age of 63 years. All of these patients showed sudden onset with severe neurologic deficits and their symptoms progressively worsened.

In the surgically treated group, involving 4 cases with internal carotid and 4 middle cerebral artery trunk occlusions, STA–MCA double anastomoses with external decompressions were carried out within 3 days of onset. The conservatively treated group consists of 5 internal carotid and 2 middle cerebral artery occlusions.

Monopolar EEGs were recorded from the bilateral central areas on the data recorder and the percent power spectrums were computed and displayed during pre-, intra-, or postadministration of agents by the special-purpose computer. Recordings of SEP were made from somatosensory hand areas 7 cm lateral and 2 cm posterior to the vertex, by averaging 100 responses with computer techniques. Electrical stimuli were applied randomly through electrodes to the contralateral median nerves by 1-msec square pulses, and intensity was adjusted to produce a small twitch of the thumb.

Angiotensin was used for increase in range from 10 to 40 mm Hg in mean arterial blood pressure (ABP) and Regitine for decrease of the same value in ABP; 200 ml 10 w/v percent glycerol solutions were administrated intravenously for decrease of intracranial pressure.

In all cases, these EEG and SEP tests have been performed within 3 days of onset, preoperatively.

Results

The Percent Power Spectrums of EEGs in Surgically Treated Cases

The changes of the percent power spectrums of EEGs were studied in induced hyper- or hypotension and glycerol administration. In cases improved after bypass, the percent powers of α waves were increased by induced hypertension, but decreased or unchanged in both slightly improved and unchanged cases. However, by glycerol administration, the percent powers of α waves were augmented in each case with slight improvement and no change (Fig. 20-1A).

Fig. 20-1B shows the correlation between changing ratios of the percent power of α waves by blood pressure changes and surgical results.

In cases with improvement, the changing ratios of the percent power were related to changes of blood pressure. However, in only one case (case 2), the changing ratio of the percent power was decreased when the different values of blood pressure change were 40 mm Hg from 20 mm Hg. It is suggested that this phenomenon might be caused by the breakthrough phenomenon[6, 7] and/or the decrease of focal CBF corresponding to augmentation of intracranial pressure. In cases with slight improvement, no change, and worsening, the ratios of the percent power were almost unchanged.

SEPs in Surgically Treated Cases

The amplitude, the N ratio, and the D/N of early negative components of SEPs were analyzed in 8 surgically treated cases. N means a negative wave. N_1 ratio is obtained from dividing N_1 amplitude in blood pressure change by that in the resting state, and D/N_1 from dividing N_1 amplitude of the affected side by that of the nonaffected side.

Fig. 20-2A shows changes of amplitude of early negative components in SEPs under resting state, induced hypertension, and glycerol administration. In 3 improved cases in which EIABs were performed, amplitudes of 2 or 3 components were increased. By glycerol administration, N_1 amplitudes were increased but N_2 and N_3 amplitudes were decreased in two cases. In cases with slight improvement and no

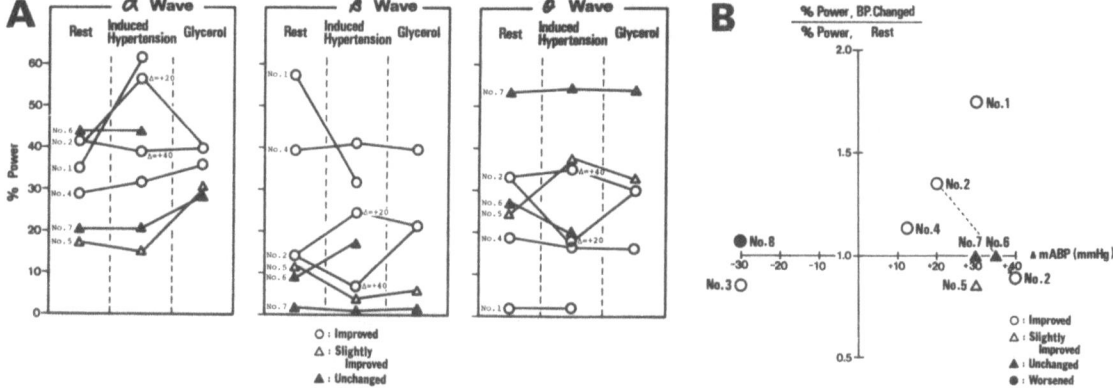

Fig. 20-1. A. Changes of percent power spectrum in induced hypertension and glycerol administration in surgically treated cases. B. Changing ratio of percent power in α wave by blood pressure change and surgical results.

change, no components of SEPs showed response and were not activated by drug administration.

Fig. 20-2B analyzes results of N_1 components in blood pressure changes. In 3 of 4 improved cases, N_1 amplitude, N_1 ratio, and D/N_1 were increased by augmenting blood pressure. In another case with no change of N_1 component by blood pressure change, only factors of N_2 and N_3 were activated. In case 2, the functional EEG and SEP tests were performed on the day after onset. In the resting state N_1 component of SEPs was not clear, but in induced hypertension and glycerol administration this component became clear. Furthermore, the change of value of blood pressure from 20 to 40 mm Hg brought decrease of N_1 amplitude and D/N_1. Thus it was estimated that this case could be improved from the hypofunction of ischemic brain by proper increase of blood supply and/or perfusion pressure.

Case Report

A 59-year-old man (case 2) was admitted to the hospital 7 hours after onset. Neurologic examinations showed right hemiparesis with drowsy consciousness on admission. Angiography revealed bilateral internal carotid artery occlusions with good collateral pathways through bilateral posterior cerebral arteries and posterior communicating arteries. The patient's condition progressively worsened to semicoma and severe hemiplegia 2 days after onset.

At this time, left-sided STA–MCA bypass with external decompression was carried out. After the bypass, moderate brain swelling and patchy low-density areas appeared in the left frontoparietal region on CT scan. However, until 14 days after onset, when right-sided STA–MCA bypass was carried out, the patient's condition remarkably improved. Hemiplegia improved to hemiparesis and consciousness changed from semicoma to alertness. At 34 days after onset, he was discharged with slight hemiparesis and aphasia.

Fig. 20-3 shows the preoperative percent power spectrums of EEGs and SEPs 2 days after onset of this case. The percent power of α wave, the N_1 amplitude, and other analyzed factors of N_1 components have been mostly activated by difference of +20 mm Hg in blood pressure and by glycerol administration.

Comparison of EEG Analysis and SEP Tests in Surgical and Nonsurgical Cases

The results of the drug-induced EEG and SEP tests were compared in surgical and nonsurgical cases (Fig. 20-4).

If the percent power of α wave and each factor of N_1 component are improved by hypertension or worsened by hypotension in cases with acute ischemic stroke, it is suggested that

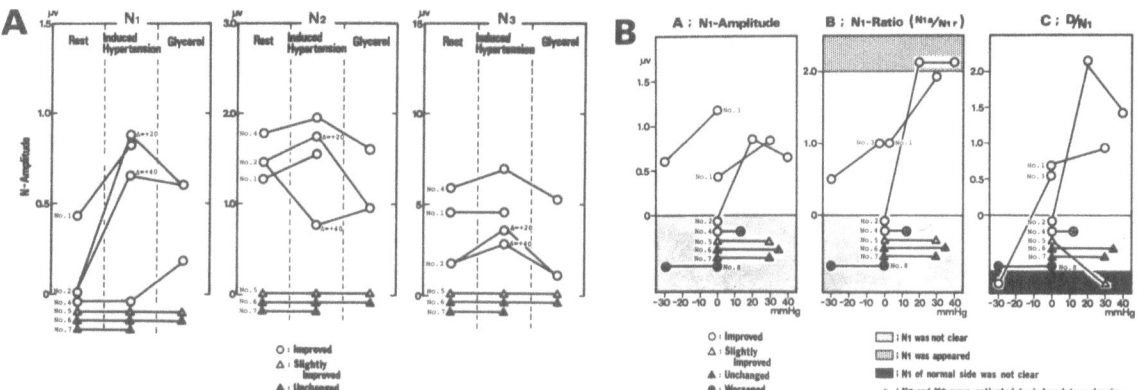

Fig. 20-2. A. Changes of amplitudes of negative early components in SEPs and surgical results. B. N_1 amplitude, N_1 ratio, and D/N_1 by blood pressure changes. N_1 ratio is obtained by dividing the N_1 amplitude in blood pressure change by that of the resting state, and D/N_1 by dividing N_1 amplitude of the affected side by that of the nonaffected side.

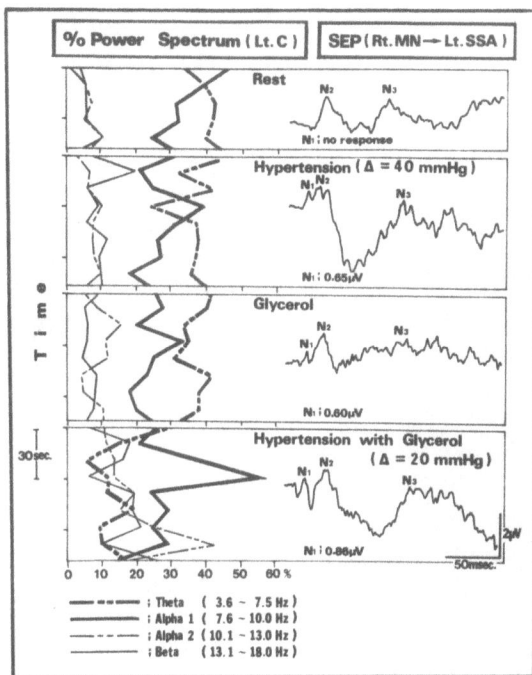

Fig. 20-3. Case 2, 59 years, male. Bilateral internal carotid artery occlusion. Preoperative EEG and SEP tests one day after onset.

ischemic brains preserve functional reversibility in increase of blood supply by reflow.

We call such cases the CBF-dependence group. In fact, 4 cases of the CBF-dependence group have been improved by the bypass surgery, but 2 nonsurgical cases of this group did not improve. The nonsurgical cases of the CBF-dependence group will be improved if increase of regional blood flow is obtained by bypass surgery.

If EEGs and SEPs are improved by glycerol administration or aggravated by induced hypertension, patients are classified to the intracranial-pressure (ICP)-dependence group.

In such cases, bypass surgery is not beneficial.

Discussion

There are many discussions about the indication of extra–intracranial arterial bypass (EIAB) but few reports about emergency EIAB for acute cerebral ischemia.

Gratzl et al.[3] performed EIAB on three pa-

tients with acute cerebral ischemia, and they reported that all patients died because of severe brain swelling in the early postoperative period.

However, Crowell et al.[1] reported beneficial effects of STA–MCA bypass for experimental acute ischemic stroke in 20 dogs, where STA–MCA bypasses were carried out about 2 hours after occlusion of the MCA root. After the bypass, the majority of animals were clinically and pathologically better than control dogs without the bypass, and hemorrhagic infarctions and damage to blood-brain barrier were more uncommon in the dogs in the surgical group than in the controls.

Furthermore, Crowell[2] described 8 of 12 cases with acute focal cerebral ischemia where neurologic improvements were obtained by EIAB in the acute stage.

From these reports, it is suggested that the EIAB is not always contraindicated for acute cerebral ischemia but could bring improvement to the function of ischemic-damaged brain if an appropriate candidate and a suitable operating time could be selected.

The principle of the drug-induced EEG and SEP test is based on utilizing the phenomenon that the increase of regional cerebral blood flow

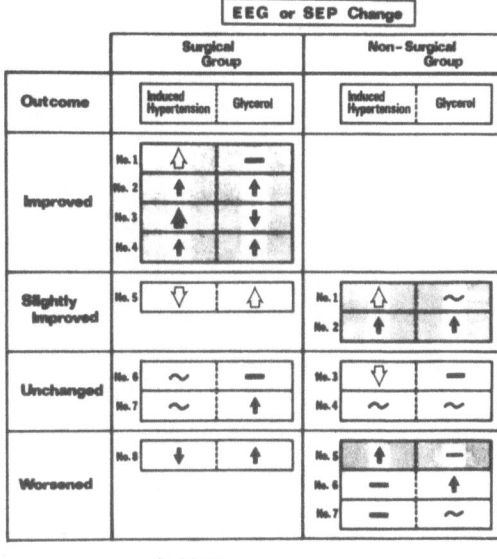

Fig. 20-4. EEG and/or SEP changes in surgical and nonsurgical groups and clinical outcome.

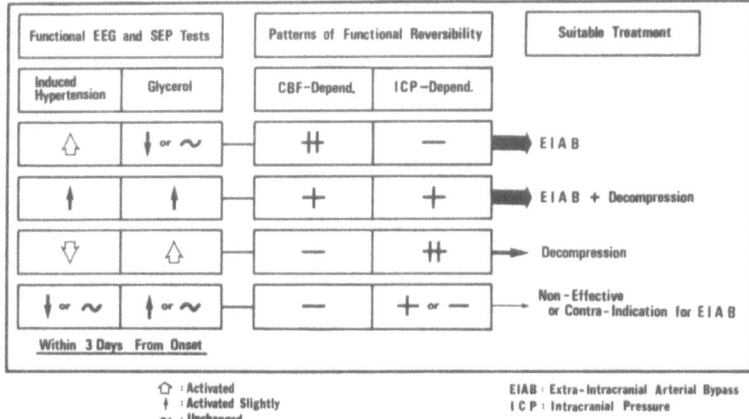

⚲ : Activated
↑ : Activated Slightly
~ : Unchanged
↓ : Worsened
⚳ : Worsened Slightly

EIAB : Extra-Intracranial Arterial Bypass
I C P : Intracranial Pressure

Fig. 20-5. Suitable treatment of acute progressive ischemic strokes based on the functional EEG and SEP tests.

on the areas of dysautoregulation could be obtained by induced hypertension. Dysautoregulations were revealed in most cases of cerebral ischemia until at least one month after onset.

Schmiedek et al.[8] studied regional cerebral blood flow (rCBF) to select suitable candidates for EIAB in 110 patients with ischemic brains. rCBF studies in their patients showed a relative regional hyperemia, paradoxical reactions of CO_2 reactivity, and focal or global loss of autoregulation within a few days after stroke. In our series, 7 conservatively treated cases with MCA occlusion had CBF examinations within 3 days of onset. In most cases, dysautoregulations were recognized in somatosensory cortexes corresponding to ischemic regions.

Accordingly, it is considered that changes of preoperative SEPs under hyper- or hypotension could estimate changes of the postreflowed function of ischemic areas even in the acute stage.

If the percent power of EEGs and the N_1 components of SEPs are activated by hypertension or worsened by hypotension, it means that the brain has the potential for functional reversibility of ischemic areas with increase of blood supply.

Such cases are classified in the CBF-dependence group.

In acute ischemic patients with progressive brain swelling, the increase of cerebral blood flow could cause increase of intracranial pressure (ICP), hemorrhagic infarctions due to high permeability of arterioles, and/or disturbances of brain function.

In such cases in this series, it was observed that EEGs and SEPs were improved by glycerol administration and worsened by induced hypertension. These cases fall in the ICP dependence group.

From the pathophysiologic aspects of the acute stage mentioned above, the suitable treatment for such cases with acute ischemic stroke could be determined.

The correlation between the patterns of functional reversibility of ischemic brain and the suitable treatment based on the drug-induced EEG and SEP tests is summarized in Fig. 20-5.

If the results of the functional EEG and SEP test show the pattern of CBF dependence, EIAB should be performed in the acute stage.

If the candidate has the components of the CBF- and ICP-dependence simultaneously, the suitable operative procedure would be EIAB plus external decompression.

In the acute ischemic stroke patient, where functional reversibility shows only the ICP-dependence pattern, external decompression would be the effective treatment.

In cases which the functional reversibility of ischemic brain is classified neither to patterns of CBF- nor ICP dependence, no treatment would be undertaken.

References

1. Crowell, R.M., Olsson, Y. Effect of extracranial–intracranial vascular bypass graft on experimental acute stroke in dogs. J Neurosurg 38:26, 1973.

2. Crowell, R.M. STA–MCA bypass for acute focal cerebral ischemia. In Microsurgery for Stroke, P. Schmiedek, editor, Springer-Verlag, New York, 1977, pp. 244–250.

3. Gratzl, O., Schmiedek, P., Spetzler, P., Steinhoff, H., Marguth, F. Clinical experience with extra–intracranial arterial anastomosis in 65 cases. J Neurosurg 44:313, 1976.

4. Ito, Z., Hen, R., Nakajima, K., Suzuki, A., Uemura, K. Selection of completed stroke patients for STA–MCA anastomosis based on measurements of somatosensory evoked potential and CBF dynamics. In Microsurgery for Stroke, P. Schmiedek, editor, Springer-Verlag, New York, 1977, pp. 177–184.

5. Ito, Z., Hen, R., Suzuki, A., Uemura, K. Prognostic factors in spontaneous recanalization of middle cerebral artery occlusion. In Fourth International Symposium on Microsurgical Anastomoses for Cerebral Ischemia, London, Canada, 1978.

6. Lassen, N.A., Agnoli, A. The upper limit of autoregulation of cerebral blood flow on the pathogenesis of hypertensive encephalopathy. Scand J Clin Lab Invest 30:113, 1973.

7. Johansson, B., Strandgaard, S., Lassen, N.A. On the pathogenesis of hypertensive encephalopathy. Cir Res (Suppl. 1) 34–35: 167, 1974.

8. Schmiedek, P., Gratzl, O., Spetzler, R., Steinhoff, H., Enzenbach, R., Brendel, W., Marguth, F. Selection of patients for extra–intracranial arterial bypass surgery based on rCBF measurements. J Neurosurg 44:303, 1976.

V

Radiology

21

Correlation of Noninvasive Doppler and Angiographic Evaluation of Extra–Intracranial Anastomoses

James I. Ausman and Fernando G. Diaz

One of the more difficult problems facing neurosurgeons involved in extracranial–intracranial anastomosis surgery is the evaluation of the function of the bypass after surgery. Angiography remains the most accurate and reliable method of determining patency of an intracranial filling by the bypass; however, this procedure cannot be used frequently to check the status of the bypass. What is needed is a noninvasive test which can be used immediately after surgery and at several intervals in the postoperative and follow-up periods and which is highly accurate in establishing the patency and function of the bypass.

This paper will compare the accuracy of the Doppler in evaluation of extracranial–intracranial bypasses in patients with the results of postoperative angiograms in each case. Our conclusion will be that the Doppler is a highly accurate qualitative test for evaluating the function of the bypass, but that false-positive results have been obtained.

Methods

Fifty-five patients who underwent 66 extracranial–intracranial arterial anastomoses in the anterior circulation were studied to compare the accuracy of the Doppler and postoperative angiography in determination of the function of the bypass.

Two basic instruments were used. The first was the Medsonics Non-Directional Doppler (Model BF4A). This instrument has a probe which is approximately 1 cm² at its tip and was initially used to determine flow in the superficial temporal artery in early bypass cases. The square configuration of the tip, however, and its relatively large size made it difficult to use in following the artery carefully to the craniectomy. For this reason a smaller pencil type of probe on the Parks Electronics Doppler was then used. The Medsonics Doppler, however, was more useful in evaluation of the posterior fossa bypass procedures because the broader tip permitted easier location of the deeply situated arteries.

The Parks Electronics Directional Doppler (806C) with a pencil probe was the instrument used in evaluation of most of the patients in this series. The pencil probe is round with a probe tip approximately 5 mm in diameter which can be maneuvered easily and can be used to follow the course of the extracranial artery to the craniectomy defect and even over the cortical surface percutaneously through the craniectomy site. This instrument has the added feature of being able to determine the direction of blood flow in the extracranial vessel.

Since the Doppler was able to detect flow in the extracranial artery, and since the extracranial artery can be followed to the craniectomy or craniotomy site and often transcutaneously over the cortical surface, it seemed reasonable to assume that if the Doppler could detect flow in the extracranial artery the anastomosis was patent. Thus, the criteria for patency of the anastomosis were established as: (1) The extracranial artery pulse could be detected by the Doppler, (2) the extracranial artery could be followed to the defect and over the cortical surface transcutaneously if a craniectomy had been performed, and (3) occlusion of the extracranial artery flow by digital compression proximal to the position of the probe would occlude the pulse in the extracranial artery and over the cortex at the craniectomy site. If these three criteria were present, the EC–IC bypass was recorded as patent. When the directional Doppler was used a fourth criterion of patency —direction of flow—could be added, but this measurement was not essential to establish patency.

All patients were studied postoperatively with the Doppler technique. In 52 of 63 anastomoses the directional Doppler could be used.

Four-vessel cerebral angiography or direct carotid or brachial angiography was used postoperatively to evaluate the function of the bypass in each case. Patency by angiography was defined as any intracranial filling occurring from the extracranial vessel used in the anastomosis.

Results

In 58 of 63 anastomoses, or 92%, the Doppler examination and cerebral angiogram indicated patency of the anastomosis.

In three anastomoses the Doppler indicated patency; however, on the angiogram only filling of the superficial temporal artery without intracranial filling could be seen. This angiographic appearance was similar to that described by Khodadad[2] in which there was slow flow through the extracranial artery but no intracranial filling. It has been suggested that this appearance is caused by extracranial artery spasm or edema.[2] In two of these three bypasses subsequent angiography indicated intracranial filling.[1] The remaining patient did not return for a follow-up angiogram to establish whether his anastomosis became patent with time.

In one additional patient the results of the Doppler were questionable and the superficial temporal artery, on angiography, seemed to be occluded. On subsequent angiograms, the Doppler definitely became positive and intracranial filling was demonstrated.

In one final case the Doppler indicated patency of the anastomosis but the angiogram revealed that an extracranial vessel which coursed over the craniectomy site was filled but no intracranial filling whatsoever was seen. This is the only case in our series with an occlusion of the EC–IC anastomosis, for an overall angiographically proved patency rate of 97%.

Thus, if the Doppler indicates patency of the anastomosis, there is at least a 92% chance that an angiogram will show intracranial filling.

In three patients who underwent double bypass procedures on the same side, the Doppler was able to distinguish each bypass in two of the three by separating out the flow over the craniectomy site for each anastomosis.

In all 53 anastomoses that could be evaluated by the directional Doppler, the direction of flow was toward the craniotomy or craniectomy site in 100% of the cases. Thus, this determination revealed that in no case did flow occur from the brain arteries out to the extracranial artery in a reverse direction.

In five of our eight cases with posterior fossa revascularization in which both Doppler evaluation and angiographic studies were performed, the Doppler and the angiogram indicated patency in all five. The quality of the Doppler determination, however, was only marginal in these cases, as the pulse disappeared when the artery coursed deeper into the posterior cervical musculature.

Discussion and Conclusion

These data indicate that the Doppler is a highly accurate means of evaluating the function of an EC–IC bypass, being accurate greater than 90% of the time in correlating with angiographic patency. It must be cautioned, however, that the Doppler will provide only a qualitative estimation of intracranial filling and that it is subject to false-positive error up to 8% of the time. Thus, although it is not 100% accurate in determining patency of EC–IC anastomosis, it is useful in determining patency indirectly with a small error. The Doppler also seems useful for posterior fossa revascularization procedures in determining anastomosis patency, but the instruments described herein do not seem to be optimal.

References

1. Ausman, J.I., Latchaw, R.E., Lee, M.C., Ramirez-Lassepas, M. Results of multiple angiographic studies on cerebral revascularization patients. In Microsurgery for Stroke. P. Schmiedek, editor, Springer-Verlag, 1977, pp. 222–229.
2. Khodadad, G. Transient postoperative occlusion of the superficial temporal–middle cerebral artery branch anastomosis: Spasm, swelling, or thrombosis. Surg Neurol 3:341–345, 1975.

22

STA–MCA Anastomosis: Detailed Analysis of Pre- and Postoperative Angiography

Richard E. Latchaw, James I. Ausman, and Myoung C. Lee

Adequate evaluation of the need for an extra–intracranial bypass procedure requires a complete preoperative analysis of the vascular status of the patient. Likewise a determination of the efficacy of the procedure necessitates an understanding of the postoperative appearance and change over time of both the surgical anastomotic circuit and the intracranial circulation. The purpose of this study is to record and analyze the angiographic findings both pre- and postoperatively in a large number of patients undergoing superficial temporal (STA) to middle cerebral artery (MCA) bypass. In particular, serial postoperative studies in this large group allow an understanding of the progressive changes that take place in both the bypass circuit and the intracranial circulation.

Materials and Methods

The patient population consisted of 40 patients with vascular occlusive disease in the internal carotid artery distribution in which a total of 45 STA–MCA anastomoses had been performed. The patients' neurologic deficits, frequency of superimposed transient ischemic attacks (TIAs), and major vascular lesions are listed in Table 22-1. The majority of the patients underwent preoperative complete cerebral angiography via transfemoral catheterization. The postsurgical studies generally consisted of transfemoral unilateral carotid angiography on the side of the anastomosis. Postoperatively, 38 of 40 patients (95%) had one angiogram, 18 of 40 (45%) had two angiograms, 4 of 10 (10%) had three angiograms, and 2 of 40 (5%) had four angiograms. The median time of the first postoperative study was 12 days following surgery; the median

Table 22-1. Patient population

1. 40 patients with 45 anastomoses	
2. Neurologic deficits	
TIAs only	6
Mild partially reversible ischemic neurologic deficit	25
Moderate partially reversible ischemic neurologic deficit	9
3. Ischemic episodes preop	
One	9
Two to three	16
Four or more	15
4. Lesions	
Unilateral internal carotid artery occlusion	60%
Bilateral internal carotid artery occlusion	23%
Siphon or MCA stenosis or occlusion	17%
5. Average time between deficit and surgery	6 months
6. Follow-up: 2–31 months, average: 20 months	

time of the second postoperative study was 5 months.

Graft Patency

Graft patency was defined as filling of the MCA branch used for anastomosis by the STA. Of the 38 patients with postoperative angiography, 34 (89%) had intracranial filling on the first postoperative study. The four cases that did not appear patent were studied 5 to 7 days after surgery; three of them had filling of the STA anastomotic branch but no visible intracranial filling. Three of the four were patent on the second postoperative study, for an overall patency rate of 97%; one case has not been restudied. In view of the patent STA branch and subsequent intracranial filling on follow-up studies, spasm at the anastomotic site on the early postsurgical angiogram may have been responsible. Thrombosis with recanalization cannot be excluded, however. None of the anastomoses became occluded over long-term observation; once patent, they remained patent.

Table 22-2. STA enlargement

I. First postoperative angiogram		
A. Enlargement relative to preop	29/36	81%
B. Degree of enlargement in these patients		70%
II. Second postop angiogram Enlargement relative to preop (two additional cases)	31/36	86%
B. Enlargement relative to first postop angio	12/18	66%
Degree of enlargement relative to first postop angio		53%
Overall enlargement relative to preop		86%
III. Three or four postop angios Progressive enlargement 8–21 months postop		50%
IV. Summary		
A. Average increase, any angiogram		83%
B. Maximum		300%
C. At least double preop size		38%
D. Decrease over time		1 patient
E. Accompanied by increased tortuosity of STA and MCA branches		

Change in STA Diameter

The changes in the postoperative diameters of the superficial temporal artery branches used for anastomosis relative to the preoperative diameters are listed in Table 22-2. Eighty-six percent of the patients with adequate pre- and postoperative studies for comparison had an enlarged STA postoperatively. Twelve of 18 patients (66%) with two or more postoperative studies had further STA enlargement on the second postsurgical study relative to the first. These 12 had an overall enlargement of 86%. Fifty percent of the patients with three or four postoperative studies had further enlargement 8 to 21 months after surgery. In summary, the average STA branch increase on any postoperative angiogram relative to the preoperative study was 83%, with a maximum increase of 300%; in 38% of the cases there was at least a doubling in size. The progressive dilatation over time is reflected in the above statistics. In

only one patient, to be discussed later, was there a decrease over time. The progressive STA enlargement was accompanied by increased tortuosity of the STA and increased diameter and tortuosity of MCA branches (Fig. 22-1).

Intracranial Vascular Filling

In an attempt to assess the contribution to intracranial filling by the bypass circuit, a diagram of the areas of perfusion by branches of the middle cerebral artery as developed by Waddington[3] was used in evaluating the sequential postoperative studies. There are six areas of MCA perfusion; the presence of filling in an area, but not the degree of filling, counted as one point. Filling of the anterior cerebral artery counted as an additional point, for a maximum of 7 points. The presence of exten-

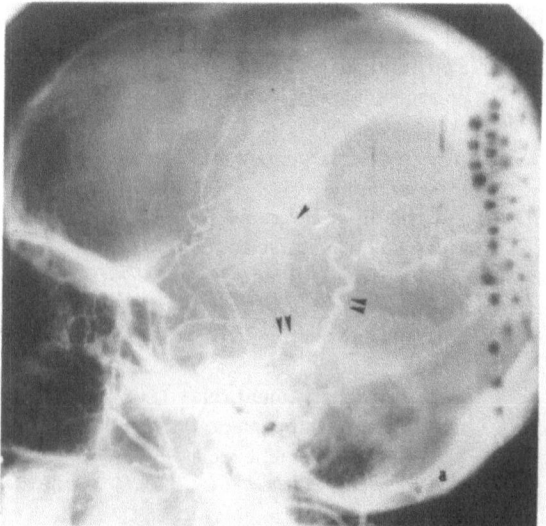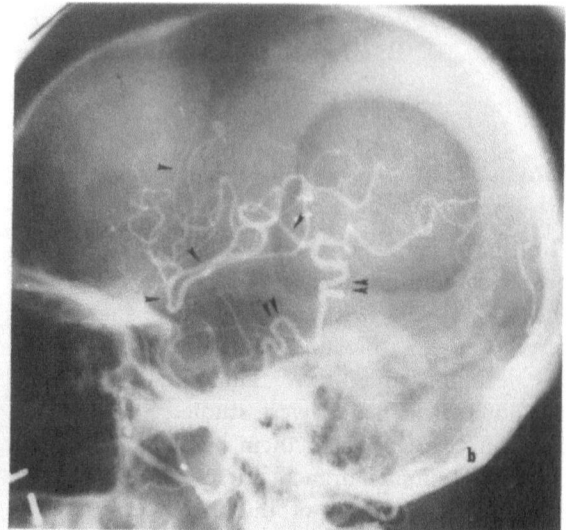

Fig. 22-1. STA–MCA bypass, with progressive STA anastomotic branch enlargement and increased tortuosity and progressive MCA branch enlargement over time. a. One month after surgery. b. Eight months after surgery.

sive collateral from the contralateral carotid and vertebral circulations on the preoperative studies made comparison with the postoperative unilateral carotid angiograms impossible. Evaluation of the sequential postoperative studies could be performed, however, by comparing the unilateral carotid injections on the side of anastomosis and analyzing the change in intracranial filling via the bypass circuit over time.

As listed in Table 22-3, 36% of the areas were filled by the surgical bypass on the initial postoperative study at a median time of 7 days following surgery. This increased to 64% of the areas by 4.5 months. This increase in intracranial filling paralleled the progressive average STA enlargement, which went from 39% to 76%. In all patients, the number of areas filled stayed the same or increased with time, with the average degree of filling almost doubling in 4 months; in no case was there a decrease. In addition, progressive filling occurred 8 to 17 months following surgery in those patients with three postoperative studies (Fig. 22-2).

The number of areas filled by the bypass circuit was dependent upon the severity of the occlusive vascular disease (Table 22-3). Fewer areas were filled in patients with a single MCA

Table 22-3. Area filling (patients with multiple angiograms)

Exam	Time	Filling	% STA
1. First postup	7 days	2.5/7 (36%)	39%
Second postop	4.5 mo	4.5/7 (64%)	76%

2. All stayed same or increased with time, filling almost doubled in 4 months
3. 2/4 with 3 postop angios continued to show increase 8–17 months postop
4. Intracranial filling increases as STA enlarges
5. Filling   Lesion

Lesion	Areas filled
A) Single middle cerebral or carotid siphon stenosis or occlusion	3/7
B) Unilateral ICA occlusion	4/7
C) Bilateral ICA occlusion	6/7

or carotid siphon stenosis or occlusion than with a unilateral internal carotid artery occlusion. Still greater was the number of areas filled in patients with bilateral internal carotid or multiple arterial sites of occlusion. In addition, the specific areas filled tended to be related to the site of anastomosis, with greater filling near the anterior parietal region, the usual site of anastomosis.

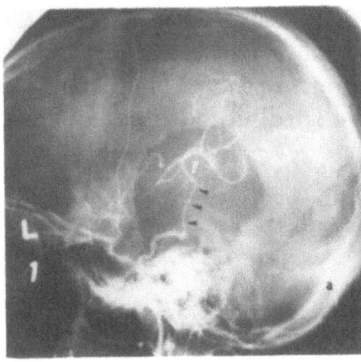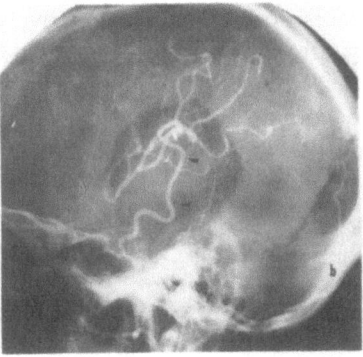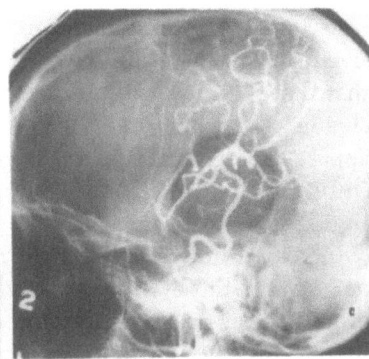

Fig. 22-2. STA–MCA bypass, with increasing MCA area filling over time. a. Seven days after surgery. b. Three months after surgery. c. Ten months after surgery.

Additional Observations

The STA anastomotic branch became compressed at the craniotomy edge in one patient with the moyamoya syndrome a number of months following operation. As found both angiographically and surgically, progressive atrophy allowed the brain to fall away from the inner table of the skull, producing compression of the bridging anastomotic artery. This was the only case in which there was a decrease in the STA branch diameter in the late postoperative period.

In two patients, a prominent degree of unilateral encephalomalacia obviated the need for increased perfusion, reflected by a lack of significant STA diameter change or increased area filling. The first patient had not had a preoperative computerized tomographic (CT) scan, but his neurologic status had not excluded operation. When he failed to show significant improvement, the CT scan was performed and demonstrated the diffuse encephalomalacia in the MCA distribution on the side of surgery. The second patient had a large area of encephalomalacia in the MCA distribution on the preoperative CT scan. A bypass procedure was performed and, while a slight initial clinical improvement, increased STA diameter, and multiple MCA areas of vascular filling were found, no further improvement occurred. Repeated CT scanning again showed the large area of encephalomalacia which prevented further improvement or angiographic change.

The takeover by the anastomotic circuit of previous collateral channels from the contra-lateral carotid or vertebral circulations was observed in a number of patients. Cross-flow from the opposite carotid was reversed in a number of cases. The findings suggested a decrease in the degree of intracranial steal from one circulation to another following bypass surgery.

Clinical Results

The clinical results of these 40 patients have been reported elsewhere[2] and hence will not be reviewed in depth. Briefly, the frequency of TIAs dropped dramatically postoperatively, with only one TIA per patient in three patients. There was no recurrent infarction over the follow-up period, averaging 20 months. There was also significant improvement in the neurologic deficit in 56% of the patients with a mild deficit before surgery and 78% of the patients with a moderate deficit.

Conclusions

Early postoperative angiography may be misleading. The lack of significant intracranial filling via the bypass may be transitory, with time necessary before a significant increase can be demonstrated. Angiography at 5 to 6 months after surgery would be more helpful.

It is difficult to assess the "adequacy" of collateral on the preoperative angiogram. The facts that the STA diameter increases progressively over time, with increasing area filling, that there is a reversal of intracranial collateral channels, and that preoperative symptoms disappear and deficits improve suggest that apparently abundant collateral on the preoperative angiogram may be inadequate.

Increased flow may occur in many patients, not just in those with marked vascular compromise and fixed neurologic deficits where there is little hope of improvement, as has been suggested by others.[1] Improvement in deficits may well occur, suggesting that relative ischemia may be present in addition to previous infarction.

Any assessment of clinical results following bypass surgery must take into account the reversal of intracranial steal. The neurologic examination is heavily weighted toward motor function. Neuropsychologic testing pre- and postoperatively may reveal more diffuse improvement in frontal and temporal lobe function secondary to increased cerebral perfusion than can be appreciated on the clinical neurologic examination.

References

1. Anderson, R.E., Reichman, O.H., Davis, D.O. Radiological evaluation of temporal artery–middle cerebral artery anastomosis. Radiology 113: 73–79, 1974.
2. Lee, M.C., Ausman, J.I., Geiger, J.D., Latchaw, R.E., et al. Clinical results of superficial temporal artery to middle cerebral artery (STA to MCA) anastomoses in ischemic stroke patients in internal carotid artery distribution. Arch Neurol (accepted for publication).
3. Waddington, M.M. Atlas of Cerebal Angiography with Anatomic Correlation, Little, Brown and Company, Boston, 1974.

23

Angiography of the External Carotid–Internal Carotid Anastomosis (EC–IC)

Allan J. Fox and John M. Allcock

Microsurgical anastomosis between external carotid and internal carotid arteries (EC–IC bypass) in patients with cerebral ischemia resulting from surgically inaccessible arterial disease has become an established procedure.[2, 5, 6, 7] To verify the bypass's effectiveness in prevention of future ischemic events, a randomized study has been set up.[3] In all reports of EC–IC bypass surgery and in the ongoing study, angiography is considered essential as part of the postoperative assessment of these patients. Radiologic evaluations of EC–IC bypasses have been done,[1] and our case material reviews some technical aspects of EC–IC angiography including difficulties of interpretation and complications.

Materials and Methods

Angiograms of 41 patients, with a total of 45 EC–IC anastomoses, were reviewed from a technical point of view. Thirty of these patients underwent EC–IC surgery as treatment for cerebral ischemia with angiographic demonstration of occlusion or inaccessible stenosis of internal carotid or middle cerebral arteries. Ten patients had giant aneurysms of the internal carotid or middle cerebral artery, where the EC–IC anastomosis was performed before surgical occlusion of internal carotid or middle cerebral artery via the Drake tourniquet or Sel-

verstone clamp.[4] In one instance an EC–IC was done in a patient with a recurrent sphenoid meningioma where there was worry that the carotid artery might have to be sacrificed at surgery, though this did not turn out to be the case.

Forty-one of the bypasses were between the superficial temporal artery and middle cerebral branches, three were from the occipital artery, and one was a venous graft from the common carotid artery.

Results

In the 30 patients who underwent operation for ischemic disease, 33 anastomoses were performed. In most of these, the EC–IC was readily evaluated postoperatively with common carotid angiography. However, in nine instances the intracranial vessels were filled at about the same time as was the anastomosis, and it was felt necessary to do selective external carotid angiography to show the EC–IC's function properly (Fig. 23-1).

In the 10 patients with giant aneurysms, 11 EC–ICs were performed. In nine cases prior to occlusion, the EC–IC had to be evaluated by selective external carotid angiography. Most of these patients underwent repeated angiography in the postoperative period. In two cases the external carotid artery supplying the anas-

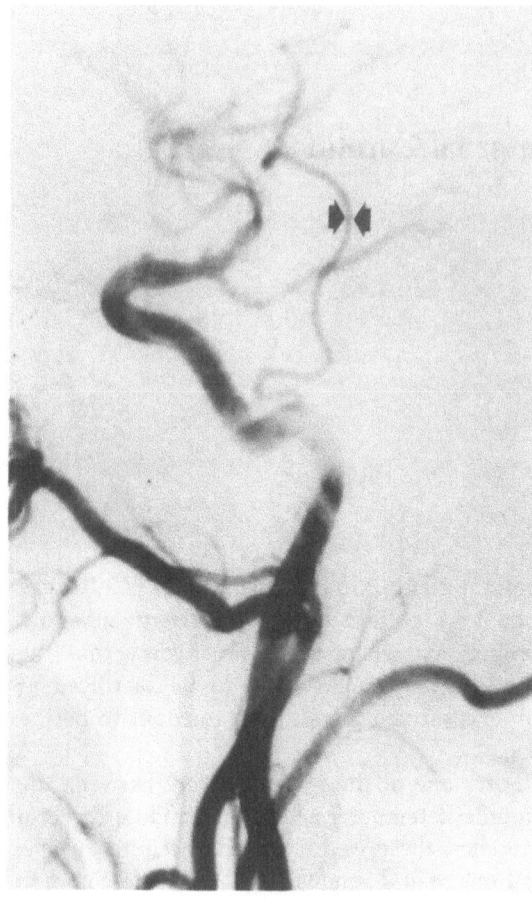

A

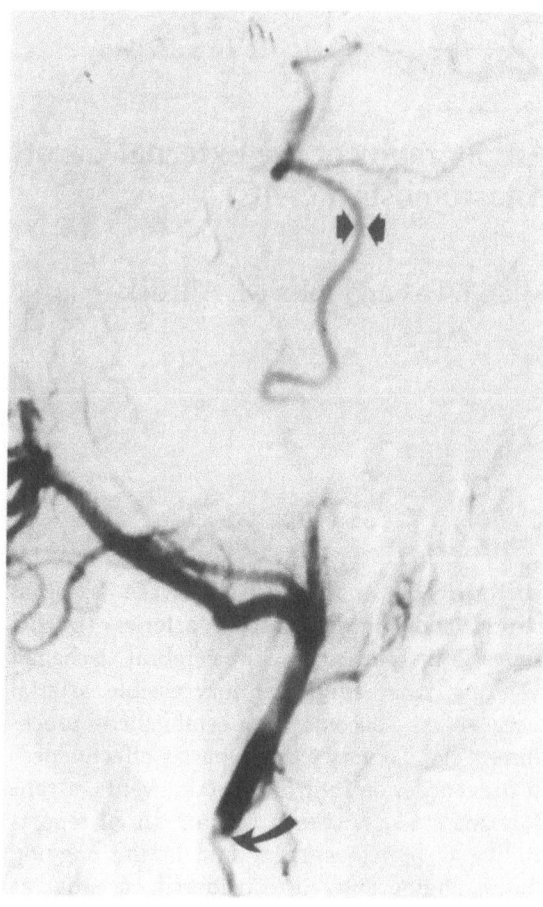

B

Fig. 23-1. A common carotid (A) and an external carotid (B) angiogram done during the same angiographic procedure. There is some spasm of the artery around the catheter (⟋) and the superficial temporal artery diameter (▶ ◀) is larger with the external study.

tomosis became occluded as a complication of angiography.

In the one case where the EC–IC was done preoperatively for a recurrent sphenoid meningioma, it was necessary to evaluate it angiographically with a selective external carotid angiogram.

In all, 19 of 45 EC–ICs were studied with selective external carotid angiography, with 11 of those 19 having both a common carotid angiogram and a selective external carotid angiogram in the same session. In comparing the diameter of the superficial temporal artery on the common carotid angiogram and the external carotid angiogram, the superficial temporal artery measured greater in size on the latter in 8 of the 11 cases. Some arterial spasm around the tip of the catheter was noted in those angiograms.

Complications

Both patients who sustained external carotid occlusion as a complication of angiography did not have any resulting neurologic deficit. The first of these was a 38-year-old woman with a giant right internal carotid bifurcation aneurysm (Fig. 23-2). She underwent an EC–IC bypass with a Drake tourniquet placed around the supraclinoid carotid artery. Subsequently, she

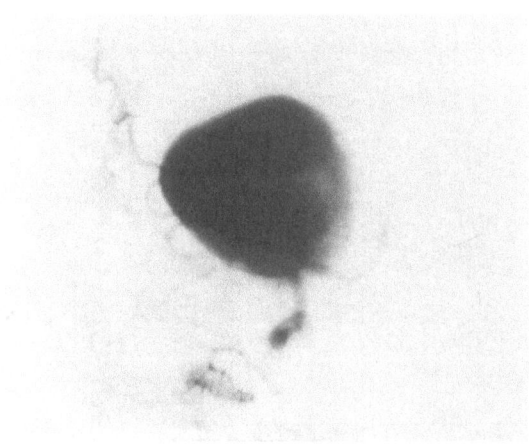

Fig. 23-2. Right internal carotid bifurcation giant aneurysm, AP projection.

underwent angiography and attempted tightening of the tourniquet. A number of times over two days repeated external carotid angiography produced intimal damage to the external carotid artery, as well as some spasm (Fig. 23-3).

One week later angiography revealed the external carotid to be occluded proximally, with excellent collaterals from the vertebral artery supplying both the superficial temporal and the middle cerebral artery (Fig. 23-4). After a follow-up of over one year, the aneurysm remains thrombosed, the EC–IC is still functioning from vertebral collaterals, and the patient is neurologically intact.

The other complication was in a 25-year-old woman with a large fusiform aneurysm of the left internal carotid artery extending to the middle cerebral artery. She underwent an EC–IC with placement of a Selverstone clamp on the cervical portion of the internal carotid artery.

Four days postoperatively, and about one day after complete tightening of the clamp, angiography was performed. Single-plane filming was done with the first series showing the head on an AP projection with excellent filling of the external carotid and the anastomosis. On subsequent lateral views the external carotid artery was occluded, owing to recoil of an inadvertently high catheter which mechanically displaced thrombus from the internal carotid stump. Immediate vertebral angiography showed excellent filling of the superficial tem-

poral and EC–IC bypass. The patient had no neurologic sequelae.

Discussion

If the middle cerebral artery branches fill at the same time from multiple sources, it is extremely difficult to show a definite angiographic picture of an EC–IC bypass. Certainly oblique tangential views and very rapid serial filming should be tried with a common carotid angiogram. However, there are instances where a selective external carotid angiogram[1] must be done even in cases of occlusive ischemic vascular disease.

Catheters often produce some local arterial

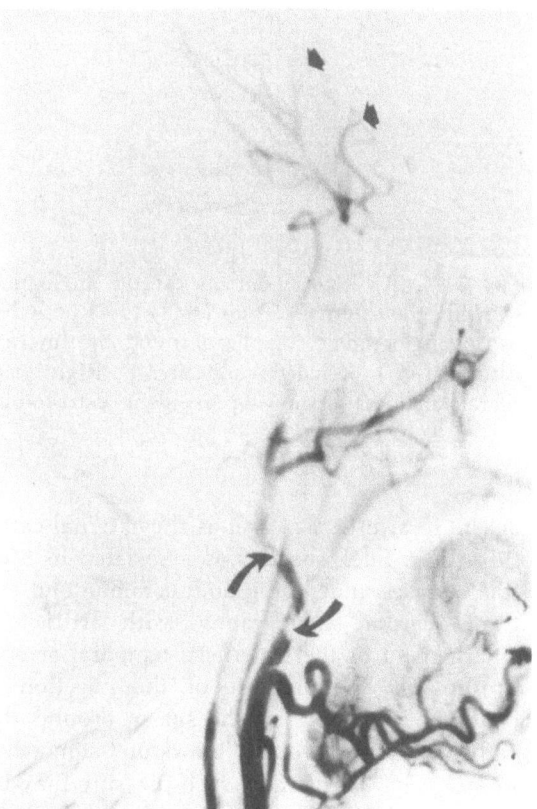

Fig. 23-3. Lateral external carotid angiogram following repeated angiography to monitor the EC–IC function during carotid artery occlusion. Intimal damage (↗) and spasm (↗) are noted in the internal maxillary artery, and excellent filling of the middle cerebral is seen (▲).

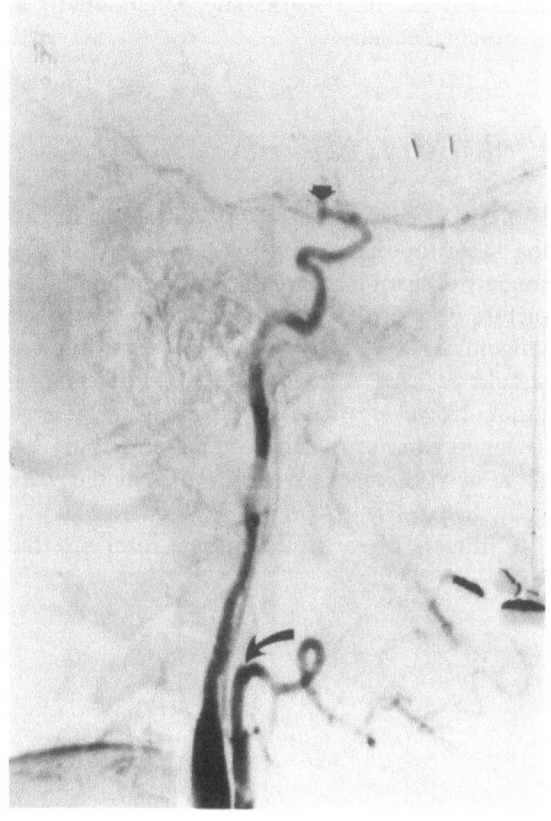

A

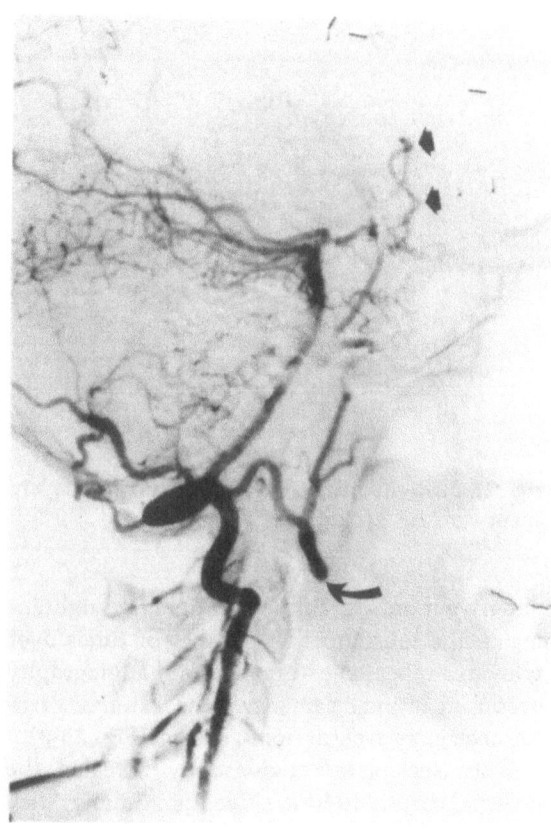

B

Fig. 23-4. A, Right common carotid angiogram showing the external carotid ( ) to be occluded as an angiographic complication and the internal carotid ( ) occluded surgically. B, Right vertebral angiogram showing excellent extracranial collaterals to the superficial temporal artery ( ) which is beginning to fill the middle cerebral artery ( ). Later films showed excellent middle cerebral filling via the EC–IC.

spasm in arteries as small as the external carotid artery. Such spasm was associated in 8 of the 11 cases undergoing both common and external carotid angiography, with artifactual enlargement of the superficial temporal artery. Presumably the pressure of the injection is confined somewhat by the spasm around the catheter, and the vessel "blows up" somewhat in size (Fig. 23-1). Also, such pressure may be transmitted through the EC–IC anastomosis to the middle cerebral branches, giving an overestimation of the effectiveness of the shunt.

Almost all reports on EC–IC studies mention the size of the superficial temporal artery.[1, 2, 5, 6, 7] However, the effect of technical factors on the size of this vessel during external carotid angiography is not mentioned. The possibility

exists, therefore, that in some instances part of the "enlargement" of the artery report is artifactual.

The first of the two complications reported here exemplifies the risk of repeated selective external carotid angiograms. In view of the potential of possible intimal damage to the small but important branch, external carotid angiography should be avoided where possible and done with the utmost care when necessary.

The second complication is different, and reiterates the principle of avoidance of high carotid catheterization in patients with abnormalities near or at the bifurcation (in this case the abnormality being thrombus in the stump of a recently occluded internal carotid artery).

The effectiveness of vertebral collaterals in both cases is reassuring.

graphic complication without neurologic sequelae.

Conclusions

In the angiography of the EC–IC bypass, external carotid angiography is sometimes necessary.

External carotid angiography on the side of an EC–IC bypass is of greater risk than usual.

External carotid angiography can give an artifactually enlarged picture of the superficial temporal artery and an EC–IC bypass.

The EC–IC bypass is being performed more and more, and angiography is essential as part of the postoperative evaluation. This review of 41 patients points out the need for selective external carotid angiography in those cases where intracranial vessels fill spontaneously at the same time as the shunt. However, 8 of 11 cases showed the superficial temporal artery to be larger on the selective external carotid angiogram than the common carotid study done during the same session. In two cases undergoing staged occlusive procedures for treatment of giant aneurysm, the external carotid artery leading to an EC–IC was occluded as an angio-

References

1. Anderson, R.E., Reichman, O.H., Davis, D.O. Radiological evaluation of temporal artery–middle cerebral artery anastomosis. Radiology 113:73–79, 1974.
2. Chater, N., Popp, A.J. Microsurgical vascular bypass for occlusive cerebrovascular disease: Current status. Adv Neurol 16:121–132, 1977.
3. McDowell, F.H. The extracranial/intracranial bypass study. Stroke 8:545, 1977.
4. Peerless, S.J., Drake, C., Ferguson, G.G. Cerebral revascularization in the treatment of giant intracranial aneurysms. Presented at Royal College of Surgeons of Canada, Annual meeting, Toronto, January 1976.
5. Reichman, O.H. Neurosurgical microsurgical anastomosis for cerebral ischemia: Five years experience. In Cerebrovascular Diseases, P. Scheinburg, editor, Raven Press, New York, 1976, pp. 311–330.
6. Sundt, T.M., Siekert, R.G., Piepgras, D.G., Sherbrough, F.W., Houser, O.W. Bypass surgery for vascular disease of the carotid system. Mayo Clin Proc 51:677–692, 1976.
7. Tew, J.M. Reconstructive intracranial vascular surgery for prevention of stroke. Clin Neurosurg 22:264–280, 1975.

24

Cortical Artery Pressure: Preoperative and Postoperative Arteriographic Findings in Patients with Internal Carotid Artery Occlusion

M. Collice, G. Scialfa, F. Valsecchi, O. Arena, and R. M. Borgia*

In ten consecutive patients with internal carotid artery (ICA) occlusion and treated by an extra–intracranial arterial bypass (EIAB) the cortical intra-arterial pressure has been measured. The results have been compared to the preoperative and postoperative arteriographic findings to evaluate (1) the significance of collateral circulation assessed by the angiographic studies and (2) the role of the pressure gradients in regard to the postoperative intracranial filling degree via the shunt.

Materials and Method

Ten patients with ICA occlusion treated by superficial temporal artery–cortical middle cerebral artery (STA–cMCA) bypass have been studied. Four demonstrated reversible ischemic attacks (RIAs) and 6 mild to moderate neurologic deficits from previous stroke (completed stroke with partial recovery = CSPR). Preoperative angiographic studies included complete 4-vessel angiography. Postoperatively only the carotid angiography of the affected side was performed. Intraoperatively blood pressure (BP) from the radial artery, STA, and proximal and distal cortical artery selected for the anastomosis was measured by means of Statham Model P23 transducers. Technique of pressure measurements was essentially as de-

scribed by Yonekawa and Yasargil.[5] External diameter of the cortical artery, usually the angular branch, varied from 1.2 mm to 1.5 mm. None of the patients presented new ischemic events in the follow-up period (average 12 months). Three of the six CSPR patients showed some neurologic improvement in the follow-up period.

Two additional patients with metastatic brain tumor have been studied as controls. In both patients pressure from the STA and the cortical branch of MCA was recorded before brain resection was performed for tumor removal.

In evaluating collaterals both the objective pathways of revascularization and the subjective degree of filling of the ischemic hemisphere were considered.

The following sources and pathways were considered: (1) contralateral ICA via the anterior communicating artery, (2) vertebrobasilar (VB) circulation via both the posterior communicating arteries and leptomeningeal anastomosis, and (3) external carotid artery (ECA) via both ophthalmic artery and meningocortical (transdural) anastomosis.

A grading system of 0, 1, 2, 3 was used to describe no, poor, fair, and good supratentorial filling from each of the three sources.

Postoperative angiographic studies were evaluated for revascularization entity. According to our method described elsewhere in these Proceedings on the lateral views of the angiograms, the MCA territory was divided into six main cortical areas and results were expressed

* Special acknowledgment for statistical advice.

in terms of number of cortical areas supplied by the bypass.

Results

Preoperative Angiographic Studies (Table 24–1)

In all ten patients occlusion of ICA at the bifurcation was observed. In eight of ten some degree of supratentorial filling from VB circulation was observed. In none did revascularization originate from all three main sources. Supratentorial filling of the affected hemisphere mainly arose from: (1) both VB and ECA circulation in three cases (group A), (2) VB circulation alone in three patients (group B), and (3) the contralateral ICA in four patients (two of whom had fair contribution from the VB circulation) (group C).

Intraoperative Pressure Measurements (Table 24–2)

When considering all the patients, mean STA pressure was found to be 78% (range 75% to 94%) of mean systemic BP.

In the two control patients mean proximal cortical BP (MPCBP) was 80.5% (range 80% to 81%) of mean systemic BP and 88.5% (range 83% to 94%) of mean STA BP.

In the ten patients with ICA occlusion MPCBP was 41% (range 15% to 73%) of mean systemic BP and 45% (range 18% to 77%) of mean STA BP. (Significant difference between the two patient groups has been disclosed, P = .025.)

In nine of ten patients MPCBP was less than 50% and 60% of mean systemic and STA BP respectively. In group A MPCBP was 35% (range 29% to 40%) of mean system BP; in group B it was 46% (range 15% to 73%), and in group C 42% (range 34% to 47%). (No significant differences among the three groups have been disclosed.) In patients with RIAs and CSPR it was 39% (range 34% to 47%) and 42% (range 15% to 73%) respectively. (No significant differences were found between the two groups.) In the three patients showing neurologic improvements after the operation, MPCBP was 15%, 29%, and 50% of systemic BP respectively.

Postoperative Angiographic Studies (Table 24–1)

The bypasses were patent in all ten patients, but a great variety of intracranial filling via the shunt was observed. In each of the three groups above considered both poor (1 to 2

Table 24-1. Clinical presentation, sources of collaterals, and supratentorial filling degree in 10 cases with ICA occlusion

Case no.	Clinical presentation	Contralateral ICA	VB	ECA	(Group)
1	RIA	0	3	3	
2	CSPR	0	2	3	(A)
3	CSPR	0	2	3	
4	CSPR	0	3	0	
5	CSPR	0	3	0	(B)
6	CSPR	1	3	0	
7	RIA	3	2	0	
8	RIA	3	0	0	
9	RIA	3	0	0	(C)
10	CSPR	3	1	0	

0, 1, 2, and 3 = no, poor, fair, and good supratentorial filling degree of the affected hemisphere.

RIA = reversible ischemic attacks.

CSPR = completed stroke with partial recovery.

Table 24-2. Intraoperative pressure measurement results in 10 patients with ICA occlusion and in 2 patients without occlusive lesions

Group	Case no.	Mean cMCA pressure (mm Hg) Proximal	Distal	% Systemic*	% STA*
A	1	30	—	36	38
	2	27	25	29	33
	3	40	—	40	42
B	4	15	—	15	18
	5	85	65	73	77
	6	50	—	50	59
C	7	30	20	42	50
	8	45	35	47	53
	9	35	27	34	36
	10	50	35	45	50
	1a	81	—	81	94
	2α	92	—	80	83

*Percentage ratio of mean proximal cMCA pressure to mean systemic and STA pressure.

1a, 2α patients with brain tumor.

Group A, B, C collateral circulation sources. A = VB and ECA circulation; B = VB circulation alone; C = ICA circulation (2 with contribution from VB circulation).

areas) and good (3, 4, 5 areas) revascularization has been observed. One of four RIA patients and four of six CSPR patients showed good revascularization (Fig. 24-1). When comparing the intracranial filling entity and pressure gradient between STA and cortical branch no significant correlations have been disclosed, although the only two patients with pressure gradient less than 30 mm Hg showed a very poor revascularization (Fig. 24-1).

Discussion and Conclusion

Bakay and Sweet[1] in 1952 succeeded in measuring the intra-arterial pressure of cortical arteries in eleven patients with brain tumor. This was found to be normally 83% of the systemic pressure. With temporary clamping of the common carotid artery the pressure dropped to 56% (range 50% to 64%) of the systemic pressure. In six patients with various types of occlusive lesions Yonekawa and Yasargil[5] found the proximal cortical MCA pressure to be 29% to 41% of the systolic systemic pressure and 34% to 54% of the systolic STA pressure.

Similar results have been reported by Ito et al.[2] in nine patients with MCA occlusion and by Mizukami et al.[4] in eleven patients with completed stroke and various types of occlusive lesions. In our ten patients with ICA occlusion cortical artery pressure was found significantly lower than in patients without occlusive lesions.

Although we have tried to correlate collat-

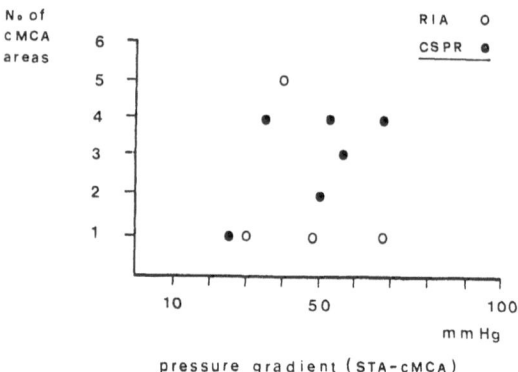

Fig. 24-1. Pressure gradient between STA and MCA cortical branch and number of MCA cortical areas supplied by the bypass in 10 cases with ICA occlusion. RIA = reversible ischemic attacks, CSPR = completed stroke with partial recovery.

eral assessment on preoperative angiographies with cortical pressure, no significant correlations have been found. For example, both the highest and lowest values of MPCBP were recorded from patients with supratentorial filling of the affected side arising from the VB circulation alone.

Also, although in patients with ICA occlusion complete filling from the contralateral ICA is usually considered the most effective type of compensation, none of our patients with this angiographic picture showed pressure values near normal or significantly higher than patients with the other types of collateral circulation sources.

Similar results were reported by Jawad et al.[3] by correlating in a very large series of patients the angiographic "collateral circulation at the circle of Willis" with the rCBF results obtained by intra-arterial [133]xenon technique both before and after ICA clamping test.

It is usually considered that after EIAB procedures the postoperative intracranial filling entity mainly reflects the pressure gradient between the donor and the recipient artery. This was only partially confirmed by our data but it must be stressed, as in this series most patients showed a relatively high pressure gradient.

Finally, in patients with neurologic deficits at the operation time, Mizukami et al.[4] reported that clinical improvements can be expected when cortical MCA pressure is 40 mm Hg or more while the outcome is poor when it is less than 40 mm Hg or 30% of the systemic BP.

We have operated on only six patients manifesting preoperative neurologic deficits and improvements have been observed in three, regardless of the MPCBP. Also, from our data it is impossible to establish whether in these patients the improvements were related to the operation rather than to the clinical course of the illness.

In conclusion, for patients with ICA occlusion the following points can be outlined:

1) In most cases some degree of supratentorial filling from the VB circulation is present.

2) In these cases cortical artery pressure is significantly lower than in patients without occlusive lesion, even though some difference from patient to patient exists.

3) Radiologic assessment of collateral circulation cannot predict the actual cortical artery pressure reduction in the individual patient. The value of collateral assessment by angiography is then poor for surgical indications. Also, this suggests that angiographic studies, which represent a potential risk for the patient, could be limited in patients with carotid symptoms to the visualization of the neck vessels and of the intracranial carotid branches. Selected catheterization of the vertebral artery could be avoided.

4) Similarly, the intracranial filling following an EIAB procedure cannot be predicted merely by looking at the preoperative angiograms.

5) Pressure gradient between donor and recipient artery is not the only factor in determining the postoperative intracranial filling via the shunt. Probably MCA anatomic configuration and metabolic request are the main factors.

6) Further and more extensive studies are necessary for establishing the significance of cortical artery pressure in regard to the postoperative clinical outcome in patients treated by an EIAB procedure.

References

1. Bakay, L., Sweet, W.H. Cervical and intracranial arterial pressure with and without vascular occlusion. Surg Gynecol Obstet 95:67–75, 1952.
2. Ito, Z., Hen, R., Nakajima, K., Suzuki, A., Uemura, K. Selection of completed stroke patients for STA–MCA anastomosis based on measurements of somatosensory evoked potential and CBF dynamics. In Microsurgery for Stroke, P. Schmiedek, editor, Springer-Verlag, New York, 1977–78, pp. 177–184.
3. Jawad, K.J., Miller, J.D., Wyper, D.J., Rowan, J.O. Measurement of CBF and carotid artery pressure compared with cerebral angiography in assessing collateral blood supply after carotid ligation. J. Neurosurg 46:185–196, 1977.
4. Mizukami, M., Kin, H., Sakuta, Y., Nishijima, M., Araki, G. Cortical arterial pressure in occlusive cerebrovascular disease and results of bypass surgery. In Microsurgery for Stroke, P. Schmiedek, editor, Springer-Verlag, New York, 1977, pp. 233–240.
5. Yonekawa, Y., Yasargil, M.G.: Extra–intracranial arterial anastomosis: Clinical and technical aspects. Results. Adv Neurosurg 3:46–78, 1977.

25

Angiographic Findings and Cross-Sectional Brain Perfusion Studies after Extra–Intracranial Arterial Bypass

M. Collice, F. Fazio, C. Fieschi, O. Arena, M. Possa, and A. Beduschi

The aims of this paper are (1) to report postoperative angiographic results obtained in a series of 40 patients treated by an extra–intracranial arterial bypass (EIAB) procedure, and (2) to describe the patterns of postoperative regional brain perfusion (rBP), as investigated in a limited series of patients, by a new method.

Material and Method

Clinical evaluation and angiograms of 40 consecutive patients treated by an EIAB procedure were reviewed. There were 31 men and 9 women with an age range of 34 to 71 (average 54) years.

Clinically 24 had had reversible ischemic attacks (RIAs), 12 had completed stroke with some degree of recovery, 2 had progressive stroke (PS), and 2 had acute completed stroke (ACS). (For RIA we intend clinical conditions usually defined as transient ischemic attack (TIA) and reversible ischemic neurologic disability.)

Preoperative angiographic diagnosis included internal carotid artery (ICA) occlusion (28 cases), intracranial steno-occlusive lesion (9 cases), and bilateral ICA occlusion (3 cases). Thirty-eight patients were treated by a single EIAB while 2 patients were treated by bilateral EIAB; thus, 42 EIAB procedures were performed in this series. As the recipient artery we used the angular artery in 50% of cases, a temporal branch in 21.5%, parietal artery in 21.5%, and a fronto-opercular branch in 7%.

All but one patient had early postoperative angiographic control of the bypass (3 to 15 days after the operation); thus 41 bypasses from 39 patients were controlled. Later control (2 to 9 months) was obtained in 15 of these patients.

Four patients, all with ICA occlusion, were studied by continuous intracarotid infusion of ^{81m}Kr and emission-computed tomography (SELO GAMMA-CT). One patient was studied before and after operation, the remaining three only postoperatively. This technique yields standard two-dimensional (2-D) images and coronal and axial sections of the regional distribution of brain perfusion, the thickness of each section being 1.8 cm. Fourteen to sixteen coronal sections and eight to ten axial sections interspaced 1.1 cm (center to center) were usually obtained for each study.

Coronal and axial sections were labeled by progressively starting from the front and the base of the skull respectively: the first coronal section will be passing across the frontal regions, approximately 3 cm from the glabella, and the first axial section across the lower part of the hemispheres approximately 3 cm from the orbitomeatal plane. (Details of the method are reported elsewhere in these Proceedings.)

Moreover, in each section the amount of brain tissue perfused was quantified by identifying on the digital (64 × 64) display the extent of the perfused area in that section. By then adding the results from all sections, the amount of brain tissue supplied by the bypass was obtained. Patients for this analysis were selected according to: (1) the postoperative angiographic intracranial filling degree via the shunt, and (2) the absence of collaterals by the external carotid artery circulation.

Results

Angiographic Study

Patency.   Early anastomosis patency was found in 36 of 41 bypasses (87.8%). Only five patients did not demonstrate any intracranial filling at the first postoperative angiographic control. Angiography was repeated on four of these five patients and patency was observed in three cases. Later patency rate of the "functioning" bypasses was 100% (11/11). Thus at the end of the angiographic follow-up patency was demonstrated in 37 out of the 39 patients (94.8%).

STA Enlargement.   Such enlargement was observed in 50% of the cases at the early control: in a few cases it was found only on the later control.

Retrograde Flow.   Development of retrograde flow from the side of the anastomosis beside the physiologic flow direction was found in 82.9% of the cases (34/41).

Intracranial Filling.   For this analysis 30 angiographies of 30 patients were reviewed and two parameters were considered: (1) the visualization, via the shunt, of the first segment of the MCA as an index of revascularization of the sylvian triangle, and (2) the cortical MCA areas supplied by the shunt. For the latter analysis cortical areas were identified by the Solomon template simplified so that only six main areas have been considered: temporal, angular gyrus, parietal, central-precentral, prefrontal and fronto-orbital (Fig. 25-1). Revascularization of the proximal segment of MCA was observed in 40% of the cases (12/30). According to the number of MCA areas sup-

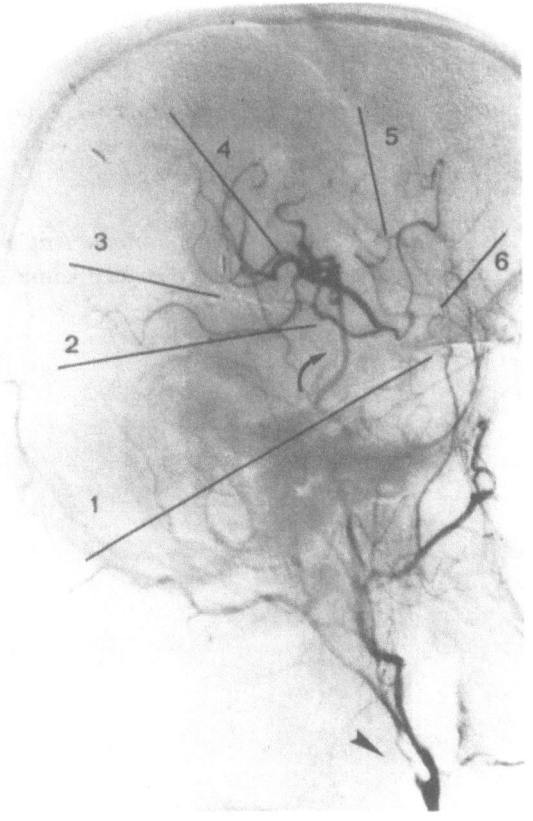

Fig. 25-1. Postoperative right common carotid angiogram from patient with right ICA occlusion. The Solomon template has been used for identifying cortical MCA areas but only 6 main areas have been considered: (1) temporal, (2) angular gyrus, (3) parietal, (4) central-precentral, (5) prefrontal, and (6) fronto-orbital. Straight arrow: ICA occlusion; curved arrow: STA. In this patient 4 cortical areas and proximal part of MCA are filled by the shunt.

plied by the bypass, patients can be divided into four groups and results expressed as follows: group I (1 area supplied by the shunt) 26.7% (8/30), group II (2 areas) 23.3% (7/30), group III (3 areas) 26.7%, group IV (4 to 6 areas) 23.3%.

Reversibility of Intracranial Steal.   The postoperative angiographic study usually consisted in the common or external carotid angiography on the side of bypass; only in a few cases was contralateral carotid or vertebral angiography performed. Evidence of a reduction of the intracranial steal from the vertebrobasilar circulation was observed in two patients, but this was never seen in the external carotid artery circulation (via the ophthalmic artery).

Enlargement of Preexisting Corticopial Anastomosis.   This phenomenon was observed in three cases.

Relationships between Postoperative Angiographic Results and Recipient Artery Choice,

Preoperative Angiographic Findings, and Clinical Conditions.   No significant correlation was found between the following parameters: postoperative intracranial filling degree, choice of the recipient artery, type of obstructive lesion, clinical presentation. Similarly, there was no correlation between intracranial filling and clinical outcome. For example, RIA patients showed a great variety of revascularization

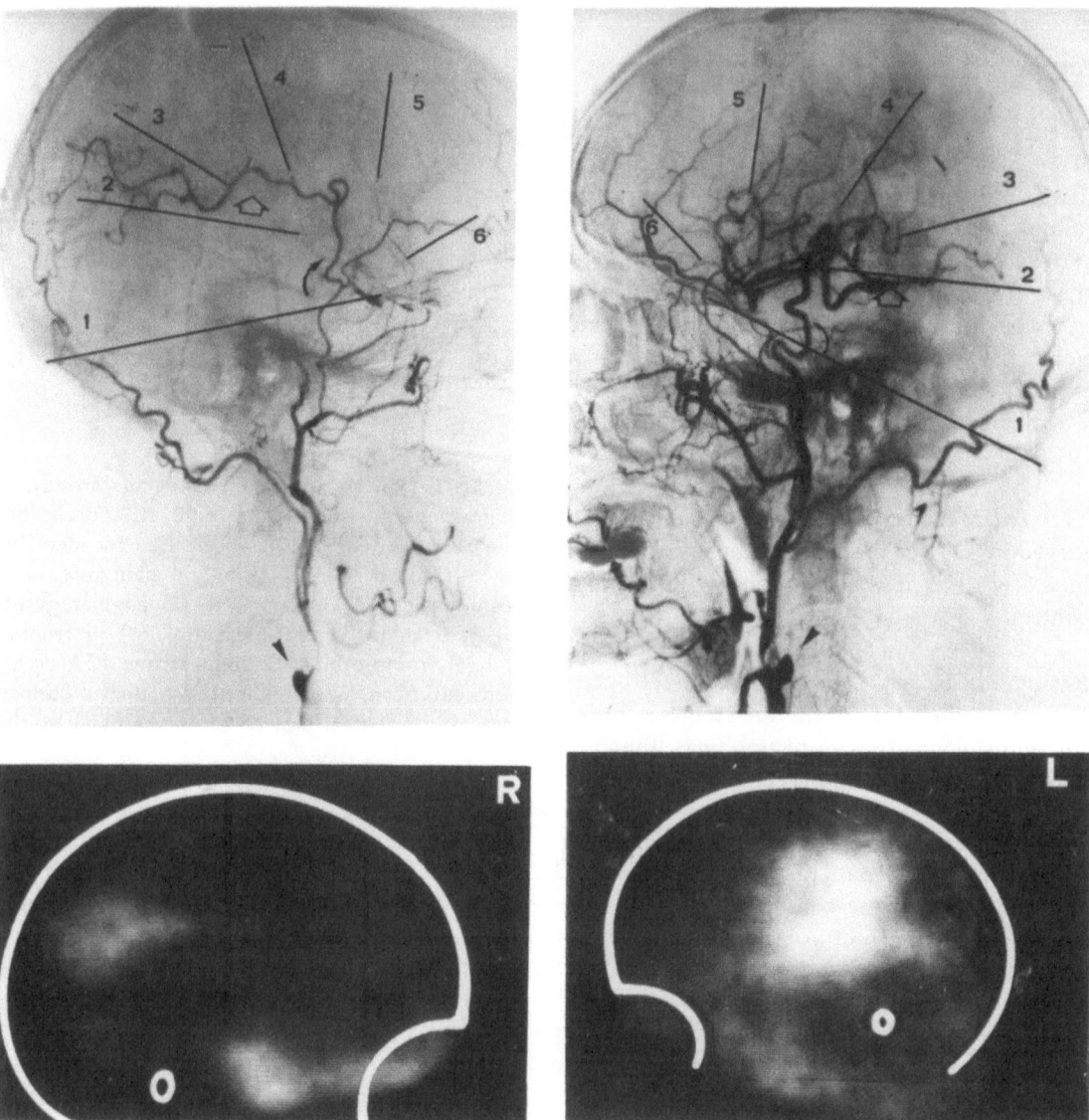

Fig. 25-2. Postoperative angiograms and postoperative static 2-D lateral views of rBP study, obtained by infusing the tracer into the common carotid artery on the bypass side. Left: Patient with 1 cortical area supplied by the bypass. Right: Patient with 4 cortical areas supplied. Both these patients exhibited ICA occlusion. Note the good correlation between angiographies and perfusion scans in terms of perfusion area extent.

patterns, but all of them (apart from two patients who had TIA) did not show further symptoms in the follow-up period (average 18 months). Patients with previous stroke showed some improvement after operation but this did not correlate with the revascularization patterns.

Postoperative rBP Results

Patients for this study were selected according to postoperative angiographic intracranial filling in order to evaluate by this new method the revascularization patterns usually obtained by an EIAB procedure. Thus one patient from each group above reported was studied.

Since all the patients were suffering from ICA occlusion without evidence of collaterals from external carotid artery circulation and the tracer was continuously infused into the common or external carotid artery on the bypass side, the brain radioactivity recorded mainly reflects the blood flow to the areas supplied by the bypass.

Bidimensional Study.   A good correlation between the postoperative angiograms and the lateral 2-D static views of the rBP study was found, that is, the size of the perfused area correlated with the number of cortical MCA areas supplied by the bypass as visualized by angiography (Fig. 25-2).

Tridimensional Study.   Tomographic rBP studies in patients of groups I and II showed areas of brain perfusion on 3 and 4 axial sections and on 4 and 6 coronal sections respectively. In both patients of groups III and IV larger areas of brain perfusion were observed on 7 axial sections and on 9 coronal sections (Figs. 25-3, 25-4, 25-5).

Groups I and II showed no definitive evidence of subcortical perfusion, blood flow being limited to cortical regions. Indeed, this was clearly shown in groups III and IV, where deep cerebral structures were perfused from the anastomosis.

The amount of brain volume perfused by the shunt was approximately 35 cm^3 and 78 cm^3 in the patients of groups I and II respectively. It was 142 cm^3 and 176 cm^3 for patients of groups III and IV. One of these four patients was also studied preoperatively by left

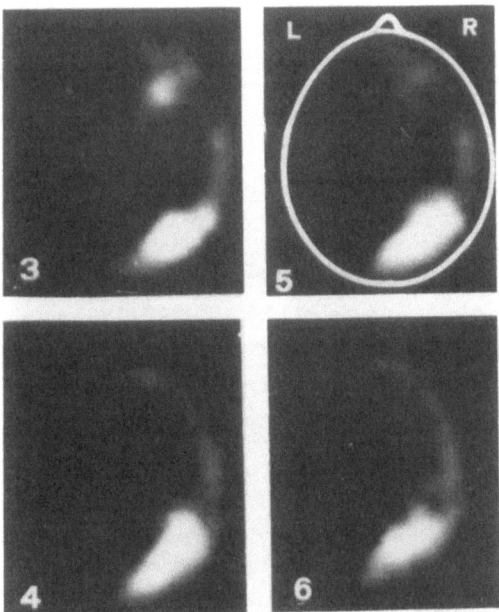

Fig. 25-3. Postoperative tomographic rBP study obtained by ^{81m}Kr continuous infusion into the common carotid artery on the bypass side. Patient with ICA occlusion and revascularization of 1 cortical MCA area. Four axial sections showing the "cortical" flow distribution. Static lateral view and angiogram from this patient are reproduced in Fig. 25-2 (left).

ICA ^{81m}Kr infusion, that is, contralaterally to the occlusion side. She was studied postoperatively by both right and left common carotid infusion. On the preoperative study, some perfusion could be shown to the right sylvian regions. On the postoperative study (obtained on the left side) there was no perfusion whatsoever to the areas corresponding to the territory of the MCA (Fig. 25-6).

Discussion and Conclusions

The results in this series of patients indicate that postoperative patency of the bypass is achieved in approximately 90% of the cases; this percentage becomes even higher if later angiographic studies are considered.

This confirms the possibility that a nonfunctioning bypass may become patent with time. Possible causes of transient postoperative occlusion of donor artery have been extensively

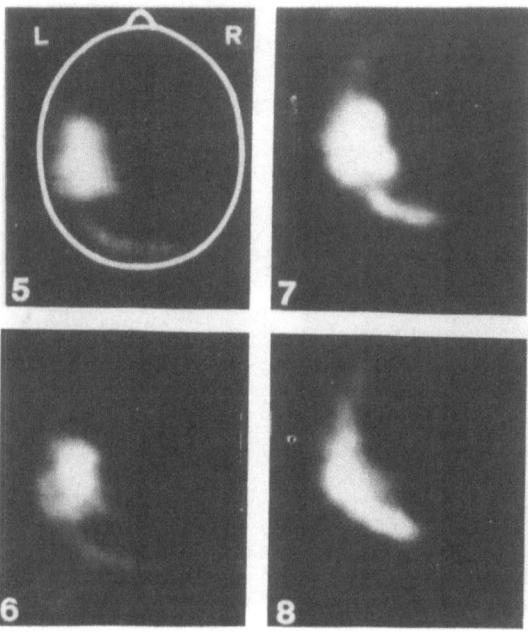

Fig. 25-4. Postoperative tomographic rBP study obtained by ⁸¹ᵐKr continuous infusion into the common carotid artery on the bypass side. Patient with ICA occlusion and revascularization of 4 cortical MCA areas. Four axial sections showing relatively large areas of brain perfusion, which is present beyond the cortical areas to deeper subcortical structures. Static lateral view and angiogram of this patient are reproduced in Fig. 25-2 (right).

studied by Khodadad,[6] who indicated the spasm of the anastomosed arteries as a major cause of temporary occlusion. The degree of intracranial filling showed a large variability from patient to patient, as first reported by Anderson.[1] Most of our patients, however, showed 2 to 3 MCA cortical areas supplied by the bypass, thus confirming the focal distribution of the revascularization patterns after such an operation. Evaluation of the revascularization entity has been usually based on qualitative judgment of the angiograms.[2] The method here described and based on both the number of the MCA areas supplied and the revascularization of the proximal segment of the MCA, offers the advantage of major objectivity, so that different series could be eventually compared. Deruty et al.,[4] in their series of 14 patients, found some correlation between intracranial filling degree and the hemodynamic insufficiency demonstrated on preoperative an-

giograms. We did not find such a correlation. Also, intracranial filling does not seem related to the choice of the cortical branch for the bypass. Finally, as reported elsewhere in these Proceedings, intracranial fillings only partially correlates with pressure gradient between STA and cMCA. Thus, according to Holbach et al.,[5] the extent of the territory supplied by the bypass seems to depend mainly on the different anatomic configurations of MCA or possibly on the metabolic request. Data in the literature on the correlations between angiographic results and clinical outcome are still controversial. Our data seems to indicate the lack of such a correlation, in keeping with most other series published.[1]

Tomographic brain perfusion studies provide unique additional information on the flow distribution inside the hemisphere. For instance, we showed that, in the patients with the best filling, perfusion is present beyond the cortical areas to deeper subcortical structures, while this is not the case in patients with more limited filling at angiography. The tomographic approach also makes it possible to assess the actual brain volume perfused by

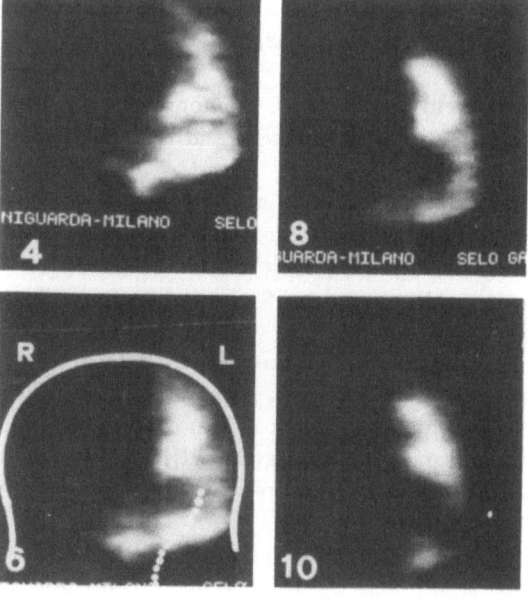

Fig. 25-5. Same case as in Fig. 25-4. Four coronal sections of tomographic rBP study. Also in these pictures there is evidence of subcortical distribution of the blood flow delivered by the shunt.

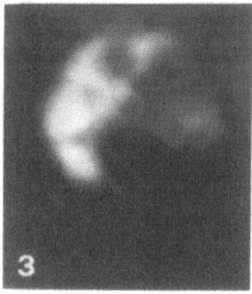 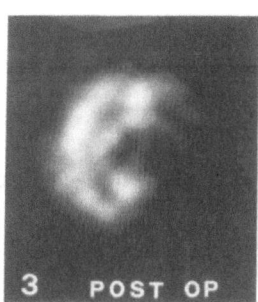

Fig. 25-6. Preoperative and postoperative tomographic rBP study obtained by intracarotid infusion of [81m]Kr from a patient with right ICA occlusion. On the preoperative axial section (left), obtained by infusing the tracer into the left ICA, some perfusion is present on the right sylvian regions. On the corresponding postoperative axial section (right), obtained by infusing the tracer into the left common carotid artery, there is no perfusion on the right MCA territory.

the blood after the bypass. This would not be possible with conventional methods of CBF measurements. Moreover, the redistribution of flow from the contralateral ICA after surgery, with a reduction of steal towards the territory of the occluded ICA, can be observed. The indirect evidence of this phenomenon has been previously provided by showing improvement of rCBF in the contralateral hemisphere following revascularization of the ipsilateral one.[3] From the clinical standpoint, however, further studies are necessary to establish if an assess-

ment of regional brain perfusion will provide important additional information for "better" management of the patient after surgery. On the other hand, these techniques might prove useful for the preoperative evaluation of patients, particularly to provide more detailed indication for surgery.

References

1. Anderson, R.E., Reichman, O.H., Davis, D.O. Radiological evaluation of temporal artery–middle cerebral artery anastomosis. Radiology, 113: 73–79, 1974.
2. Ausman, J.I., Latchaw, R.E., Lee, M.C., Ramirez-Lessepas, M. Results of multiple angiographic studies on cerebral revascularization patients. In Microsurgery for Stroke, P. Schmiedek, editor, Springer-Verlag, New York, 1977, pp. 220–229.
3. Austin, G., Laffin, D., Hayward, H. Microcerebral anastomosis for the prevention of stroke. In Microneurosurgery, H. Handa, editor, Igaku Shoin, Tokyo, pp. 47–67.
4. Deruty, R., Lecuire, J., Dechaume, J.P., Bret, Ph. Angiographic features of the cortical extra–intracranial anastomosis. In Microsurgery for Stroke, P. Schmiedek, editor, Springer-Verlag, New York, 1977, pp. 218–221.
5. Holbach, K.H., Wassmann, H., Bodosi, M., Bonatelli, A.P. Superficial temporal–middle cerebral artery anastomosis for internal carotid occlusion. Acta Neurochir 37:201–217, 1977.
6. Khodadad, G. Transient post-operative occlusion of the superficial temporal–middle cerebral artery branch anastomosis: Spasm, swelling or thrombosis. Surg Neurol 3:341, 1975.

26

Morphologic and Functional Correlates in Transient Cerebral Ischemia

P. Schmiedek, V. Olteanu-Nerbe, O. Gratzl, E. Kazner,
and F. Marguth

As the two extreme entities of clinical cerebral ischemia, we have transient cerebral ischemia (TIA) on the one side and the completed stroke syndrome (CS) on the other. The essential criterion for this classification, which also includes various other terms such as prolonged reversible cerebral ischemia (PRIND) and progressive stroke (PS), is based on the temporal profile of presenting neurologic symptoms following an ischemic event in the brain. Thus, in a completed stroke the resulting neurologic deficit is more or less definite and represents a stabilized condition. It is generally accepted and well documented in the literature, particularly since the introduction of CT scanning, that a completed stroke is associated with irreversible structural damage of the brain tissue.[1, 4] In contrast to this, the complete reversibility of neurologic symptoms within 24 hours, which by definition is characteristic of transient cerebral ischemia, would, at least theoretically, imply that there are no lasting functional or structural sequelae detectable within the brain beyond the given time period after an attack. Previous reports on this question, using either measurement of regional cerebral blood flow (rCBF) or CT scanning, have shown inconsistent results. Thus, Skinhøj et al. found focal rCBF abnormalities only during the first 1 to 4 days following a TIA,[11] whereas permanent CBF abnormalities are documented in other studies.[7, 12] In the present paper, a combined diagnostic approach was used employing cerebral angiography, CT scanning, and rCBF studies with the aim of detecting any persistent structural or functional changes in the brain of patients clinically exhibiting TIAs.

Clinical Material and Methods (Table 26–1)

The study concerned 20 patients who according to a careful inquiry demonstrated a history of TIA in the territory of one internal carotid artery. There were 5 females and 15 men, ranging in age from 18 to 70 years with a mean of 49 years. The neurologic manifestation of TIAs disclosed a wide spectrum of symptoms with pure sensory attacks without disturbances of motor function and patient reporting of transient episodes of combined sensory and motor dysfunction. In one patient the only manifestation was aphasia without sensory or motor involvement. Eight patients had only one TIA, 7 patients had 2 to 4 previous attacks, and 5 patients reported multiple TIAs. The duration of symptoms was less than one hour in 11 cases. Two patients reported a complete reversibility of symptoms within 24 hours. The interval between the last TIA and the time they were studied varied from one week to three months, with a mean of about five weeks.

In addition to cerebral angiography, which was performed via the transfemoral approach, all patients were examined with the CT

Table 26-1. Clinical data of 20 patients with TIA

Patient no.		Age	Sex	Neurologic manifestation	Total no. of TIAs	Duration of last TIA
1	Z.J.	55	M	weakness L leg	1	10 hr
2	R.F.	54	M	numbness R side, aphasia	1	30 min
3	K.K.	55	M	R hemiparesis	1	20 min
4	S.M.	57	M	numbness L arm	2	3 hr
5	M.H.	43	F	L hemiparesis	4	3 hr
6	T.R.	40	M	aphasia	1	2 hr
7	H.K.	47	M	L hemiparesis	2	10 min
8	B.W.	53	M	L hemiparesis	1	24 hr
9	W.U.	18	M	weakness R arm, aphasia	1	10 min
10	R.F.	49	M	numbness R hand, aphasia	1	20 min
11	C.G.	55	M	numbness and weakness L leg	multiple	20 min
12	S.U.	53	F	weakness A arm, aphasia	multiple	2 hr
13	G.H.	54	M	L hemiparesis	3	1 hr
14	S.A.	51	F	L hemiparesis	1	24 hr
15	E.H.	54	M	L hemiparesis	3	30 min
16	B.R.	49	F	numbness L arm	3	10 min
17	W.R.	28	M	weakness L leg	multiple	2 hr
18	F.T.	43	M	L hemiparesis	multiple	10 min
19	M.P.	70	M	L hemiparesis	2	10 min
20	S.T.	48	F	numbness R hand, aphasia	multiple	10 min

scanner, without using contrast enhancement, however. Measurement of rCBF was done with the intra-arterial xenon-133 injection method.[3] Isotope clearance was recorded by 16 small scintillation detectors arranged over the symptomatic hemisphere. The details of this technique have been previously described in detail.[8]

Results (Table 26–2)

Angiography

Nine patients had normal angiograms. Except for one patient with angiographic signs of generalized artherosclerotic brain vessel disease, all others had evidence of definite stenosis or obstruction of cerebral arteries. Internal carotid artery lesions were found in three cases. In seven patients the lesions were located within the middle cerebral artery distribution, four of them showing middle cerebral artery stenosis. A second angiogram in a 43-year-old woman revealed partial recanalization of a middle cere-

bral artery occlusion which had been demonstrated on her angiogram three weeks earlier.

CT Scanning

Thirteen of the 20 patients of this study had normal CT scans. The CT scan gave positive diagnostic information in seven patients. Two patients had areas of hypodensity within the cortical brain tissue suggestive of cerebral infarction. A so-called strategic infarction, which has been previously defined as a small, circumscribed area of low absorption value within the deep structures of the symptomatic hemisphere, was noticed in four patients.[9] The last patient had only indirect evidence of cerebral ischemia, showing enlargement of the ventricular system and slight cortical atrophy.

rCBF Studies

The highest percentage of positive results were obtained by rCBF studies, with only three

Table 26-2. Results of angiography, CT, and rCBF in 20 patients with TIA

Patient no.	Angiography	CT	rCBF	Bypass
1	MCA–BO	infarct	FR	
2	normal	normal	normal	
3	normal	infarct	FR	
4	ISA–SS	atrophy	RFR	+
5	MCA–O (R)	normal	FR	+
6	normal	normal	FR	
7	SVD	normal	RFR	+
8	MCA–BO	infarct	SGR	
9	normal	normal	normal	
10	normal	infarct	MGR	
11	ICA–O	normal	RFR	+
12	MCA–S	normal	FR	+
13	MCA–S	normal	FR	+
14	normal	infarct	FR	
15	normal	normal	RFR	+
16	normal	normal	normal	
17	ICA–SS	infarct	RFR	+
18	MCA–S	normal	FR	+
19	MCA–S	normal	FR	+
20	normal	normal	FR	

ICA–O = internal carotid artery occlusion; ICA–SS = internal carotid artery siphon stenosis; MCA–O = middle cerebral artery occlusion; MCA–S = middle cerebral artery stenosis; MCA–BO = middle cerebral artery branch occlusion; (R) = recanalized.

FR = focal reduction of CBF; RFR = relative focal reduction of CBF; MGR = moderate general reduction of CBF; SGR = severe general reduction of CBF.

+ Extra–intracranial bypass performed.

cases showing a normal CBF. Ten patients had a CBF pattern which has been termed focal reduction of CBF and which is defined as a normal hemispheric flow except for a specific ischemic focus with subnormal flow values in at least three adjacent measuring areas.[8] Relative focal reduction, which means a focal abnormality of CBF in addition to a hemispheric decrease of flow, was demonstrated in five patients. Thus, the majority of positive rCBF findings consisted of focal or predominantly focal lesions. More severe abnormalities were seen in two patients, one with a moderate general reduction, the other with a severe general reduction of CBF.

Comparative Analysis

The comparative analysis (Figs. 26-1, 26-2) of the three methods with regard to accuracy in detecting positive findings in patients with TIAs demonstrated the CT scan to be the least sensitive method, followed by cerebral angiography and the rCBF method. When cerebral angiography and the CT scan were taken together, 13 out of 20 patients were found to have morphologic abnormalities of either the cerebral vasculature or the brain tissue itself. In three cases with abnormal CT scans, angiography was reported to be normal. Of 17 cases with positive rCBF findings, seven were found to have abnormal CT scans and four had positive results on all three examinations. In three cases with positive rCBF findings, both cerebral angiography and the CT scan were normal.

In an attempt to find out whether the number or duration of previous TIAs had any effect on the rate of positive diagnostic findings, both factors were correlated separately with the results of angiography, CT scanning, and rCBF studies (Fig. 26-3). As a result it was found that it is not possible to predict with certainty

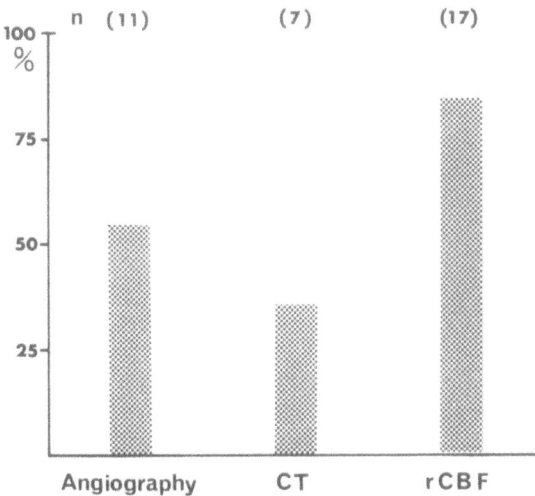

Fig. 26-1. Percentage of positive findings obtained by angiography, CT, and rCBF in 20 patients with transient cerebral ischemia.

the rate and degree of functional or morphologic abnormalities in the brain from the number or duration of ischemic episodes. A patient with one TIA of only short duration can have a positive angiogram, an infarction on the CT scan, and a clearly abnormal CBF result, whereas another patient with multiple TIAs of longer duration may have a normal angiogram and a normal CT scan.

Case Reports

Case 1 (Fig. 26–4)

A 55-year-old man was admitted to the hospital 10 weeks after he had a TIA on his left side with marked weakness in his leg which had lasted for about 10 hours. Following his complete recovery, he was asymptomatic and did not experience any further ischemic episodes. His neurologic examination was normal on admission, with no residual focal neurologic signs. Cerebral angiography was performed and demonstrated a middle cerebral artery branch occlusion on the right side. On his CT scan a large infarction area was found within the distribution of the inferior and posterior middle cerebral artery. In addition to the sharply circumscribed area of cavitation, there was an enlargement of the lateral ventricles. An rCBF study was done on his right side, showing very low flow values over the temporo-occipital region with normal or near-normal flow values over the rest of the hemisphere. When the study was repeated during CO_2 inhalation only the nonfocal areas exhibited the expected flow increase, with no reactive flow increase over the infarction area. Since these findings were interpreted as suggestive of a complete cerebral infarction with full functional compensation, bypass surgery seemed to be not justified and the patient was discharged from the hospital.

Case 17 (Fig. 26–5)

A 28-year-old man had 10 episodes of transient weakness in his left leg over a 6-month period prior to admission to the hospital. Each of the attacks had lasted for about 1 to 2 hr. He had been asymptomatic for the last three weeks. On right cerebral angiography a marked internal carotid artery siphon stenosis

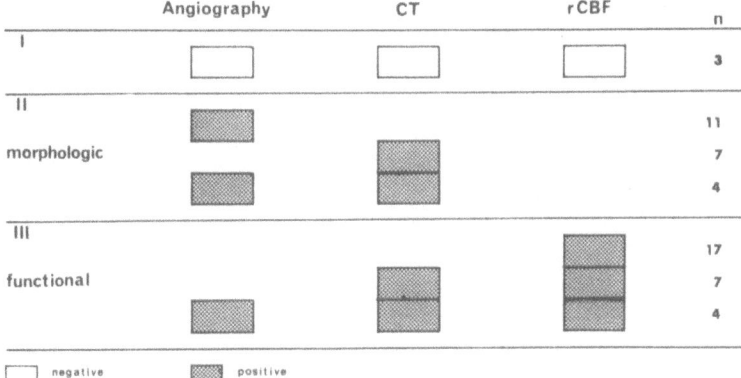

Fig. 26-2. Comparative analysis of positive findings obtained by angiography, CT, and rCBF in 20 patients with transient cerebral ischemia.

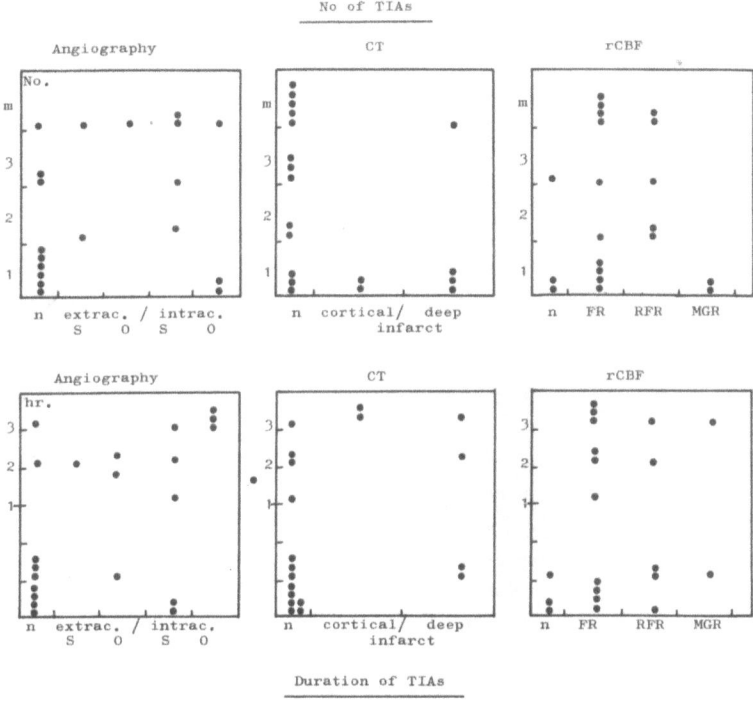

Fig. 26-3. Correlation of number (above) and duration (below) of ischemic episodes with results of angiography, CT and rCBF. n = normal; extrac. S/O = extra-cranial vessel stenosis/occlusion; intrac. S/O = intracranial vessel stenosis/occlusion; FR = focal reduction of CBF; RFR = relative focal reduction of CBF; MGR = moderate general reduction of CBF.

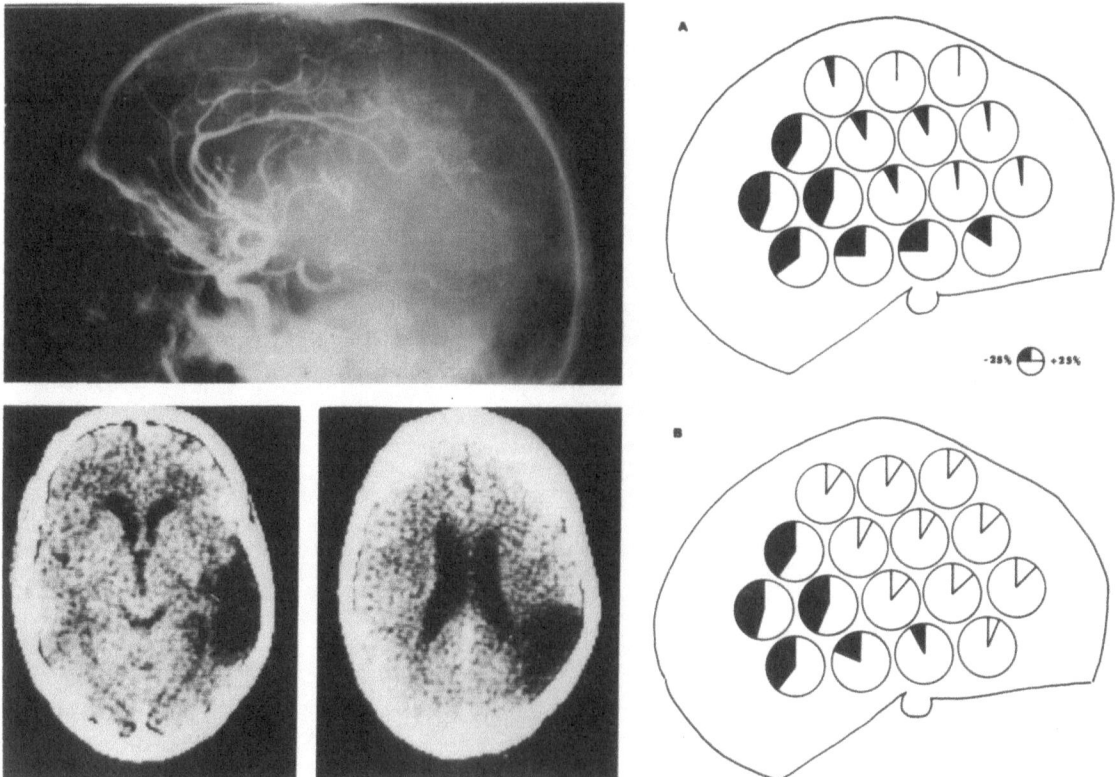

Fig. 26-4. Case 1. For details see text.

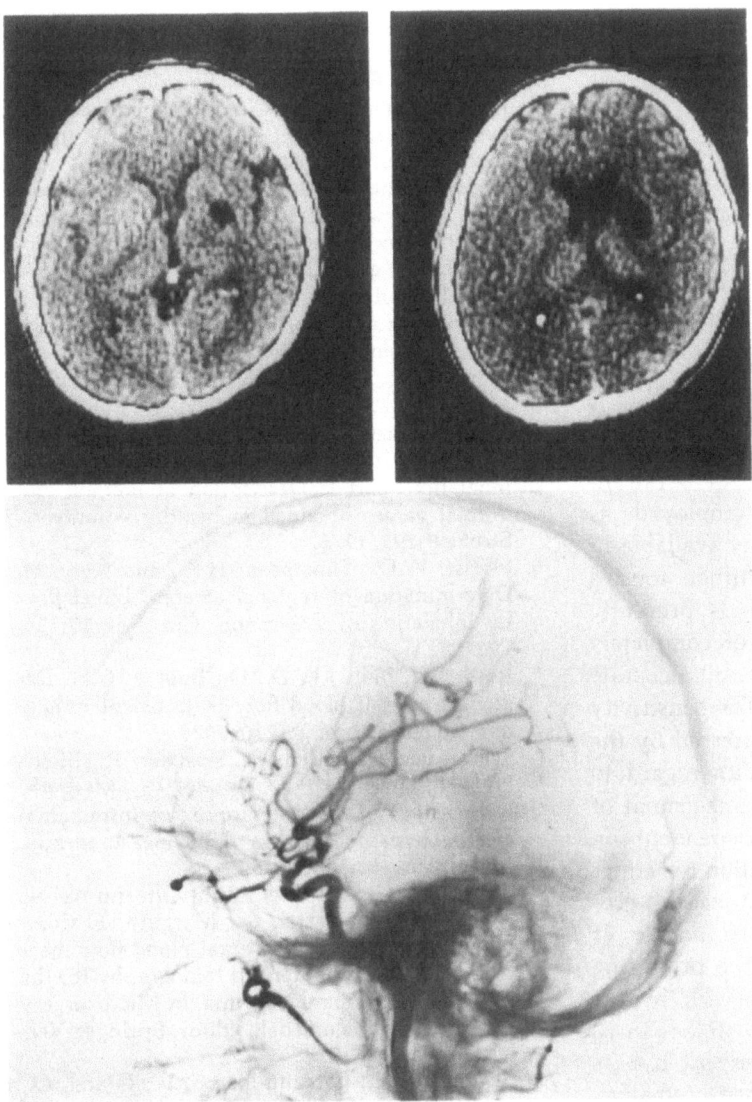

Fig. 26-5. Case 17. For details see text.

was demonstrated. The CT scan revealed a well-demarcated area of low absorption values deep in his right hemisphere. The rCBF study showed a relative focal reduction type of cerebral ischemia. In view of these results and his history of multiple TIAs, an extra–intracranial arterial bypass operation was done on the right side. The patient has remained asymptomatic over the last 12 months following surgery.

Discussion

From the evidence provided in this study it seems to be relevant to emphasize that tran-

sient cerebral ischemia has to be considered as a purely descriptive clinical definition. The term transient therefore is correct only with regard to the complete reversibility of focal neurologic symptoms within a 24-hr period. It does not mean, however, that the functional and structural integrity of the brain remains unaffected beyond this time limit. On the contrary, the present study showed permanent morphologic changes in seven patients as a result of previous TIAs. Even more striking was the finding of lasting functional abnormalities as reflected by rCBF studies in 17 patients of this series. It is unknown whether these changes of CBF are indeed permanent or could have been reversible over a longer period of time. The latter possibility, however, seems to be unlikely because the asymptomatic interval from the last ischemic episode was in the range of five weeks. Therefore, it must be assumed that the critical level to the actual vulnerability of the brain tissue is not the same as that which guarantees a normal neurologic function of the brain. The brain obviously can accommodate to a considerable reduction in flow and nevertheless continue to function at a normal rate.

The question then arises as to which are the clinical implications of this concept. First of all, this question would affect the diagnostic approach to patients with TIAs. Cerebral angiography should be routinely employed, as should CT scanning which is now available in most places. The ambiguous attitude toward the use of rCBF measurements is presently changing with the introduction of completely atraumatic techniques which permit accurate and rapid collection of data.[5, 6] The sensitivity of this technique is once again stressed by the results of the present study. With regard to therapeutic considerations, the management of patients with TIAs is largely dependent on angiographic findings. The indication for either vascular surgery or a revascularization procedure seems to be no longer a matter of debate, particularly in view of the promising results that have been obtained with bypass surgery.[2] Postoperative follow-up studies in 10 patients of this series who underwent bypass surgery revealed that all of them remained asymptomatic to date. Therapeutic concepts remain, however, controversial for those patients with TIAs who have normal cerebral angiograms. This, however, will be the subject of a separate communication.[10]

References

1. Davis, K.R., Taveras, J.M., New, P.F.J., Schnur, J.A., Roberson, G.H. Cerebral infarction diagnosis by computerized tomography. Am J Roentgengol 124:643, 1975.

2. Gratzl, O., Schmiedek, P., Spetzler, R., Steinhoff, H., Marguth, F. Clinical experience with extra–intracranial arterial anastomosis in 65 cases. J Neurosurg 44:313, 1976.

3. Hoedt-Rasmussen, K., Sveinsdottir, E., Lassen, N.A. Regional cerebral blood flow in man determined by intra-arterial injection of radioactive inert gas. Circ Res 18:237, 1966.

4. Kinkel, W.R., Jacobs, L. Computerized axial transverse tomography in cerebrovascular disease. Neurology 26:924, 1976.

5. Meyer, J.S., Ishihara, N., Deshmukh, V.D., Naritomi, H., Sakai, F., Hsu, M.-C., Pollack, P. Improved method for noninvasive measurement of regional cerebral blood flow by 133-xenon inhalation. Part I: Description of method and normal values obtained in healthy volunteers. Stroke 9:195, 1978.

6. Obrist, W.D., Thompson, H.K., and King, H. Determination of regional cerebral blood flow by inhalation of 133-xenon. Circ Res 20:124, 1967.

7. Rees, J.E., Bull, J.W.D., Du Boulay, G.H. Regional cerebral blood flow in transient ischaemic attacks. Lancet 2:1210, 1970.

8. Schmiedek, P., Gratzl, O., Spetzler, R., Steinhoff, H., Enzenbach, R., Brendel, W., Marguth, F. Selection of patients for extra–intracranial arterial bypass based on rCBF measurements. J Neurosurg 44:303, 1976.

9. Schmiedek, P., Lanksch, W., Olteanu-Nerbe, V., Kazner, E., Gratzl, O., Marguth, F. Combined use of regional cerebral blood flow measurement and computerized tomography for the diagnosis of cerebral ischemia. In Microsurgery for Stroke, P. Schmiedek, editor, Springer-Verlag, New York, 1977.

10. Schmiedek, P., Olteanu-Nerbe, V., Gratzl, O., Leschem, D., Marguth, F. Extra–intracranial arterial bypass surgery for cerebral ischemia in patients with normal cerebral angiograms. Chapter 41, this volume.

11. Skinhoj, E., Hoedt-Rasmussen, K., Paulson, O.B., Lassen, N.A. Regional cerebral blood flow and its autoregulation in patients with transient focal cerebral ischemic attacks. Neurology 20:485, 1970.

12. Wong, E., Bull, J.W.D., Du Boulay, G.H., Marshall, J., Russel, R.W., Symon, L. Regional cerebral blood flow in completed strokes and transient ischemic attacks. Neurology 23:949, 1973.

VI

Technical Aspects

27

In-Situ Dissections of Brain with Emphasis on the Blood Supply at the Base of the Brain

Margaret M. Waddington

The purpose of this presentation is to illustrate the anatomy of the circle of Willis and origin of the arteries at the base of the brain in relation to the skull, cranial nerves, and brain by in-situ dissection with serial photographs and segmental resection of the brain. In the original presentation, colored photomicrographs of the specimens and line drawings to clarify the anatomy were used. In the printed presentation, only line drawings are submitted because the colored photomicrographs did not reproduce well in black and white.

It is hoped that this approach will impart a three-dimensional concept of this rather complex anatomy in a way not previously shown and thus facilitate the surgical approach in case of aneurysmal surgery or when microsurgical bypass procedures come under consideration. The dissections were carried out over a span of several years and were done at the Rutland Hospital, Rutland, Vermont on routine autopsy material.*

The next five illustrations are close-up views of a chiasmal dissection.

Because the posterior cerebral artery might become an implant site for possible bypass procedures, special interest may exist for the normal anatomy of it, and for this reason it will be summarized here. The basis for the findings are 50 hemispheric dissections. The anterior temporal artery of the posterior cerebral artery, in 60% of specimens, originates proximally prior to the division of the posterior cerebral artery into the medial and lateral branches. In 22% of dissections, this vessel originated as the first major branch of the lateral branch of the posterior cerebral artery. In 18% of specimens there was no well-defined anterior temporal artery coming from the posterior cerebral artery; rather, the temporal pole, in those instances, was entirely supplied by branches coming from the middle cerebral artery.

The middle temporal artery of the posterior cerebral artery is inconstant, present only as a clearly definable vessel in 20% of specimens. It may either originate as a separate vessel off the posterior cerebral artery prior to the major division into medial and lateral branches or, probably more commonly, constitutes one of the multiple bifurcations of the lateral branch. It is, however, in that circumstance, very difficult to know if it is a genuine middle temporal artery or indeed just one of the multiple divisions.

As for the medial branch of the posterior cerebral artery, it always divides into the calcarine branch and the parieto-occipital branch. These two vessels are constant.

*Dr. Philip G. Merriam, Chairman of the Department of Pathology, kindly assisted in the dissections and photography of the material. Without his generosity and enthusiasm in granting free access to his laboratory, this project would not have come about.

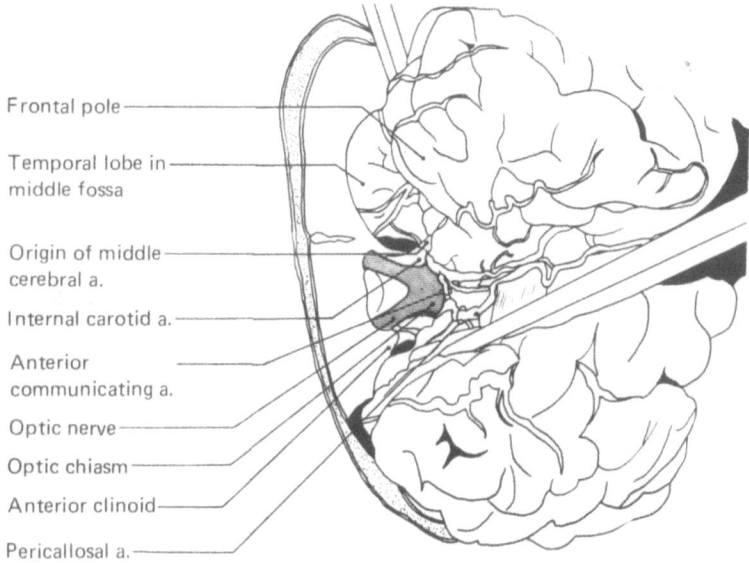

Frontal pole

Temporal lobe in middle fossa

Origin of middle cerebral a.

Internal carotid a.

Anterior communicating a.

Optic nerve

Optic chiasm

Anterior clinoid

Pericallosal a.

Fig. 27-1. Brain specimen in situ with skull particularly lowly resected at the base allowing maximal exposure of the frontal lobes. After removal of the dura, the frontal lobes were spread apart to show the relation of the internal carotid arteries and pericallosal arteries to optic nerve and chiasm. Proximal portion of corpus callosum is also exposed.

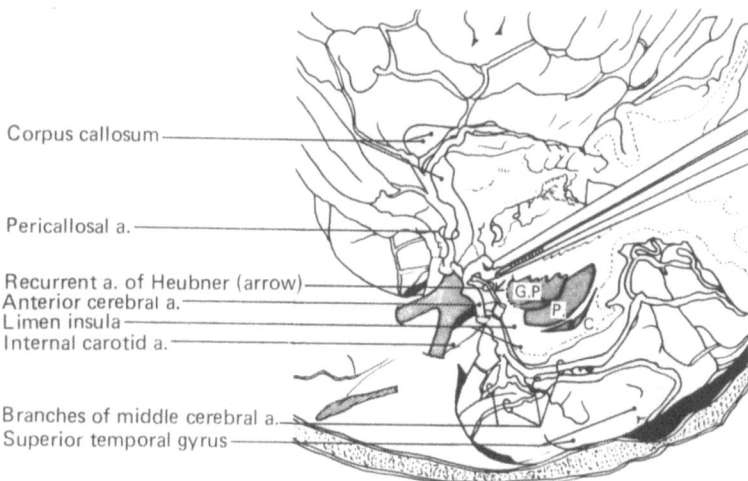

Corpus callosum

Pericallosal a.

Recurrent a. of Heubner (arrow)
Anterior cerebral a.
Limen insula
Internal carotid a.

Branches of middle cerebral a.
Superior temporal gyrus

Fig. 27-2. Same specimen with left frontal lobe removed and forceps on stump of left pericallosal artery. The right pericallosal artery is seen in semilateral projection. Origin of left middle cerebral artery, as well as its course around the limen insulae, can be seen. Several branches are running on the superior surface of the temporal lobe in the depth of the sylvian fossa. G.P. = globus pallidus; P. = putamen; C. = claustrum.

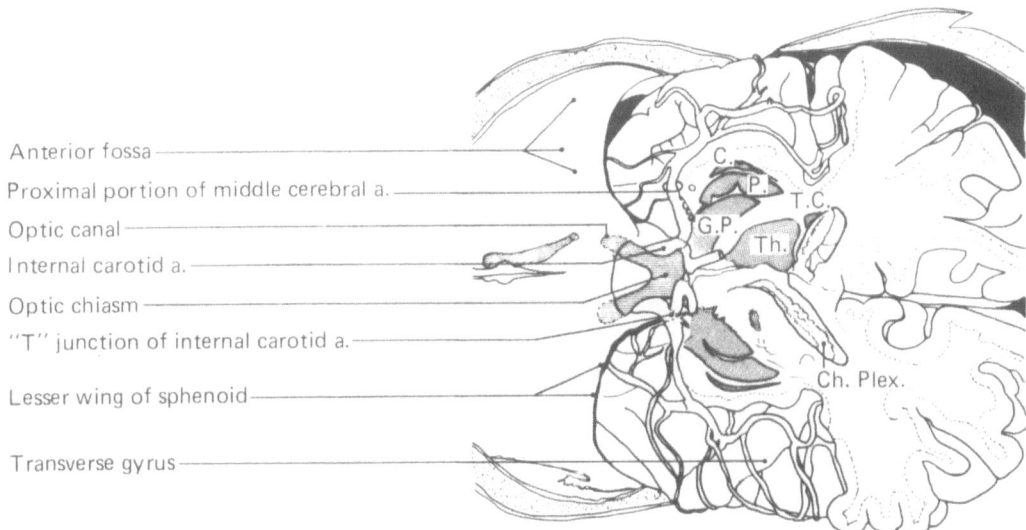

Anterior fossa

Proximal portion of middle cerebral a.

Optic canal

Internal carotid a.

Optic chiasm

"T" junction of internal carotid a.

Lesser wing of sphenoid

Transverse gyrus

Fig. 27-3. Both frontal lobes resected, exposing the middle cerebral arteries as they are usually seen in a vertex angiographic projection. C. = claustrum; G.P. = globus pallidus; P. = putamen; Th. = thalamus; T.C. = tail of caudate nucleus; Ch. Plex. = choroid plexus.

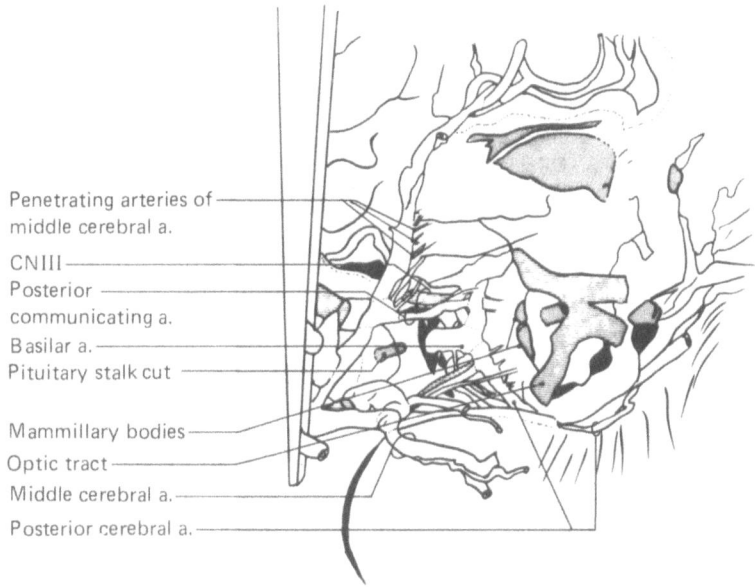

Penetrating arteries of middle cerebral a.

CNIII

Posterior communicating a.

Basilar a.

Pituitary stalk cut

Mammillary bodies

Optic tract

Middle cerebral a.

Posterior cerebral a.

Fig. 27-4. Same specimen with optic nerves cut and deflected posteriorly and left temporal lobe removed exposing the left posterior cerebral artery. Note relationship to optic tract and tentorium.

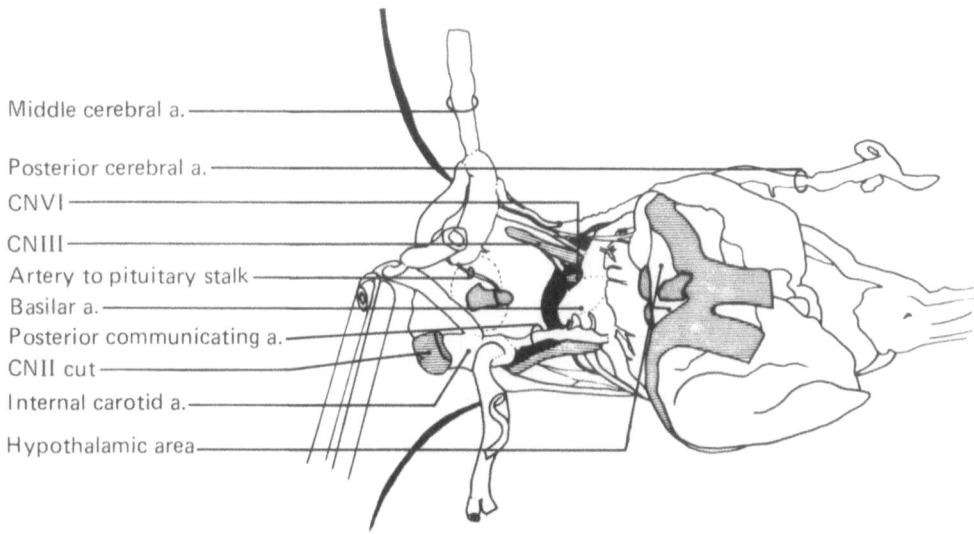

Middle cerebral a.
Posterior cerebral a.
CNVI
CNIII
Artery to pituitary stalk
Basilar a.
Posterior communicating a.
CNII cut
Internal carotid a.
Hypothalamic area

Fig. 27-5. Above specimen with both temporal lobes removed and brain stem retracted posteriorly exposing hypothalamic area, pituitary and circle of Willis in situ, as well as terminal portion of basilar artery. Note cranial nerves III and VI in relation to circle of Willis.

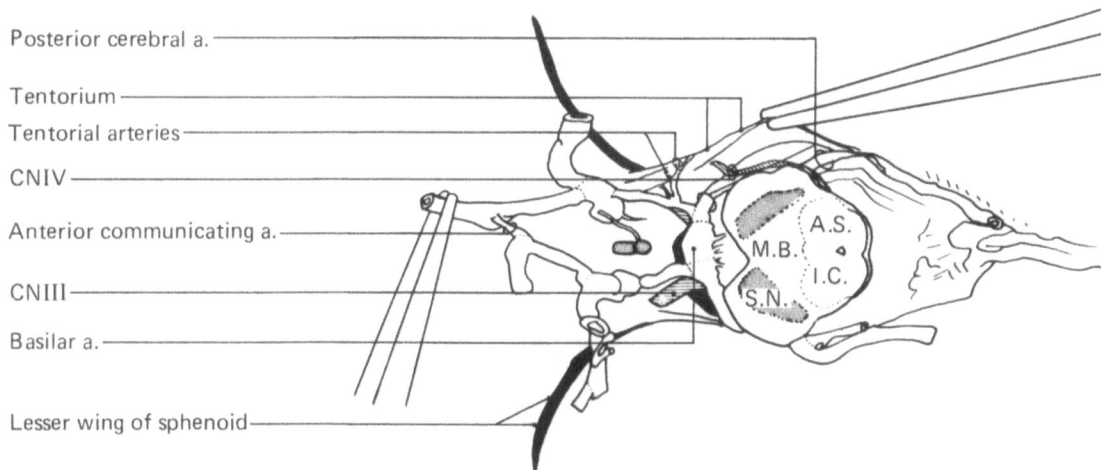

Posterior cerebral a.
Tentorium
Tentorial arteries
CNIV
Anterior communicating a.
CNIII
Basilar a.
Lesser wing of sphenoid

A.S.
M.B.
I.C.
S.N.

Fig. 27-6. Brain stem sectioned at the level of the midbrain. The tentorium is retracted exposing cranial nerve IV beneath the tentorium and superior to the posterior cerebral artery. M.B. = midbrain; S.N. = substantia negra; A.S. = aqueduct of sylvius; I.C. = inferior colliculi.

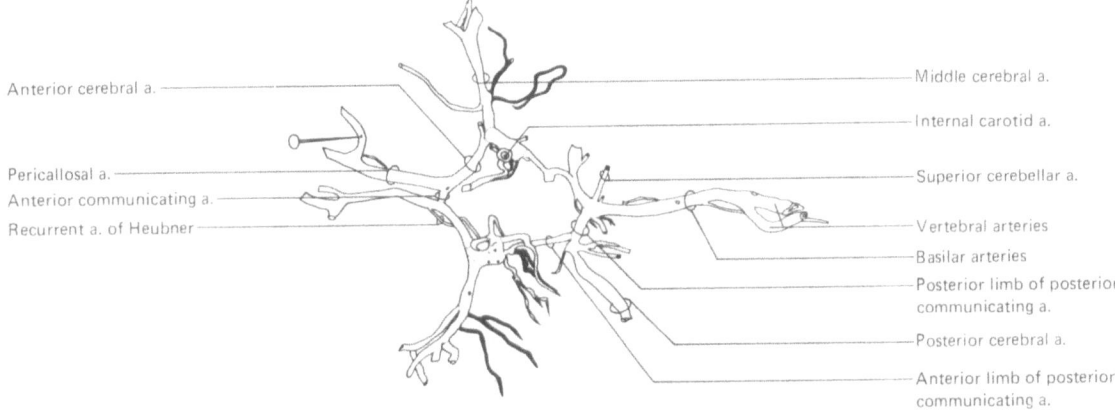

Anterior cerebral a.

Pericallosal a.
Anterior communicating a.
Recurrent a. of Heubner

Middle cerebral a.

Internal carotid a.

Superior cerebellar a.

Vertebral arteries
Basilar arteries
Posterior limb of posterior communicating a.
Posterior cerebral a.
Anterior limb of posterior communicating a.

Fig. 27-7. Standard dissection of circle of Willis after removal from cranial vault and brain.

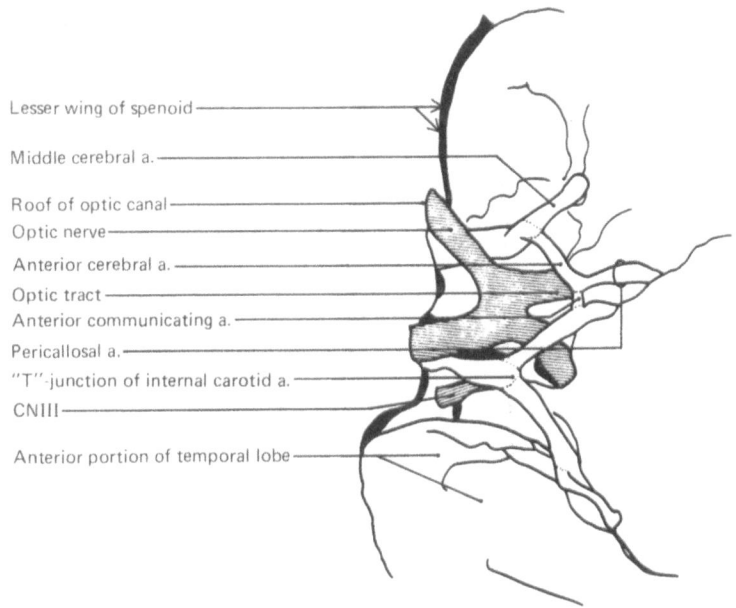

Lesser wing of spenoid

Middle cerebral a.

Roof of optic canal
Optic nerve

Anterior cerebral a.

Optic tract
Anterior communicating a.

Pericallosal a.

"T"-junction of internal carotid a.

CNIII

Anterior portion of temporal lobe

Fig. 27-8. Frontal lobes retracted in situ exposing T junction of internal carotid artery and optic chiasm.

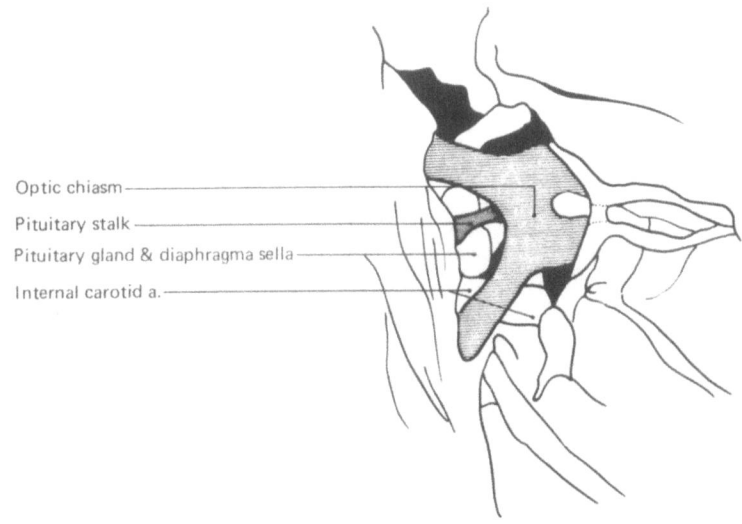

Optic chiasm
Pituitary stalk
Pituitary gland & diaphragma sella
Internal carotid a.

Fig. 27-9. With posterior retraction of brain, pituitary stalk and pituitary gland are visible. Note X formed by optic nerve and internal carotid artery lying inferiorly.

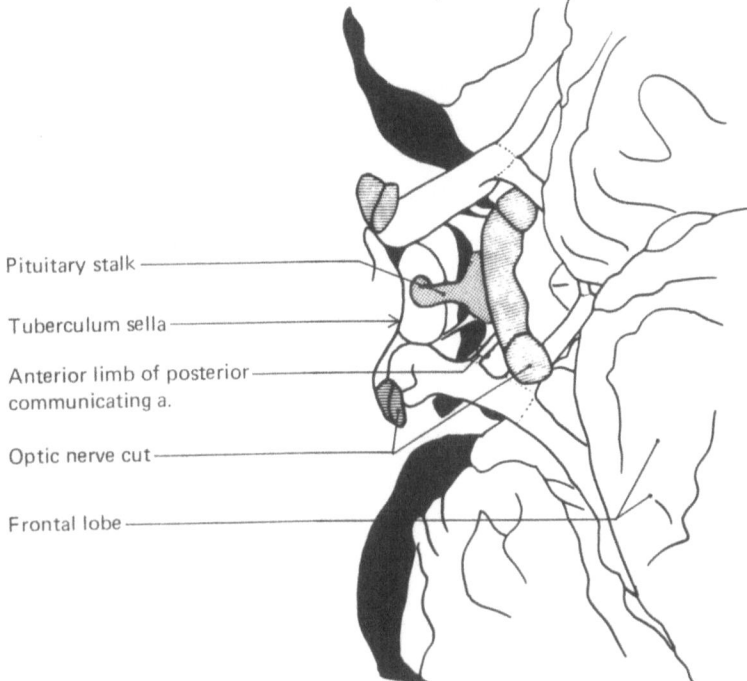

Pituitary stalk
Tuberculum sella
Anterior limb of posterior communicating a.
Optic nerve cut
Frontal lobe

Fig. 27-10. Optic nerves cut proximally and brain retracted posteriorly showing origin of pituitary stalk, hypothalamic area, and proximal origin of posterior communicating arteries off the internal carotid artery.

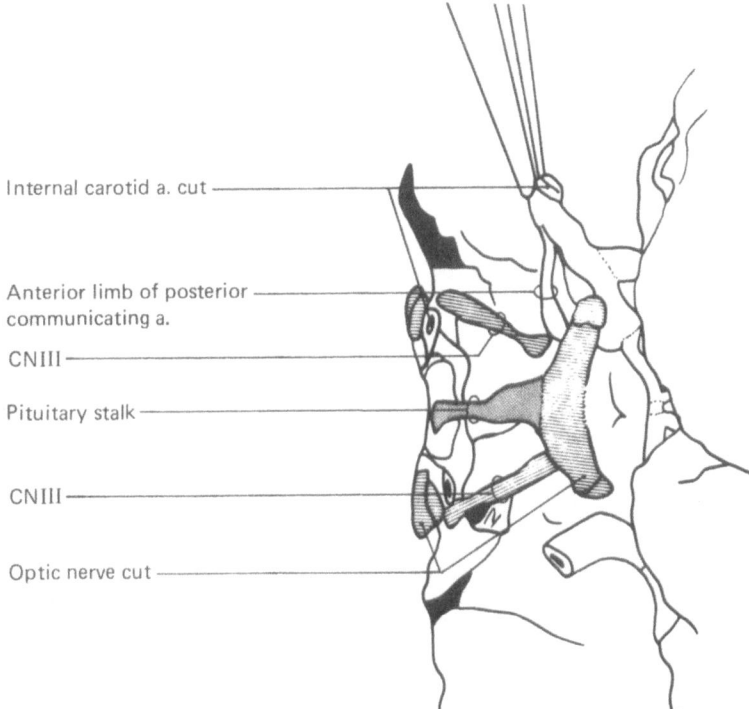

Internal carotid a. cut

Anterior limb of posterior
communicating a.

CNIII

Pituitary stalk

CNIII

Optic nerve cut

Fig. 27-11. Carotid artery sectioned proximally and retracted, exposing cranial nerve III.

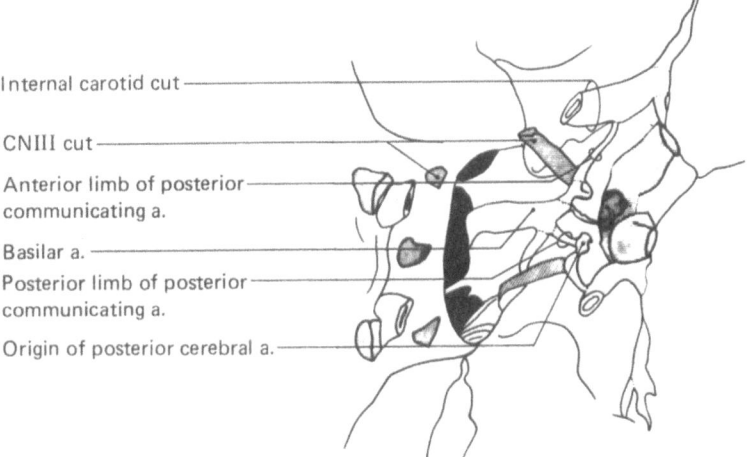

Internal carotid cut

CNIII cut

Anterior limb of posterior
communicating a.

Basilar a.

Posterior limb of posterior
communicating a.

Origin of posterior cerebral a.

Fig. 27-12. Pituitary stalk sectioned, exposing basilar artery and posterior portion of circle of Willis.

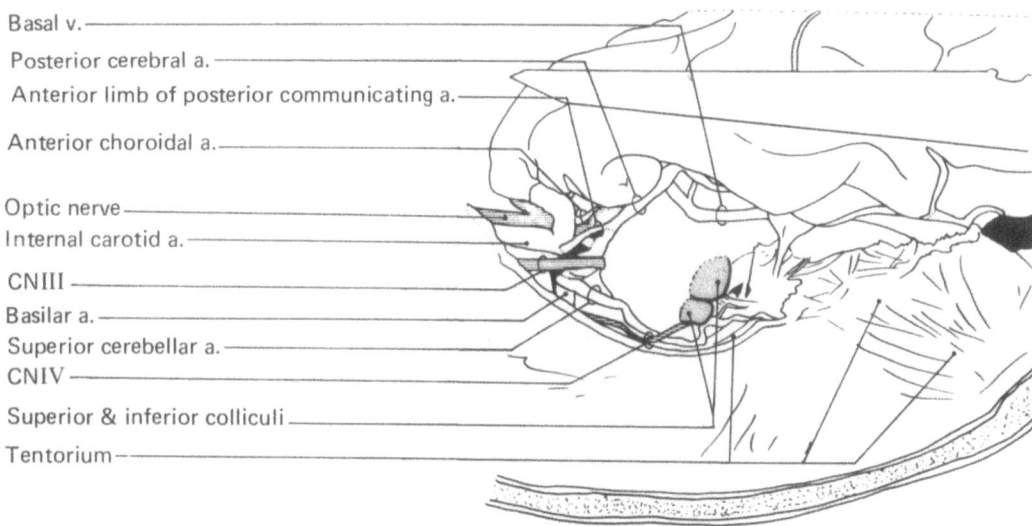

Basal v.
Posterior cerebral a.
Anterior limb of posterior communicating a.
Anterior choroidal a.
Optic nerve
Internal carotid a.
CNIII
Basilar a.
Superior cerebellar a.
CNIV
Superior & inferior colliculi
Tentorium

Fig. 27-13. Lateral approach to the brain stem by retraction of the right temporal lobe superiorly exposing cranial nerve III, cranial nerve IV, midbrain area, tentorium, and nearby arteries.

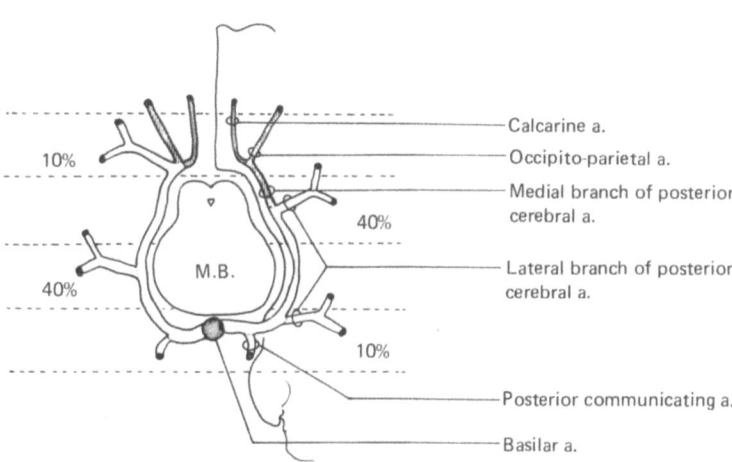

10%
40%
M.B.
40%
10%

Calcarine a.
Occipito-parietal a.
Medial branch of posterior cerebral a.
Lateral branch of posterior cerebral a.
Posterior communicating a.
Basilar a.

Fig. 27-14. Diagrammatic illustration of the division of the posterior cerebral artery into medial and lateral branches.

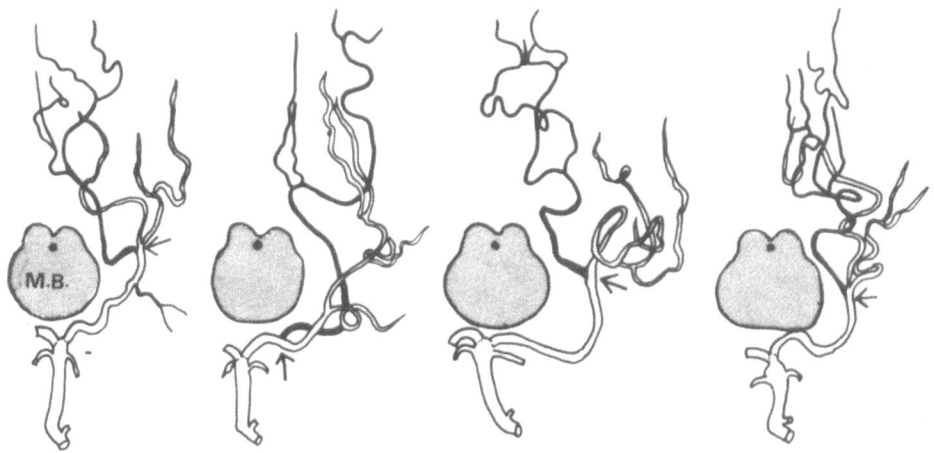

Fig. 27-15. Tracings from vertebral angiograms (AP views). The arrows point to the division of the posterior cerebral artery into medial and lateral branches. The medial branch is in solid black. From left to right, the first figure shows a late bifurcation, the next figure an extremely proximal bifurcation close to the origin off the basilar artery, and the next two figures the more common variants present in 80% with division along the lateral aspect of the brain stem. M.B. = midbrain.

28

Successful Adhesive Repair of Middle Cerebral Arteriotomy in Primates*

R. M. Crowell, R. B. Morawetz, T. H. Jones, C. F. Kieck, S. Hayashi, S. FitzGibbon, and U. de Girolami

The use of tissue adhesives in experimental[2, 5, 6, 16, 18-20] and clinical[1, 5, 7, 8, 15, 17] neurovascular surgery has been widely reported. Most reports have described extracranial vascular repair and intracranial aneurysm coating. Intracranial arteriotomy repair with tissue adhesives has rarely been reported.[1]

Experimental and clinical studies have shown ethyl cyanoacrylate (Aron Alpha) to be a particularly promising agent.[5, 11, 13, 20] Attractive features include rapid polymerization, easy application, and high tensile strength. Pathologic studies have shown persistence of the material at three years, normal healing, and virtually no inflammatory response in a variety of tissues including brain. Studies of Aron Alpha** in our laboratory have demonstrated good patency for longitudinal arteriotomy closure in rat carotid arteries. In these animals, minimal tissue reaction was observed on histopathologic and ultrastructural study. A recent report has indicated, however, tissue toxicity in cats from some samples of Aron Alpha.[4, 6] Only limited toxicologic data for Aron Alpha is available for primates, particularly with reference to major intracranial arteries.

We now report the long-term results of successful arteriotomy closure with Aron Alpha in the middle cerebral artery (MCA) of three Macaca irus monkeys.

Methods

Three macaque monkeys (Macaca irus), unselected for sex and weighing 3 to 5 kg, were used for these studies. We carried out transorbital MCA arteriotomy and closure with Aron Alpha. After one year of survival, we performed angiography, cerebral blood flow studies, and neuropathologic evaluation.

Surgery

Under general anesthesia (pentobarbital), monkeys underwent exenteration of the orbit and microsurgical exposure of the middle cerebral artery (MCA)[10] (Fig. 28-1). The MCA was carefully freed of arachnoid for about 1 cm distal from the carotid bifurcation. Scoville aneurysm clips were placed proximally and distally on the exposed MCA segment. A broken razor blade was used to make a 2-mm longitudinal arteriotomy. A small amount of bleeding occurred during the procedure because of retrograde flow through the intact MCA perforating branches. Arterial edges were coapted with slight eversion. A shunt was not used because of the confined area. Aron

*Supported in part by Teacher-Investigator Award NS-1101 (to Dr. Crowell) and a Stroke Center Grant from the National Institute of Neurological and Communicative Disorders and Stroke.

**Aron Alpha, Toagosei Chemical Industry Co. Ltd., Tokyo; distributed by Vigor Co., Division of B. Jaslow and Sons, Inc., New York, N.Y. 10010; supplied by Wm. A. Klinger and Son, 826 Sylvan, Milwaukee, Wisconsin, 52317.

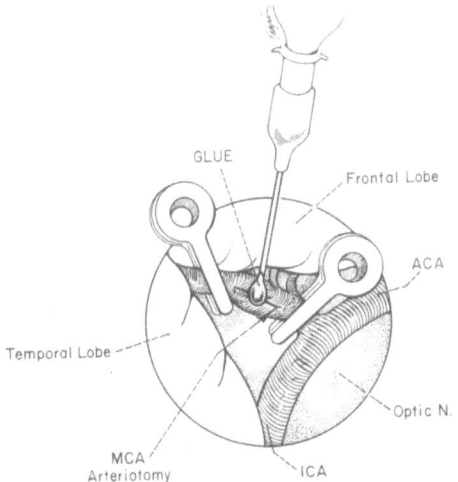

Fig. 28-1. Surgical technique. Transorbital approach to middle cerebral artery allows arteriotomy repair with tissue adhesive. Tuberculin syringe and 27-gauge needle permit precise application of 2 to 3 tiny droplets.

Alpha was applied to the arteriotomy. Using a tuberculin syringe with a 27-gauge needle, we applied 2 or 3 tiny drops of Aron Alpha to the arteriotomy site. After 3 to 5 minutes of polymerization, Scoville clips were removed. A piece of Gelfoam was placed over the craniectomy at the orbital apex, which was then sealed with dental cement. Soft tissue was closed with 4-0 silk sutures.

Neurologic Examination

After recovery from surgery, animals were examined in their cages for evidence of neurologic deficit.

Angiography

About one year after surgery, animals underwent transfemoral right carotid angiography. Under pentobarbital anesthesia, the left femoral artery was exposed and a preformed 2-gauge catheter was inserted. Under fluoroscopic control, the catheter was positioned in the internal carotid artery. After injection of 2 to 3 cc 70% Renografin, submental vertex and lateral magnified films were taken at 1-sec intervals over a 5-sec period. Subtraction

processing was carried out for detailed film analysis.

Local Cerebral Blood Flow Studies

Just after angiography, monkeys underwent stereotactic placement of platinum-iridium electrodes.* Two electrodes were placed in each hemisphere, one in posterior frontal gray matter and one in posterior white matter. Electrodes were made of 70% platinum and 30% iridium wire 0.010 inch in diameter, and coated with Teflon except for the terminal 2 mm. A femoroaortic catheter was inserted for blood pressure monitoring. A saphenous vein catheter was also introduced for infusions. Animals were placed in a primate restraining chair.

On the day following stereotaxis, unanesthetized animals underwent CBF studies. The hydrogen clearance method[14] was used to determine local CBF under control conditions and after administration of phenylephrine, trimethaphan, and CO_2.

Neuropathologic Examination

After completion of CBF studies, animals were anesthetized with pentobarbital. Transcardiac perfusion was accomplished either with 10% phosphate buffered glutaraldehyde (animal #3) or with 3% glutaraldehyde in cacodylate buffer (animals #1 and #2). The brain was removed, and both MCAs were excised together with adjacent brain from their origins out beyond the first bifurcation. The vessels from animal #3 were allowed to fix in formalin for 4 days, embedded whole in paraffin, then serially sectioned at 7-μm intervals and alternately stained with hematoxylin and eosin and elastic tissue/van Gieson stains. Selected sections were stained with phosphotungstic acid/hematoxylin, Holzer, and Masson stains. The vessels from animals #1 and #2 were cut transversely into 1-mm blocks and then were allowed to fix for 4 hours in glutaraldehyde. The specimens were then transferred to cacodylate buffer and embedded in plastic. Blocks were

*Rhodes Medical Instruments, Woodland Hills, California.

sectioned at 1-μm intervals, and sections were stained with toluidine blue. All brains were embedded whole in celloidin after severing the brain stem and cerebellum, and serial horizontal sections were stained with hematoxylin and eosin, cresyl violet, and Loyez (myelin), as previously described.

Results

During arterial surgery, cross-clamping times were 1 hour, 30 minutes, and 40 minutes. Animal #3 developed a right orbital abscess 10 months after surgery. This was drained and treated with systemic penicillin and streptomycin and local neomycin ointment.

Neurologic Status

During the follow-up period, all three animals remained neurologically intact.

Angiography

In all three monkeys, the MCA was patent without evidence of stenosis or aneurysmal dilatation (see Fig. 28-2). In satisfactory basal projections, available in two cases, the operated and unoperated sides could not be distinguished.

Local Cerebral Blood Flow Studies

Suitable local CBF determinations were obtained in cases #1 and #2. Operated and unoperated hemispheres showed similar basal flow and autoregulation characteristics (Table 28-1). After MCA repair with Aron Alpha, the two hemispheres showed similar increases in CBF response to inspired 7% CO_2. On both sides, gray and white CBF exceeded 200% of control (ipsilateral gray 200%, white 230%; contralateral gray 210%, white 280%).

Pathology

Gross Findings.   After removal of the brain in animal #3, it was clear that the infection was confined to the orbit; dense fibrosis excluded infection from the intracranial space. In all three cases, we observed fine adhesions overlying the MCA. Careful inspection of the MCA under the surgical microscope revealed

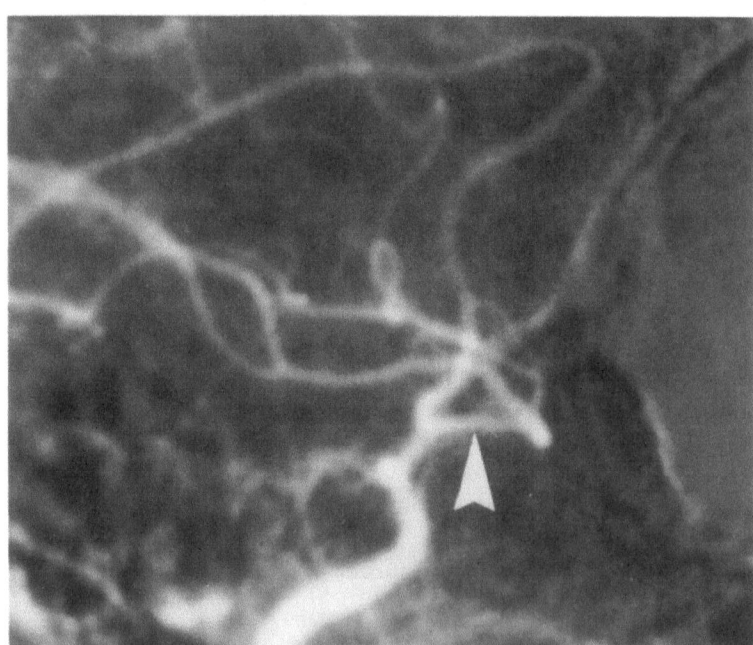

Fig. 28-2. Angiography. Right internal carotid angiogram of animal #2 shows patency at arteriotomy site (arrow). There is no narrowing or aneurysm formation.

Table 28-1. Preserved autoregulation after right MCA repair with ECA*

			93	105	120
	MABP (mm Hg)		93	105	120
(M1)	CBF (ml/100 g/min)	R gray	54	63	58
		white	21	21	22
		L gray	51	52	48
		white	42	46	38
	MABP (mm Hg)		73†	105	128
(M2)	CBF (ml/100 g/min)	R gray	28	50	56
		white	9	26	29
		L gray	48	98	96
		white	12	15	17

*Note that operated and control hemispheres maintain stable autoregulated CBF values except when marked hypotension † depresses CBF on both sides.

no irregularities, stenosis, or aneurysmal dilatation. The brains were normal.

Microscopic Findings. Serial sections through all three brains showed no evidence of abnormality. Neural tissue adjacent to the arteriotomy site (animal #3) showed no evidence of astrocytic proliferation, gliosis, or connective tissue reaction (Fig. 28-3). Histologic sections embedded in Epon demonstrated the arteriotomy site (Fig. 28-5). The internal elastic lamina was severed, and the gap between the severed ends was filled with smooth muscle cells. The adventitia showed moderate connective tissue proliferation with occasional foreign body giant cells around the adhesive mass. The vessel was patent throughout and somewhat wider in caliber at the arteriotomy site than in the contralateral MCA (Figs. 28-4, 28-5). The arteriotomy site was identified by demonstrating an interruption of the internal elastic lumen for approximately 10% of the artery circumference. In specimens embedded in plastic, the smooth muscle cells had all but disappeared, and the wall of the vessel was made up of acellular (presumably collagen) tissue. The intima was somewhat thickened,

and the lumen was lined by one or more rows of endothelial cells (Fig. 28-5). Ultrastructural studies of these vessels are in progress.

Discussion

Tissue adhesives have seemed promising for intracranial vascular surgery.[1, 5, 8, 15, 20] In 1956, Dutton reported the successful coating of an intracranial aneurysm with methylmethacrylate.[7] Experimental arteriotomies have also been closed with tissue adhesive.[2, 16, 19] Numerous adhesives have been investigated, including methylmethacrylate,[18] methyl-2-cyanocrylate (Eastman 910),[18, 20] Biobond,[17, 18, 20] and Aron Alpha.[5, 11, 18, 20]

Several problems have arisen with tissue adhesives. Methylmethacrylate, being hydro-

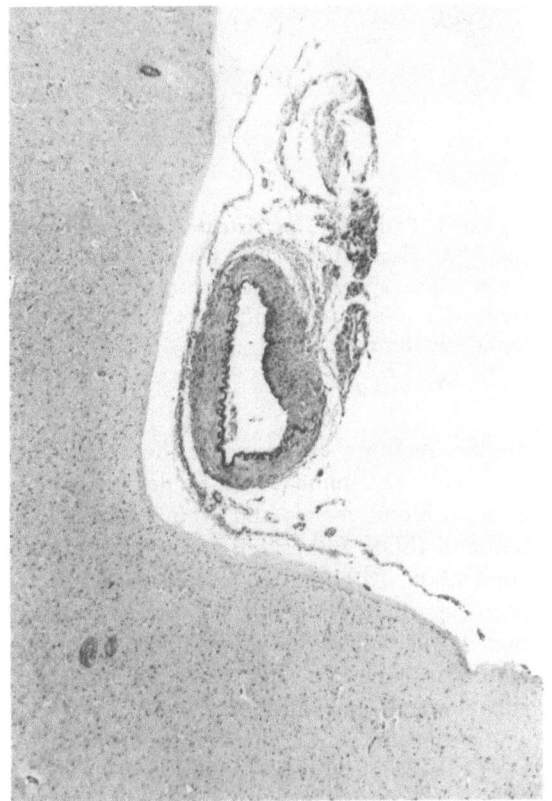

Fig. 28-3. Pathology: patency and minimal reaction. Animal #3, elastic tissue/van Gieson stain, × 15. Minimal leptomeningeal reaction is seen around a patent middle cerebral artery and normal overlying brain.

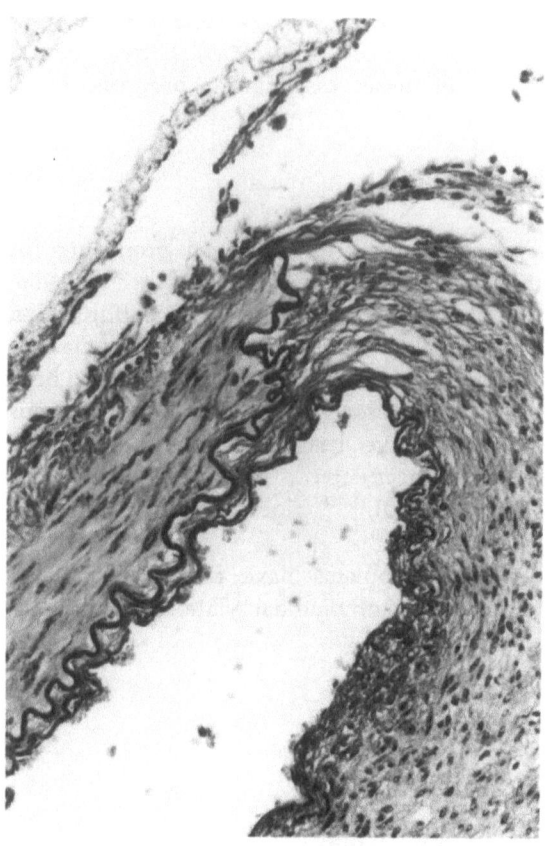

Fig. 28-4. Pathology: persistent Aron Alpha. Animal #3, elastic tissue/van Gieson stain, × 40. Aron Alpha appears as clear space just above artery wall. Note interruption of internal elastic lamina at top right.

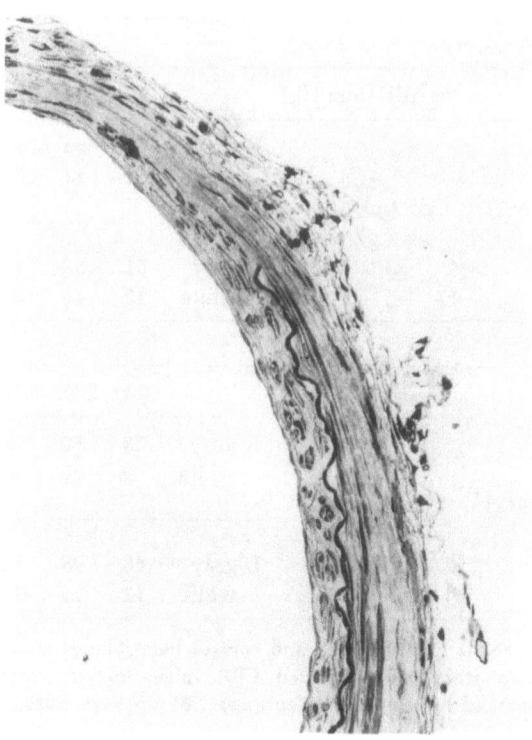

Fig. 28-5. Pathology: vascular healing. Animal #1, plastic embedding, toluidine blue stein, × 125. Note interruption of internal elastic lamina at top, thinning of vascular wall, and loss of smooth muscle cells.

phobic, requires air drying of the agent. Eastman 910 was found to be biodegradable and toxic to blood vessels and brain tissue.[3, 9, 18, 20] Biobond (EDH Adhesive) requires complicated application. Although no related neoplasm has been reported in the clinical situation, it is said that tissue adhesives cause fibrosarcomas in laboratory animals after 12 to 20 months of subcutaneous implantation.[12]

A promising new adhesive, ethyl cyanoacrylate (Aron Alpha), was introduced in 1965.[11, 13] This is a slightly viscous agent that polymerizes in 2 to 3 minutes in the presence of moisture. These properties permit accurately controlled application through a 27-gauge needle. A minimal cellular and macrophage response has been noted. The agent has an excellent adhesive strength, withstanding ten-

sion of up to 8200 g at 10 days and intraluminal pressures as high as 390 mm Hg.[16] It is not biodegradable, remaining intact in chronic experiments at one year. Experimental and clinical reports have indicated little reaction to the adhesive by blood vessels and brain tissue.[5, 20] Recently, however, Diaz et al.[6] reported that Aron Alpha refrigerated for five years caused marked inflammatory and degenerative changes in arterial wall and adjacent nervous tissue.

Earlier surgical reports dealt with successful sealing and anastomosis of extracranial vessels. Carton's early work showed that intracranial arteriotomies can be sealed with Eastman 910 monomer;[1, 2] however, this agent has proven toxic. Shintani et al.[16] sealed arteriotomies in 1-mm rabbit vessels, using microsurgical technique and a combination of stay sutures and Aron Alpha. Our earlier work on rat carotid artery (unpublished) showed that Aron Alpha without sutures or special instruments can yield successful sealing of arteriotomies with good patency. In rat carotid arteriotomies sealed with restricted Aron Alpha, gradual dilatation (with occasional aneurysm formation) occurred over time. In the present study, short MCA arteriotomies did not lead to aneurysm formation or to vascular occlusion. One year following arteriotomy the vessel wall contains a fibrous scar with lack of union between edges of severed internal elastic lamella and diminution of smooth muscle cells.

Our results indicate excellent functional results after MCA arteriotomy closure with Aron Alpha: neurologic examination, CBF studies, and angiography were indistinguishable from normal one year after adhesive repair.

In our pathologic studies of rat carotid artery and monkey MCA, adverse effects of Aron Alpha have not been seen. Aron Alpha has stimulated a minimal cellular subarachnoid reaction, with a few microphages and some giant cells present. The Aron Alpha has persisted intact up to 12 to 15 months. In monkey MCA, loss of smooth muscle cells and interruption of the internal elastic lamina at the arteriotomy site resulted in the formation of a fibrous scar in the wall of the vessel. This scar maintained the integrity of the vascular wall and led to minimal dilatation. Total restoration of intima occurred with moderate thickening and no significant luminal obstruction. The adjacent brain tissue showed no reaction to the glue. Neoplastic change was not observed.

Aron Alpha possesses, therefore, a number of properties favorable for clinical intracranial arterial repair. If individual samples of the material could be screened to eliminate toxic batches, perhaps clinical application could be recommended. Further experimental studies are clearly needed before the agent can be safely used in the operating room on a routine basis.

Conclusion

In three monkeys, short MCA arteriotomies were closed with ethyl cyanoacrylate (Aron Alpha). After one year follow-up, neurologic studies were normal, angiography showed wide patency in all three cases, and blood flow studies appeared normal. Pathologic examina-

tion showed widely patent vessels, persistence of the Aron Alpha, minimal arterial dilatation, and a fibrous scar in the vascular wall.

References

1. Carton, C.A., Heifetz, M.D., Kessler, L.A. Patching of intracranial internal carotid artery in man using a plastic adhesive (Eastman 910 adhesive). J Neurosurg 19:887–896, 1962.
2. Carton, C.A., Kessler, L.A., Seidenberg, B., Hurwitt, E.S. Experimental studies in surgery of small blood vessels. II. Patching of arteriotomy using a plastic adhesive. J Neurosurg 18:188–194, 1961.
3. Coe, J.E., Bondurant, C.P., Jr. Late thrombosis following the use of autogenous fascia and a cyanoacrylate (Eastman 910 monomer) for the wrapping of an intracranial aneurysm. J Neurosurg 21:884–886, 1964.
4. Chou, S.N. Use of cyanoacrylates. J Neurosurg 46:266, 1977.
5. Chou, S.N., Ortiz-Suarez, H.J., Brown, W.E., Jr. Technique and material for coating aneurysms. Clin Neurosurg 21:182–193, 1974.
6. Diaz, F.G., Mastri, A.R., Chou, S.N. Neural and vascular tissue reaction to aneurysm-coating adhesive (ethyl-2-cyanoacrylate). Neurosurgery 3:45–49, 1978.
7. Dutton, J.E.M. Intracranial aneurysm. A new method of treatment. Br Med J 2:585, 1956.
8. Handa, H., Ohta, T., Kamijyo, Y. Encasement of intracranial aneurysms with plastic compounds. Prog Neurol Surg 3:149–192, 1969.
9. Hoppenstein, R., Wesiberg, D., Goetz, R.H. Fusiform dilatation and thrombosis of arteries following the application of methyl 2-cyanoacrylate (Eastman 910 monomer). J Neurosurg 23:556–564, 1965.
10. Hudgins, N.R., Garcia, J.H. Transorbital approach to the middle cerebral artery of the squirrel monkey: A technique for experimental cerebral infarction applicable to ultrastructural studies. Stroke 1:107–111, 1970.
11. Inou, T., Masi, S., Mizuno, K., Ota, K. A new adhesive for vascular surgery. J Int Coll Surg 44:241–252, 1965.
12. Laskin, D.M., Robinson, I.B., Weinmann, J.P. Experimental production of sarcoma by methyl methacrylate implants. Proc Soc Exp Biol Med 87:326–332, 1954.
13. Ota, K., Mori, S., Koike, T., Inou, T. Blood vessel repair utilizing a new plastic adhesive. Experimental and clinical studies. J Surg Res 5:453–462, 1965.
14. Pasztor, E., Symon, L., Dorsch, N.E.C., et al. The hydrogen clearance method in assessment of blood flow in cortex, white matter, and deep nuclei of baboons. Stroke 4:556–567, 1973.

15. Selverstone, B., Ronis, N. Coating and reinforcement of intracranial aneurysms with synthetic resins. Bull Tufts N Engl Med Cent 4:8–12, 1958.

16. Shintani, A., Zervas, N.T., Kuwayama, A. Rapid microvascular repair using plastic adhesive. Stroke 3:34–40, 1972.

17. Sugar, O., Tsuchiya, G. Plastic coating of intracranial aneurysms with "EDH-adhesive." J Neurosurg 21:114–117, 1964.

18. Tsuchiya, G., Sugar, O., Yashon, D., Hubbard, J. Reactions of rabbit brain and peripheral vessels to plastics used in coating arterial aneurysms. J Neurosurg 28:404–416, 1968.

19. Weinstein, P.R., Wilson, C.B. Nonsuture closure of small vessel arteriotomies. Surg Forum 20:447–449, 1969.

20. Yodh, S.B., Wright, R.L. Experimental evaluation of four synthetic adhesives for possible treatment of aneurysms. J Neurosurg 26:504–510, 1967.

29

A New Technique for the End-to-Side Anastomosis Between Small Arteries

C. A. F. Tulleken, P. Hoogland, and J. Slooff

The construction of an end-to-side anastomosis between arteries of small caliber, as in the extra–intracranial bypass procedure, will take, in experienced hands, about 25 to 40 minutes. During this period the receiving cortical artery is occluded. Since this artery is part of the leptomeningeal collateral circulation system, normally no local ischemia develops.

For an end-to-side anastomosis in the more proximal portion of one of the three main cerebral arteries (anterior, middle, and posterior cerebral) this occlusion period is much too long, since collateral flow at this level is insufficient.

The use of an intraluminar shunt, as in carotid endarterectomy, is technically difficult in vessels of this caliber and a sufficient flow can seldom be established.

We experimented with a new technique for end-to-side anastomosis between small arteries, in our experiments the carotid arteries of the rat (diameter 0.8 to 1 mm). This technique has the advantage of a very short occlusion time in the receiving artery.

Technique (Fig. 29–1)

The artery which receives the end-to-side anastomosis is dissected free, but care is taken to leave the adventitia intact. The distal portion of the artery used for the anastomosis is prepared as shown in Fig. 29-1. The distal

opening of this artery is enlarged by a longitudinal cut with a straight microscissors.

With about ten interrupted sutures of 10.0 Ethylon, which pass through all the layers of the donor artery but only through the adventitia of the receiving artery, the end-to-side

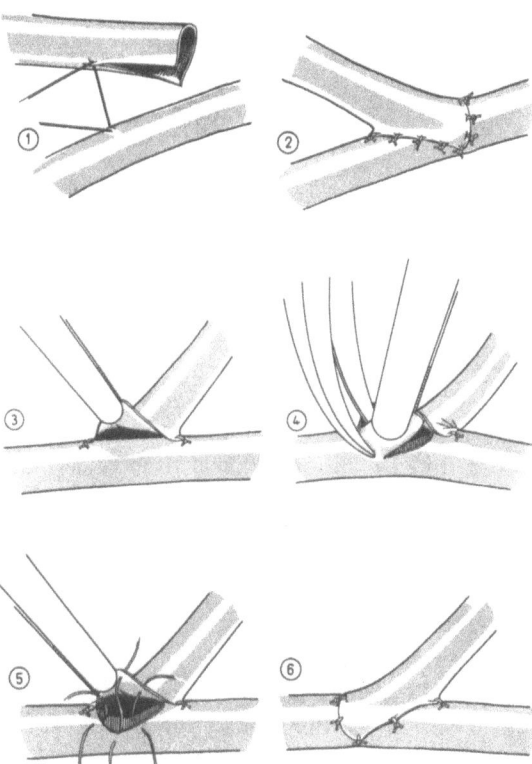

Fig. 29-1. Different stages of the new end-to-side anastomosis.

anastomosis is constructed for three quarters of its circumference. During this part of the procedure the lumen of the receiving artery remains patent and the flow in the artery is, therefore, undisturbed.

When the needle is inadvertently introduced into the lumen of the receiving artery, brisk bleeding occurs but can be easily controlled by gentle tamponade with Surgicel.

After completion of the end-to-side anastomosis for three quarters of its circumference, the receiving artery is then occluded by two microclips on both sides of the anastomosis.

With a microforceps the wall of the receiving artery is grasped inside the anastomosis, and with a curved microscissors a hole is cut which just fits in the anastomosis. The site of the anastomosis is now flushed with a solution of heparin in saline (0.25 ml heparin in 10 ml saline) and the anastomosis is completed with three sutures of 10.0 Ethylon, which pass through all the layers of the receiving and the donor artery. The clips are removed and gentle tamponade with Surgicel is exerted for 3 to 5 minutes at the site of the constructed anastomosis.

With some experience, the occlusion time of the receiving vessel necessary to complete the anastomosis is 5 to 7 minutes.

Methods and Materials

Acute Experiments

White Wistar rats weighing between 250 and 400 g, of both sexes, were used for the experiments. General anesthesia was introduced by an intraperitoneal injection of a solution of pentobarbital sodium in saline (1 ml pentobarbital in 5 ml saline), 0.5 ml per 100 g body weight. If necessary additional injections of this solution were given.

In a group of 25 rats acute experiments were performed till the technique described above was finally proved to be successful, at least up to one hour after completion of the anastomosis, when the animal was sacrificed.

Different types of end-to-side anastomoses were made: (1) part of the left common carotid (CCA) was used as a bypass on the right CCA;

(2) the left CCA was proximally ligated, cut, and connected end to side to the right CCA; (3) a CCA of one rat was taken out and connected end to side to both CCAs of another rat.

Chronic Experiments

In a group of 15 rats chronic experiments were performed to check the patency of this new type of end-to-side anastomosis on the long run.

In a group of 5 rats the left CCA was proximally ligated and cut, and connected end to side to the right CCA. In a group of 6 rats, the left CCA was partially taken out and used as a bypass on the right CCA using the new technique for one end-to-side anastomosis and the routine technique for the other. In another group of 4 rats the left CCA was used as a bypass on the right CCA, utilizing the new technique for both end-to-side anastomoses.

The animals were sacrificed between 6 hours and 3 months after the operation. The anastomoses were studied in four different ways: (1) inspection when the animal was still alive (pulsations, direction of flow) (all animals); (2) angiography (9 animals); (3) inspection of the anastomosis site at autopsy after opening of the arteries, with the aid of the operating microscope (all animals); (4) histologically (3 animals).

Results

(N.B. In 4 rats which were operated on for a chronic experiment, the anastomosis became, by a technical error, occluded in the immediate postoperative phase and the animals were sacrificed.)

In the first group (5 rats), the animals were sacrificed after 6 hours, 16 hours, 48 hours, 72 hours, and 23 days.

Inspection when the animals were still alive showed good pulsations and a normal direction of flow in each animal. Angiography was performed in three animals (48 hours, 72 hours, 23 days) and the anastomosis was shown to

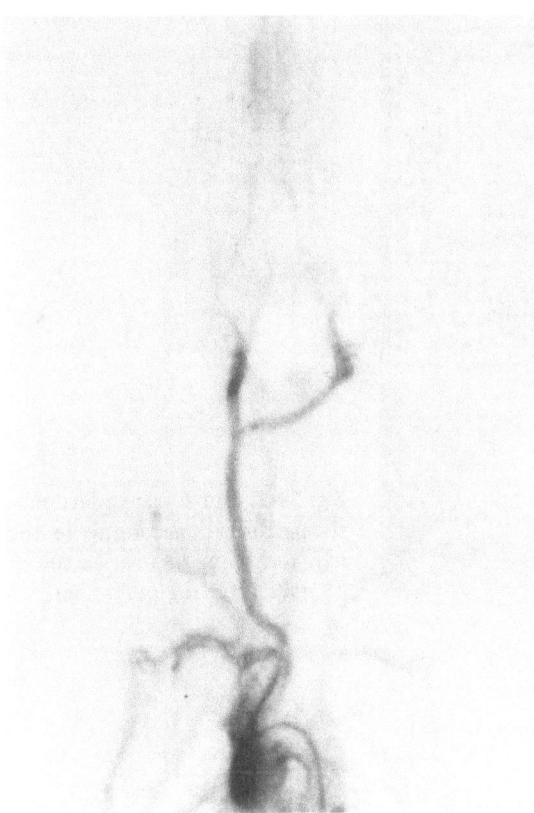

Fig. 29-2. Angiography performed 23 days after operation, where left common carotid artery is connected end to side to the right CCA utilizing the technique described in this communication.

be nicely patent (Fig. 29-2). Inspection of the anastomosis with the aid of the operating microscope at autopsy showed in each animal a patent anastomosis without any thrombus formation (Fig. 29-3).

In the second group (6 rats) the right CCA was ligated between the two anastomoses. The animals were sacrificed after 12 hours, 28 hours, 10 weeks, and 3 months (2 ✕).

Inspection during life showed good pulsations distally from the bypass and normal direction of flow in each animal. Angiography was performed in four animals (72 hours, 10 weeks, 3 months (2 ✕)) (Fig. 29-4). Inspection in autopsy with the operating microscope disclosed nicely patent anastomoses, without thrombus formation either on the proximal or on the distal anastomosis. Histologic examination was performed in two rats, which were sacrificed 10 weeks and 3 months postop-

eratively (Fig. 29-5). The dissected vessel was embedded in paraffin wax, cut in serial sections, and stained with hematoxylin and eosin and elastin/van Gieson. At the cardial site of the constructed anastomosis some intimal fibrosis was seen (Fig. 29-5(1)). This extended to the area where the incoming vessel was sutured (Fig. 29-5(2)) and disappeared gradually (Fig. 29-5(3, 4)). In none of the sections could occluding thromboses be found.

In the third group (4 rats), the right CCA was ligated between the two anastomoses. The animals were sacrificed after 8 hours, 48 hours, 8 days, and 5 weeks.

Inspection when the rat was still alive showed good pulsations distally from the bypass and a normal direction of flow in 3 of the 4 animals. In one rat (sacrificed after 48 hours) pulsations were noted in the bypass, but distally no pulsations were present, indicating an occlusion of the distal anastomosis. At autopsy a thrombus mass was found in the distal anastomosis and the proximal anastomosis was patent, without any sign of thrombus formation.

Angiography was performed in two rats. The bypass was shown to be patent in these animals.

Inspection of the anastomoses at autopsy with the microscope disclosed patent anastomoses, without any thrombus formation in the remaining three animals. Histologic examination of the anastomoses was performed in the rat which was sacrificed after 5 weeks. No thrombus was found at the anastomosis sites and the histologic findings were about the same as those shown in Fig. 29-5.

Discussion

The new technique for end-to-side anastomosis between arteries of small caliber described in this communication has the advantage of a very short occlusion period of the receiving artery: 5 to 7 minutes. As a consequence, this type of anastomosis can possibly be performed on the more proximal portion of the cerebral arteries where collateral flow is insufficient and therefore occlusion for a longer period of time is contraindicated.

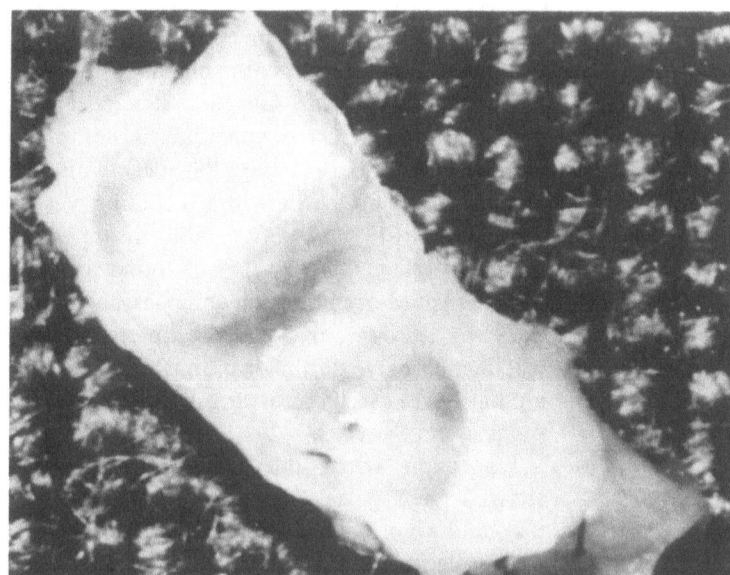

Fig. 29-3. End-to-side anastomosis performed according to the new technique in a rat sacrificed 23 days after the operation.

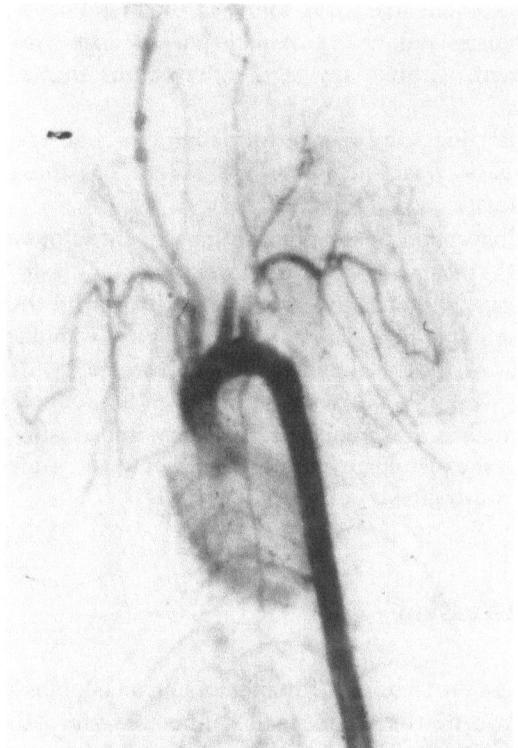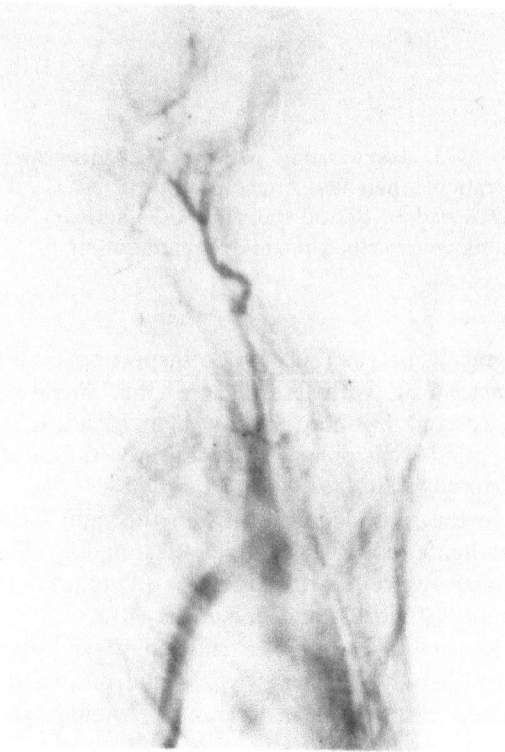

Fig. 29-4. Angiography (AP and lateral projections) performed 3 months after the operation, where left CCA is used as a bypass on the right CCA, which is ligated between the two anastomosis sites. The proximal end-to-side anastomosis is made with the new technique, the distal one with the routine technique.

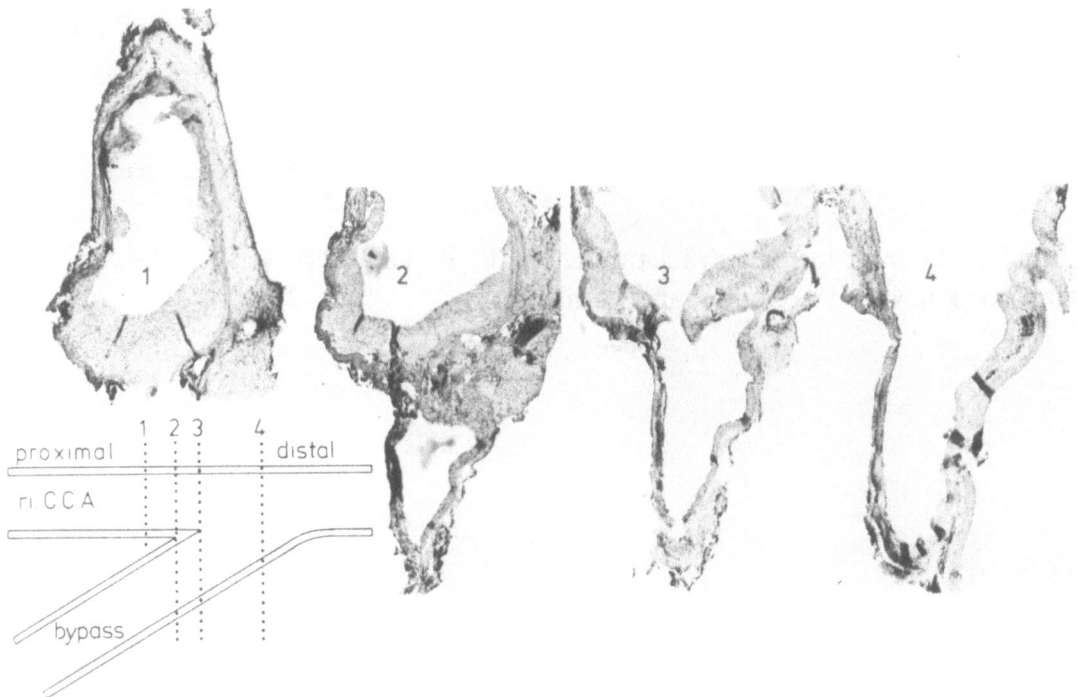

Fig. 29-5. Histologic examination of anastomosis 3 months postoperatively. 1. One-sided intimal fibrosis near the sutures, H & E × 40. 2. Suture area: intimal fibrosis in the receiving vessel, H & E × 40. 3–4. Area where the vessels are sutured, H & E × 40.

The experiments were started purely as a technical exercise and without much hope of obtaining a patent anastomosis, since at the site of the anastomosis the three layers of the receiving artery are exposed to the blood stream. A thrombogenic influence by adventitia and media was expected, but, to our surprise, when the operation was correctly performed no thrombus developed and the anastomosis remained nicely patent, as could be shown by angiography, at autopsy, and by histologic examination.

30

Safe Microclip Occlusive Force for Temporary Vascular Occlusion*

Manuel Dujovny, Norman Wackenhut, Ranjit K. Laha, Nir Kossovsky,
Debra Nelson, Carl W. Gomes, and Louis Leff

A need for refined techniques and instrumentation is becoming more apparent with the widespread application of microvascular procedures in neurosurgery. Commercially available microvascular clips currently recommended for temporary small artery occlusion have been substantially improved over the miniature aneurysm clips available previously. Nevertheless, some of these specially designed clips inflict considerable endothelial damage when applied temporarily to small arteries. To date, there are no standard guidelines for atraumatic vascular occlusion; even the minimal force necessary to occlude a small vessel is not known empirically. In our study we evaluated several commercially available temporary microclips in an attempt to determine the mechanism responsible for endothelial damage.

Materials and Methods

Fifty Sprague-Dawley rats, weighing between 350 and 500 g, were divided into five groups. The animals were anesthetized with pentobarbital (40 mg/kg intraperitoneally) followed by subcutaneous administration of 0.4 mg atropine. The ventral side of the neck was shaved and the carotid arteries were exposed

*Research supported by Grants-in-aid from the American Heart Association.

bilaterally through a midline incision. The right common carotid artery of each rat was dissected and occluded for one hour with the following temporary clips: group A, Acland; group B, Kleinert-Kutz; group C, Biemer; group D, Variangle; group E, Yasargil.

Following removal of the clips, blood flow was restored for 20 minutes. The left common carotid was used as the control. After placement of proximal and distal ligatures, the carotid arteries were excised under the Zeiss OPM 1 operating microscope ($\times 25$), opened longitudinally, and gently washed with Ringer's solution. The opened arteries were fixed with buffered 2% glutaraldehyde (pH 7.2) for five minutes, and stored in the same solution for 24 hours. The specimens were then dehydrated by serial passage through 30, 50, 75, and 95% ethanol. Preparation of the specimen for scanning electron microscopy included critical point drying with CO_2 for complete dehydration. Each specimen was then mounted on a circular aluminum stub and coated with gold palladium 100 to 400 Å thick in a vacuum chamber. The endothelial surfaces were examined at $\times$ 40 to 16,000 using a scanning electron microscope.[2] According to the technique described by Leffingwell, all specimens were later rehydrated and stained with H & E in preparation for light microscopy.[8]

The following criteria were considered when evaluating endothelial damage: displacement, flattening, disruption, fracture, swelling, crater and thrombus formation, and lesion location and configuration (corner mirror or transverse).

Results

The 50 control specimens showed a uniform architecture of fine longitudinal ridges and folds, measuring about 15 μm wide. Their smooth undulations comprised a "normal" pattern.

The specimens occluded for one hour with the temporary vascular clips presented endothelial damage of corner mirror or transverse configuration. The corner mirror lesions comprised damaged paired endothelial regions, situated across one another on the vessel diameter. The transverse lesions comprised two parallel lesions, oriented perpendicular to the artery and the endothelial ridge. Varying layers of endothelial damage, consisting of flattening, distortion of the endothelial folds, frac-

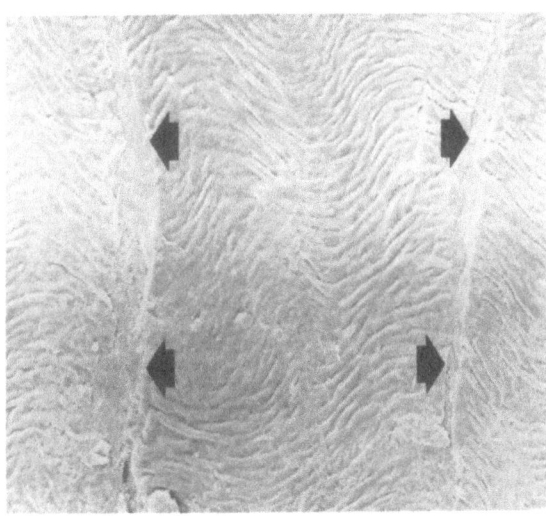

Fig. 30-2. Transverse lesion of two parallel grooves marking the boundaries of the clip blades.

ture, crater formation, and thrombus, were observed in all specimens (Figs. 30-1 to 30-3). The findings are summarized in Table 30-1.

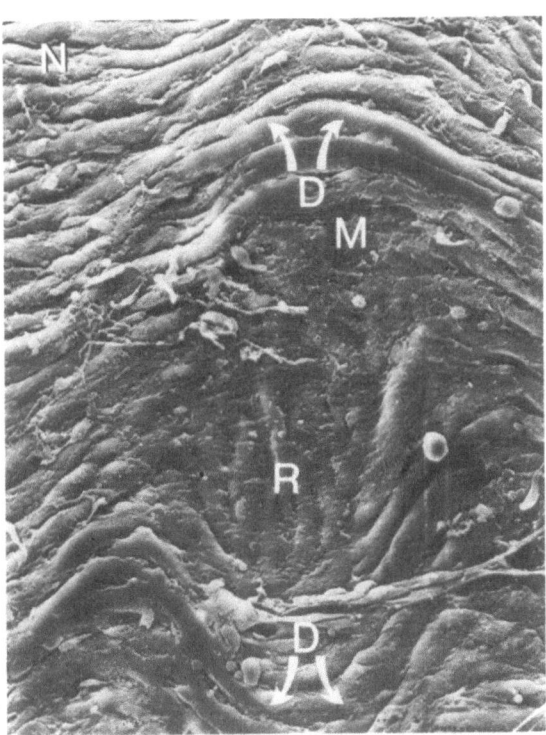

Fig. 30-1. Corner mirror lesion. Note displacement (D) and rearrangement (R) of endothelial ridges. M = missing patch where media is exposed, N = normal pattern.

Discussion

Although there are a number of commercially available clips for vascular occlusion, none is truly suitable for temporary use. The miniature aneurysm clips, originally intended for temporary use, apply too much force and result in severe endothelial and medial lesions with a positive threat for postoperative thrombosis.[1, 3, 5, 6, 9]

The newer temporary microclips, though said to apply considerably less pressure during occlusion, may still cause substantial endothelial damage and vessel thrombosis. The possible mechanisms of such damage are related to one of two clip lever designs: the pivot type or the alpha type. The pressure exerted on the vessel by these clips is not uniform along the blade. A corollary of Archimedes' law states that for a lever system the force exerted by the lever is inversely proportional to the distance from the fulcrum, i.e., $f = k/l$ where k is a work constant of proportionality. Thus, the force exerted by the blade near the fulcrum is much greater than the force exerted at the tips.

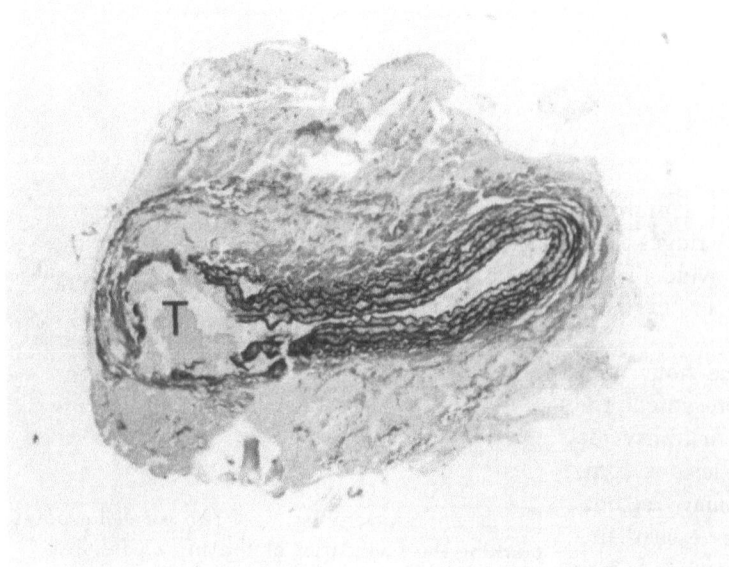

Fig. 30-3. Low-power photomicrograph showing aneurysmal lesion caused by destruction of the media. Note thrombus (T) which contains a small fragment of elastica. Verhoeff van Gieson's stain, × 32

The severity of endothelial lesions is therefore partially proportional to the proximity of the vessel to the fulcrum.

The configuration of the temporary clip producing transverse or corner mirror lesions was of particular interest. While the transverse lesions seemed to conform to the edge of the clip blades, the corner mirror lesions appeared at the points where the occluded vessel was folded sharply over itself.

Using a finite element technique, the stresses in a vessel wall from clipping action were determined by mathematical analysis. A computer simulation was modeled on a three-layered vascular ellipse. Vessel material properties suggested by Wiederhield et al.[10] and adapted by Hrico[7] were employed in a computer library program, PLNESS, available at the University of Pittsburgh Computer Center (Table 30-2).

Two types of clipping pressures were investigated. The first was a uniform compressive load of 2×10^6 dynes per unit width (simulating parallel closing clip jaws), with a simulated internal blood pressure of 120 mm Hg (Fig. 30-4). The second was a compressive load varying linearly from 2.5×10^6 dynes per unit width to 5×10^5 dynes per unit width (simu-

Table 30-1. Comparison of vascular injury with microclips

Clip	Acland	Kleinert-Kutz	Biemer	Variangle	Yasargil
Corner mirror lesion	6	7	4	8	6
Transverse lesion	4	3	6	10	4
Endothelium displacement	10	10	10	10	10
Endothelium flattening	10	10	10	10	10
Endothelium fracture	6	5	4	1	6
Crater	3	7	8	0	9
Thrombus	6	7	8	4	10

Table 30-2. Material properties

	Instantaneous Young's modulus $E \frac{dynes}{sq\ cm}$	Poisson's ratio (v)
Collagen A	50×10^6	0.48
Smooth muscle	30×10^6	0.48
Collagen B	5×10^6	0.48

lating a lever design clip) with an internal pressure of 120 mm Hg (Fig. 30-5).

In both instances, the calculated shear forces were very high at the points where the radius of curvature was the smallest. The analysis indicated that the inner layer of a vessel which is closest to the fulcrum receives the greatest amount of stress, and thus is most susceptible to damage.

There are several factors contributing to the adverse effects of the clips. Serrated blade clips with low closure force exert high pressure along the serrations. Another important factor is the rate of jaw closure during vessel occlusion. A rapid closure can cause greater insult to the endothelium, even though the static force of the blades might be very low.

Based on our observations of the injurious effects of excessive clamping pressure, an attempt was made to determine (1) the minimal occlusion force (MOF) necessary to occlude a blood vessel and (2) the relationship between

occlusion force and minimal endothelial damage.

The parameters considered for this purpose were vessel size, blood pressure, blade contact area, and vessel elasticity. The force that a clamp must exert to occlude small vessels comprises two components: it opposes (1) the internal blood pressure (BP) immediately under the clamp face and (2) the pressure on the area immediately adjacent to the clamp. The first force component is easily evaluated if it is assumed that the vessel circumference does not change as it is occluded. The flattened width thus becomes one half the vessel's interior circumference. The area under the clamp is then one half π times the inside diameter times the clamp width. This area multiplied by the internal blood pressure yields the force component for area 1 (Fig. 30-6); therefore:

$$F_1 = \frac{\pi}{2} D_i W_c BP$$

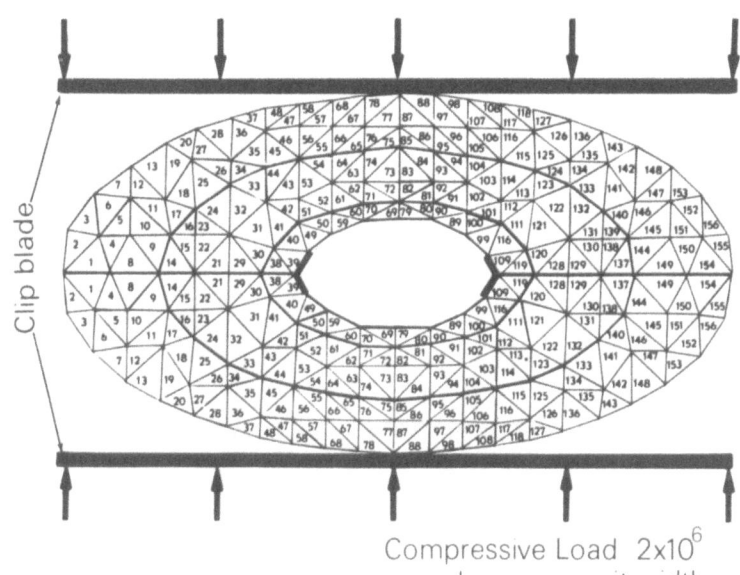

Clip blade

Compressive Load 2×10^6
dynes per unit width

Fig. 30-4. Finite element analysis of a vessel being occluded by a uniform parallel load. Critical stress regions are elements 38, 39, 109, and 119.

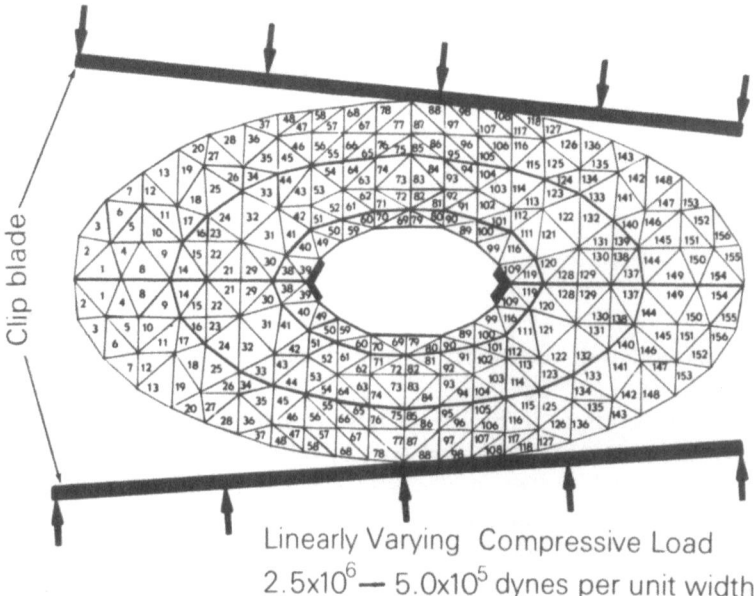

Linearly Varying Compressive Load

$2.5 \times 10^6 - 5.0 \times 10^5$ dynes per unit width

Fig. 30-5. Finite element analysis of a linearly increasing lever-type load. Greatest stress was on the inner boundary where the vessel folded over itself proximal to the fulcrum at elements 109 and 119.

The second force component opposes the pressure acting on the area immediately adjacent to the clamp (area 2). The magnitude of this second force is dependent upon the geometric shape of this region of the vessel when occluded, which in turn is related to the vessel's material properties. It can be shown that the force in the adjacent region is:

$$F_2 = \frac{\pi}{2} D_i^2 M BP$$

where BP is the internal blood pressure, D_i is the inside vessel diameter, and M, the shape factor, represents the number of diameters away from the clamp site that the vessel has

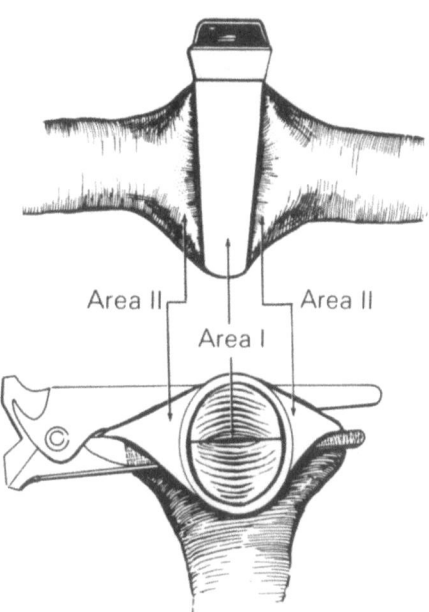

Fig. 30-6. Vessel wall deformation during clip application.

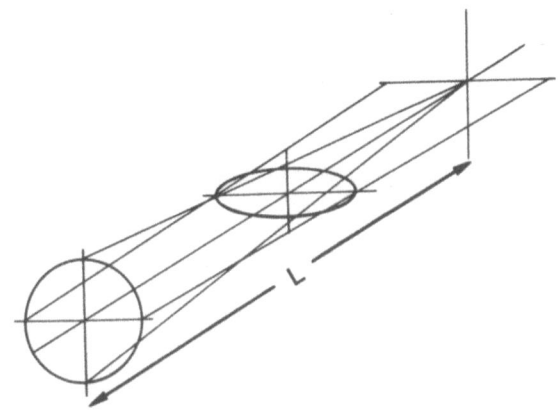

Fig. 30-7. The cross-sectional view of a clipped vessel progresses from a circle through an ellipse into a line at the clip blades. L is the distance from the clip edge to the point on the vessel where the cross section is restored to a circle.

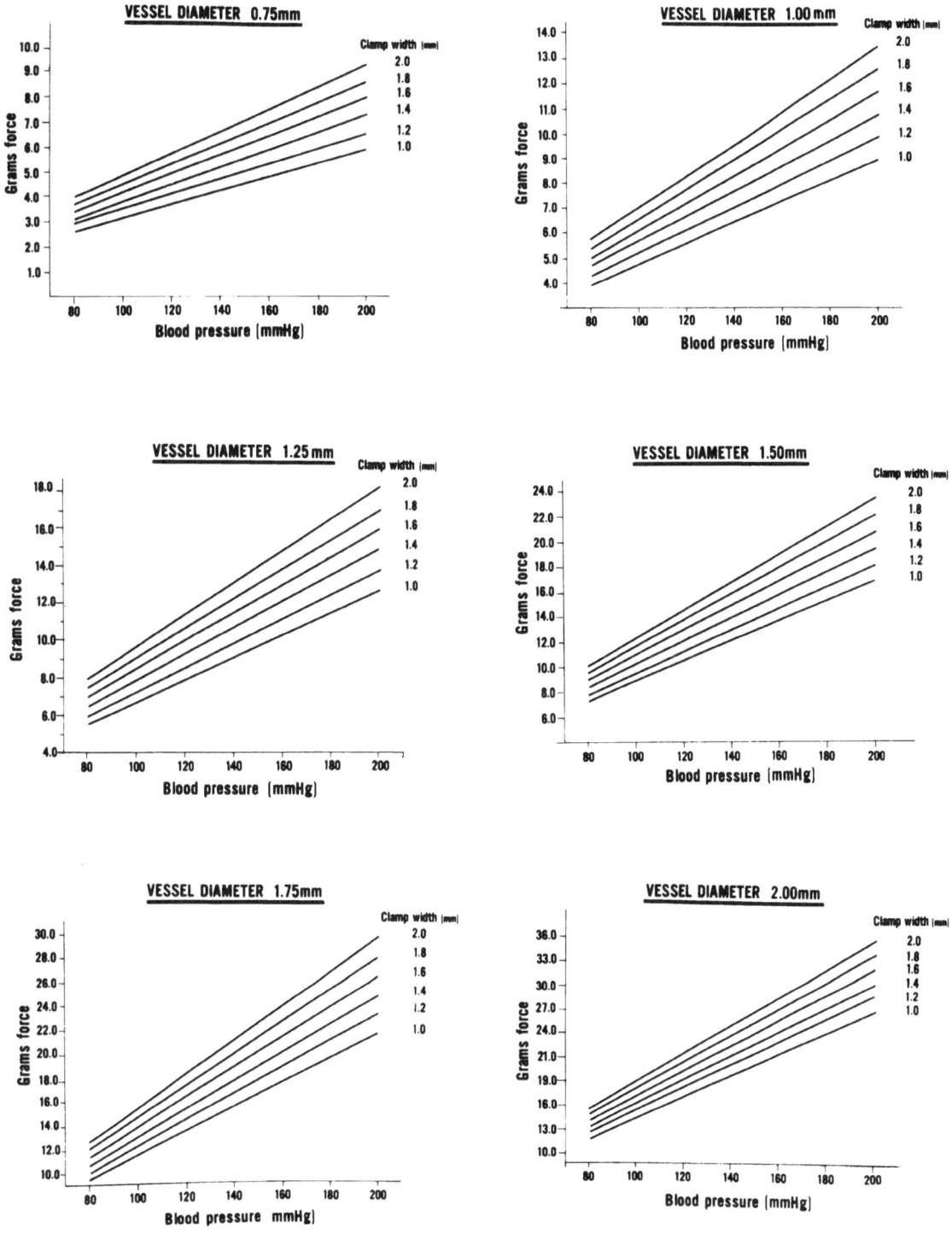

Fig. 30-8. Computer-generated theoretical minimum occlusion force (MOF) graphs for a variety of vessel diameters, blood pressures, and clamp blade widths.

regained its normal cylindrical shape. The shape factor can be expressed by:

$$M = \frac{L}{D_1}$$

where L is the distance from the clamp site to the point where the vessel regains its normal circular shape (Fig. 30-7). In a vessel that is pliable, the shape factor will be small because the vessel will remain cylindrical shape close to the clamp site, and the second force component will be insignificant. The shape factor, M, should be a function of blood pressure, vessel diameter, and material properties. The two force components can be combined to yield the total force necessary to occlude a blood vessel:

$$MOF = F_1 + F_2 = BP\,\frac{\pi}{2}\,D_1\,W_c + D_1^2\,\frac{\pi}{2}\,M$$

This equation models the problem more accurately than was possible with the law of Laplace.[3, 4]

By varying the diameter (D_1), the clamp width (W_c), and the blood pressure (BP), theoretical minimal occlusion force values were computer generated with M conservatively estimated as 1.0 (Fig. 30-8). With a variable-force clamp gauge (VFCG) similar MOF data were obtained in the abdominal aorta of the rat and the carotid artery of the guinea pig.

We found that the MOF varies according to the vessel diameter and blood pressure. For each vessel diameter (1.6 mm, 1.8 mm, 2 mm, 2.2 mm, and 2.4 mm), the MOF correlated linearly with blood pressure. The close relationship between theoretical and experimental results is shown in Fig. 30-9.

Our investigation showed that temporary vessel occlusion can be safely accomplished by applying only a minimal occlusion force. Occluding a vessel for periods up to one hour causes mild endothelial flattening and distortion, and forces of 50 g or more than MOF cause irreversible endothelial fracture and thrombus formation.

Acknowledgments

We thank George M. McManus for his scanning electron microscope expertise. We also thank the Department of Medical Media of the Veterans Administration Hospital of Pittsburgh, Pennsylvania.

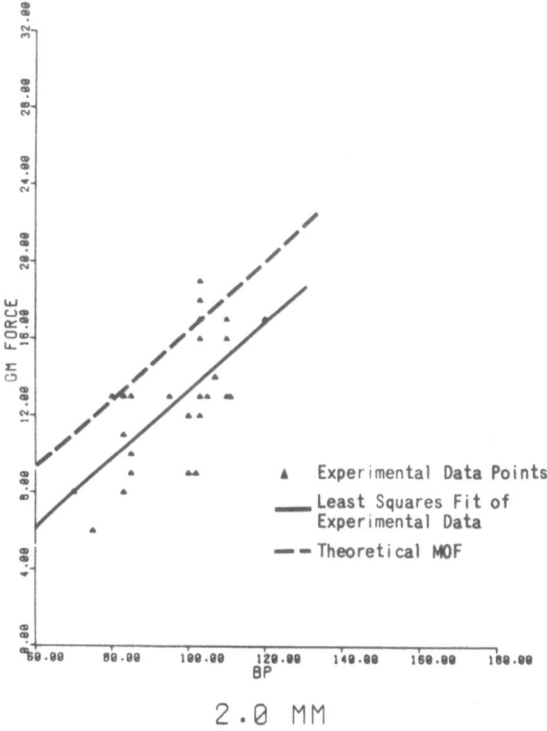

2.0 MM

Fig. 30-9. Correlation between experimental data and theoretical MOF calculations.

References

1. Dobson, R.E., Tagashira, Y., Chu, W.F. Acute ultrastructural changes in the middle cerebral artery due to the injury and ischemia of surgical clamping. Can J Neurol Sci 3:23–27, 1976.
2. Dujovny, M., Laha, R.K., Barrionuevo, P.J. Endothelial changes secondary to use of a Fogarty catheter. Surg Neurol 7:39–41, 1977.
3. Dujovny, M., Osgood, C.P., Barrionuevo, P.J., Perlin, A., Kossovsky, N. SEM evaluation of endothelial damage following middle cerebral artery occlusion in dogs. J Neurosurg 48:42–48, 1978.
4. Early, C.B., Fink, L.H. Some fundamental applications of the law of Laplace in neurosurgery. Surg Neurol 6:185–189, 1976.
5. Fox, J.L. Vascular clips for the microsurgical treatment of stroke. Stroke 7:489–500, 1976.
6. Gertz, S., Rennel, M.L., Forsea, M.S., Kawa-

mura, J., Sunaga, T., Nelson, E. Endothelial cell damage by temporary arterial occlusion with surgical clips. J Neurol 45:514–519, 1976.

7. Hrico, G.J. Finite element computer program for plane strain or plane stress analysis. Unpublished M.S. Thesis, Department of Mechanical Engineering, School of Engineering, University of Pittsburgh, 1976.

8. Leffingwell, H.A. Fossil polymorphs. In Principles and Techniques of Scanning Electron trand, New York, 1974, Vol. 2, pp. 150–162. Microscopy, M.A. Hayat, editor, Van Nos-

9. Thurston, J.E., Buncke, H.J., Chater, N.L., Weinstein, P.R. A study of microarterial damage and repair. Plast Reconstr Surg 57:197, 1976.

10. Wiederhielm, C.A., Kobayashi, A.S., Stromberg, P.D., Woo, S.L.Y. Structural response of relaxed and constricted arterioles. J Biomech 1:259–270, 1968.

31

The Influence of Adventitial Tissue to Healing Processes Following Microsurgical Interventions on Small Vessels

R. Meyermann, M. Nishikawa, and M. G. Yasargil

Since the development of microvascular surgery by Jacobson and Suarez,[6] a great number of technical details have been introduced to avoid the obstruction of the reconstructed vessel wall after operation. One of these is the complete removal of connective and adventitial tissue before the vessel wall is sutured. Sometimes clinical observations of patients who had undergone an extra–intracranial arterial bypass operation (EIAB operation) have demonstrated that there is a better postoperative anastomotic function if the superficial temporal artery (STA) was left embedded in connective tissue before being anastomosed to the middle cerebral artery (MCA). On the other hand, the successful treatment of patients suffering from cerebral ischemia has increased the number of patients selected for operation but has also increased the number of patients with very small arteries of the cerebral cortex. Thus STA–MCA anastomoses have to be performed using branches of MCA which may approach the minimal diameter for reliable patent anastomoses.[4] Therefore, all technical details have to be examined to determine if there is anything which facilitates the microsurgical procedure on the one hand but on the other has an unfavorable influence on the subsequent healing process, for the healing process is very important for the long-term result.

Experimental studies concerning the histology and ultrastructure of microvascular surgical anastomoses have not taken these problems into account.[1, 2, 8, 9, 14] Other studies of morphologic changes of the vessel wall following traumatic lesions examine only the tunica intima, sometimes the tunica media, but never the influence of the injured adventitial tissue over the intimal reaction.[3, 5, 7, 11, 15]

Material and Methods

In 3-month-old rats the adventitial tissue, including the vasa vasorum of the common carotid artery, was stripped off. Following this procedure the carotid artery was severed and end-to-end anastomosis was performed by means of microsurgical techniques.[16] This treatment was carried out on only one vessel of the animal. On the other side the adventitial tissue also was removed from the common carotid artery; however, the vessel was not severed. Always three of the animals treated this way were examined 1, 2, 4, 8, and 12 weeks after microsurgical intervention. The vessels taken out were neither fixed by perfusion nor washed out, in order to avoid artificial removal of loosely adhering coagulum. The material was fixed in buffered formalin (pH 7.4), embedded in paraffin, and cut into serial sections. Hematoxylin-eosin, azan, and elastic/van Gieson stains were prepared from these sections.

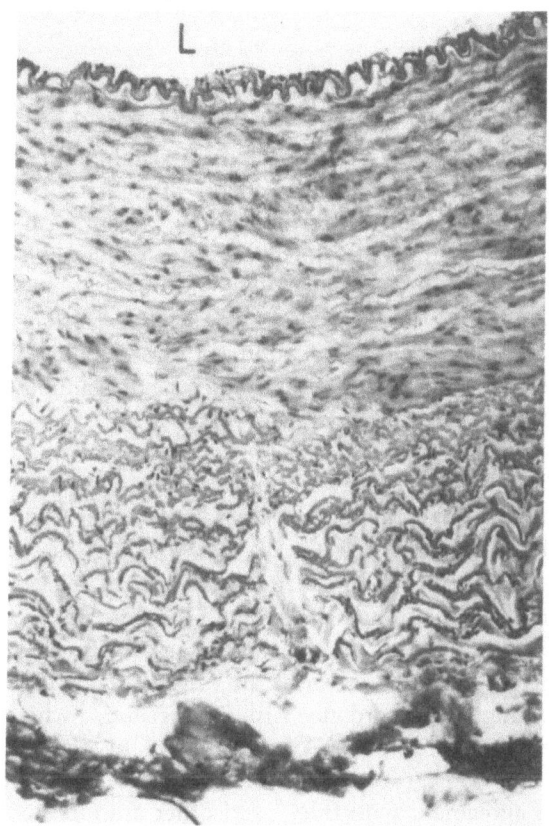

Fig. 31-1. Cross section of the common carotid artery of a 2-month-old rat. The adventitia is interlaced by small vessels, to supply the media. The intima consists of only one layer of endothelial cells. L = arterial lumen. H & E, × 140.

Results

In a normal carotid artery the cross section shows surrounding adventitial tissue of nearly the same extent as that of the inner layers of the vessel wall (Fig. 31-1). Small blood vessels pass this tissue toward the media. The adjacent media is bordered by an external elastic lamina. Inside the media five or more elastic laminae can be seen. The intima consists of an internal elastic lamina and one layer of endothelial cells. In the longitudinal section the elastic laminae of the media are not arranged in continuous layers. Capillaries in the media are absent.

Within one week after removing the entire adventitial tissue, the outer layer of the media undergoes necrosis. No nuclei are stainable (Fig. 31-2). Only in some regions can pyknotic cells be detected. At that time this part of the

vessel wall consists of collagen, elastic material, and necrotic material. The intima reacts by thickening. The interior of the vascular lumen shows no changes; however, in some regions it is lined by a tissue substitute consisting of several layers of cells. The adventitia is only partially substituted for by cicatricial tissue.

If end-to-end anastomosis is carried out at the time of stripping the adventitial tissue, only collagen, elastic material, and necrotic cells constitute the ends of the vessel wall connected by sutures (Fig. 31-3). The interior of the anastomosis is lined by one or two cell layers. Only necrotic material supports the anastomosis because scar tissue has not replaced the adventitial tissue in this part of the sutured vessel wall.

Two weeks after microsurgical intervention none of the operated anastomoses had healed definitively. Even in cases where the cut end of the vessel wall was embedded in scar tissue, the removed adventitia was not completely replaced by scar. However, the interior of the anastomosis is regularly lined by hyperplastic intima. Even four weeks after operation, the

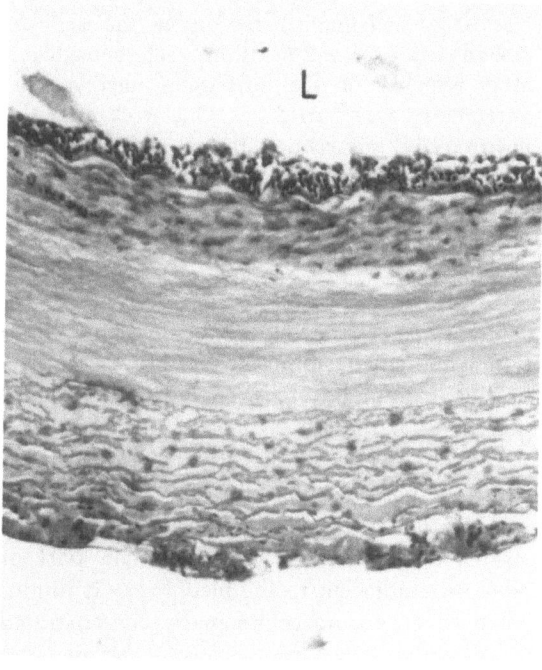

Fig. 31-2. Cross section of the common carotid artery of a 2-month-old rat. One week after removal of adventitia, the outer layers of the media undergo necrosis. The intima is marked by several layers of cells. L = arterial lumen. H & E, × 140.

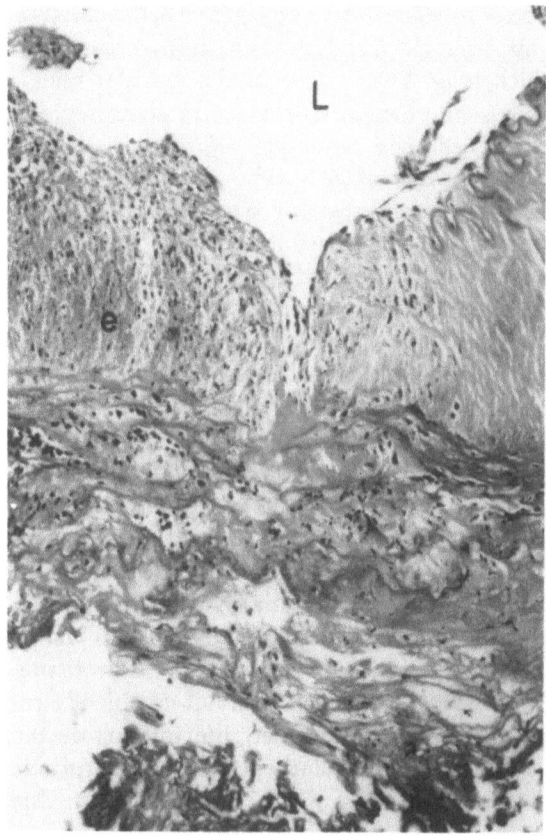

Fig. 31-3. Longitudinal section of the common carotid artery of a 2-month-old rat. Immediately after removal of the adventitia, microvascular anastomosis was carried out. One week after this microsurgical intervention, the cut ends of the vessel are partially necrotic. L = arterial lumen; e = necrotic area filled with erythrocytes. H & E, × 140.

examined vessels demonstrate the same situation whether anastomosed or not. A complete healing cannot be observed during the entire period.

Four to twelve weeks after removal of adventitial tissue and following microsurgical intervention the treated vessel wall demonstrates the same changes. The main part of adventitia adjacent to the media cells is diminished. Even so, no cells can be demonstrated in the outer layers of the media and in some parts of the anastomosed ends of the vessel. The intima shows thickening by five to ten cell layers. Collagen interlaces this tissue connecting the cut end of the vessel wall, as in cases where the anastomosis has been performed.

Discussion

The findings about the histologic changes of microvascular anastomoses following removal of adventitial tissue show an important influence of adventitial tissue on the other parts of the vessel wall. After removal of adventitia a varying number of layers of the media cells undergo necrosis, the extent presumably depending on how far the adventitial tissue has been removed. In fact, none of the examined vessels has lost the external elastic lamina through the microsurgical removal of adventitia, but there is no possibility of standardizing the stripping of adventitial tissue. In this way only a large number of operated vessels can give a significant result.

The intima reacts partially by intimal thickening. This intimal thickening seems to be dependent on the width of necroses inside the media, but this is only an impression. This finding is in accordance with Staubesand,[12] who reported the pattern of reaction of myocytes inside the media of lump-loaded vessel walls. In agreement with Buck[8] and other authors he described the immigration of myocytes into the subendothelial space of the intima. When the adventitia is removed, the vessel wall is weakened and the unaffected part tries to compensate for the weakness by intimal thickening. The degree of intimal thickening appears to be the same after microsurgical anastomosing. However, the necrotic areas in the vessel walls after microsurgical intervention have a much higher extension than those of the vessels in the control group. Additionally, the lost adventitia is only partially replaced by scar tissue. Presumably, this last fact makes it possible to detect necroses inside the media over a long time. However, in this experiment the demonstrated necroses cannot be differentiated from media necroses following microsurgical suturing as described by many authors.[1] Indeed Acland described trimming off the adventitia before anastomosing the cut end of the vessel, but necroses were also described by authors who refrained from trimming off the adventitia.[8] To differentiate the factors causing necroses, new experiments are necessary. Particularly, examinations have been carried out with microsurgical techniques which avoid or decrease the necessity of sutures.

The demonstrated results can be summarized to indicate that the removal of adventitia has a prolonged effect on the healing process of microsurgically anastomosed vessels. Occluding of STA–MCA anastomoses after a long period of good function can be explained by this technical detail, in addition to other components. This is even more evident in cases with cortical cerebral vessels of small diameter, because reducing the flow inside the vessel supports intimal thickening.[10, 13] Also, there is no doubt that prolonged media necrosis can advance intimal thickening.

Summary

Microsurgical anastomosing of small vessels with a diameter less than 1 mm is facilitated by trimming off the adventitial tissue of the anastomosing vessel. Therefore this technical procedure might be examined to determine whether the facilitation of microsurgical intervention influences the healing process. The influence of adventitia was studied by removing the tissue from the common carotid artery of the rat as far as possible. After this, microsurgical end-to-end anastomosis was performed. The morphologic changes were studied 1, 2, 4, 8, and 12 weeks after operation by light microscopic methods and compared to the changes in controls. The results indicate that trimming off the adventitia induces necrosis within the media and prolongs the healing process. Because in EIAB operation very often anastomoses have to be performed on vessels with a diameter as small as 0.7 mm, the deterioration of the healing process following microsurgical procedure is greater than the benefits derived from removal of adventitial tissue.

References

1. Acland, R.D., Trachtenberg, L. The histopathology of small arteries following experimental microvascular anastomoses. Plast Reconstr Surg 59:868–875, 1977.
2. Baxter, Th.J., O.'Brien, B.Mc.C., Henderson, P.N., Bennett, R.C. The histopathology of small vessels following microvascular repair. Br J Surg 59:617–622, 1972.
3. Buck, R.C. Intimal thickening after ligature of arteries. An electron-microscopic study. Circ Res 9:418–426, 1961.
4. Chater, N., Spetzler, R.F., Tonnemacher, K., Wilson, Ch.B. Microvascular bypass surgery; Part I: Anatomical studies. J Neurosurg 44: 712–714, 1976.
5. Glagov, S., Ts'ao, Ch. Restitution of aortic wall after sustained necrotizing transmural ligation injury; Role of blood cells and artery cells. Am J Pathol 79:7–30, 1975.
6. Jacobson, J.H., Suarez, E.L. Microsurgery in anastomoses of small vessels. Surg Forum 11: 243–245, 1960.
7. Knieriem, H.-J., Bondjers, G., Björkerud, S. Electron microscopy of intimal plaques following induction of large superficial mechanical injury (transverse injury) in the rabbit aorta. Virchows Archiv Pathol Anat 359:267–282, 1973.
8. Meyermann, R., Kletter, G. Causes of stenoses and embolic occlusion in microsurgical anastomoses (experimental study). In Advances in Neurosurgery, Vol. 2, Klug, et al., editors, Springer-Verlag, Berlin, 1975.
9. Meyermann, R., Kletter, G. Ultrastructural findings after microsurgical interventions on the carotid artery of the rat. Acta Neurochir 35:71–83, 1976.
10. Meyermann, R., Kletter, G., Koos, W.Th. Morphologic changes after vascular microanastomoses as a function of the technique used. In Microsurgery for Stroke, P. Schmiedek, editor, Springer-Verlag, New York, pp. 123–127, 1977.
11. Schwartz, S.M., Stemermann, M.B., Benditt, E.P. The aortic intima. II. Repair of the aortic lining after mechanical denudation. Am J Pathol 81:15–42, 1975.
12. Staubesand, J. Intra- und extrazelluläre Lysosomen bei myozytärer Reaktion der Arterienwand. Med Welt 28:1470–1474, 1977.
13. Stehbens, W.E. Pathology of the Cerebral Blood Vessels. C.V. Mosby, St. Louis, 1972.
14. Stolte, M. Morphologische Analyse der Koronarchirurgie. Gerhard Witzstrock, Baden-Baden, 1975.
15. Webster, W.S., Bishop, S.P., Geer, J.C. Experimental aortic intimal thickening. I. Morphology and source of intimal cells. Am J Pathol 76: 245–264, 1974.
16. Yasargil, M.G. Microsurgery Applied to Neurosurgery. Georg Thieme Verlag, Stuttgart, 1969.

32

Ultrastructural Control of Small Vessels Following Microsurgical Intervention by Tissue Adhesion with Fibrin*

R. Meyermann, A. Anyai, G. Kletter, and C. Pini

The microsurgical anastomosing operation on vessels less than 1 mm in diameter is based on 8 to 10 interrupted sutures. Although many resources were developed for adapting the ends of the vessels, this fundamental principle has not changed since microvascular surgery was introduced into surgery.[1-5] On the other hand, microvascular surgery has advanced experiments with adhesive techniques to avoid damaging of the vessel wall by sutures or sharp pins. First Carton and co-workers[2] tried methyl-2-cyanoacrylate in vascular surgery. However, this glue causes local necroses.[4] Additionally it has toxic side effects on the cerebral tissue, so that the application of methacrylate in microvascular anastomoses for cerebral ischemia is impossible.

Fibrin for tissue adhesion was introduced to peripheral neurosurgery first in 1940 by Young and Medawar.[11] Because of the success achieved by gluing nerve anastomoses with blood coagulation substances, this technique was attempted in microvascular surgery.[6] These experiments resulted in a decrease of adapting sutures. Only two sutures were necessary to fit together the cut ends of a 1-mm vessel (the left carotid artery) of 2-month-old rats. Histologic examinations showed a healing process, which is in agreement with follow-up studies after microvascular anastomoses by interrupted sutures. However, there is no narrowing of the arterial lumen by cicatricial tissues after gluing the anastomoses, as has been described with sutured anastomoses.

Because intimal thickening calls into question the long-term results of microvascular anastomoses, the gluing operation technique seems to be an improvement in microvascular surgery. To understand the different reactions of the vessel walls after gluing or suturing, the adhesive operation technique was performed and the vessel wall was studied by histologic and electron microscopic methods.

Gluing Material and Technique

The gluing material we used is a fibrinogen concentrate (Fibrinkleber-Human-Immuno) produced from human blood plasma with an average of 110 mg coagulable material per 1 ml solution. Before application the deep-frozen concentrate was slowly heated to body temperature. The highly viscous solution was applied in a quantity of 5 to 8 μl. With subsequent dripping of an equal amount of thrombin solution, the fibrinogen was caused to coagulate. The thrombin solution was composed of 500 IU of thrombin (Topostasin) dissolved in 1 ml of Ringer's solution. The high thrombin concentration accelerated the clotting time to 8 to 10 sec.

*Supported by IMMUNO GmbH, Heidelberg, FRG.

Operation Technique

The rats were anesthetized by ether. Additionally 0.05 ml of an atropine solution was applied intraperitoneally. The left common carotid artery was dissected under the operating microscope. After proximal and distal clipping with microclips the vessel was cut transversely and two sutures were applied at 180°. Afterwards the unsutured parts of the cut ends of the vessel were slightly adapted by forceps and the wall was glued by dripping fibrinogen concentrate and the thrombin solution on the vessel. Fifteen seconds after this procedure the forceps was taken away. Approximately 3 min after gluing, first the distal and then the proximal microclips were opened and removed. The operation field was closed layer by layer. The postoperative survival was 1 hour to 16 weeks.

Ultrastructural Methods

In all animals the circulatory system was perfused with 2.5% glutaraldehyde solution. Afterwards the common carotid arteries on both sides were exposed under the operating microscope, severed peripherally at the common carotid artery bifurcation and at a distance of 5 mm centrally from the anastomoses. The specimens were fixed in 2.5% isotonic glutaraldehyde solution for 4 hours and then postfixed in 1% osmium tetroxide for one hour. Finally the material was embedded in Araldite after dehydration in an ascending alcohol sequence. Sections of 1-μm thickness were stained with toluidine blue. Ultrathin layers were examined by electron microscopy, counterstained with lead citrate and uranyl acetate. The sections were made along the course of the vessels.

Results

Immediately after the operation the intima has lost the endothelial cell layer (Fig. 32-1A). Only parts of the reticular basal membrane can be demonstrated, partially covered by thrombocytes within one hour (Fig. 32-1B). This state can be observed up to three days after operation. Inside the aggregation of thrombocytes which narrow the arterial lumen at the anastomosing point, fibrin can be seen only sporadically. Within the intima no migration of smooth muscle cells can be demonstrated. Gaps of the internal elastic lamina are filled with collagen, cytoplasmic processes of media myocytes, and cell detritus, and are covered by platelets regularly (Fig. 32-1C). Sometimes necrotic endothelial cells can be observed. Between the reticular basement membrane and the loosened cytoplasm, thrombocytes are found (Fig. 32-2). The media does not differ markedly from a normal unoperated vessel wall.

After three days the space between the cut ends of the vessel wall is filled by granulation tissue (Fig. 32-3A). Fibroblasts produce collagen fibers which can be demonstrated by collagen fibrils inside intracytoplasmic vacuoles. Now smooth muscle cells begin to migrate into this part of the anastomosis, also. They show signs of increased metabolism such as pinocytosis, enlarged endoplasmic reticulum, and sometimes diminishing of myofilaments (Fig. 32-3B). Ten to fourteen days after operation the healing process is complete. The interior of the arterial lumen is covered by endothelial-like cells. The cell layers are closed. All the junctions of the endothelial cells over the internal elastic lamina as well as over the space between the cut ends of the vessel are accentuated by cytoplasmic processes overlapping the junctions (Fig. 32-4A). The cytoplasmic membrane is marked by numerous pinocytotic vesicles. Inside the cytoplasm an extended Golgi apparatus can be demonstrated in the perinuclear space (Fig. 32-4B). Occasionally the cytoplasm wears specific organelles of endothelial cells. Cut ends of the elastic lamellae are also covered by these endothelial-like cells (Fig. 32-4B).

In some parts several cell layers are found over the intact internal elastic lamina. The deeper layer consists of smooth muscle cells defined by basal membrane, myofilaments, enlarged endoplasmic reticulum, and localization of the organelles in the perinuclear space. The intercellular space is filled with collagen fibers, undefined electron-dense material, and extracellular lysosomes.

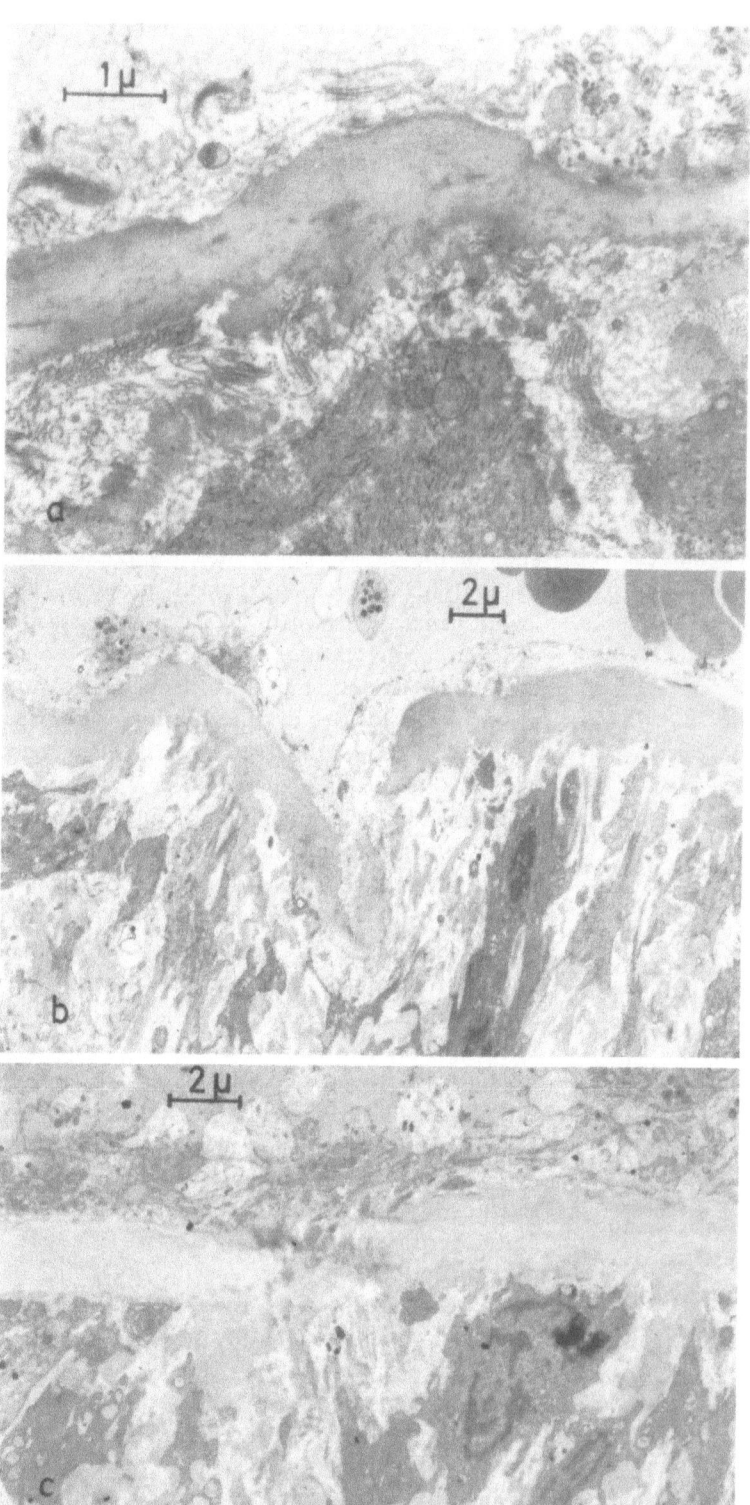

Fig. 32-1. Common carotid artery of a 2-month-old rat 1 hour after microsurgical intervention. a. Lacking endothelial cells, the reticular basement membrane is interspersed by collagen fibrils and cell detritus. Uranyl acetate, × 16 000. b. The reticular basement membrane is partially covered by platelets. Uranyl acetate, × 4275. c. The reticular basement membrane is completely covered by platelets. Fibrin is lacking. Uranyl acetate, × 5700.

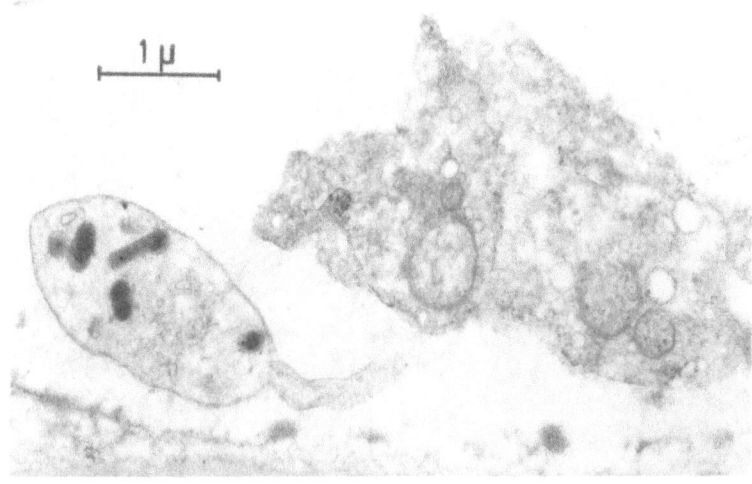

Fig. 32-2. Common carotid artery of a 2-month-old rat 10 hours after operation. Between reticular basement membrane and necrotic endothelial cell the process of a platelet can be seen. Uranyl acetate, × 20 000.

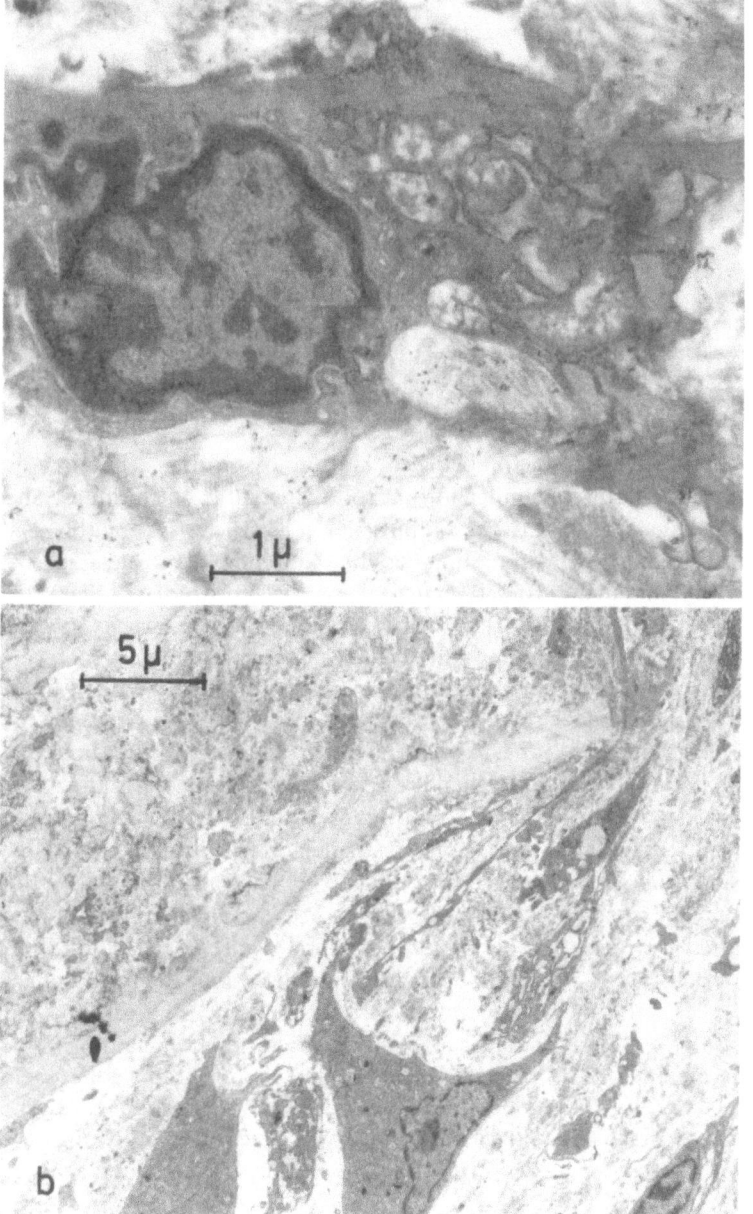

Fig. 32-3. a. Common carotid artery of a 2-month-old rat 4 days after operation. Fibroblast of a scar tissue between the cut ends of the vessel, containing collagen fibrils. Uranyl acetate, × 16 800. b. Common carotid artery of a 2-month-old rat 9 days after operation by adhesive technique. Migration of so-called media myocytes into the scar tissue between the cut ends of the vessel. Uranyl acetate, × 3800.

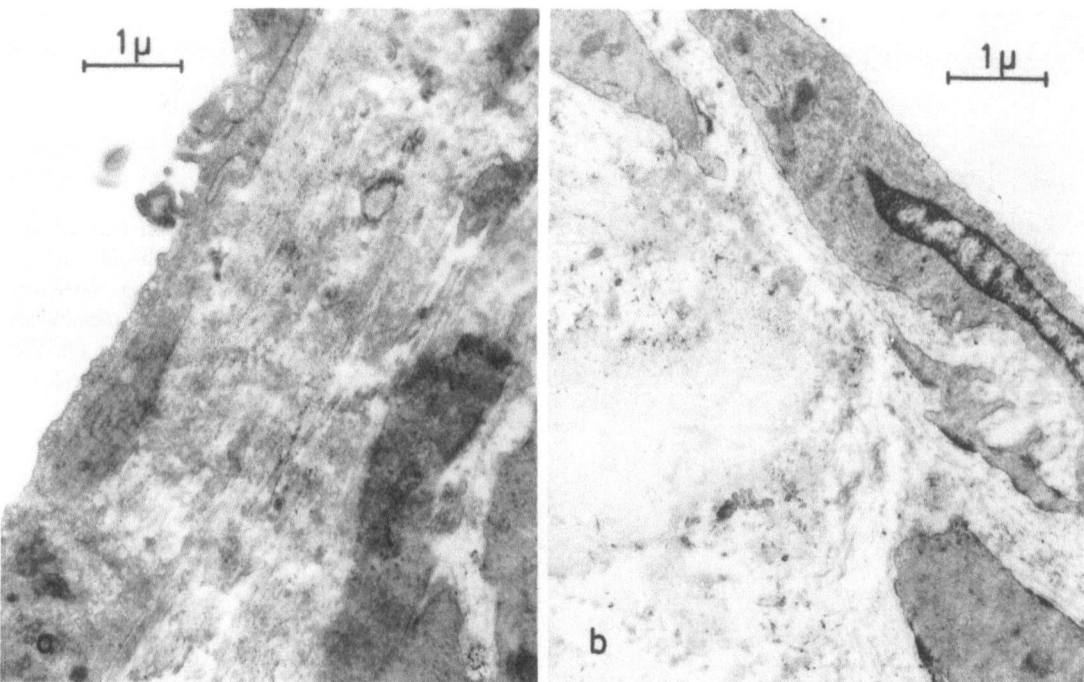

Fig. 32-4. a. Common carotid artery of a 2-month-old rat 2 weeks after operation by adhesive technique. The scar tissue is covered by a closed endothelial cell layer. Uranyl acetate, × 16 000.

b. Common carotid artery of a 5-month-old rat 3 months after operation. The cut ends of the elastic lamella are covered by a monolayer of endothelial cells. Uranyl acetate, × 16 000.

Between the cut ends of the internal elastic lamina the intact endothelial cell layer is supported by smooth muscle cells arranged like palisades (Fig. 32-5). Endothelial cells and smooth muscle cells are separated by reticular basal membrane material. The other cells of the scar tissue are arranged in cell layers too, although sometimes they are unarranged. In the last case cells are more active, characterized by enlarged rough endoplasmic reticulum and vacuoles filled with granular material (Fig. 32-3B). These cells are only partially surrounded by a basal membrane. The intercellular space contains parts of elastic material. The adventitial tissue is constructed by extensive bundles of collagen fibrils interlaced by fibroblasts. No residues of glue can be detected.

Discussion

The healing process of vessels with a diameter of less than 1 mm following microsurgical an-astomosing operation by gluing technique is similar to that following suture technique.[8] The loss of endothelial cells is caused by the manipulation at the cut ends of the vessel by forceps, microcannulas, and needles. Dilatation of the vessel wall produces necroses of the endothelial cells, as described above. However, after completion of the healing process there are some remarkable differences from micro-anastomoses following suture technique. It is true that the reaction of the media is the same in both. However, the extent of the intimal thickening is smaller after adhesive than after suture technique. This can be explained by the fact that sutures are lacking. Sutures cause folding of the vessel wall, so that first the arterial lumen is narrowed and then the impact of blood flow is reduced within the formed sinuses, which causes intimal thickening once more.[10] This can be supported by histologic control of the operated vessels[6] (Fig. 32-6). The most significant observation was an intact endothelial cell layer showing no evidence of

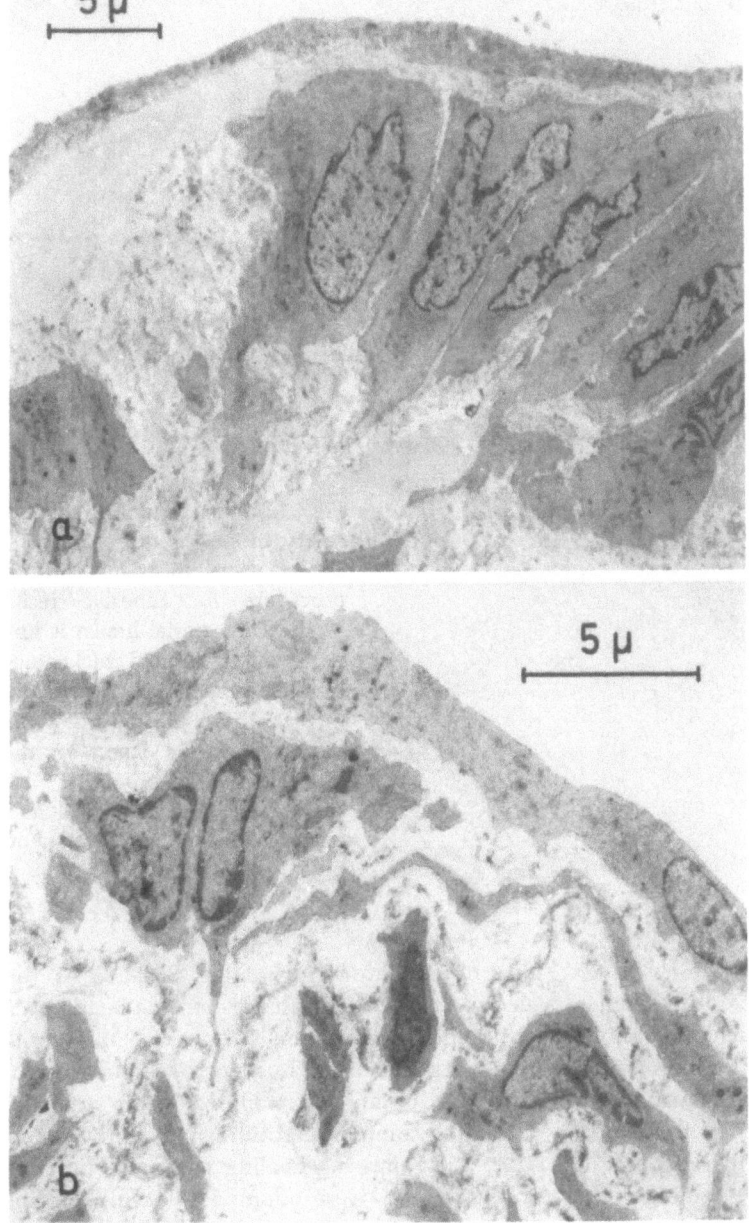

Fig. 32-5. Common carotid artery of a 2-month-old rat 2 weeks after operation by adhesive technique. The closed endothelial cell layer is supported by palisade-like media myocytes. a. Uranyl acetate, × 2850. b. Uranyl acetate, × 3325.

the site of closure. A single cell cannot be distinguished from endothelial cells of untreated vessel walls by morphologic methods. Increased numbers of pinocytotic vesicles and cytoplasmic processes can also be observed in endothelial cells of stressed vessel walls. The number of specific organelles of endothelial cells has not increased.

These findings are in contrast to ultra-structural changes following microsurgical anastomoses by suture technique.[9] In this case the interior of the arterial lumen is covered by a gapped cell layer. These cells are sometimes completely surrounded by reticular basal membrane material, so that this material is in contact with the blood stream. Gluing technique in microvascular surgery is the method of best preservation. Additionally, in extra–

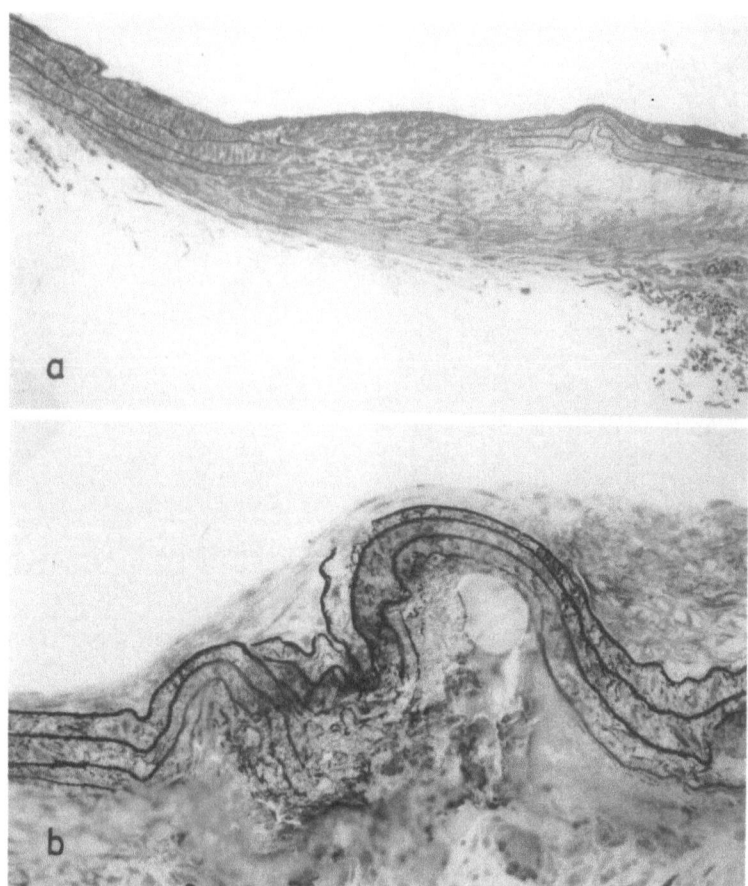

Fig. 32-6. a. Common carotid artery of a 2-month-old rat 14 days after microanastomosis procedure by adhesive technique. The arterial lumen is not narrowed by intimal thickening. Toluidine blue, × 140. b. Common carotid artery of a 2-month-old rat 14 days after microanastomosis procedure by folding of the vessel wall and intimal thickening. Toluidine blue, × 140.

intracranial arterial bypass operation (EIAB operation) these techniques give the chance to perform anastomoses if such operations by suture technique seem to be impossible because of small cortical vessels or short stump of the extracranial vessel. However, this study cannot completely explain why the vessel wall reacts in a different manner after gluing technique.

Summary

Since the pioneering of microsurgical anastomosing procedure by Jacobson and Suarez,[5] the technique of adapting the ends of the vessels is based on 8 to 10 interrupted sutures. However, even the finest suture material causes a foreign body reaction. Additionally, many authors[8] reported media necroses following interrupted suture technique. Because of the success achieved by gluing nerve anastomoses with blood coagulation substances, this technique was introduced into microvessel surgery.[6] Fifty end-to-end anastomoses were married out in the common carotid artery of the rat to study the following healing process. The ends of the vessels were adapted by using Fibrin-kleber-Human, a cryoprecipitated fibrinogen, polymerized by means of thrombin added simultaneously.

The ultrastructurally studied healing process does not differ significantly from the other healing processes of an injured vessel wall. However, this technique avoids necrotic areas inside the vessel wall and diminishes the internal thickening, narrowing the arterial lumen. The endothelial coat of the vessel is better preserved than in sutured anastomoses. To date, there is no explanation of these differences.

References

1. Acland, R.D. Microvascular anastomosis: A device for holding stay sutures and a new vascular clamp. Surgery 75:185–187, 1974.
2. Carton, C.A., Kessler, L.A., Seidenberg, B., Hurwitt, E.S. Experimental studies in surgery of small blood vessels: II. Patching of arteriotomy using a plastic adhesive. J Neurosurg 18:188–194, 1961.
3. Carton, C.A., Kobayashi, T., Cagungun, J., Pineda, T. A nonsuture ring anastomotic method for small vessel surgery: Laboratory studies. In Microsurgical Anastomoses for Cerebral Ischemia, G. Austin, editor, Charles C Thomas, Springfield, pp. 68–98, 1976.
4. Cobbett, J.R. Microvascular surgery. Surg Clin North Am 47:521–542, 1967.
5. Jacobson, J.H., Suarez, E.L. Microsurgery in anastomosis of small vessels. Surg Forum 11:243–245, 1960.
6. Kletter, G., Matras, H., Chiari, H., Dinges, N., Witzmann, A. Comparative evaluation of conventially sutured and clot-sutured microsurgical anastomoses. In Microsurgery for Stroke, P. Schmiedek, editor, Springer-Verlag, New York, pp. 149–153, 1977.
7. Matras, H., Braun, F., Lassmann, H., Ammerer, H.P., Mamoli, B. Plasma clot welding of nerves (experimental report). J Maxillofac Surg 1:236–240, 1973.
8. Meyermann, R., Kletter, G. Ultrastructural findings after microsurgical interventions on the carotid artery of the rat. Acta Neurochir 35:71–83, 1976.
9. Meyermann, R., Wismann, H., Kletter, G. Morphometric approach to fine structured changes in the intima of the common carotid artery of the rat following microsurgery. In Microsurgery for Stroke, P. Schmiedek, editor, Springer-Verlag, New York, pp. 128–134, 1977.
10. Stehbens, W.E. Pathology of the Cerebral Blood Vessels. C.V. Mosby, St. Louis, 1972.
11. Young, J.Z., Medawar, P.B. Fibrin suture of peripheral nerves. Measurement of the rate of regeneration. Lancet 239:126–128, 1940.

33

Comparative Evaluation of Microvascular Arterial Graft: Arterial Autograft versus Human Umbilical Artery Graft*

H. Maximilian Mehdorn, Philip R. Weinstein, Jeannette J. Townsend, and Norman L. Chater

Several authors have reported their experiences with autografts suitable for the microvascular, extracranial–intracranial (EC–IC) arterial bypass procedure. The radial artery autograft has been used most frequently,[1, 3, 6] although the use of the saphenous vein has been reported in some instances.[11] Clinical experience with these graft materials has been successful over the short term—although the experience in coronary artery bypass surgery, where these grafts have been used for longer intervals, raises questions about their long-term patency.[2, 4, 7] Indeed, a recent paper has shown rather poor patency rates after a long-term follow-up of animals receiving venous graft material.[8] To date, no microvascular graft material has been available on an "on-shelf" basis.

In an experimental model, we used glutaraldehyde-denatured and ethanol-preserved human umbilical artery (HUA) as microvascular graft material, and compared our results to those achieved with arterial autograft material (AA). For anatomic reasons, we decided to use the cat carotid artery as the recipient vessel for the HUA and the AA.

Seventy-six segments of HUA (3 to 5 cm long) and 19 segments of AA (1 to 5 cm long),

both of which had an internal diameter of 1 to 2 mm, were microsurgically interposed into the carotid arteries of 58 cats. The details of surgery have been reported elsewhere.[9]

At intervals ranging from a few days to a few weeks after operation, transfemoral catheter angiography of the aortic arch and the carotid arteries was performed to examine the graft patency (Fig. 33-1). At intervals of 10 days to 8 months after surgery, the grafts were removed after in-vivo perfusion fixation with glutaraldehyde, and were prepared for light microscopy and for scanning and transmission electron microscopy (SEM/TEM).

The patency rate for AA was 100%, whereas the patency rate for the HUA was greater than 80% during the first few weeks after surgery and decreased to 45% after more than three months.

On histologic examination of the AA, both the autograft and the host artery appeared viable (Fig. 33-2). In rare instances, signs of devitalization of the host artery were apparent close to the anastomotic site, where its media became thinner and eosinophilic (Fig. 33-3). This might have been a consequence of the severe damage caused by the heavy-weight clips that were used. There was very little reactive change at the anastomotic site although, occasionally, foreign body cells were found close to the suture material. The majority of AAs showed a moderate amount of dense connective tissue covered by a thin layer of endothelial-like cells. Only one anastomotic site

*Supported in part by the Herzstein Fund, the Robert Benjamin Fund, and the G. Irwin Medical Research Fund (University of California, San Francisco), by United States Veterans Administration Hospital Research Project Grant No. 9285, and by a grant from the Office of Naval Research, Contract No. 00014-76-C-0486.

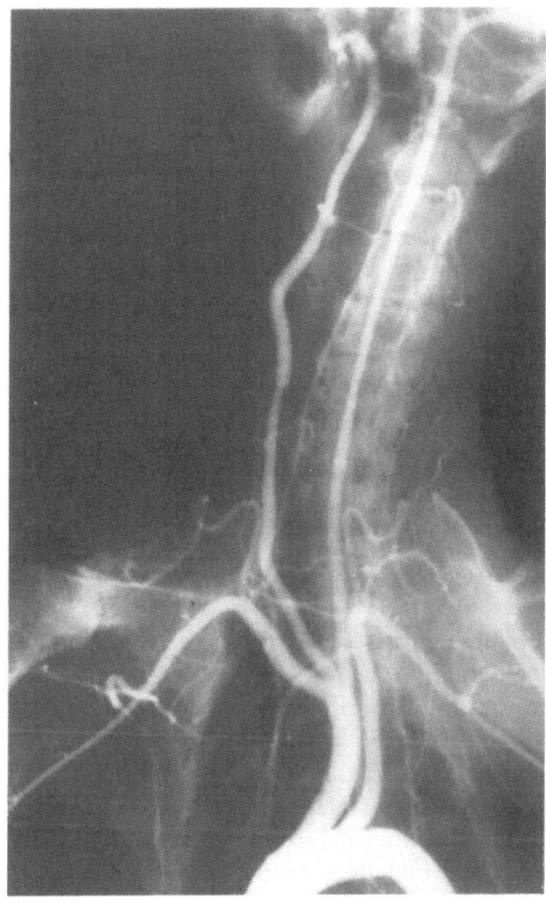

Fig. 33-1. Transfemoral catheter angiography showing two interposed grafts: right carotid artery with slightly redundant umbilical artery graft, left carotid artery with interposed arterial autograft (segment of the right carotid artery 2 cm long). Three weeks after surgery.

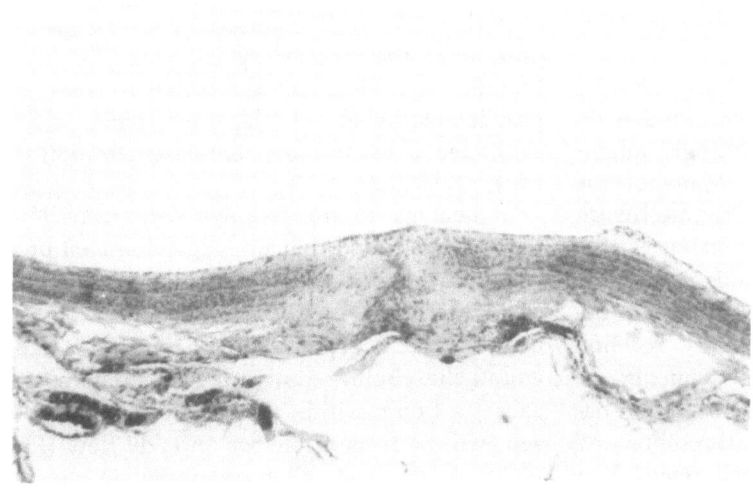

Fig. 33-2. Anastomosis between carotid artery and arterial autograft. Note: It is difficult to distinguish between host artery and graft. Hematoxylin-eosin. Two months after surgery.

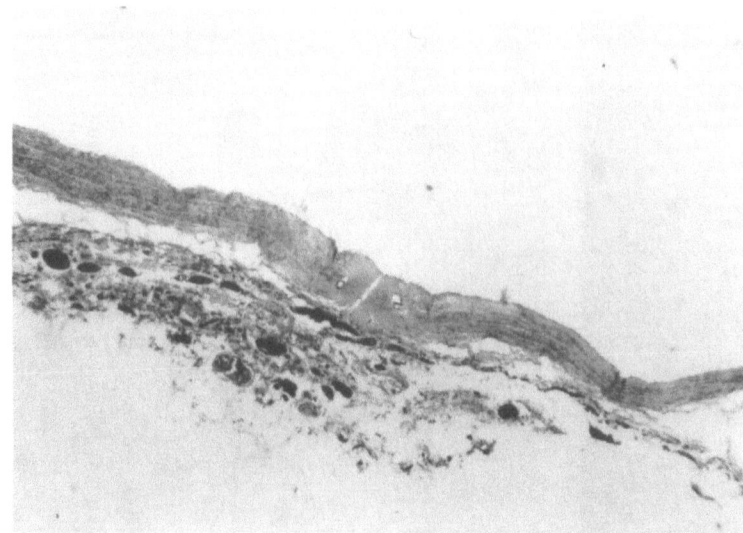

Fig. 33-3. Anastomosis between carotid artery and arterial autograft. Note: Autograft (right part of the picture) shows thinning of the media. Hematoxylin-eosin. Three months after surgery.

showed some subendothelial proliferation of fibroblast-like cells. This finding occurred in an autograft which, at the time of angiography and subsequent removal two weeks after surgery, was found to be in severe spasm, permitting very little blood flow. The difficulty in this case certainly was related to surgical problems encountered when major retraction of the severed artery necessitated our using an autograft 1 cm long to bridge a gap of 3 to 4 cm between the two stumps of the host artery.

SEM showed rapid reendothelialization of the graft surface. A single layer of endothelial-like cells covered the subendothelium (Fig. 33-4 A, B).

Histologic evaluation of the HUA showed that most of these graft were surrounded, in varying degrees, by subacute to chronic inflammatory infiltrate (Fig. 33-5 A). Many of the cells appeared to be reacting to the meshwork surrounding the graft. In some instances, the inflammatory cells invaded the graft tissue (Fig. 33-5 B). There appeared to be a correlation between the amount of inflammatory reaction surrounding the graft and its tendency to thrombosis. There was no strict correlation between the histologic age of the thrombus and the interval between surgery and removal of the graft; in other words, in several grafts thrombosis must have occurred weeks to months after the graft had been implanted. This observation correlates well with the clini-

cal finding that some grafts were patent at angiography, one to several weeks after surgery, but were occluded when angiography was performed again at later dates.

In patent vessels, a consistent histologic pattern was found: a subintimal proliferation of fibroblasts extended from both proximal and distal anastomotic sites into the graft, and this proliferation was covered by one to several layers of flat, endothelial-like cells (Fig. 33-6). Mononuclear cells with granular cytoplasm were attached to the luminal surface in areas that were not covered by the pseudoendothelial cells (Fig. 33-7). SEM showed that these cells grew from the host artery and over the anastomotic site (Fig. 33-8). Isolated areas of pseudoendothelial cells also were found, which suggested a blood-borne endothelialization of the graft (Fig. 33-9).

In analogy to the findings with respect to the AA, we found that the subendothelial proliferation—which depends on the surrounding cellular reaction—markedly determines whether or not an HUA graft remains patent. This subendothelial proliferation at the anastomotic site causes a bump within the lumen which, by itself, will be responsible for an eddy flow (Fig. 33-10 A, B). The cell types found in the reactive tissue around the graft suggest that this tissue is mainly of infectious and immunologic etiology. One must consider that the HUAs used in this experiment were not sterile, and

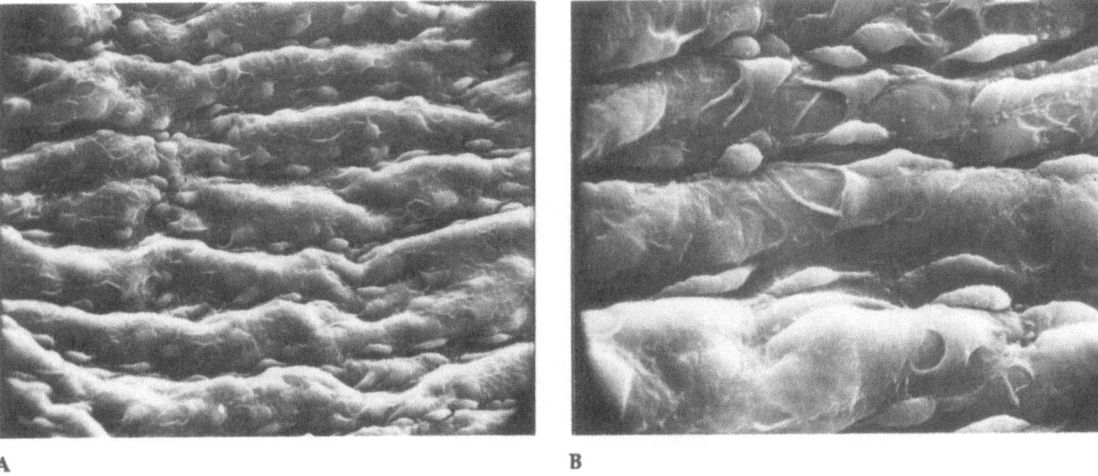

A   B

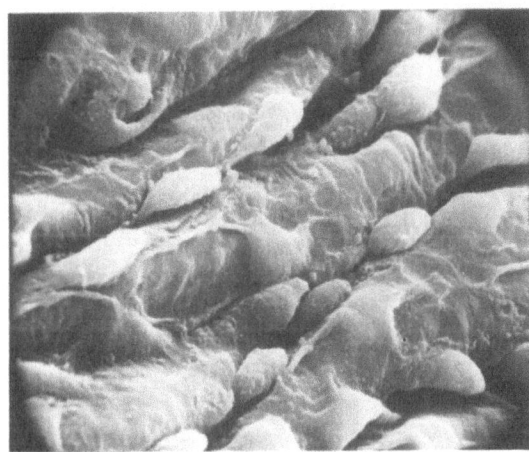

C

Fig. 33-4. Reendothelialization of arterial autograft 2 months after surgery; A. × 600, B. × 1560; C. × 2400. Note transitional phases between blood cells and endothelial cells.

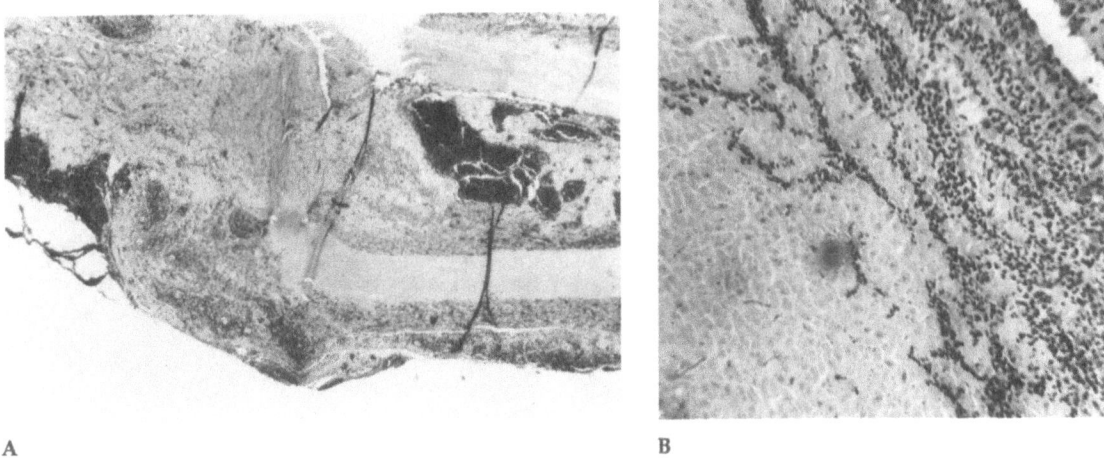

A   B

Fig. 33-5. Cellular reaction surrounding the implanted human umbilical artery graft. A. Subacute infiltrate mainly close to sutures and meshwork. B. Acute invasion of cells into the graft wall.

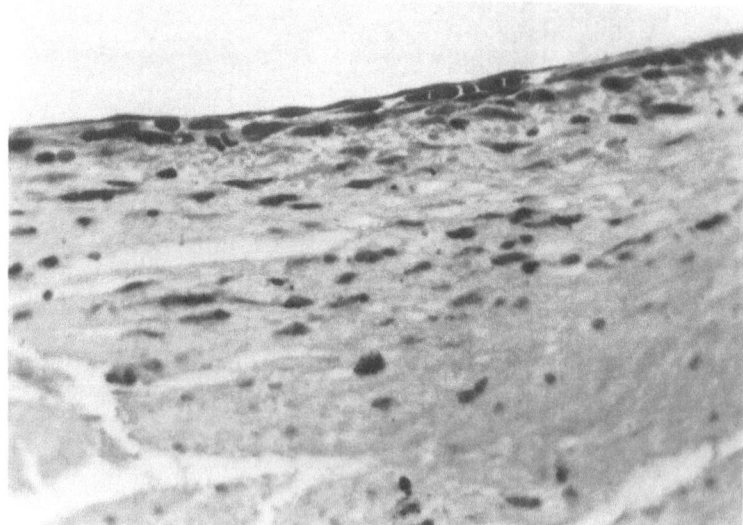

Fig. 33-6. Endothelialization of umbilical artery graft, 3 months after surgery. Hematoxylin-eosin.

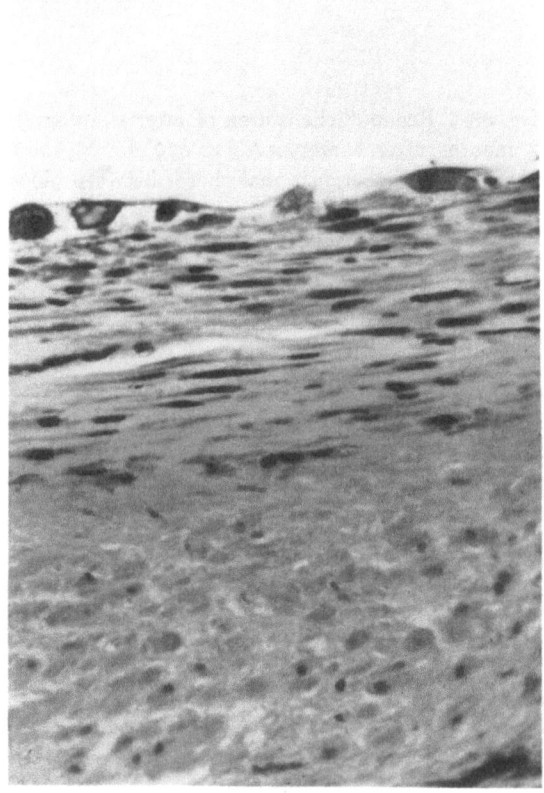

Fig. 33-7. Endothelialization of umbilical artery graft, 3 months after surgery. Note white blood cells (monocytes, phagocytes) beginning to form "endothelial lining." Hematoxylin-eosin.

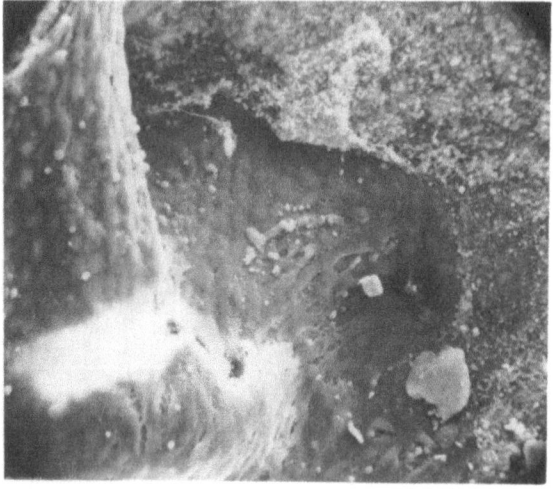

Fig. 33-8. "Endothelial lining cells" growing over the anastomotic site (bottom of Fig.: suture). Flow from right to left, distal anastomosis, 12 days after surgery. × 270.

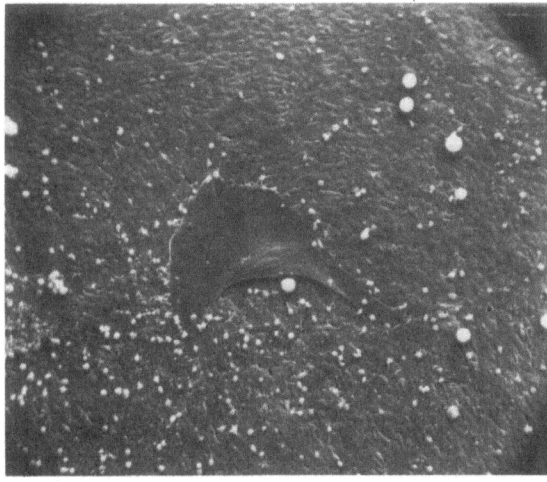

Fig. 33-9. Isolated "endothelial lining cell" on a layer of flattened, nonthrombogenic platelets, 7 weeks after surgery. × 600.

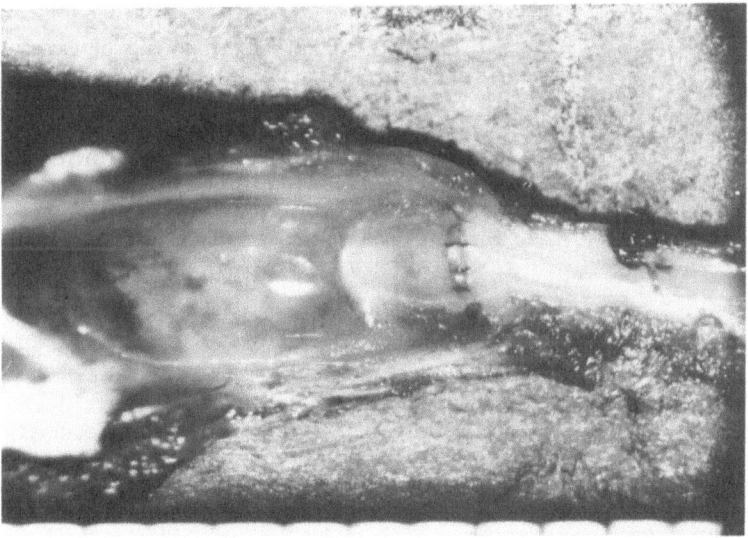

A

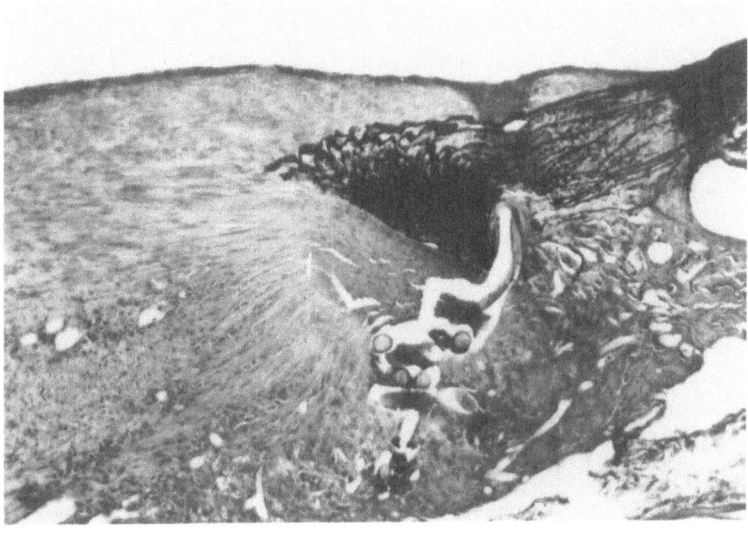

Fig. 33-10. Proximal anastomosis 3 to 4 months after surgery. Right, carotid artery; left, umbilical artery graft. A. Note bump caused by subendothelial proliferation. Bottom, rule in mm. B. Elastic-van Gieson.

B

that—since they were implanted into cats—they acted as xenografts. The problem of sterility has been overcome since we completed these experiments, and the problems of a xenograft are not encountered when the HUA is implanted into human beings. Immunologic studies of similarly denatured human umbilical veins[5] showed that they no longer represent a source of major antigenicity.

Considering the data obtained in our studies, we suggest that arterial (or, similarly, venous) autografts may be used during the EC–IC bypass procedure when the patient can tolerate the time-consuming processes of preoperative angiography to identify a suitable vessel and dissection. We also suggest that the use of the HUA might be a safe alternative when the patient's vessels are not considered suitable for use as autografts, as well as when a readily available microvascular graft is needed for patients undergoing emergency EC–IC arterial bypass operation for acute stroke.

References

1. Ausman, J.I., Nicoloff, D.M., Chou, S.N. Posterior fossa revascularization: Anastomosis of vertebral artery to PICA with interposed radial artery graft. Surg Neurol 9:281–286, 1978.
2. Brody, W.R., Kosek, J.C., Angell, W.W. Changes in vein grafts following aortocoronary bypass induced by pressure and ischemia. J Thorac Cardiovasc Surg 64:847–854, 1972.
3. Chater, N.L. Personal communication, 1976.
4. Curtis, J.J., Stoney, W.S., Alford, W.C., Burrus, G.R., Thomas, C.S., Jr. Intimal hyperplasia. A cause of radial artery aorto-coronary bypass graft failure. Ann Thorac Surg 20:628–635, 1975.
5. Dardik, H., Ibrahim, I.M., Sprayregen, S., Dardik, I.I. Clinical experience with modified human umbilical cord vein for arterial bypass. Surgery 79:618–624, 1976.
6. Epstein, M.H., Liebrock, L., Long, D.M. The anatomy of the so-called "middle cerebral artery trifurcation" and its potential for extracranial–intracranial bypass. Presented at the Meeting of the Congress of Neurological Surgeons, New Orleans, 1976.
7. Karayannacos, P.E., Hostetler, J.R., Bond, M.G., Kakos, G.S., Williams, R.A., Kilman, J.W., Vasko, J.S. Late failure in vein grafts: Mediating factors in subendothelial fibromuscular hyperplasia. Ann Surg 187:183–188, 1978.
8. Khodadad, G. Eight-year followup of experimental carotid-middle cerebral and carotid-basilar arterial bypass grafts and anastomoses. Neurosurgery 2:246–251, 1978.
9. Mehdorn, H.M., Weinstein, P.R., Townsend, J.J., Chater, N.L. Human umbilical artery as a source of small diameter vascular grafts. 46th Meeting of the American Association of Neurological Surgeons, New Orleans, April 23–27, 1978.
10. Peerless, S.J. Comment on: Cerebral revascularization: Common carotid to distal middle cerebral artery bypass (Story, J.L., Brown, W.E., Eidelberg, E., Arom, K.V., Stewart, J.R., in Neurosurgery 2:131–135, 1978). Neurosurgery 2:134, 1978.
11. Story, J.L., Brown, W.E., Eidelberg, E., Arom, K.V., Stewart, J.R. Cerebral revascularization: Common carotid to distal middle cerebral artery bypass. Neurosurgery 2:131–135, 1978.

34

Patency, Blood Flow, and Histologic Response in 2- to 3-mm Arterial Autografts*

Philip R. Weinstein, H. Maximilian Mehdorn, and David A. Telles

Extra–intracranial arterial bypass (EC–IC) for augmentation of collateral blood flow in patients with symptomatic intracranial occlusive vascular disease is usually performed by anastomosis of either the superficial temporal or occipital scalp arteries to a cortical branch of the middle cerebral artery using the end-to-side technique. Under special circumstances, an alternative procedure can be utilized consisting of subcutaneous implantation of a vascular graft from the external carotid artery (ECA) to a cortical branch of the middle cerebral artery (MCA) by performing end-to-side anastomosis at both sites.[10, 19] Indications for ECA-to-MCA bypass grafting include arteriographic evidence of inadequate diameter scalp artery or absence due to previous trauma or craniotomy. In addition, some patients, such as those who require internal carotid artery (ICA) or MCA ligation during treatment for intracranial aneurysm or tumor, may require greater initial collateral blood flow which can be provided only by a larger-diameter bypass graft. Finally, should indications be established for revascularization surgery in acute cerebrovascular insufficiency, availability of a somewhat-larger diameter vascular graft which could be more rapidly inserted would be of value.

Clinical reports indicate that saphenous or cephalic vein grafts have been utilized in the past.[10, 19] However, clinical and experimental studies of results of arterial interposition of small-diameter vein grafts indicate that subintimal hyperplasia and medial fibrosis may lead to progressive stenosis and occlusion of such graft material.[1, 11, 18] Results of previous work in our laboratory indicate that long-term patency cannot be expected with 2-mm diameter synthetic graft material.[21] Extensive experimental evaluation of antigenically denatured human umbilical artery heterografts implanted in cat carotid arteries indicates that only a 40% long-term patency rate can be expected with 5-cm-long segments.[13] Umbilical artery grafts 10 to 15 cm in length were found to thrombose within 2 hours after implantation in dog carotid arteries, suggesting possible mechanical or chemical thrombogenic effects of endothelial damage or glutaraldehyde tanning during graft preparation. Alternative graft harvesting and preparation techniques are currently under study.

Our initial results indicated that a 100% patency rate could be expected following interposition of 2-mm diameter arterial autografts 5 cm in length in the cat common carotid artery examined at intervals of up to 6 months. Histologic studies indicated that satisfactory survival of the vessel wall could be expected. Scanning electron microscope (SEM) studies documented satisfactory endothelial regeneration. Accordingly, it was felt that evaluation of long-term patency and histologic response in 2- to 3-mm arterial autografts suitable for use in ECA–MCA bypass surgery (by virtue

*Work supported by Veterans Administration Research Grant #MRIS 9285.

of 15- to 20-cm length) should be evaluated. In addition, it was felt that blood flow studies would be helpful to document adequate function of such grafts and to investigate their capacity to enlarge with demand for increased collateral blood flow.

Methods

Twenty adult mongrel dogs were sedated with ketamine hydrochloride and Acepromazine and anesthetized with intravenous pentobarbital. Endotracheal intubation was accomplished and respiration assisted when necessary. Through a vertical midline anterior cervical incision the common carotid arteries were exposed bilaterally. Using the Zeiss operating microscope and microsurgical technique the vessels were isolated, taking care to protect and preserve surrounding adventitia. The left common carotid artery (CCA) was exposed from the clavicle to the CCA bifurcation, a distance measuring between 15 and 19 cm depending on the size and the weight of the dog. The right CCA was isolated from its adventitia over a 3- to 4-cm segment of its midportion. Occurrence of dissection-induced vasospasm was occasionally noted which could be reversed by topical application of 1% lidocaine solution. The left CCA was then ligated and severed proximally and distally, and the graft lumen was irrigated with heparinized saline solution, 200 units/ml, using a blunt 18-gauge needle. The graft was then temporarily immersed in a bowl of heparinized saline.

Microvascular occlusion clips with 40-g opening pressures were applied to the right CCA, which was then severed with microscissors. Right CCA vessel stump lumens were likewise irrigated with heparinized saline solution. Each vessel stump was observed to retract a distance of 3 to 5 cm. If necessary, an additional 2- to 3-cm segment of the right CCA was trimmed and discarded to make room for the interposition graft. Although the graft also retracted somewhat, it was observed to expand to its original length after blood flow was restored.

End-to-end anastomoses were married out at 16 and 24 × magnification, using 10-0 mono-filament nylon interrupted sutures on a 100-μm needle. Twelve to eighteen sutures were required. Microclips were removed and blood flow was reestablished after air was flushed from the graft. Bleeding from the suture line was controlled by temporary application of cotton pledgets or placement of an additional suture. All anastomoses were carefully inspected under the operating microscope and animals were excluded from the study if postoperative stenosis at the anastomotic site was observed. Both the graft and recipient vessels were kept moistened or immersed in saline solution throughout the surgical procedure.

External vessel diameters were measured before removal and after implantation of grafts in all animals, and graft lengths were recorded. Electromagnetic blood flow determinations were carried out after initial exposure of the recipient vessel and after graft implantation using a Statham SP2204 flowmeter and 2.5- to 3.5-mm diameter probes. The incisions were closed and initial postoperative patency was verified with daily palpation and Doppler ultrasonic flowmeter auscultation.

Arteriograms were carried out by percutaneous transfemoral catheterization of the aortic arch for injection of 10 ml of 60% Renografin in some animals at intervals of 1 day to 6 weeks after graft implantation. Animals were anesthetized and the grafts were reexplored for final verification of patency and blood flow determinations before sacrifice for graft removal at intervals of 1 day to 6 months. Vessels were prepared for histologic and SEM examination by in-vivo transaortic perfusion fixation with Karnovsky's fixative* solution after prior saline flush of all blood from the grafts. Recipient vessels were clamped 3 cm proximal and distal to the graft anastomoses during fixative perfusion to prevent backflow of blood cells within the vessel lumens.

Vessels were prepared for SEM by longitudinal section of 2-cm segments obtained at each anastomotic site, from the center of the graft and from a point on the graft 3 cm away from each anastomosis. Specimens were subjected to critical-point drying and gold impregnation for scanning on an ETEC AutoScan

---

*Formaldehyde-glutaraldehyde fixative of high osmolarity for use in SEM studies.

electron microscope. Adjacent vessel segments were prepared for histologic study using hematoxylin-eosin and elastic/van Gieson stains. Prior arteriograms were not performed on animals prepared for study by SEM.

Results

Graft Dimensions

Vessel lumen diameter measurements indicated that all grafts fell within the 2.0- to 3.5-mm range. Prior to removal, donor vessels measured 16 to 19 cm in length with an average of 17 cm.

Patency

There was no postoperative thrombosis of the grafts. Each graft remained patent at the time of arteriography and reexploration prior to sacrifice. Six animals were sacrificed between 1 and 18 days, three at 1 month, four at 3 months, and seven at 6 months (Table 34-1). During surgical reexploration of the grafts, minimal fibrosis was found surrounding the vessels. Evidence of bleeding from the anastomotic site or postoperative infection was not found. Graft surfaces and adventitial vascularity appeared identical on parent and graft vessels.

Arteriograms

CCA arteriograms demonstrated satisfactory graft perfusion even when vessel curves or kinks were present because of excess graft length. In a few animals, slight dilatation of

the graft was observed by comparison with parent-vessel diameter and arteriographic diameters in unoperated controls. However, in most cases, both parent vessel and graft appeared to have dilated slightly. This finding was confirmed by comparison of postoperative arteriograms with preoperative control studies obtained in three dogs. Stenosis of grafts was not observed arteriographically even at sites of anastomosis (Fig. 34-1).

Blood Flow

Electromagnetic blood flowmeter determinations indicated that control CCA flows were 75 to 150 ml/min, with an average of 125. Measurements repeated one month postoperatively in six dogs demonstrated increases of 30 to 60% with flows of 200 to 275 ml/min, presum-

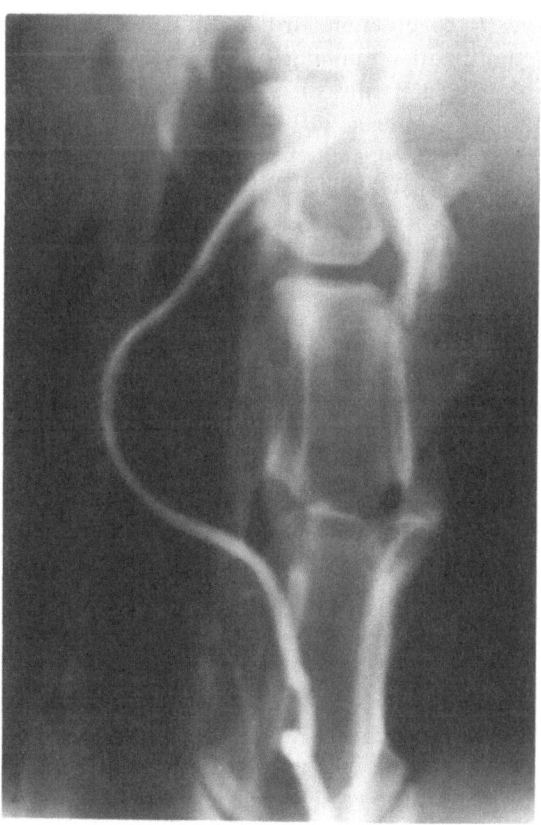

Fig. 34-1. Right common carotid arteriogram in dog 1 week after autograft implant. Satisfactory perfusion without evidence of stenosis is demonstrated.

Table 34-1. Patency of canine common carotid artery autografts

Duration	Number
1–18 days	6/6
1 month	3/3
3 months	4/4
6 months	7/7
Total	20/20 = 100%

ably in response to demand for collateral blood supply after ligation of the opposite CCA. Graft blood flow measured at 6 months following implant averaged 195 ml/min.

Histology

At 1 and 6 days after implant considerable patchy endothelial necrosis and loss of intimal continuity were observed. Regeneration occurred between 3 and 6 weeks. The intimal layer was reconstituted at 3 months. There was no evidence of late subendothelial fibrosis causing graft stenosis at 6 months. At 1 and 6 days after implant histologic examination of the grafts consistently demonstrated preservation of most of the media layer except at the anastomotic sites. In two animals focal necrosis of muscularis cells and disruption of elastic lamellae were seen, possibly due to mechanical injury of the vessel wall by forceps or adventitial vessel coagulation. In two animals diffuse circumferential thinning of the media with loss of the outer muscularis layers was seen (Fig. 34-2). In some graft specimens formation of vacuoles and patchy necrosis of muscle cells in the external 2 or 3 layers of the muscularis were observed. These changes were not seen in the parent vessels of these animals. At 3 weeks external muscularis layers in some specimens exhibited an amorphous hyalinized appearance with some evidence of fibroblastic proliferation. From 6 weeks to 3 months fibrous replacement of the outer muscularis layers was occasionally observed, with preservation of elastic lamellae. No evidence of muscle cell regeneration was seen in the media even in the 6-month specimens.

Satisfactory healing by fibrosis of the entire media occurred at all anastomotic sites. Small suture granulomas were seen. There was no evidence of false aneurysm formation.

Diffuse hemorrhage seen in the adventitial layer in specimens at all time intervals was consistent with the expected effects of surgical dissection for vessel removal and was reduced in specimens dissected after rather than before glutaraldehyde perfusion. Despite the fact that donor vessels were isolated and removed as free grafts, thrombosis of adventitial microvasculature was rarely seen. At 10 days inflamma-

tory and granulation response was seen within the adventitial layer with formation of multiple capillaries, and early fibrosis was evident at 3 weeks. Between 6 weeks and 3 months the adventitial microvasculature appeared to have been reconstituted even though fibrosis had completely replaced the normal adventitial areolar tissue components.

No significant histologic differences were observed between segments obtained from proximal, distal, or central segments of the grafts.

Scanning Electron Microscopy

Diffuse patchy sloughing of the graft and parent-vessel endothelial layer with adherence of platelets to exposed subendothelium and internal elastica was observed at 24 hours. An unexpected finding was that of small islands of intact, preserved endothelium seen in the center of the graft (Fig. 34-3). In addition, small focal areas of cellular proliferation were observed in the 24-hour specimens, suggesting that pseudointima formation by proliferation of myointimal cells or reaction of preserved endothelial cells may begin shortly after endothelial necrosis caused by the surgical procedure (Fig. 34-3).

SEM examination of anastomotic sites at 24 hours revealed needle puncture sites filled with platelet plugs and small clumps of fibrin-laced thrombus adherent to the suture line. Loss of endothelium and minimal intimal damage due to temporary clip application were seen on both proximal and distal segments of the parent vessels.

At 6 days following graft implantation SEM examination revealed marked reduction of platelet aggregates and disappearance of thrombus material. Denuded intimal surfaces close to the anastomotic sites were partly covered by small reactive or proliferating endothelial cells which appeared to cross the suture line into the graft from both proximal and distal parent vessel stumps (Fig. 34-4). Proliferation or reaction of endothelial cells was also seen, but to a lesser extent, in segments obtained from the center of the graft. An intermediate degree of neoendothelial proliferation was observed in graft segments located 3 cm away from each suture line.

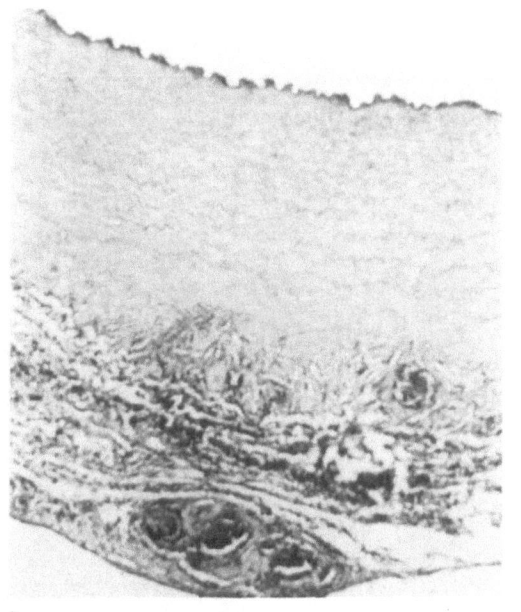

Fig. 34-2. Histology. A. Cross section of control dog CCA specimen obtained after microsurgical dissection and ligation of the vessel showing well-preserved intima and media with patent adventitial microcirculation. H & E stain, × 30. B. Cross section of dog CCA autograft specimen obtained 10 days after implant showing diffuse thinning of the media with loss of nuclei and cellular detail despite preservation of the elastic lamellae. H & E stain, × 25. C. Cross section of autograft obtained 3 months after implant showing focal atrophy of the media, with fibrosis and granulation response in its outer third. Intimal cells are present, and adventitial necrosis is noted. H & E stain, × 25.

A

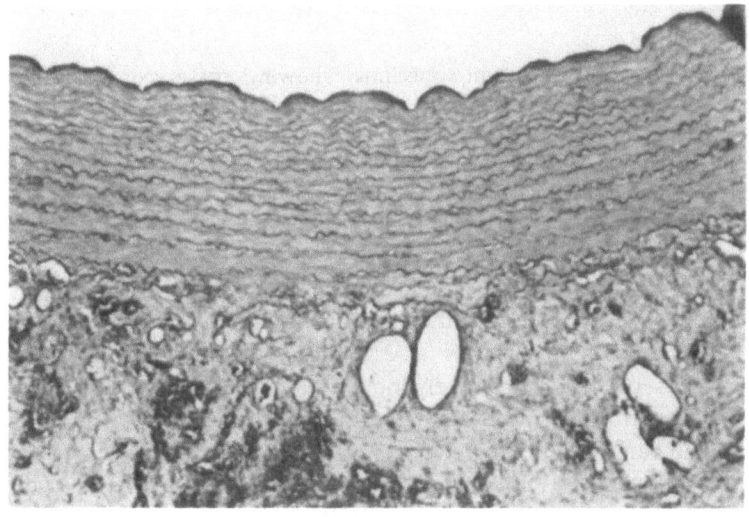

B

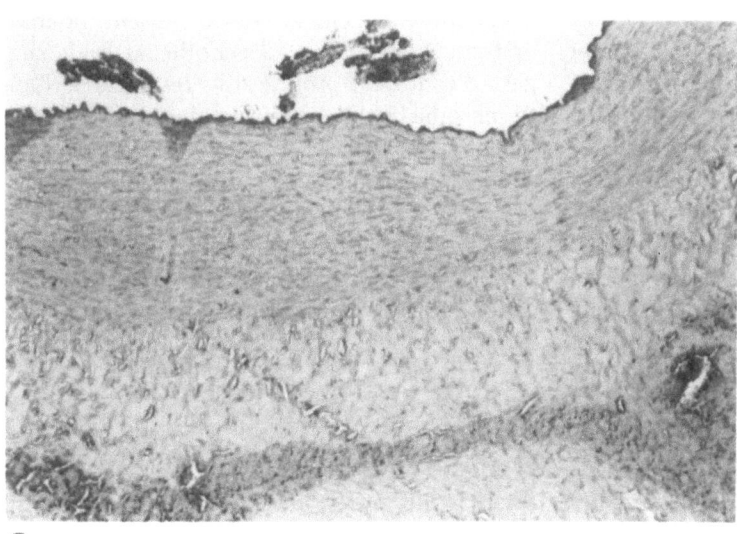

C

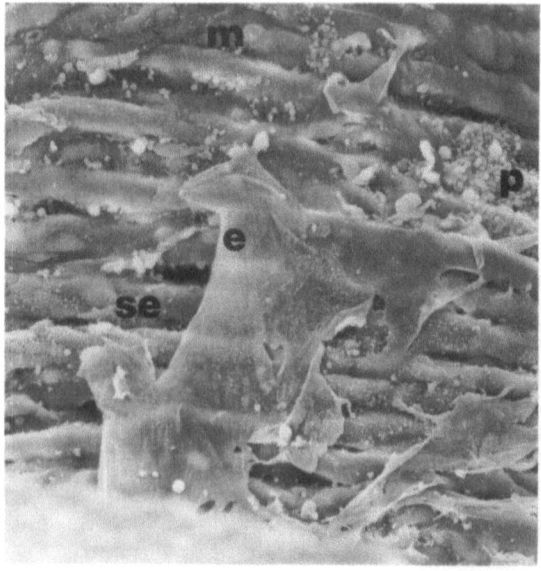

A

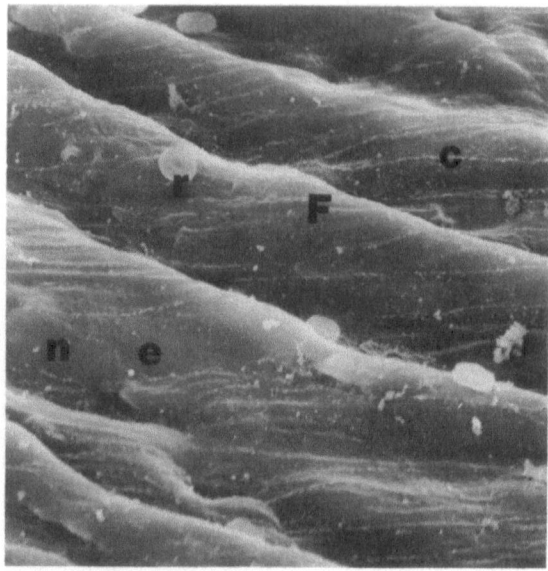

B

Fig. 34-3. A. SEM photograph of dog CCA auto-graft near proximal suture line removed 24 hours after implant showing endothelial necrosis (e), platelet clumps (p) adherent to exposed subendo-thelium (se), and proliferating myointimal calls (m). × 300. B. SEM photograph of center segment, 24-hour specimen showing preserved endothelial cell layer (e), oriented obliquely across corrugated intimal folds (F) of internal elastic layer. Note nucleus (n), cell border (c), and red blood cells (r). × 1000.

The normal corrugated appearance of en-dothelial folds was preserved to a greater extent in the parent vessels than in segments of the grafts adjacent to anastomoses (Fig. 34-4). More centrally located graft luminal surfaces were less flattened. A more normal pattern of intimal folds was reconstituted in the 3-week specimens.

Luminal surfaces of grafts examined 3 weeks after implantation showed variable patterns of endothelial regeneration. In most cases a pseudointima of small fusiform cells with prominent nuclei and indistinct cell borders had completely covered the graft and parent vessel lumina (Fig. 34-4A). However, in one specimen areas covered with an entirely normal endothelial layer were present in proximal and distal but not central graft segments (Fig. 34-5). This finding in a single animal may re-flect a greater degree of initial endothelial preservation at the time of grafting with only minimal damage due to vessel wall ischemia since most 3- and even 6-month specimens continue to exhibit a predominantly immature neoendothelial surface pattern.

Endothelial regeneration was considered complete at 3 months after graft implant, but an entirely normal luminal surface was never observed even in grafts harvested at 6 months. Persistent irregularities in surface contour were observed in association with distorted endo-thelial fold patterns adjacent to some suture lines. Crowding of nests of small immature neoendothelial cells at sites of absent, oblique, or transversely oriented endothelial folds sug-gested continued proliferative response perhaps to chronic intimal trauma due to flow tur-bulence. However, occasional observation of similar phenomena in the center of grafts har-vested at 3 and 6 months suggests that surgical damage to underlying subendothelium, internal elastica, and media may prevent ultimate re-constitution of normal intimal surfaces.

Discussion

Previous experimental studies of microvascular arterial autografts have not provided the in-formation needed for evaluation of long-term

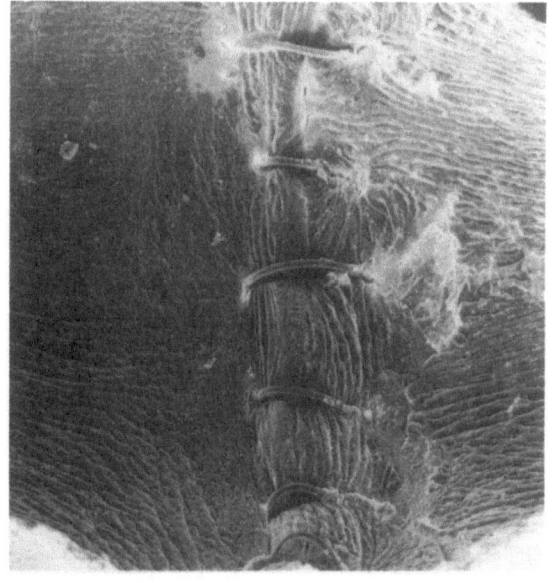

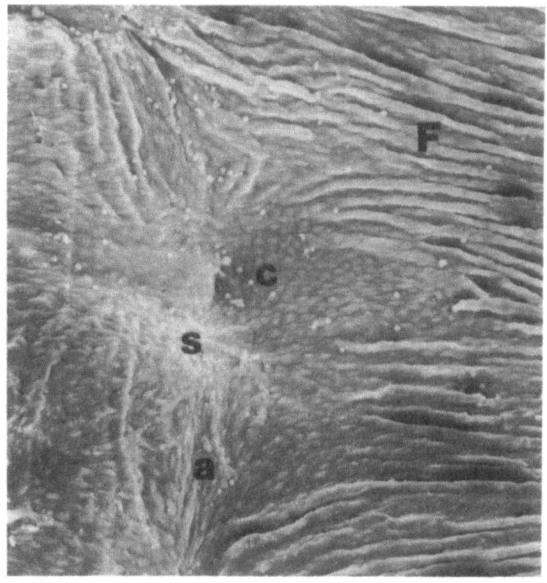

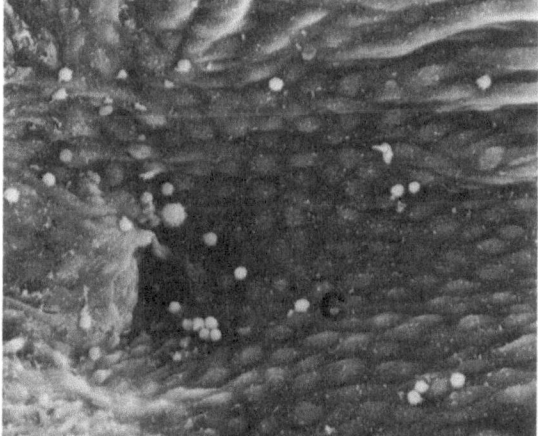

Fig. 34-4. A. SEM photograph of anastomosis 6 days after surgery. Note intimal laceration by center suture. × 40. B. Suture crater (c) in another proximal anastomosis 6 days after graft implant. Small fusiform cells of neoendothelial layer cover anastomotic site (a), suture (s), and folds (F), which are preserved in the parent vessel to the right but lost in the graft to the left. × 100. C. Magnified view of suture crater in B. showing cellular detail of reconstituted neointimal surface. × 300.

patency in vessels of dimensions suitable for EC–IC in patients.[21] Although immunologic rejection of homologous transplanted tissue is not a problem with autografts and long-term tissue preservation is not required as it is with cadaver-donated vessels, maintainance of postoperative patency, restoration of cellular viability, and restoration of adequate blood flow in long segments of arteries 2 to 3 mm in diameter completely isolated from their adventitial blood supply have not been demonstrated previously.[15, 17, 20] Implantation of 1- to 3-mm diameter canine saphenous arteries as CCA–MCA bypass autografts resulted in only 30 to 60% patency rates, possibly because of anatomic and technical problems related to the animal model and to the relatively low blood flows observed.[9, 12, 23] Accordingly, a patency rate of 82% was reported in a study of canine CCA autografts 3 to 4 mm in diameter and 12 cm in length.[4] Anastomoses were not performed with the operating microscope in that

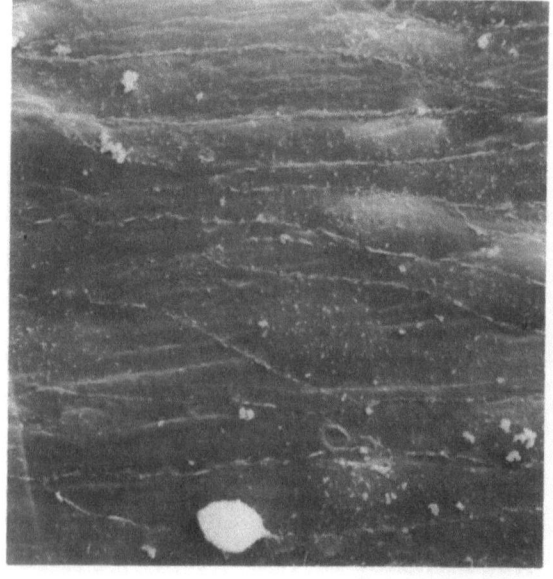

A

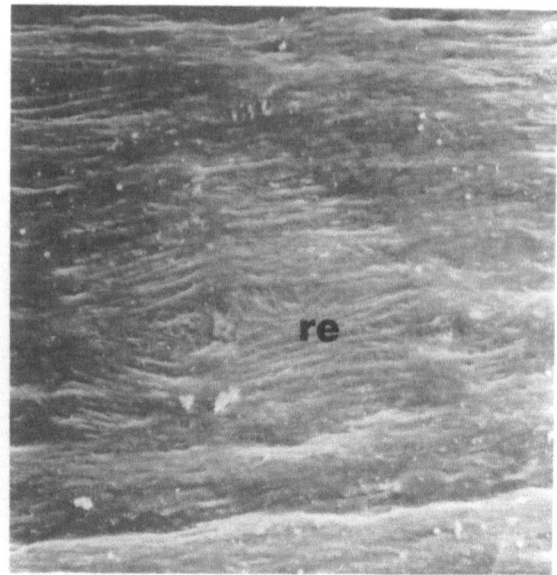

B

Fig. 34-5. A. SEM photograph of normal endo-thelial surface in 3-week graft specimen 3 cm away from the distal anastomosis. × 1600. B. Center segment of same 3-week specimen showing patch of pseudo- or reactive endothelium (re) covering depression in subendothelium surrounded by nor-mally preserved intimal surface. × 200.

study. Use of microsurgical technique resulted in 100% patency rates of 1.5- to 2.0-mm diam-eter rabbit arterial autografts at 3 months but grafts measured only 1 to 3 cm in length.[6] Satisfactory clinical results have been reported for coronary, aortoiliac or peripheral vascular autografting procedures using shorter segments of radial and femoral arteries as donor ves-sels.[5, 22] Our experimental results now indi-cate that satisfactory long-term patency might be expected in microvascular arterial autografts suitable in diameter and length for use in ECA–MCA bypass surgery.

Although canine CCA external vessel diam-eters varied from 2.5 to 4.0 mm, the average was 3.0 mm; internal diameters averaged 2.5 mm. These measurements correspond well with those of the distal radial artery at the wrist in man, which has been used successfully for EIAB.[21] Therefore the dog CCA seems to be an acceptable model for the purposes of this study. The radial artery provides a graft of sufficient length for ECA–MCA bypass and can be removed safely when a brachial arterio-gram demonstrates adequate collateral supply to the hand via the ulnar artery. A larger proxi-mal diameter of 4 to 5 mm would present no problems with end-to-side anastomosis to the ECA.

Arteriograms and blood flow studies per-formed during this experiment indicate slight graft dilatation and moderate flow increases. Our results thus suggest that such small vessel arterial autografts are capable of enlarging with the demand for increased collateral blood flow created by ligation of the contralateral CCA. This is an important requirement of grafts used for ECA–MCA bypass which may not be ful-filled by prosthetic grafts. Progressive graft stenosis or thrombosis due to pseudointimal hy-perplasia or subendothelial fibrosis often ob-served with vein or prosthetic grafts[1, 2, 7, 21] was not found to narrow the lumen or reduce blood flow in any of the animals studied. Aneurysmal graft dilatation occasionally seen following arterial interposition of vein grafts did not occur in this study, indicating, as ex-pected, that the thicker arterial walls may be more likely to remain viable and maintain their tensile strength.[3] Wound or graft infection which may complicate prosthetic or homolo-gous vascular grafting operations did not occur, and antibiotics were not administered to the animals in this study.[14]

Results of the histologic examinations of the grafts indicate that isolation, removal, and reimplantation of 17- to 19-cm-long small artery segments during a 1- to 2-hour operative procedure do not result in extensive necrosis of the arterial wall. We were interested to observe in many animals little, if any, significant difference between the histologic appearances of the graft and parent vessels. Although necrosis and later fibrosis of the outer media layers were seen in some specimens, preservation of the entire muscularis seen in others suggests that intraluminal blood circulation can provide sufficient nutrition to metabolically support the entire media following surgical interruption of adventitial blood supply. This could occur either by diffusion or by capillary circulation within the vessel wall.[8]

Another interesting observation was that of lack of thrombosis and preservation of adventitial vessels and vaso vasorum seen 24 hours after implantation of the grafts. The expected surgical obliteration of adventitial microvasculature did not occur despite complete isolation and removal of the graft artery. A surprising degree of endothelial preservation was also observed in the center of these grafts as compared to vessels examined in our previous autograft studies.[13] We have noted complete endothelial loss in 2- to 5-cm-long segments of 1- to 2-mm diameter arterial autografts in rats and cats. Identical surgical technique, keeping grafts immersed in balanced saline solution to prevent drying, has been utilized in all experiments.

Despite our finding of 100% patency rate, including the seven dogs sacrificed at 6 months, SEM studies indicated that the endothelial cell layer, although reconstituted within 3 weeks, does not resume its normal appearance even 6 months after surgery. Observation of patches of entirely normal endothelium in 24-hour and 3-week specimens probably reflects areas of cellular preservation at the time of autograft surgery. The significance of these persistent morphologic abnormalities in the graft endothelium is unknown, and further longer-term studies of patency and endothelial response in 17- to 19-cm-long microvascular arterial auto-

grafts will be required to resolve this question.[16]

Conclusion

A 100% patency rate in canine common carotid artery autografts 3.0 mm in diameter and 17 to 19 cm in length up to 6 months after operation is reported. Results of angiographic and blood flow studies document satisfactory function of the grafts. Histologic and SEM studies demonstrate preservation of the media, reconstitution of endothelium, and fibrosis of adventitia. When required, arterial autografts may provide a satisfactory conduit for clinical ECA–MCA bypass surgery.

References

1. Bannister, A.M., Mundy, L.A., Mundy, J.E. Fate of small diameter cervical veins grafted into the common carotid arteries of growing rabbits. J Neurosurg 46:72, 1977.
2. Bannister, C.M., Mundy, L.A., Mundy, J.E. Comparative merits of autogenous arterial and venous bypass grafts as alternatives to direct arterial anastomosis. In Microsurgery for Stroke, P. Schmiedek, editor, Springer-Verlag, New York, 1976.
3. Barner, H.B., DeWeese, J.A., Schenk, E.A. Fresh and frozen homologous venous grafts for arterial repair. Angiology 17:389, 1966.
4. Brown, R.B., Huggins, C.E., Koth, D.R. An experimental re-evaluation of the problem of small vessel replacement. Surgery 43:63, 1958.
5. Carpentier, A., Guermonprey, J.L., Deloche, A., Frechette, C., DuBose, C. The aorto-to-coronary radial artery bypass graft. Ann Thorac Surg 2:111, 1973.
6. Crowell, R.M., Yasargil, M.G. Experimental microvascular autografting. J. Neurosurg 31:101, 1969.
7. DeWeese, J.A., Rob, C.G. Autogenous venous bypass grafts five years later. Ann Surg 174:346, 1971.
8. Heck, A.F., Hasuo, M., Furuse, M., Brock, M., Dietz, H. Distribution of serum protein labeled with Evans blue in the walls of extra- and intracranial blood vessels of the cat. Atherosclerosis 23:227–238, 1976.
9. Khodadad, G. Extracranial–intracranial bypass grafts. J Neurol Neurosurg Psychiatry 35:522, 1972.
10. Lazar, M.L., Clark, K. Microsurgical cerebral

214   Philip R. Weinstein, et al.

revascularization: Concepts and practice. Surg Neurol 1:355, 1973.

11. Malone, J.M., Gervin, A.S., Kischer, C.W., Keown, K., Moore, W.S. Venous fibrinolytic activity and histology with distention. Clin Res 26:250, 1978.

12. Maroon, J.C., Donaghy, R.M.P. Experimental cerebral revascularization with autogenous grafts. J Neurosurg 38:172, 1973.

13. Mehdorn, H.M., Weinstein, P.R., Townsend, J.J., Chater, N.L. Comparative evaluation of microvascular arterial grafts: Arterial autograft vs. human umbilical artery graft. Chapter 33, this volume.

14. Moore, W.S., Swanson, R.J., Campagna, G., Bean, B. The use of fresh tissue arterial substitutes in infected fields. J Surg Res 18:229, 1975.

15. Nicholas, G.G., DeMuth, W.E., Graham, W.P. Preservation of venous tissue. J Surg Res 20: 221, 1976.

16. Parks, L.C., ter Haar, A.M., Williams, G.M. Biological significance of endothelial repopulation in allografted vessels. Surg Forum 23:290, 1972.

17. Perloff, L.J., Reckard, C.R., Rowlands, D.T., Barker, C.F. The venous homograft: an immunological question. Surgery 72:961, 1972.

18. Rimm, A.A., Blumlein, S., Barboriak, J.J., Anderson, A.J., Walker, J.A., Johnson, W.D. The probability of closure in aortocoronary vein bypass grafts. JAMA 236:2637, 1976.

19. Tew, J.M., Jr. Reconstructive intracranial vascular surgery for prevention of stroke. Clin Neurosurg 22:264, 1975.

20. Vickery, C.M., McCombs, H.L., Warren, R. Experimental small artery grafts in dogs treated with immunosuppressive drugs. N Engl J Med 272:325, 1965.

21. Weinstein, P.R., Chater, N.L., Peters, N.D., Popp, A.J. Evaluation of 2-mm arterial grafts for extra- to intracranial bypass in occlusive cerebrovascular disease. In Microsurgery for Stroke, P. Schmiedek, editor, Springer-Verlag, New York, 1976.

22. Wylie, E.J. Vascular replacement with arterial autografts. Surgery 57:14, 1965.

23. Yasargil, M.B., Donaghy, R.M.P. Micro-vascular surgery. Report of First Conference. C.V. Mosby, St. Louis, 1967.

35

Arterial Dilatation and Augmentation of Blood Flow in Experimental Arteriovenous Fistulas*

Philip R. Weinstein, H. Maximilian Mehdorn, Robert F. Spetzler, and David A. Telles

Augmentation of cerebral blood flow has been documented following extra–intracranial (EC–IC) anastomosis for bypass of occlusive intracranial vascular lesions.[5] However, in some cases bypass graft enlargement with extensive perfusion of cerebral vessels is not observed on postoperative arteriograms. Several factors influencing graft enlargement and perfusion through the bypass can be identified:

1) Initial diameter of the graft vessel

2) Presence of arteriosclerosis in the graft and recipient vessel

3) Technical accuracy of the anastomosis

4) Initial diameter of the recipient cortical vessel

5) Pressure gradients and resistance determining runoff in the recipient cerebrovascular bed (need for augmentation of collateral blood flow)

Pre- and postoperative arteriographic measurements of EC–IC graft diameters are of uncertain significance, since some cases have demonstrated a lack of correlation with clinical results. At present, no information is available regarding the relationship between arteriographically measured lumen diameter and flow through microvascular grafts. Furthermore, little information is available regarding biomechanical factors limiting arterial dilatation, vessel wall injury or hypertrophy with increasing blood flow, and length of time required for

maximum adaptation of microvascular grafts to increased flow loads. The purpose of this study is to investigate some of these factors by examination of vascular response to increased blood flow through experimental arteriovenous fistulas (AVF).

Methods

Rats, cats, and dogs were used to obtain a vessel diameter range of 1, 2, and 3.5 mm, respectively.

1) Rat AVF. Using microsurgical technique and 10-0 suture at $\times$ 24 under the Zeiss operating microscope, an end-to-side anastomosis was performed attaching the femoral artery to an elliptical incision in the femoral vein in 50 rats (Fig. 35-1). Animals were reexplored surgically at intervals of up to 6 months postoperatively for verification of patency by inspection, measurement of graft diameters, and histologic studies, including scanning electron microscopy (SEM).

2) Direct AVF. Using microsurgical technique, end-to-side anastomosis between the common carotid artery (CCA) and jugular vein (JV), creating a direct AVF, was performed in 20 dogs and 8 cats. CCA external diameters were measured before and after anastomosis by surgically isolating the vessel from surrounding connective tissue, leaving adventitia intact, and placing the vessel inside circumferential flowmeter probes with diameters known to within

*Work supported by funds from United States Veterans Administration Research Office MRIS 9214.

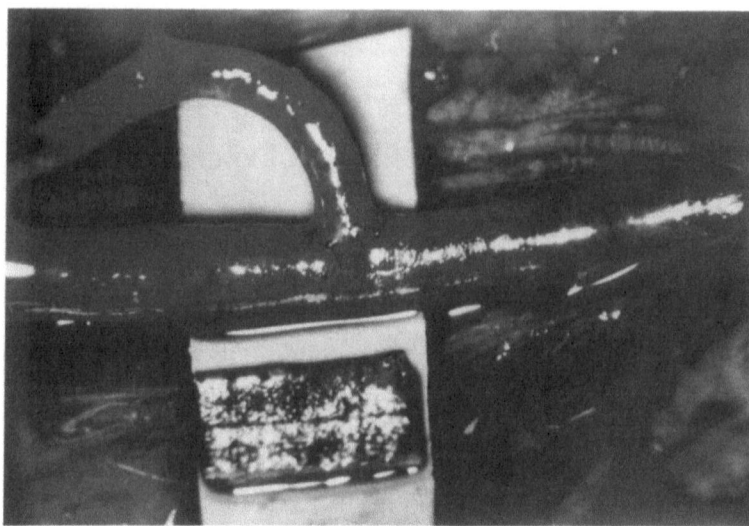

Fig. 35-1. Photograph through the operating microscope at × 16 magnification of end-to-side anastomosis creating a femoral arteriovenous fistula in the rat. Artery measures 1 mm and the vein 3 mm in diameter.

0.5 mm. Following 1% lidocaine irrigation to reverse vasospasm, electromagnetic flowmeter CCA blood flow determinations were made with a Statham SP 2204 flowmeter before and after anastomosis and at the time of surgical reexploration, 1 to 6 weeks later. Graft artery diameters were again recorded at reexploration.

3) Indirect AVF. End-to-end microsurgical anastomosis between the rostral stump of the transected left CCA and the caudal stump of the left JV was performed in 30 cats and 6 dogs. The caudal CCA stump and rostral JV stump were ligated. In this indirect fistula blood flows up the left CCA, through the anterior communicating artery, and down through the AVF, passing across the resistance of the intracranial circulation (Fig. 35-2). External diameter and electromagnetic blood flow determinations were obtained from both CCAs before and after anastomosis and at reexploration 1 to 3 weeks postoperatively.

Carotid arteriograms were obtained by percutaneous transfemoral catheterization of the aortic arch in cats and dogs preoperatively, at the time of direct or indirect AVF construction, and in conjunction with later surgical reexploration (Fig. 35-3). Width of contrast columns was measured on each CCA arteriogram with calipers at the midportion of the vessel under study. Correction for radiographic magnification was computed.

Systemic arterial blood pressure (SABP) was

monitored through a femoral artery catheter during all blood flow measurements. Minor variations of 10 to 44 mm Hg in SABP induced by intravenous phenylephrine did not significantly alter CCA flow; therefore, flow correction for such SABP variations was not deemed necessary.

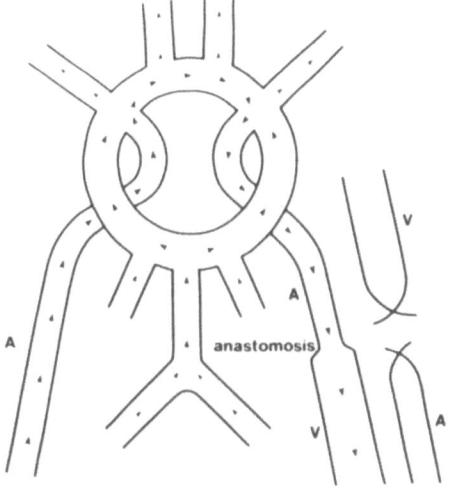

Fig. 35-2. Diagram of indirect AVF model after end-to-end anastomosis between the left rostral anastomosis (direct AVF). Note 80% stenosis of the circle of Willis down the left internal carotid. The AVF is fed in part by the right CCA where changes in blood flow and vessel diameter are measured.

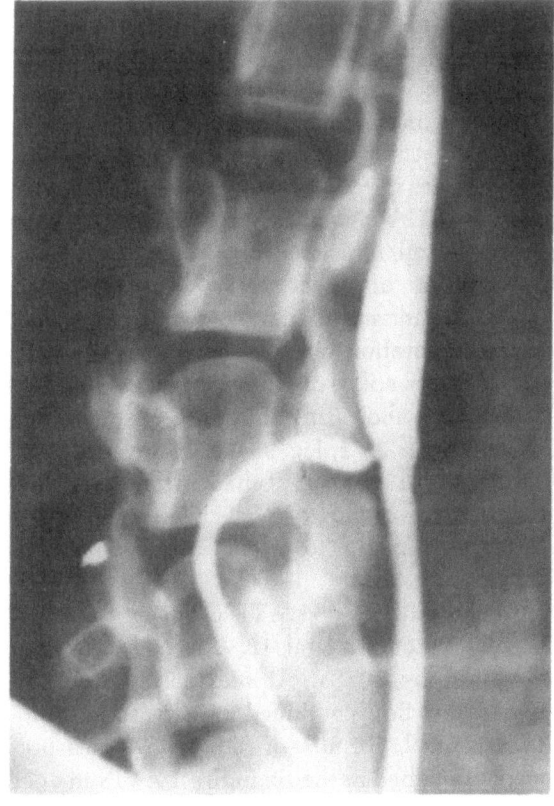

A

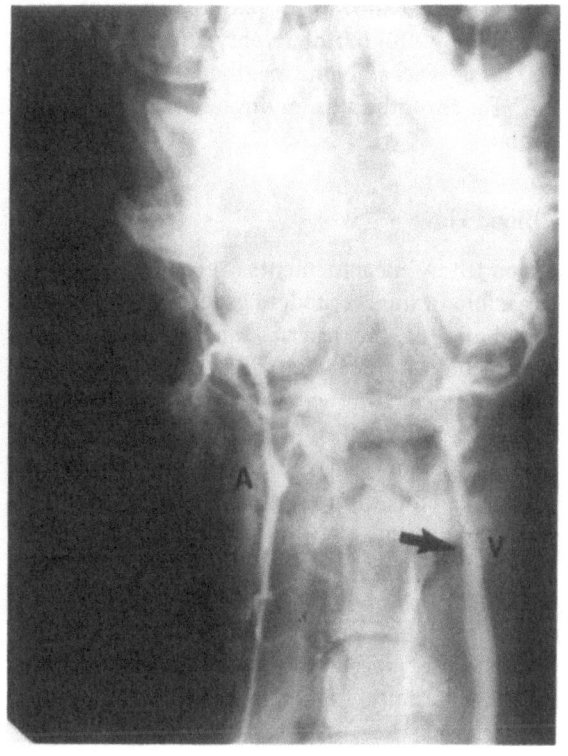

B

Fig. 35-3. A. Right CCA arteriogram obtained 3 weeks after end-to-side canine carotid–jugular anastomosis (direct AVF). Note 80% stenosis of CCA just proximal to the fistula and bidirectional perfusion in the vein which has dilated rostrally and narrowed caudally. In this animal control CCA flow of 94 ml/min increased to 764 ml/min immediately after AVF construction. At the time of arteriography 3 weeks later, a flow of 123 ml/min was recorded, perhaps reduced by arterial stenosis due to intimal hyperplasia seen histologically and on SEM studies. B. Arteriogram obtained 3 weeks after left end-to-end feline carotid–jugular anastomosis (indirect AVF). Contrast opacifies right common carotid artery (A), anastomosis (arrow), both intracranial internal carotids and left CCA–JV fistula (V).

AVFs were preserved for removal via an in-vivo transaortic (rats) or brachiocephalic (cats and dogs) infusion, saline rinse, followed by perfusion with Karnovsky's fixative. Vessels were prepared for histologic examination with hematoxylin-eosin and elastic/van Gieson stains. Lumen surfaces of vessels were prepared by critical-point drying after dehydration with alcohol and gold impregnation for scanning on an ETEC AutoScan SEM. Because of the risk of intimal damage, angiography was not performed prior to perfusion of specimens to be used in SEM studies.

Results

Patency

In 50 rat anastomoses a 100% patency rate was verified by reexploration at intervals of up to 6 months. Similarly, in the cat direct AVF model no postoperative thromboses were discovered at reexplorations done at intervals of up to 3 weeks. In the cat indirect AVF model an 80% patency rate was found, that is, of thirty animals only six were shown to have thrombosis of the fistula when reexplored at intervals of up to 3 weeks. The dog direct AVF series showed a patency rate of 95% with only one out of twenty thrombosed after 3 to 6 weeks. None of the six dog indirect AVFs thrombosed, giving a 100% patency rate.

Blood Flow

Blood flow measurements were not technically feasible in the rat model because of small initial diameter of the arteries and failure of AVF construction to induce later graft dilatation. However, qualitative assessment of blood flow through the AVF was attempted by observation of changes in the amount of venous distention and filling with red arterial blood before, during, and after application of a temporary vascular clip to the femoral artery. Diameter of the feeding artery and flow through the AVF appeared to have remained the same or decreased at the time of reexploration, especially in the animals explored at 3 months or later.

In cats CCA blood flows of 15 to 50 ml/min (control) were observed following initial exposure of the vessel. Measurements obtained following completion of the direct CCA to JV anastomoses averaged 363% increase, or 125 ml/min (Table 35-1). When repeated measurements were obtained 1 to 3 weeks postoperatively, average blood flow remained relatively unchanged with respect to control, but in one cat flow had increased to 845%.

In the indirect cat AVFs flow measurements obtained from the contralateral CCAs revealed an immediate 91% postoperative increase with a 181% increase found at 1 week. AVF flows measured on the anastomosed CCA were 18% less than control initially with variable increases seen 1 to 3 weeks postoperatively.

Initial CCA blood flows in twenty dogs were 75 to 150 ml/min (control). Immediately after construction of direct AVFs in twelve dogs, blood flow increased an average of 581%. During reexploration at 3 weeks after surgery values were still 121% over control but had dropped to about one third the postoperative values (Table 35-1, Fig. 35-3). At 6 weeks postoperatively 1 dog's AVF had thrombosed and another had stenosed to such an extent that flow was too low to measure electromagnetically.

In the indirect dog AVF group initial postoperative contralateral CCA blood flow had increased by 105%. At reexploration 1 to 3 weeks later flow continued to increase to 278% over control. Results of serial flow measurements obtained in the six indirect AVFs in dogs showed more consistent changes than those obtained in the cat series. Comparison between flow measurements in cat and dog direct and indirect AVFs is shown in Fig. 35-4 and Table 35-1.

External Vessel Diameter

In-vivo measurements of external diameter of the artery feeding the AVFs showed no discernible change in 50 rats at the intervals of re-

Table 35-1. Blood flow (ml/min)

		P OP 1 hour		P OP 1 to 3 weeks	
	Control	Average	Percent change	Average	Percent change
Direct					
Dogs	112	769	587%	248	121%*
Cats	27	125	363%	98	263%
Dogs & Cats			504%*		154%*
Indirect					
Dogs	152	311	105%	422	178%
Cats	21	40	91%	59	181%
Dogs & Cats			99%*		179%*

*Percentage calculations weighted for number of animals studied.

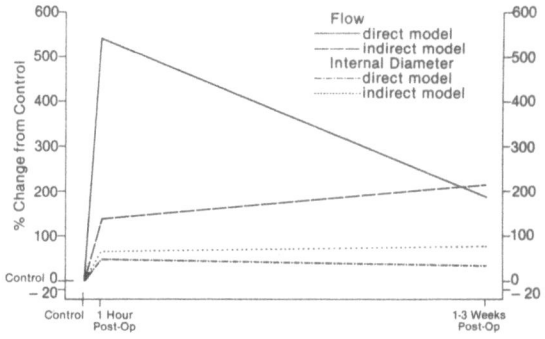

Fig. 35-4. Comparison of average percentage change from control in blood flow measured electromagnetically and internal vessel lumen diameter measured arteriographically 1 hour and 1 to 3 weeks after construction of direct and indirect arteriovenous fistula. Note marked initial increase in direct AVF flow followed by later decline, while gradual progressive flow increase is observed with indirect AVFs. Slight dilatation of the feeding artery is observed only in the indirect model.

increase in contralateral CCA was observed initially, while reexploration showed an additional 12% increase.

Luminal Diameter

Both dogs and cats revealed a trend toward initial and progressive increase in luminal diameters of the AVF feeding arteries in the indirect model and initial increase followed by decrease in the direct model as estimated by measurements of intravascular contrast column width (Table 35-3). In direct AVFs arteriograms showed diffuse narrowing of that portion of the feeding artery which had been dissected prior to anastomosis. In the indirect AVF model both dogs and cats evidenced a consistent diameter increase up to 3 weeks postoperatively. Although some variations were noted, average postoperative diameters were 7 to 54% greater than those of controls.

Blood Flow Versus Vessel Diameter

exploration. In the cat direct AVFs enlargement of up to 0.5 mm was seen immediately after the fistulas were established, with some animals showing a slight increase at reexploration 1 to 3 weeks later. In the cat indirect AVF model similar results of contralateral CCA measurements were observed (Table 35-2). Direct AVFs in dogs resulted in an average initial increase of 0.5 mm or 12% in external arterial diameters immediately postoperatively with slight additional increase seen at 3 weeks. In the dog indirect AVF series an average of 4%

In six small cats average control CCA external diameter was 2.0 mm in association with average arteriographic contrast column width of 1.4 mm and blood flow values of 25 ml/min measured simultaneously. In six large dogs average control CCA external diameters of 3.5 mm corresponded with arteriographic measurements of 3.0 mm and blood flows of 147 ml/min. In one dog CCA external and arteriogram

Table 35-2. External diameter (mm)

| | Control | P OP 1 hour | | P OP 1 to 3 weeks | |
		Average	Percent change	Average	Percent change
Direct					
Dogs	3.46	3.85	12%	3.88	12%
Cats	2.10	2.20	5%	2.50	19%
Dog & Cats			11%*		13%*
Indirect					
Dogs	4.10	4.25	4%	4.75	16%
Cats	1.90	2.20	16%	2.12	12%
Dogs & Cats			10%*		14%*

*Percentage calculations weighted for number of animals studied.

Table 35-3. Internal diameter (mm)

		P OP 1 hour		P OP 1 to 3 weeks	
	Control	Average	Percent change	Average	Percent change
Direct					
Dogs	2.94	3.06	4%	2.56	−13%
Cats	1.40	1.50	7%	1.80	29%
Dogs & Cats			5%*		− 1%*
Indirect					
Dogs	3.10	3.30	7%	4.00	29%
Cats	1.30	1.90	46%	2.00	54%
Dogs & Cats			27%*		42%*

*Percentage calculations weighted for number of animals studied.

diameters were 5.0 and 4.2 mm in association with the highest control blood flow value of 190 ml/min. In a smaller dog external and arteriogram diameters of 3.0 and 1.9 respectively were measured with a flow of 53 ml/min observed.

When blood flow changes were compared with external and internal vessel diameter measurements, no correlation was found for direct AVFs. For example, an average initial blood flow increase of 431% was observed in three direct dog AVFs immediately after anastomosis while arteriographic arterial lumen diameters increased an average of only 4%. However, in another dog the initial postoperative arterial diameter increased from 2.7 to 3.1 mm at 3 weeks while blood flow decreased from 1000 to 459 ml/min, whereas in another animal a similar postoperative flow decrease was associated with a lumen diameter decrease from 2.4 to 2.1 mm. Only indirect AVFs in both dogs and cats showed a consistent correlation between contralateral CCA diameters and blood flow. Internal diameter of the anastomosed CCA of indirect AVFs was not proportional to the retrograde blood flow it received. For example, the arteriographic diameter of the anastomosed CCA decrease from an average of −19% from control postoperatively to −23% at 1 week, while flow increased from 12% to 47% over control for the same period. However, on the contralateral side the average arteriographic diameter increased 7% over control postoperatively to 29% at 1 week, and there was a simultaneous increase in blood flow from 82% to 114% over control during the same period.

Histology and Scanning Electron Microscope (SEM) Studies

Direct AVFs. Histologic studies of the direct AVFs in the rat, cat, and dog revealed evidence of mild to moderate subintimal fibrosis and endothelial hyperplasia with varying degrees of stenosis, more on the arterial than on the venous side of the fistulas. These changes were not observed until 3 to 6 months postoperatively in the rats, but were present and more extensive at 1 to 3 weeks than at 1 to 2 days in the cats and dogs. No evidence of damage or hyperplasia in the muscularis layers of the arterial media relating to dilatation caused by experimentally induced increase in blood flow was observed. However, in some animals atrophy and fibrosis of the muscular layer of veins were seen.

SEM studies confirmed the histologic findings of intimal and subintimal hyperplasia in the direct AVFs, which were more extensive in the arteries and at the site of anastomosis than in the veins. Initial loss and later reconstitution of an irregular neoendothelial cell layer at the anastomotic site were observed. Significant persistent distortion and irregularity of the subendothelial surface configuration with formation of polyps, flaps, and ledges were also seen (Fig. 35-5 A, B). Loss of normal corrugated fold patterns with irregular foci of marked endothelial immaturity and hyperplasia in both arteries and veins was observed (Fig. 35-5 C). Deposition of platelet aggregates, fibrin strands, and microthrombi was noted to persist at 2 weeks. A smooth carpet of reconstituted flat polygonal endothelial cell monolayer was never observed at the anastomotic site or in the adjacent artery, although relatively normal venous endothelium was seen 1 cm from the anastomosis in some specimens at 3 weeks (Fig. 35-5 D).

In some specimens more severe polypoid subintimal and endothelial hyperplasia was observed just proximal to the suture line, resulting in preocclusive stenosis of the artery in one dog and thrombosis in another. Most rat specimens studied 6 months after construction of the AVF showed artheromatous plaques in the veins at sites of polypoid subendothelial hyperplasia opposite the arterial anastomosis, presumably related to chronic intimal trauma and degeneration.

Indirect. Histologic and SEM studies of the indirect AVFs demonstrated more abnormalities in the veins than in the arteries, a finding just opposite to the results in the direct AVF studies. Mild to moderate subintimal hyperplasia and medial fibrosis in the arterialized veins were noted. A more normal pattern of venous endothelial regeneration was observed which differed little in cats and dogs. Striking abnormalities were seen on SEM studies of the contralateral CCA specimens, which showed platelet deposition, reactive endothelial hyperplasia, and patchy intimal necrosis present at 2 days and still persistent at 1 to 3 weeks. However, histologic studies showed no damage or hyperplasia in the media. Arteries feeding the indirect AVFs appeared to be more dilated with straightened internal elastica folds than those feeding direct AVFs.

Examination of the anastomotic sites showed marked subendothelial and medial proliferative cellular reaction often exceeding the expected foreign body response to suture material. Intraluminal projection of organized thrombus or redundant vessel wall may have contributed to stenosis in some specimens, although serial measurements of blood flow through the AVFs indicated that progressive increases had occurred despite this narrowing.

Discussion

Flow of blood through small arteries depends largely upon resistance when pressure, volume, and viscosity remain constant. Since resistance is varied mainly by changes in vascular lumen diameter, considerable attention has been devoted in the neurosurgical literature to comparison of initial and postoperative caliber of EC–IC bypass grafts. This experimental study of vessel diameter and flow in experimental AVFs is intended to investigate the significance of these clinical observations.

We studied hemodynamic and histologic response to the construction of experimental AVFs in three different animals (rats, cats, and dogs) in order to compare results in arteries of varying sizes which were superficial in location and therefore easy to expose without risk of surgical complications. Species differences in vascular physiology were not considered to be significant for the purposes of this study, but variations in animal size, weight, cardiac output, and blood pressure are important factors.

The direct AVF model was selected so that blood flow changes, biomechanical limitations to arterial dilatation, and morphologic effects could be evaluated after end-to-side arterial anastomosis into an extremely low-pressure and low-resistance circulatory bed where maximum potential flow augmentation might occur through the fistula. This system does not accurately model the end-to-side artery anastomosis used clinically to EC–IC bypass, but it does provide an opportunity to study vascular response to a need for increased blood flow. For comparison with these results, the indirect AVF model provides data obtained under circumstances whereby blood in one CCA flows through the circle of Willis into an efferent venous fistula constructed in the opposite proximally ligated CCA.

Initial patency rates were 100% in rats, cats, and dogs. The AVF thromboses observed in cats and dogs all occurred between 3 and 6 weeks postoperatively and were clearly related histologically to stenosis of the artery and/or vein due to subintimal thickening rather than to inaccurate suture technique. Therefore our results confirm that satisfactory patency can be expected when precise microvascular technique

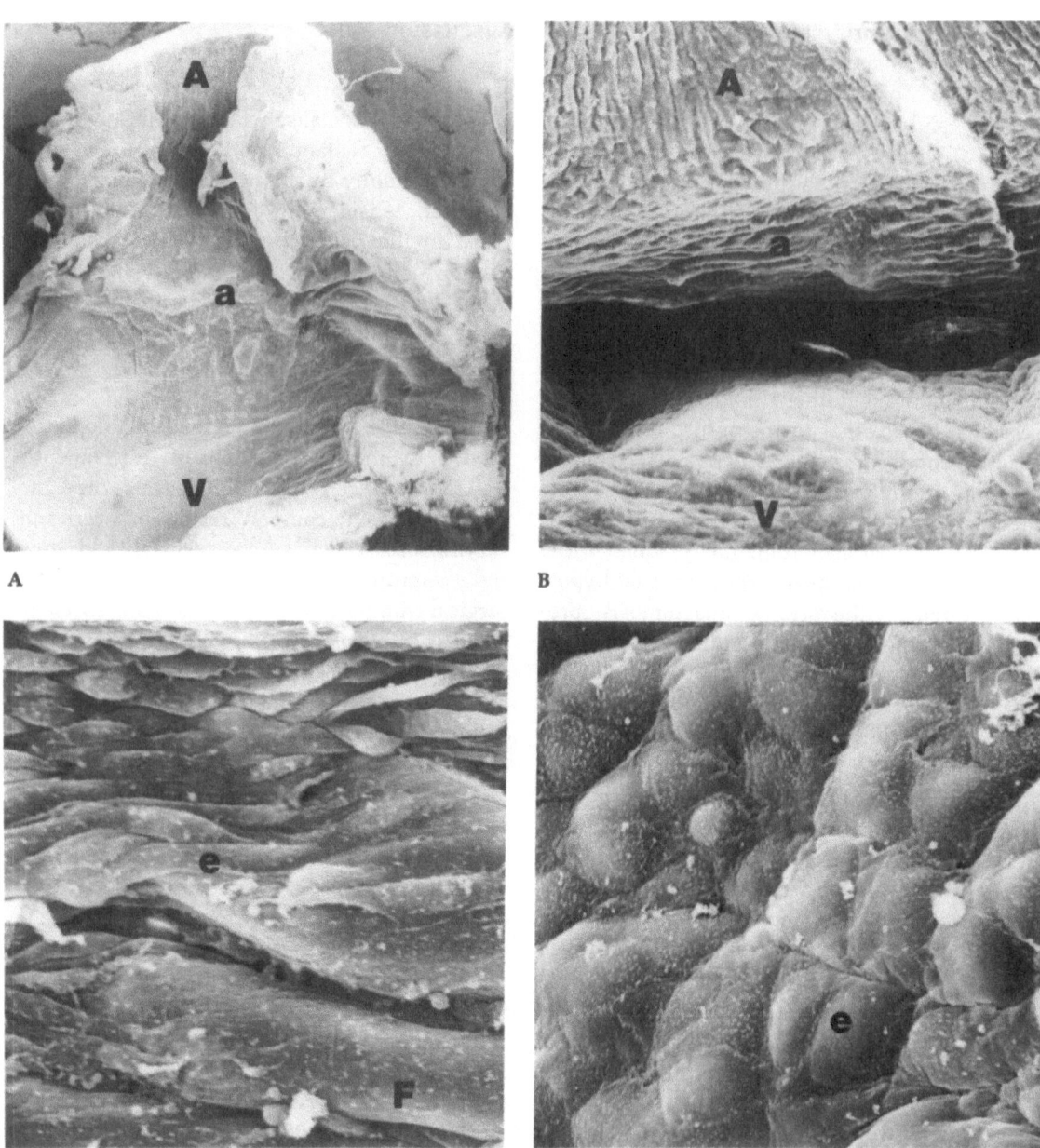

Fig. 35-5. A. SEM photograph of end-to-side anastomosis (a) of CCA (A) to JV (V) 3 weeks after surgery. Note irregular endothelial bunching and subendothelial projections on luminal surface. Stenosis and mural thickening of the artery are observed. × 10. B. At higher magnification covering of arterial (A) and venous (V) surfaces with small swollen neoendothelial cells is observed.

× 70. C. Arterial lumen surface shows marked irregularity with discontinuity of endothelial cell monolayer (e) and disorganization of endothelial folds (F). × 1000. D. Venous luminal surface is covered with foreshortened plump neoendothelial cells (e) showing much less distortion and discontinuity than the artery.

is utilized for end-to-side anastomosis with external diameters of donor or graft vessel ranging from 0.75 to 4.0 mm. Moreover, a donor-to-recipient vessel diameter ratio often equal

to 1:2 or 1:3, which is the reverse of that observed clinically in EC–IC bypass, did not adversely influence initial patency in the direct AVF model. Our observations in rats do suggest that graft vessels of 1 mm or less in diameter preoperatively cannot be expected to enlarge with increased blood flow after surgery. These findings have been confirmed by preliminary results of recent experiments in which a 1-mm diameter thyroid branch of the CCA failed to enlarge in dogs after anastomosis to the JV with distal CCA ligation. Flows of less than 10 ml/min were observed and late thrombosis of the AVF occurred.

Control CCA measurements in cats indicated that blood flows of only 15 ml/min were observed in 1.5-mm arteries and 20 to 50 ml/min in 2-mm vessels. Flows of 75 to 125 ml/min can be expected in 3-mm dog CCAs and 4- to 5-mm arteries in larger dogs may carry control flows of 150 to 195 ml/min. Accordingly, use of 2.5- to 3.5-mm grafts should be considered for clinical application in EC–IC bypass patients requiring immediate substitution for a major intracranial vessel where higher flow rates are needed. Comparison with human cerebral arterial diameters and flows is presented in Table 35-4.

Perhaps the most unexpected finding in this study was the observation of a combined average of over 500% initial increase in blood flow through direct AVFs in cats and dogs. Despite the relative inaccuracy of electromagnetic flowmeter determinations, the dramatically increased flow values of well over 500 ml/min recorded after direct canine CCA to JV anastomoses cannot reasonably be attributed to errors of measurement alone. The flowmeter used has been shown to result in standard deviations of ± 5% for flows under 100 ml/min with 1- to 2-mm flow probes, flows under 300 ml/min with 25- to 30-mm probes, and up to 1000 ml/min with 3.5-mm probes. Ob-

servations of venous distention and rapid, often bidirectional, flow of arterialized blood through the fistulas were considered to be compatible with results of electromagnetic recordings. Also consistent with our findings are documented blood flows greater than 250 to 300 ml/min in human radial arteries (average 3 mm in diameter), routinely used in side-to-side radial arteriovenous shunts constructed clinically for renal dialysis.[4]

Cardiac output measurements indicate that values of 900 to 2700 can be expected in 8- to 12-kg animals.[3] Since in our study dog weights averaged 15 to 35 kg and cats weights 4 to 8 kg, we can assume that direct AVF blood flows observed could have represented approximately 30% of the animals' cardiac output. Cardiac failure was not observed postoperatively. Cerebral blood flow in humans normally represents 20% of cardiac output.

Our results indicate that an arterial graft 2 to 3 mm in diameter is anatomically and physiologically capable of carrying blood flows of 250 to 400 ml/min into an experimental AVF. Theoretically, such flow rates could functionally replace the human internal carotid (350 ml/min and 3.7- to 4.5-mm external diameter) or middle cerebral (100 to 125 ml/min and 1.8- to 3.1-mm diameter) arteries. A graft 1 to 2 mm in diameter could carry flows of 75 to 240 ml/min. Superficial temporal and occipital arteries usually fall in the 1- to 2-mm diameter range.

Unexpectedly, the finding of maximum blood flow augmentation immediately following direct AVF construction with no change or decrease in flow at the time of reexploration contradicts clinical experience with postoperative arteriograms in EC–IC bypass patients. We had

Table 35-4. Clinical correlation of experimental arterial external diameter and blood flow data

	Carotid artery diameter	Control blood flow	Human anatomical equivalent
Cat	1–2 mm	15– 50 ml/min	Cortical branch, middle cerebral artery (MCA)
Dog	3 mm	75–125 ml/min	Main trunk, MCA
Dog	4–5 mm	150–195 ml/min	Approaches internal carotid artery diameter (3.7–4.5 mm) and flow (350 ml/min)

anticipated finding relatively low initial AVF flows with progressive increase to be recorded as the feeding vessel to the AVF dilated over a period of several weeks. However, our results indicate that in the direct model high AVF flows occur initially, with gradual later decrease. This could be caused by increased central venous pressure, decreased cardiac output and/or progressive stenosis at the anastomotic site, and atrophy of the arterialized vein. Later improvement in EC–IC bypass blood flow, as reported in clinical studies, may be due to resolution of vasospasm, removal of platelet aggregates and microthrombi from anastomotic sites, or resistance in the recipient cerebral circulatory bed rather than to the maturation and dilatation of the graft itself.[5] The progressive increase in flows seen in the indirect AVFs is probably a more accurate model of the clinical situation.

Of considerable importance was the observation that size and weight of the experimental animal and resulting initial preoperative feeding arterial diameter, rather than the capacity for expansive delayed arterial dilatation at some time after AVF construction, determined the level of maximum flows achieved through the arterial grafts. Thus, while maximum AVF feeding arterial flows of 200 to 250 ml/min were recorded in cats, flows of 600 to 1000 ml/min were measured in dogs. The role of other factors, such as individual animal or species differences in cardiac output, was not assessed in these experiments but has been reviewed in clinical studies of patients with radial artery AVFs constructed for renal dialysis.[6]

Although a trend toward increase of both external vessel diameter and arteriographic contrast column width was observed postoperatively, no mathematical relationship between blood flow and vessel diameter was found in these studies. As expected, Poiseuille's law: flow = $\Delta P \, r^4/8 \, nl$,* which relates laminar nonpulsatile flow of a homogenous liquid through a rigid tube across a known constant pressure differential to the fourth power of its radius, did not apply. Accordingly, in the indirect model, where a higher resistance was present

*P = pressure, n = viscosity, l = length, r = radius.

in the circulation distal to the vessel under study, there was a more consistent correlation between increases in contralateral CCA blood flow and internal diameter. Dilatation of EC–IC bypass grafts and intracranial arteries feeding arteriovenous malformations in the clinical situation may thus be promoted by the presence of a circulatory bed with greater resistance and higher opposing pressure. Our findings of less extensive flow increase but more predictable feeding vessel dilatation in the indirect AVF model would be consistent with such an interpretation. Further comparative studies with these two models are needed.

Failure of the feeding artery to enlarge progressively after construction of direct AVFs also suggests that attempts to obtain larger scalp vessels for EC–IC anastomosis by preliminary creation of a superficial temporal artery arteriovenous shunt using an adjacent scalp vein several weeks prior to bypass might not succeed. Such a technique has been proposed, but clinical trials have not been reported.

Finally, lack of correlation between repeated external and/or arteriographic luminal diameter measurements and simultaneous electromagnetic blood flow determinations in the same animals suggests: (1) inaccuracy in external diameter measurements (± 0.5 mm) and/or flow values (± 5 to 10%) are responsible; (2) vasospasm, vessel wall edema, or adventitial fibrosis interfered with accuracy of measurements; (3) central venous pressure, cardiac output, and blood pressure variations and adaptations may have introduced significant error; (4) external or luminal diameter differences of 1 mm or less observed by intraoperative measurement or serial arteriography may not, in fact, represent significant differences in blood flow through microvascular grafts. Therefore findings on early postoperative arteriograms in EC–IC bypass patients should be interpreted cautiously.

The histologic and SEM findings of impaired endothelial regeneration and proliferative response to chronic intimal trauma are consistent with the hemodynamic effects of high flow and turbulence reported in other experimental studies of arteriovenous shunts.[8, 9] After end-to-side CCA to JV anastomosis in sheep, intimal tears, dissection, subintimal or mural thrombus formation, and degenerative atheromatous changes were seen, especially on the venous side of the anastomosis. Intimal thickening, medial degeneration, and irregular enlargement with occasional aneurysmal dilatation of the arteries was observed. Arteriosclerosis and intimal thickening have also been observed in venous grafts after arterial interpositioning.[1, 2, 10] Injury to endothelium of venous grafts after experimental distention at arterial pressure has also been reported.[7] Our SEM studies of specimens obtained at 24 and 48 hours after end-to-side anastomosis showed similar evidence of venous endothelial tearing and disruption. No unusual early arterial damage was seen, although later specimens showed significant reactive, proliferative, and stenotic changes while the venous side of the AVF appeared to normalize, perhaps through decreasing blood flows. Further long-term morphologic studies of end-to-side EC–IC arterial anastomosis, including examination of specimens obtained from autopsy of bypass patients, will be required to determine whether or not progressive stenosis due to hemodynamic stress will interfere with long-term patency and blood flow.

Our findings of less extensive histologic and SEM evidence of arterial wall damage in the end-to-end indirect AVF model suggests that abnormal intraluminal hemodynamic stresses are more extensive after end-to-side anastomosis and after construction of a direct high-flow fistula. Observation of extensive endothelial damage and reaction without evidence of abnormality in the media or late decrease in blood flow in the opposite unoperated CCA of the indirect AVF animals suggests that significant but less damaging hemodynamic stresses are applied in small arteries which undergo sudden increases in blood flow subsequent to rapid onset of demand for collateral circulation. It would appear unlikely that arterial distention due to dilatation rather than to intraluminal hemodynamic stress is responsible. The extensive chronic reactive and hypertrophic intimal changes observed at the site of anastomosis were more severe in the direct AVFs and appeared consistent with sustained trauma due to turbulence and hemodynamic stress.

Summary

Blood flow through experimental arteriovenous fistulas depends more on initial feeding artery diameter and construction of shunt directly into a low pressure recipient vessel than on capacity of the feeding artery to undergo progressive dilatation over an extended period of time. Maximum blood flows of 250 ml/min can be expected through 2-mm diameter arterial grafts (cat CCA) while flows as high as 600 to 1000 ml/min are observed through 3- to 4-mm diameter grafts (dog CCA). Variations of 1 mm or less in intraoperative external vessel diameter measurements and postoperative arteriographic lumen diameter estimates may not correlate with proportional differences in blood flow through microvascular grafts. Chronic turbulence-related intimal damage at sites of experimental end-to-side arteriovenous microvascular anastomosis can lead to progressive stenosis and decrease in blood flow in this model. Intimal damage, resultant intimal proliferation, and hypertrophy appeared to be much less serious problems in the end-to-end anastomosis. Microvascular grafts and recipient vessels 1 mm or less in diameter may fail to enlarge with demand for increased blood flow or develop progressive stenosis in relation to increased hemodynamic stresses.

References

1. Bannister, C.M., Mundy, L.A., Mundy, J.E. Comparative merits of autogenous arterial and venous bypass grafts as alternatives to direct arterial anastomosis. In Microsurgery for Stroke, P. Schmiedek, editor, Springer-Verlag, New York, 1976.
2. Beebe, H.G., Clark, W.F., DeWeese, J.A. Atherosclerotic change occurring in an autogenous venous arterial graft. Arch Surg 101: 85–88, 1970.
3. Brescia, M.J., Cimino, J.E., Appel, K., Hurwich, B.J. Chronic hemodialysis using venipuncture and a surgically created arteriovenous fistula. N Engl J Med 275:1089–1902, 1966.
4. Detweiler, D.K., Buchanan, J.W., Gregin, G.F., Hill, J.D. The beagle as an experimental dog. In Heart, A.C. Andersen, editor, Iowa State University Press, Ames, 1970.
5. Gratzl, O., Schmiedek, P., Spetzler, R., Stein-

hoff, H., Marguth, F. Clinical experience with extra–intracranial arterial anastomosis in 65 cases. J Neurosurg 44:313–324, 1976.

6. Johnson, G., Jr., Blythe, W.B. Hemodynamic effects of arteriovenous shunts used for hemodialysis. Ann Surg 171:715–723, 1970.

7. Malone, J.M., Gervin, A.S., Kischer, C.W., Keown, K., Moore, W.S. Venous fibrinolytic activity and histology with distention. Clin Res 26:250, 1978.

8. Stehbens, W.E. Blood vessel changes in chronic experimental arteriovenous fistulas. Surg Gynecol Obstet X:327–338, 1968.

9. Stehbens, W., Karmody, A. Venous atherosclerosis associated with arteriovenous fistulas for hemodialysis. Arch Surg 110:176–180, 1975.

10. Vlodaver, Z., Edwards, J.E. Pathologic changes in aortic–coronary arterial saphenous vein grafts. Circulation 44:719–728, 1971.

36

The Effect of Heparin on the Patency Rate of Autogenous Vein Grafts Inserted into the Arterial System of Rats

Carys M. Bannister and Sonia A. Chapman

In earlier experiments we found that in rats jump grafts made from autogenous veins with diameters of about 1 mm had very poor patency rates.[1] It was our opinion that a major factor leading to the blockage of the grafts is the net-like construction of the venous internal elastic lamina which provides scanty cover for the numerous collagen fibers lying in the subendothelial layer once the endothelium is lost. Exposure of the strongly thrombogenic collagen to the blood stream is followed by deposition of fibrin and platelets on its surface, and rapidly leads to occlusion of the vessels.

In spite of this, veins remain an attractive means of carrying blood from proximal arteries to the ischemic cortex when branches of the external carotid artery are unavailable for direct artery-to-artery anastomosis. It is, therefore, of interest to investigate further the sequence of events leading to the blockage of vein grafts, and the effect of heparin on them.

Grafts were made in nine albino rats by anastomosing 1-cm lengths of cervical veins to the common carotid arteries. After blood had flowed through the grafts for 5, 15, 30, or 60 minutes, the grafts together with a few millimeters of adjacent artery were excised and fixed in 2.5% buffered glutaraldehyde. The specimens were then passed through graded solutions of acetone and critically point dried before being coated with gold in a splutter coater. They were examined and photographed with a Cambridge Stereoscan S4–10.

The two grafts examined at 5 min were patent, but at 15 min only one out of three was patent, at 30 min one of two was patent, and at 60 min both grafts were occluded.

Scanning electron microscopy of the 5-min grafts showed that, although the arterial and venous endothelium was damaged, there were no platelets or fibrin on the luminal surface of the artery (Fig. 36-1A), and on the vein there was only a thin sheet of fibrin on the surface near the anastomosis (Fig. 36-1B). Elsewhere in the graft there were occasional platelets and a few strands of fibrin (Fig. 36-1C). At 15 min, there were only a few strands of fibrin and some platelets on the luminal surface of the artery at the sites of endothelial damage. However, the anastomotic lines were almost obscured by thick wads of fibrin (Fig. 36-2A), and near the anastomoses the surface of the graft was covered by a meshwork of fibrin with red blood cells entangled in it (Fig. 36-2B). Where the endothelium of the graft was intact there were only a few red blood cells lying on its surface (Fig. 36-2C). At 30 min, the numbers of platelets sticking to the damaged arterial endothelium were small, but the anastomotic lines were now totally obscured by wads of fibrin which extended for a short distance into the graft (Fig. 36-3A). Along the length of the graft parts were covered by a fibrin meshwork with entangled red blood cells, and on others very large numbers of platelets had been laid down (Fig. 36-3B). Where the endothelial damage was less severe, few platelets had been laid down but white blood cells

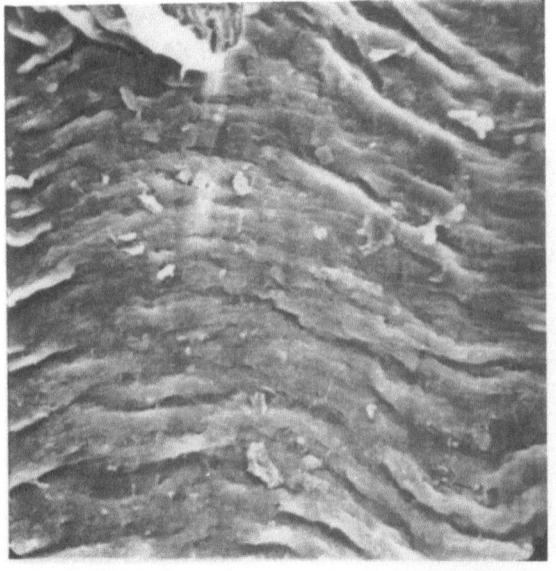

A

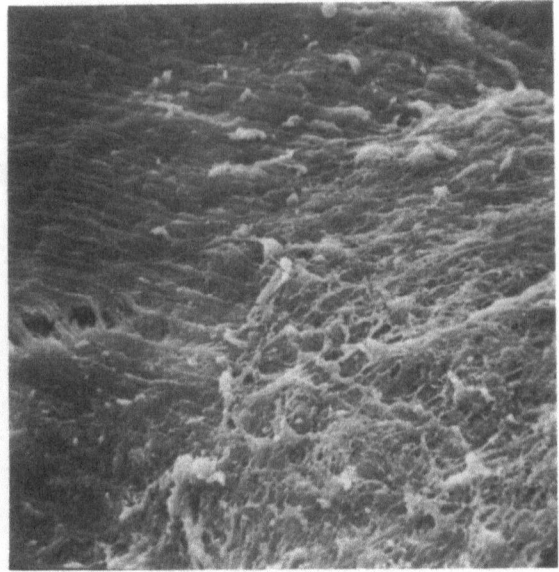

B

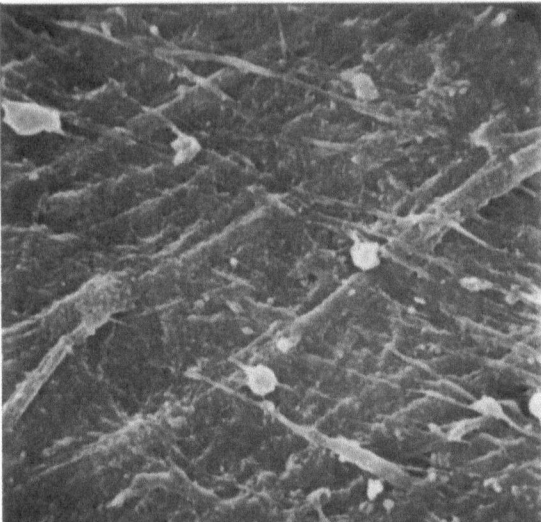

C

Fig. 36-1. Photomicrographs of a vein graft 5 min after blood had started to flow through it. A. Luminal surface of the adjacent artery showing endothelial damage but no adherent platelets or fibrin. × 500. B. Vein graft near anastomosis showing a thin layer of fibrin on the luminal surface. × 1050. C. Vein graft away from the anastomosis showing occasional platelets and strands of fibrin on the luminal surface. × 5400.

were present among them (Fig. 36-3C). In other areas where the endothelial damage consisted only of swelling of the cells, microvilli, and occasional holes in the endothelial layer, a few scattered platelets were present adhering mainly at the sites of the endothelial holes (Fig. 36-3D). Clotting prevented a detailed examination of the 60-min grafts.

Arterial endothelial damage excites little response, but venous endothelial damage, particularly at the anastomotic lines, causes fibrin to be deposited in increasing amounts, so that eventually the blood flow through the grafts is impeded. Within an hour after the blood is allowed to enter the grafts, clotting of stagnant blood trapped in the grafts caused them to be completely occluded (Fig. 36-4).

Heparin acts by neutralizing thrombin and factor X (probably also factors XII, XI, and IX) and affects platelet adhesiveness. Given

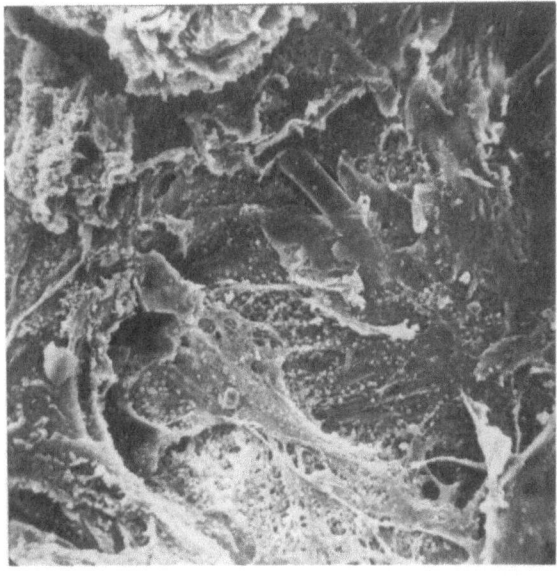

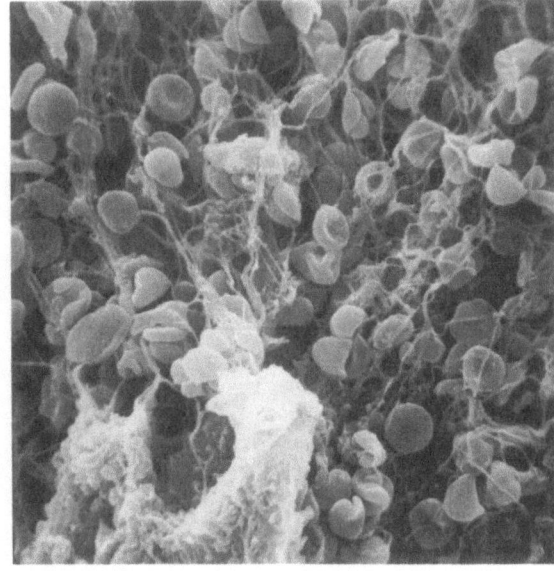

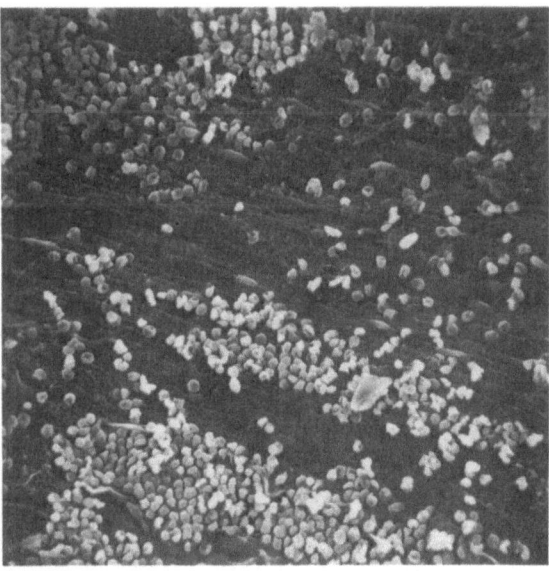

Fig. 36-2. Photomicrographs of a vein graft 15 min after blood had started to flow through it. A. One of the anastomoses almost covered by wads of fibrin. × 210. B. Luminal surface of the vein graft near the anastomosis covered by a meshwork of fibrin with entangled red blood cells. × 2100. C. Part of vein graft where the endothelium is intact and there are only red blood cells on its surface. × 530.

subcutaneously to rats it was ineffective; however, if heparin in dosages of 5 units per 100 g of body weight were given intravenously half an hour before completion of the operation and a solution of heparin was used to wash out the veins before grafting, it prevented the occlusion of 8 grafts examined 5, 15, 30, or 60 minutes after blood was allowed to flow through them. These grafts were prepared for scanning electron microscopy.

Scanning electron microscopy of the 5-min graft showed that there were a few platelets and some strands of fibrin adhering to the damaged endothelium of the artery. They were also present at the sites of anastomosis and along the length of the graft (Fig. 36-5). At 15 min, the arterial surface again had only a few platelets and strands of fibrin. At the anastomoses (Fig. 36-6A) and along the length of the graft there were only a few scattered platelets in spite of extensive endothelial damage (Fig. 36-6B). The 30- and 60-min grafts

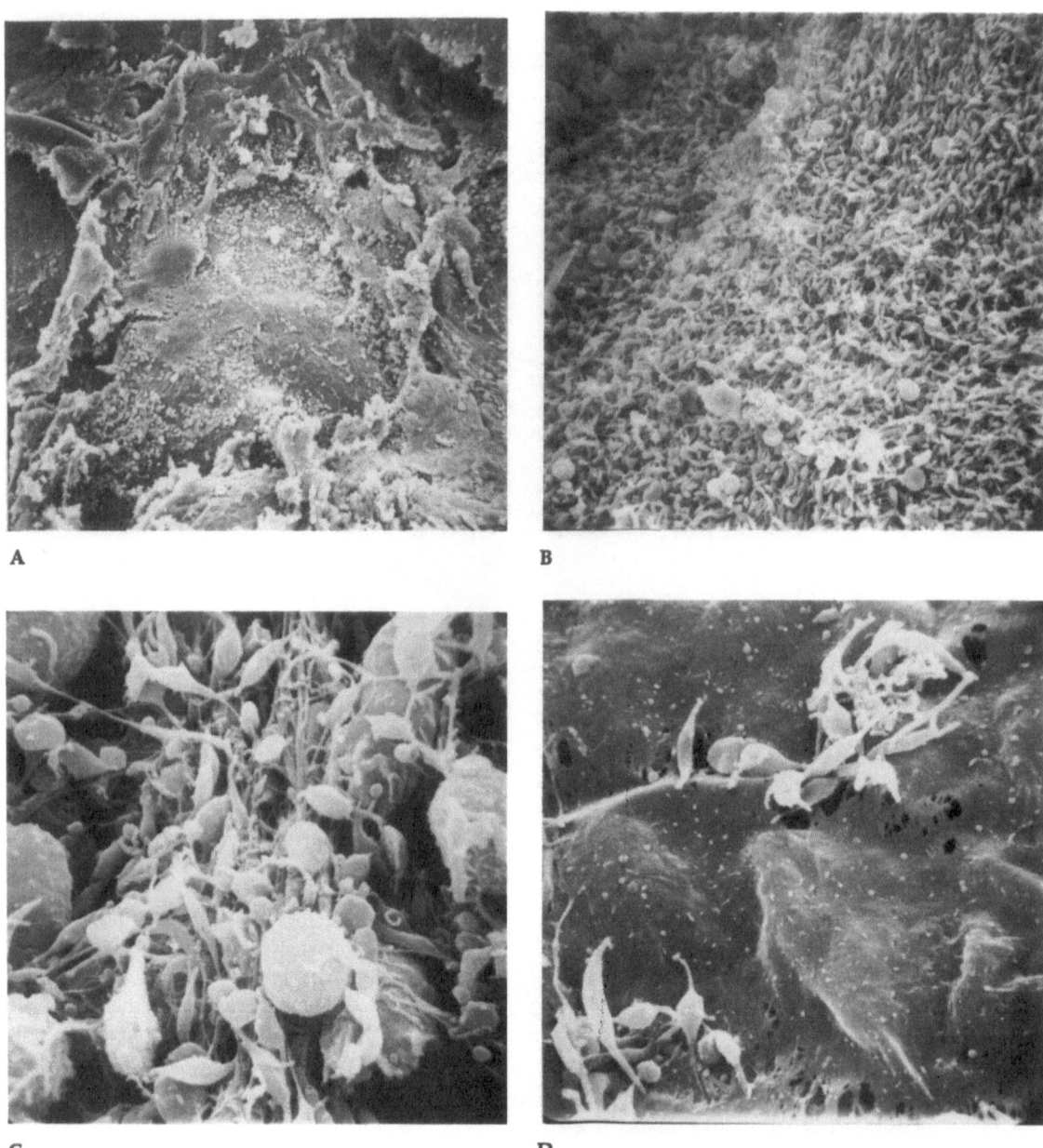

Fig. 36-3. Photomicrographs of a vein graft 30 min after blood had started to flow through it. A. One of the anastomoses obscured by wads of fibrin. × 210. B. Vein graft near an anastomosis covered by enormous numbers of platelets. × 1050. C. Another part of the vein graft covered by fewer plate-lets and white blood cells. × 250. D. An area of the vein graft less severely damaged; there are holes in the endothelium with platelets grouped around them. The endothelial cells have microvilli on them. × 5250.

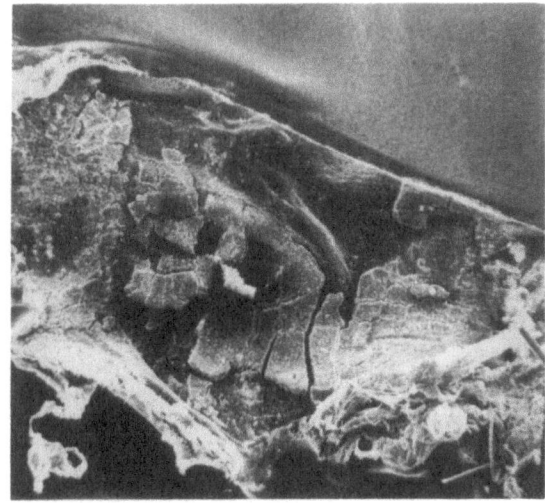

Fig. 36-4. Photomicrograph of a vein graft 15 min after blood had been allowed to flow through it, showing clotting of blood trapped in the graft. × 21.

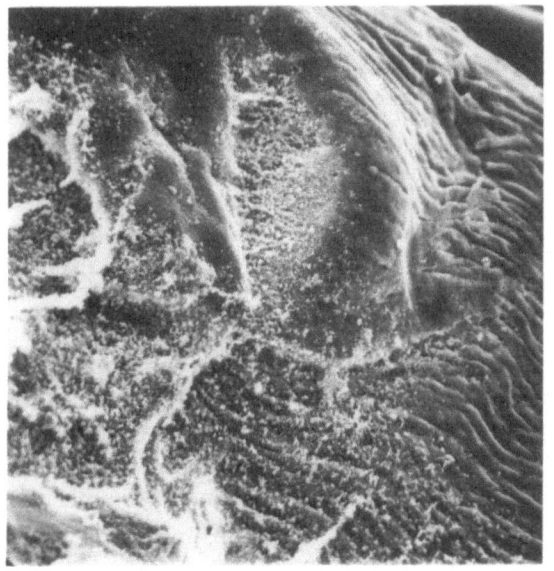

A

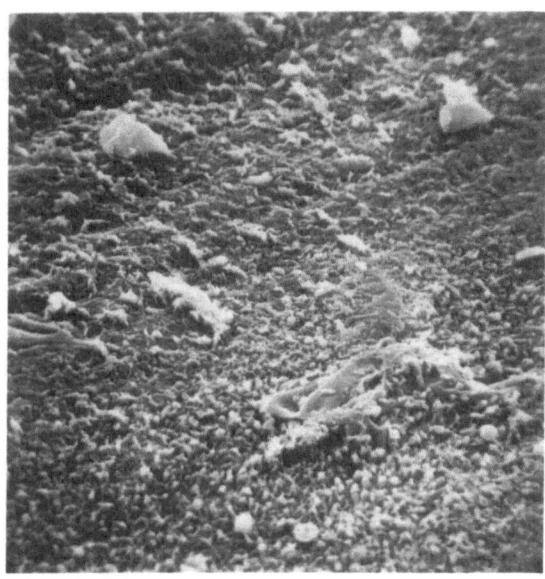

B

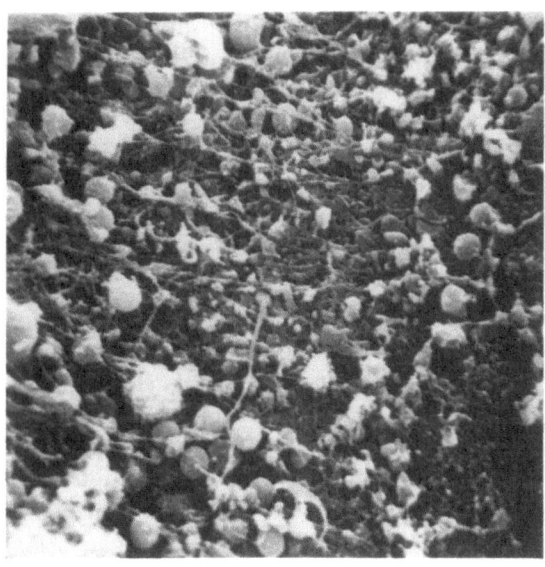

C

Fig. 36-5. Photomicrographs of a vein graft made after heparin had been given intravenously and 5 min after blood had been allowed to flow through the graft. A. Luminal surface of the artery adjacent to one of the anastomoses showing a few platelets and some fibrin adhering to the endothelium. × 210. B. Luminal surface of the vein graft near the anastomosis showing a thin layer of fibrin and platelets. × 1050. C. Same area of the graft under increased magnification showing strands of fibrin and platelets. × 2100.

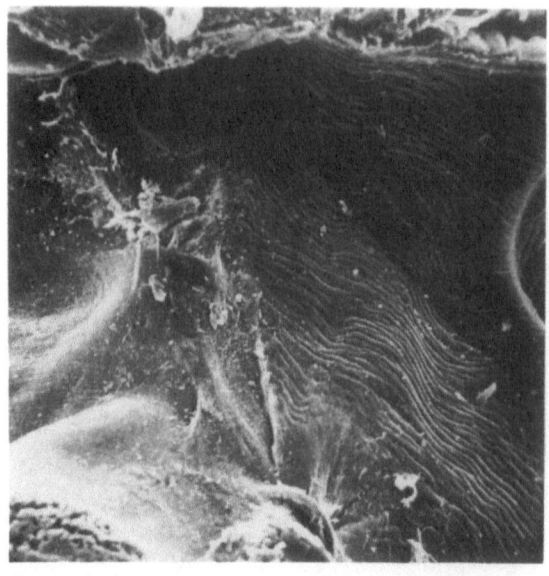

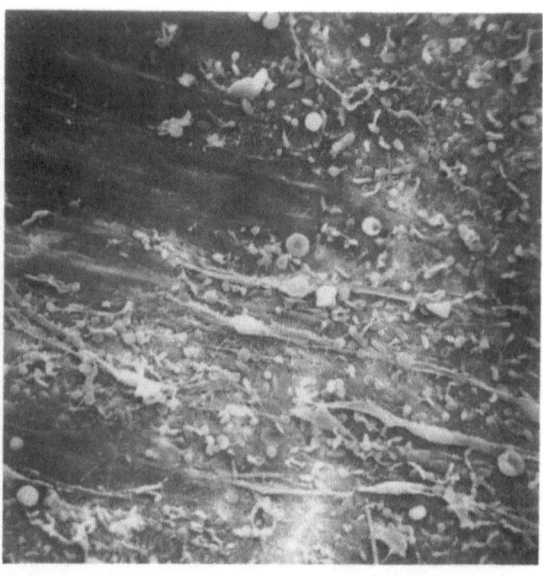

A

B

Fig. 36-6. Photomicrographs of a vein graft made after heparin had been given intravenously and blood had been allowed to flow through the graft for 15 min. A. One of the anastomoses showing very little fibrin. × 105. B. Part of the vein graft showing extensive endothelial damage but only a few platelets adhering to the luminal surface. × 1100.

showed essentially the same appearance as the 15-min ones.

Heparin significantly reduces the amount of fibrin formed on the anastomotic lines and along the lengths of the grafts. It also limits the numbers of platelets deposited, and allows the vein grafts to remain patent for at least an hour. But the half-life of heparin given intravenously is only 1½ to 2 hours, and endothelium heals slowly, during which time potentially thrombogenic material is exposed to the blood stream. It was not possible, however, to give the rats repeated doses of intravenous heparin. Nevertheless it was decided to follow the progress of grafts made in rats who had received a single dose of heparin half an hour before the completion of their operations and in whom heparin had been used to wash out the veins before grafting. Eight grafts were made and were examined between 1 and 11 weeks later; all except the graft examined at 7 weeks were patent. The patent grafts were prepared for scanning electron microscopy.

Scanning electron microscopy of the 1-week graft showed that considerable regeneration of the arterial endothelium was taking place (Fig. 36-7A). Many of the arterial endothelial cells were swollen, and these cells extended up to the anastomotic line (Fig. 36-7B). There was no fibrin at the anastomoses, but a part of the graft was covered by a fibrin meshwork with red blood cells entangled in it, and another part was covered by a thin layer of fibrin with platelets on its surface (Fig. 36-7 C, D). No regenerating venous endothelial cells were seen, probably because they were covered by fibrin. At 2 weeks arterial endothelial regeneration was still in progress, and many of the cells had microvilli on them (Fig. 36-8A). In the graft venous endothelial regeneration was now seen, and many cells in these areas had microvilli (Fig. 36-8B). Prominent bridging structures were present joining some of the venous endothelial cells (Fig. 36-8C). Here and there along the graft a few platelets and strands of fibrin were present. At 3 weeks regenerating arterial endothelial cells were again seen, and cells close to the anastomoses were swollen. In the graft the venous endothelial cells were also regenerating. Large numbers of white blood cells were present, many of them congregated at the edges of areas denuded of endothelium (Fig. 36-9A). Some of the white blood cells appeared to be acting as scavengers (Fig.

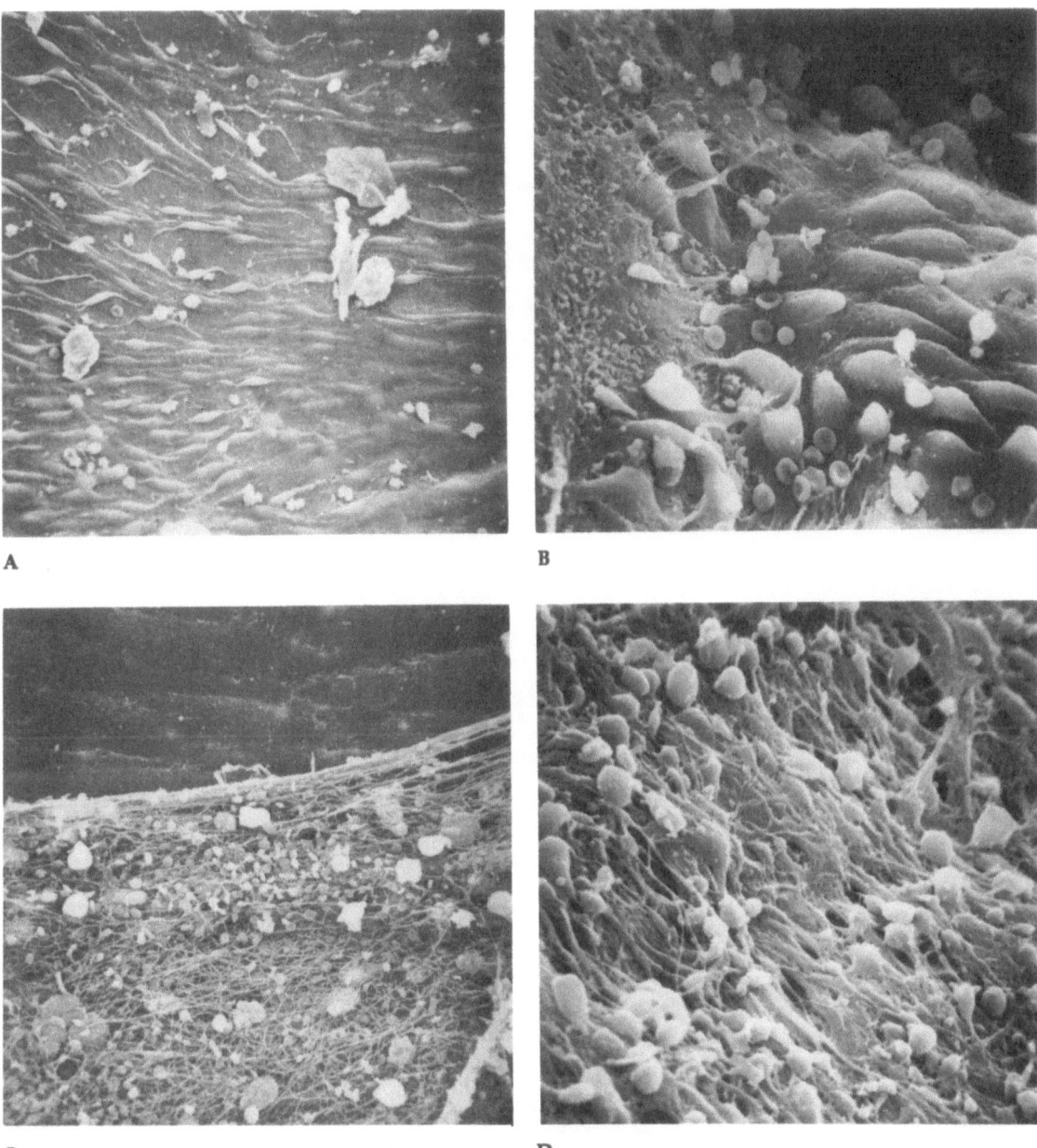

A

B

C

D

Fig. 36-7. Photomicrographs of a vein graft made after heparin had been given intravenously and examined 1 week later. A. Endothelial regeneration occurring in the artery adjacent to one of the anastomoses. × 530. B. Many of the arterial cells are swollen and these extend up to the anastomotic line. × 1100. C. Part of the luminal surface of the vein graft is covered by a meshwork of fibrin with entangled red blood cells. × 1100. D. Another part of the vein graft is covered by a thin layer of fibrin and platelets. × 5400.

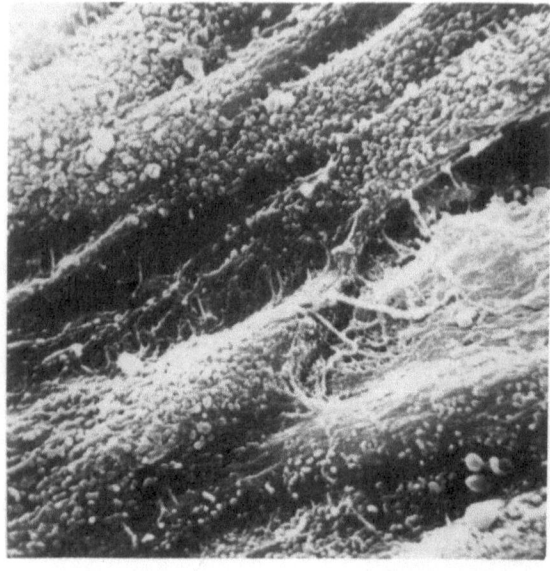

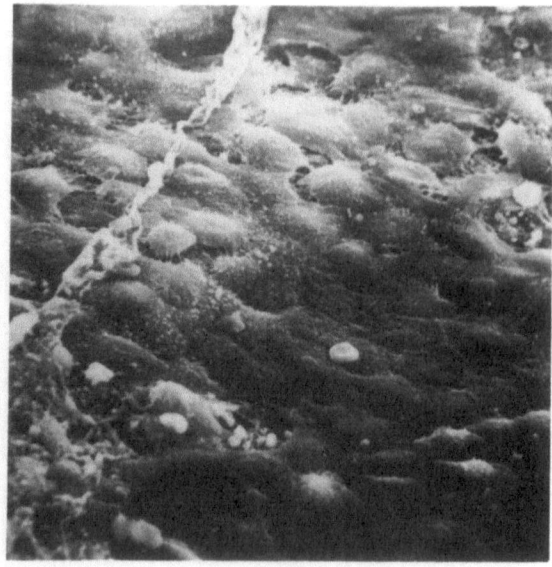

A

B

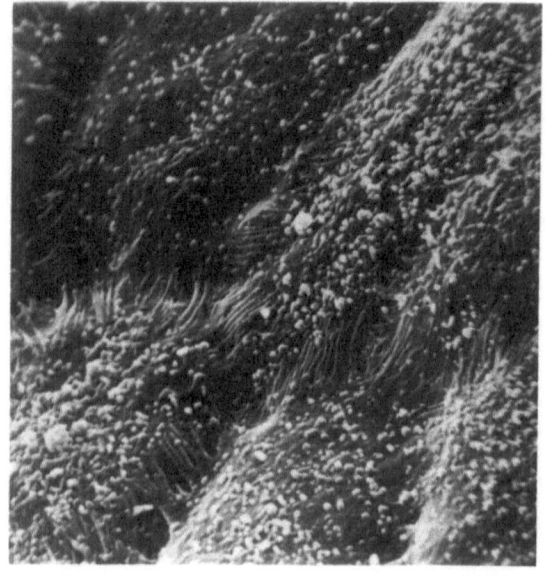

C

Fig. 36-8. Photomicrographs of a vein graft made after heparin had been given intravenously and examined after 2 weeks. A. Regeneration of the arterial endothelium is occurring close to the anastomoses. Many of the cells have microvilli on them. × 5400. B. The venous endothelium is also regenerating. × 1100. C. Many of the venous endothelial cells have prominent structures bridging adjacent cells. Many cells have microvilli. × 5400.

36-9B). At 5 weeks, regeneration of the arterial endothelium was complete although many cells were swollen. In the graft venous endothelial regeneration was still in progress, in places beneath persisting patches of fibrin (Fig. 36-10A). White blood cells were again present on the endothelial surface in areas where endothelialization was incomplete (Fig. 36-10B). Many venous endothelial cells had microvilli on them. By 11 weeks venous endothelial regeneration appeared to be complete.

Dirrenberger and Sundt[3] and Fishman et al.[4] have shown that arterial endothelium after injury regenerated completely in about 10 days, though Christensen and Garbarsch[3] showed that the process could take much longer. In our specimens arterial healing was complete only after 5 weeks, and the venous endothelium of the graft took longer, about 10 weeks. Throughout this time tissue other than endothelium was exposed to the blood stream but no fibrin was seen other than that laid down

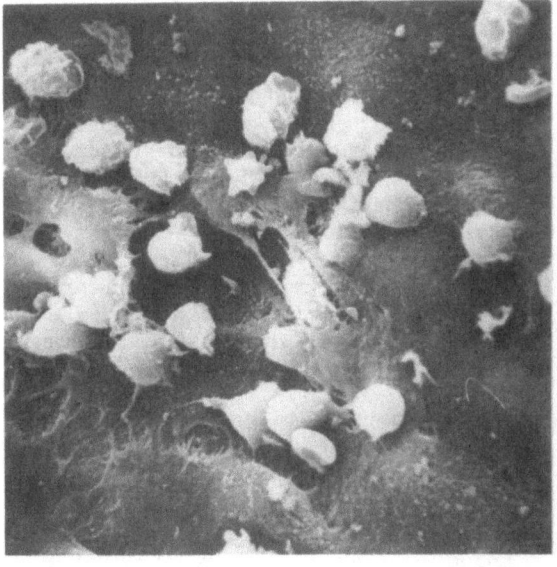

A

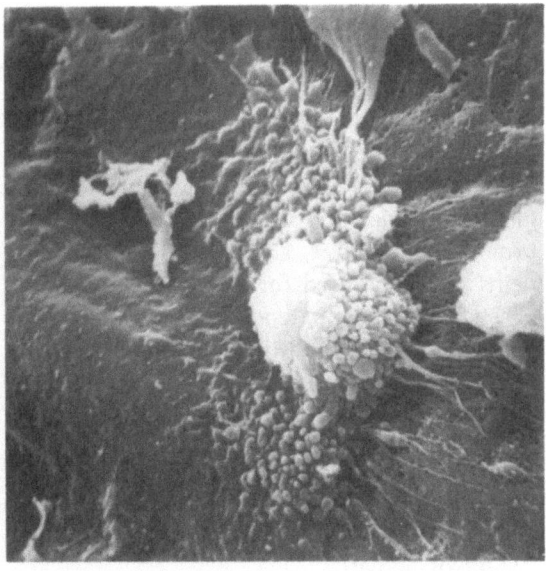

B

Fig. 36-9. Photomicrographs of a vein graft made after heparin had been given intravenously and examined 3 weeks later. A. On the luminal surface of the vein graft white blood cells are present at the edges of areas denuded of endothelium. × 2150. B. Some of the white blood cells appear to be acting as scavengers. × 5400.

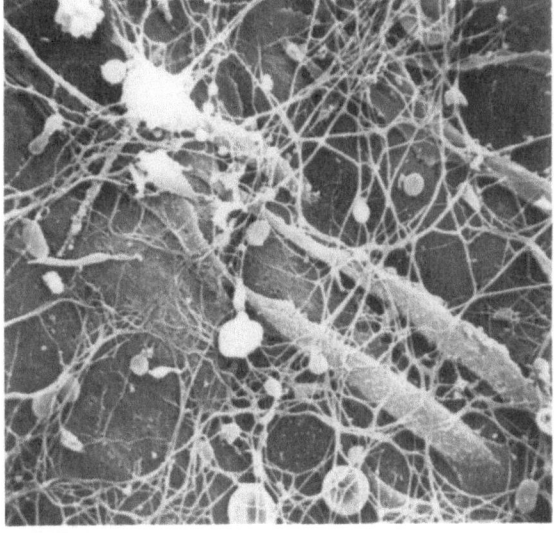

A

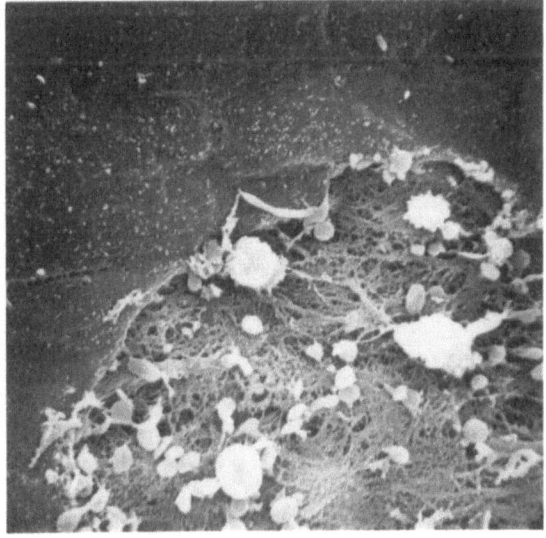

B

Fig. 36-10. Photomicrographs of a vein graft after heparin had been given intravenously and examined 5 weeks later. A. Venous endothelial regeneration is still occurring, in places beneath persisting fibrin meshwork. × 2200. B. White blood cells are also still present at the edges of areas denuded of venous endothelium. × 2200.

during the first hour after blood started to flow through the graft; only occasional newly deposited platelets were seen lying on the surface of the graft in areas denuded of endothelium. It appears, therefore, that within a very short time exposed subendothelial tissues in both arteries and veins lose their ability to promote thrombosis, so that if small-diameter veins are to be used for jump grafts one way of ensuring their patency is to wash out the veins to be grafted with a solution and give heparin intravenously half an hour before operation, and then continuing the heparinization for the immediately ensuing few hours; long-term heparinization is not necessary.

Acknowledgment

We wish to express our sincere thanks to Professor Peter Yates for making it possible for us to carry out this work.

References

1. Bannister, C.M., Mundy, L.A., Mundy, J.E. Comparative merits of autogenous arterial and venous bypass grafts as alternatives to direct arterial anastomosis. In Microsurgery for Stroke, P. Schmiedek, editor, Springer-Verlag, New York, 1977, pp. 105–118.
2. Collatz Christensen, B., Garbarsch, C. Repair in arterial tissue. A scanning electron microscopic (SEM) and light microscopic study on the endothelium of rabbit thoracic aorta following a single dilitation injury. Virchows Arch Pathol Anat 360:93–106, 1973.
3. Dirrenberger, R.A., Sundt, T.M. Carotid endarterectomy. Temporal profile of the healing process and effects of anticoagulation therapy. J Neurosurg 48:201–219, 1978.
4. Fishman, J.A., Ryan, G.B., Karnovshy, M.J. Endothelial regeneration in the rat carotid artery and the significance of endothelial denudation in the pathogenesis of myointimal thickening. Lab Invest 32:339–351, 1975.

37

The Quantitative Assessment of the Effect of Antiplatelet Drugs on Thrombosis in Microvascular Anastomoses*

G. G. Ferguson, M. L. Bream, and R. B. Philp

The effect of various antiplatelet drugs on the patency of microvascular anastomoses in a laboratory model using the rat has been studied. The objectives were threefold: (1) to test the usefulness of microvascular anastomosis as an animal model of thrombosis, as no entirely satisfactory model exists,[1] (2) to develop a quantitative measure of thrombosis with which to compare the antithrombus activity of the drugs, as considerable controversy exists on the basis of prior model experiments and clinical trials as to their efficacy,[2] and (3) to determine if enhanced microvascular patency was possible using single intravenous bolus injection of the drugs during the anastomosis procedure itself.

The rationale for the study was as follows. A low, but definite, incidence of thrombosis at the site of anastomosis occurs in clinical microvascular surgery.[4] The exposure of subendothelial collagen at the site of microvascular anastomosis is a stimulus for platelet adhesion and aggregation and is possibly a more physiologic model of thrombosis than are many of the experimental models used to date.[3]

Materials and Methods

Seventy-two male Wistar rats were assigned randomly to one of six treatment groups: saline, polyethylene glycol, aspirin, sulfinpyra-

zone, dipyridamole, or VK744. Saline and polyethylene glycol were the vehicle controls for sulfinpyrazone and aspirin respectively, while VK744 is an experimental analog of dipyridamole. All drugs were given at a dose of 100 mg/kg body weight.

A rigidly standardized end-to-end anastomosis of the common carotid artery using interrupted stitches of 10-0 monofilament nylon suture (S&T 14V33) was used as the model. The test drug was injected into the femoral vein before the placement of the seventh suture in each case. Blood was allowed to flow through the anastomosis for exactly 30 minutes, at the end of which time the artery was clamped and fixed in situ with 10% buffered formalin.

Serial sections 7 μm thick were taken along a 2- to 3-mm segment of artery centered on the anastomosis and stained in phosphotungstic acid hematoxylin (PTAH). This stain differentiated red blood cells, which were stained blue, from platelets, which were stained pink. The total luminal area of each cross section of artery, with that portion of the lumen that was thrombosed, was estimated using a microscope eyepiece grid containing 100 squares. The ratio obtained was converted to a percentage and the process was repeated for all sections. In this way a profile of the percentage of thrombosis along the length of the artery relative to the site of the anastomosis could be obtained for each arterial segment.

Using this histologic technique the effect of the drugs in reducing the maximum thrombosis

*Supported by a grant from the Ontario Heart Foundation.

(the greatest percentage of thrombosis seen in any section along the artery) and the total volume of thrombus in an arterial segment was assessed. As well, a correlation between the visual assessment of patency at the time of surgery and the histologic assessment of patency was made.

Results

Maximum Thrombosis

Table 37-1 compares the effect of the various agents on mean maximum thrombosis. Saline and polyethylene glycol were associated on the average with a maximum thrombosis of 70%. Aspirin and sulfinpyrazone significantly reduced the maximum thrombosis in comparison to their respective controls ($p < .001$). Dipyridamole and VK744 had no effect.

Total Volume of Thrombus—Thrombus Profile

The ability of each drug to reduce the total volume of thrombus as revealed by the thrombus profiles is compared in Figs. 37-1 through 37-3. For each graph the percentage of thrombosis ± 1 SEM is plotted as a function of distance along the artery. Each graph depicts the mean thrombosis at distances along the artery relative to the beginning of the suture line and the direction of blood flow. In the case of the

Table 37-1. Mean maximum thrombosis for each treatment group (expressed as percentage of cross-sectional area of vessel occluded)

Treatment	n	Mean maximum thrombosis (%)	SEM
Saline	11	68.6	7.4
Polyethylene glycol	12	71.2	9.0
ASA	11	25.9*	4.8
Sulfinpyrazone	11	30.0**	6.5
Dipyridamole	11	62.0	9.1
VK744	12	67.8	9.4

  *ASA significantly different from polyethylene glycol control $p < 0.001$.

  **Sulfinpyrazone significantly different from saline control $p < 0.001$.

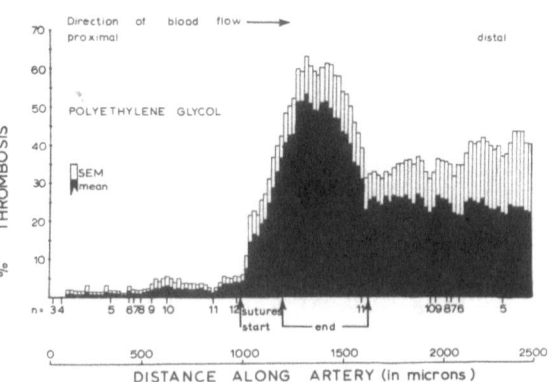

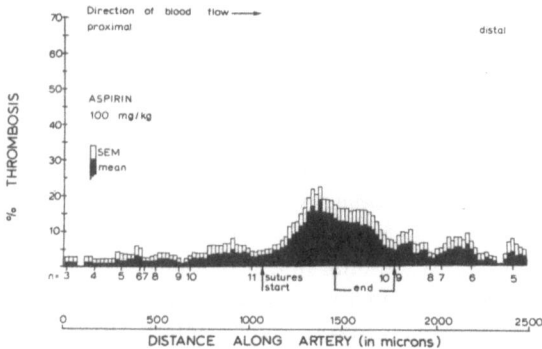

Fig. 37-1. Graphs comparing the thrombus profiles for polyethylene glycol (top) and aspirin (bottom). Polyethylene glycol was the vehicle control for aspirin. On all of the graphs, n represents the number of arteries from which the mean calculation was made. See text for description.

control agents, polyethylene glycol (Fig. 37-1) and saline (Fig. 37-2), there was a large volume of thrombus beginning within 200 to 300 mm of the beginning of the suture line and extending downstream. By contrast, aspirin (Fig. 37-1) and sulfinpyrazone (Fig. 37-2) produced a dramatic reduction in the volume of thrombus in comparison to their respective controls. Dipyridamole and VK744 (Fig. 37-3) had no significant effect.

Visual Assessment of Patency

A comparison of the apparent patency of an anastomosis as determined by visual inspection at the time of surgery and the true status of the anastomosis as determined histologically revealed that visual assessment did not reliably

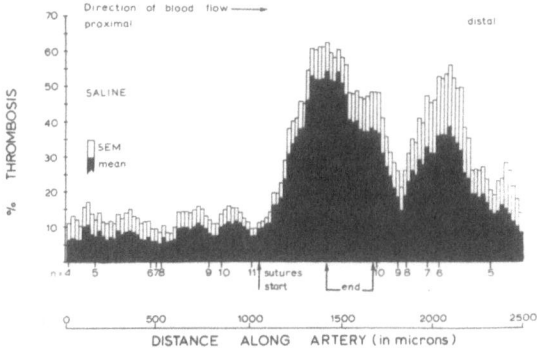

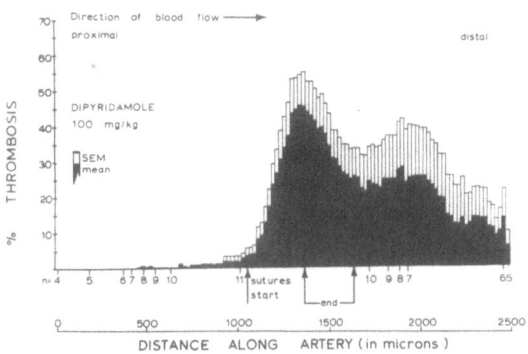

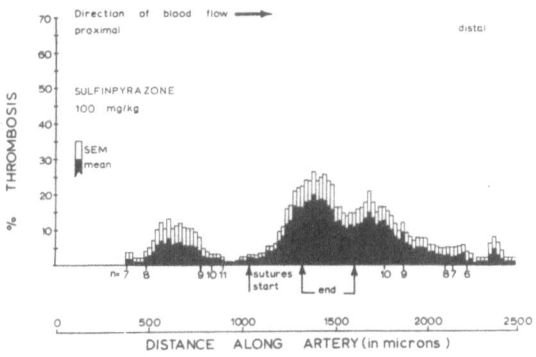

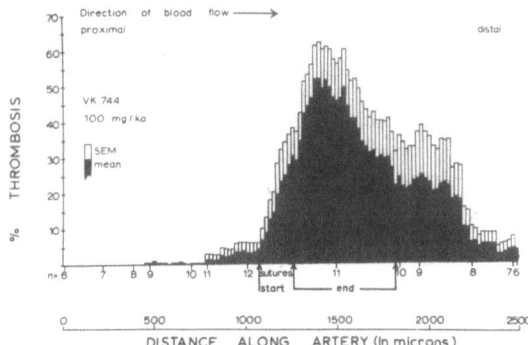

Fig. 37-2. Graphs comparing the thrombus for saline (top) and sulfinpyrazone (bottom). Saline was the vehicle control for sulfinpyrazone.

Fig. 37-3. Graphs comparing the thrombus profiles for dipyridamole (top) and VK 744 (bottom).

predict patency. Anastomoses that appeared patent (based on pulsation, color, and filling) could be shown to have extensive and sometimes occlusive thrombi in the lumina.

Conclusions

The following conclusions are drawn from these experiments:

1) Microvascular anastomosis is a useful animal model for the experimental study of thrombosis and antiplatelet drugs.

2) A quantitative method for the assessment of the antithrombotic effect of antiplatelet drugs has been developed and utilized.

3) Both aspirin and sulfinpyrazone are effective in reducing the maximum thrombosis at any one point and the total volume of thrombus associated with a microvascular anastomosis, when given as a single high-dose intravenous bolus during surgery. Dipyridamole and VK744 are ineffective.

4) Visual assessment of the patency of an anastomosis is unreliable.

5) The use of aspirin or sulfinpyrazone would appear to be a reasonable pharmacologic adjunct in clinical microvascular surgery.

References

1. Didisheim, P. Animal models useful in the study of thrombosis and anti-thrombotic agents. Prog Hemost Thromb 1:165–179, 1972.
2. Gallus, A.S., Hirsh, J. Anti-thrombotic drugs: Part II. Drugs 12:132–157, 1976.
3. Rosenbaum, T.J., Sundt, T.M. Thrombus formation and endothelial alterations in microarterial anastomoses. J Neurosurg 47:430–441, 1977.
4. Sundt, T.M., Siekert, R.G., Piepgras, D.G., Sharbrough, F.W., Houser, O.W. Bypass surgery for vascular disease of the carotid system. Mayo Clin Proc 51:677–692, 1976.

38

Relationship of Internal Carotid Artery Stump Pressure to STA–MCA Bypass Function

Jack M. Fein

The hemodynamic value of the superficial temporal artery–middle cerebral cortical artery (STA–MCA) microanastomosis may vary from one patient to the next. The quality of the microsurgical technique employed is especially important to the success of the bypass graft. The end-result may also be related to intrinsic factors such as the caliber of the donor and recipient arteries,[3] the standing pressure gradient between these vessels,[15] and the metabolic demands of the ischemic brain for energy-rich nutrients.[6]

Qualitative techniques such as postoperative angiography[1] and quantitative measurements of regional cerebral blood flow[11] have described the local circulatory changes in juxtaposition to the bypass graft. In patients with multiple unilateral or multiple bilateral occlusive lesions a bypass graft may have a more distant effect on cerebral hemispheric perfusion pressure which can influence the risks related to a second lesion.

The occurrence of multiple occlusive lesions usually requires staged intracranial and extracranial revascularization procedures. Under these circumstances the contribution of a bypass graft to internal carotid artery (ICA) stump pressure and hemispheric collateral blood pressure can be measured. This has been accomplished in 12 patients to date. The results suggest that in patients with bilateral internal carotid artery occlusive disease and a competent circle of Willis the protective effect of a bypass graft may extend to regions of the brain not immediately contiguous to the bypass.

Intraoperative Measurement Techniques

Of the 60 patients in our series, 12 underwent STA–MCA bypass graft for bilateral occlusive cerebrovascular disease. The end-to-side microanastomosis was performed as an onlay bypass graft through a 1.0- to 1.2-cm arteriotomy which utilized 25 to 35 #10-0 Ethilon sutures on a BV-5 needle.[7] In the immediate postoperative period the patency of the bypass was assessed using both Doppler sonography and postoperative angiography. The craniotomy incision was healed and swelling receded 10 days to 2 weeks later, at which time carotid endarterectomy was performed.

Carotid procedures were done under halothane anesthesia with careful monitoring of arterial blood pressure and blood gases. Spectral frequency analysis of the EEG and internal carotid artery stump pressure measurements were used to evaluate the need for an internal shunt during endarterectomy. This stump pressure was measured through a 18-gauge needle in the common carotid artery connected to a Statham PV-23 transducer. Transient ligation of the common carotid artery produced a drop in mean arterial blood pressure. This decreased further in 11 of the 12 patients when the external carotid artery was also temporarily ligated and denotes reversal of flow in the external carotid artery. After this "stump" pressure level was achieved, the STA graft pulse was obliterated percutaneously. Any change in ICA stump pressure was again recorded. The difference in the first and second stump pressures was referred to as the collateral graft pressure (CGP). The arterial PCO_2 was then increased approximately 10 mm Hg by decreasing the minute volume and the stump pressure was again measured before and after percutaneous compression of the graft. In one patient with traumatic aneurysm secondary to a gunshot wound, the stump pressure measurements in the internal carotid artery were made before and after the ipsilateral STA–MCA microanastomosis.

In all of these patients the patency of the bypass, the number of middle cerebral branches, and the pattern of collateral filling were determined with angiography, which was performed 1 to 10 days postoperatively.

Results

Seven patients had an initial STA–MCA bypass graft on the side of a completely occluded internal carotid artery followed in 10 days to 2 weeks by contralateral endarterectomy for an internal carotid stenosis. In six of these patients preoperative angiography demonstrated a patent anterior communicating artery with cross filling toward the hemisphere ipsilateral to the occlusion. At the time of carotid endarterectomy there was evidence in all six of some contribution to internal carotid stump pressure from the previously placed bypass graft. In one patient (case 10) there was no preoperative cross filling, and no evidence of postoperative contribution of the collateral graft pressure to contralateral stump pressure.

In four patients (cases 6, 7, 9, 12) in whom a bypass graft was performed for stenosis of the middle cerebral artery there was no transmission of collateral graft pressure to the opposite hemisphere.

There was a general correlation between the mean collateral graft pressure and the degree of filling observed on the arteriogram in patients with bilateral internal carotid disease. Collateral graft pressure between 5 to 12 mm Hg was associated with filling of 1 to 3 middle cerebral branches, and collateral graft pressures greater than 15 mm Hg were associated with filling of the entire middle cerebral circulation. In patients with middle cerebral stenosis (cases 6, 7, 9, 12) or an incompetent circle of Willis (case 10) there was no relationship between the degree of collateral filling seen on the angiogram and the collateral graft pressure.

Illustrative Cases

Case 1—M.N.   Left Internal Carotid Occlusion, Right Internal Carotid Stenosis

A 60-year-old white male was in good health until 2 weeks prior to admission when he developed weakness in the left arm and leg which resolved within 2 days. On examination a decreased left carotid pulse and a low-pitched bruit over the right carotid artery were noted. The left superficial temporal pulse was 3+ and the right 2+. ODM −O.D. 80/40, O.S. 40/20. The CT scan was normal. Static ^{99m}Tc scan was normal. A dynamic brain scan disclosed poor flow in both carotid arteries, but especially on the left.

Transfemoral cerebral angiography disclosed a high-grade localized stenosis of the right common carotid artery (Fig. 38-1) with intracranial filling of both A2 segments through a patent anterior communication artery (Fig. 38-2). There was a complete occlusion of the left internal carotid artery with minimal intracranial filling through the left ophthalmic artery (Fig. 38-3).

It was elected to increase the collateral circulation of the dominant left cerebral hemisphere prior to right carotid endarterectomy. A left STA–MCA anastomosis was carried out using a temporal cortical artery. A postoperative arteriogram (Fig. 38-4) disclosed filling of 3 or 4 inferior sylvian branches.

A right carotid endarterectomy was performed 2 weeks later. Mean arterial blood pressure measurements were made in the common carotid artery (Table 38-1).

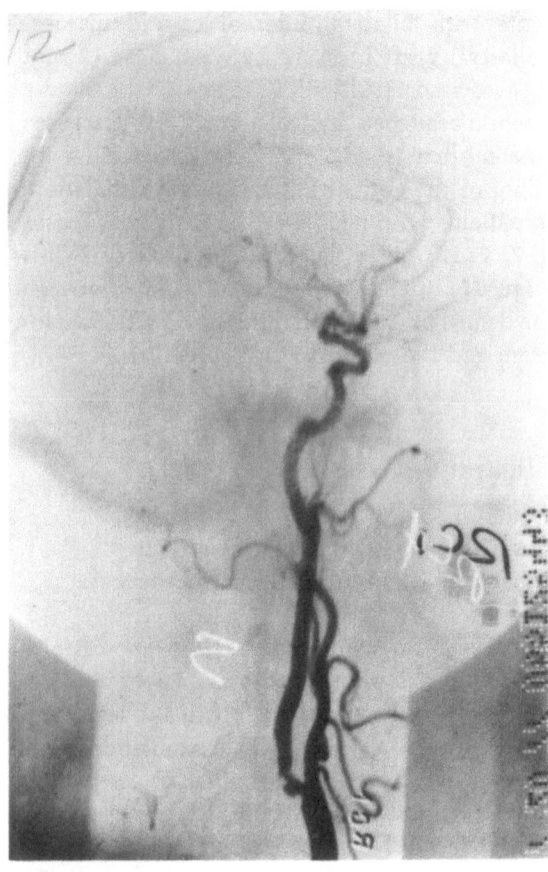

Fig. 38-1. Lateral angiogram film (case 1) showing high-grade stenosis of right internal carotid artery, covered by ulcerated and stenotic plaque.

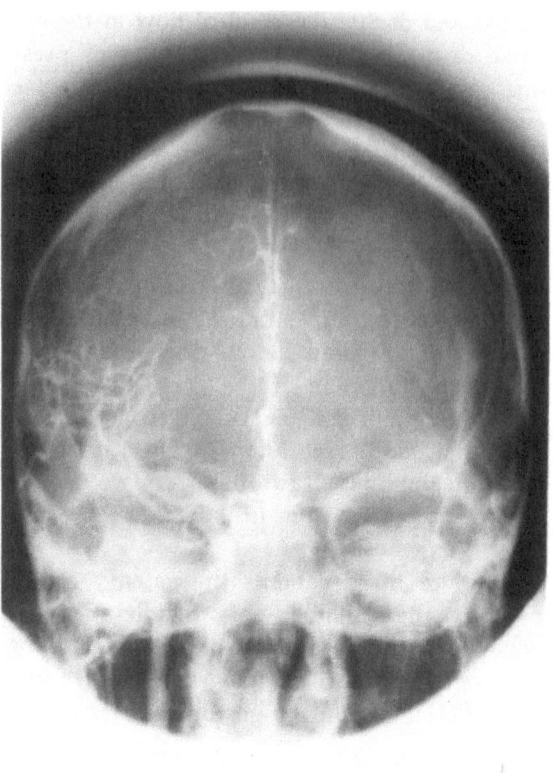

Fig. 38-2. AP angiogram (case 1). There is cross-filling from right to left despite the stenosis illustrated in Fig. 38-1.

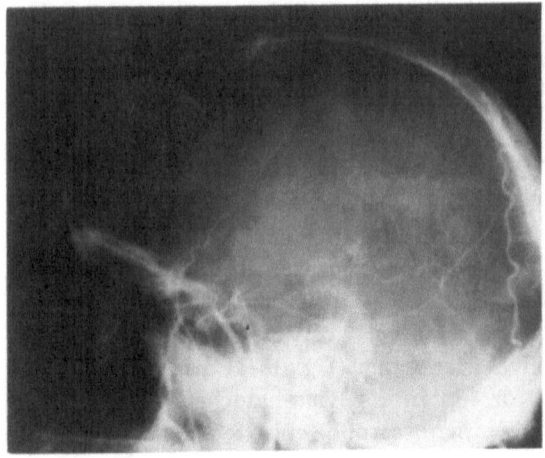

Fig. 38-3. Preoperative left carotid angiogram showing supraclinoid occlusion with some retrograde ophthalmic collateral filling.

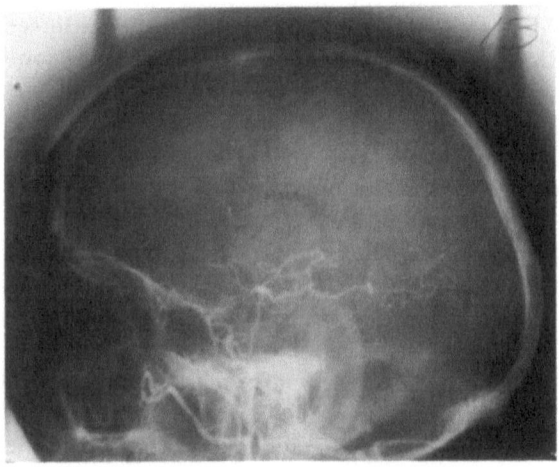

Fig. 38-4. Postoperative angiogram (case 1) demonstrates filling of inferior sylvian branches.

Table 38-1. Mean arterial pressure measurements, case 1

Pressure	APCO$_2$	Unclamped	C.C. clamp +	(S$_1$) E.C. clamp + STA	(S$_2$) COMPR =	CGP
Common (below lesion)	32	100	70	50	37	13
	42	100	65	50	35	15
Internal (above lesion)	32	100	90	53	40	13
	42	100	85	53	35	20
Postendarterectomy	32	100	90	50	40	10
	42	100	80	45	32	13

The arterial pressure gradient across the stenosis was measured with a second 18-gauge needle in the internal carotid artery above the lesion. The common carotid artery was then clamped below the needle. The external carotid artery was clamped and the stump pressure was recorded (S$_1$). Finally the STA graft was compressed percutaneously and the new stump pressure (S$_2$) was recorded.

The difference $S_1 - S_2 =$ collateral graft pressure (CGP).

The pressure gradient ($\sim$20 mm Hg) across the stenotic plaque was effectively eliminated by the operation. The drop in pressure with external carotid clamping indicates reversal of flow in the external carotid artery, despite a contribution to right internal carotid artery stump pressure of 20% by the graft. CO$_2$-induced vasodilation was associated with a relative increase in CGP contribution. This suggests that as the contralateral internal carotid artery approaches an ideal conducting system the CGP is transmitted with minimal decrement.

Case 4—R.C. Right Internal Carotid Pseudoaneurysm, Ipsilateral Bypass Graft

A 59-year-old white man was shot in the region of the right neck, sustaining a temporary loss of consciousness and a mild left hemiparesis which resolved within 5 days. Plain radiographs disclosed that the bullet lodged in the right anterior cervical triangle, and carotid arteriography disclosed a pseudoaneurysm of the right internal carotid artery at the level of C1-C2 (Fig. 38-5). The right posterior cerebral artery filled from the right posterior communi-

cating artery and there was no significant left-to-right cross-filling.

Approximately 2 weeks after this episode an attempt was made to ligate the right internal carotid artery. Stump pressure measurements (Table 38-2), however, demonstrated that this

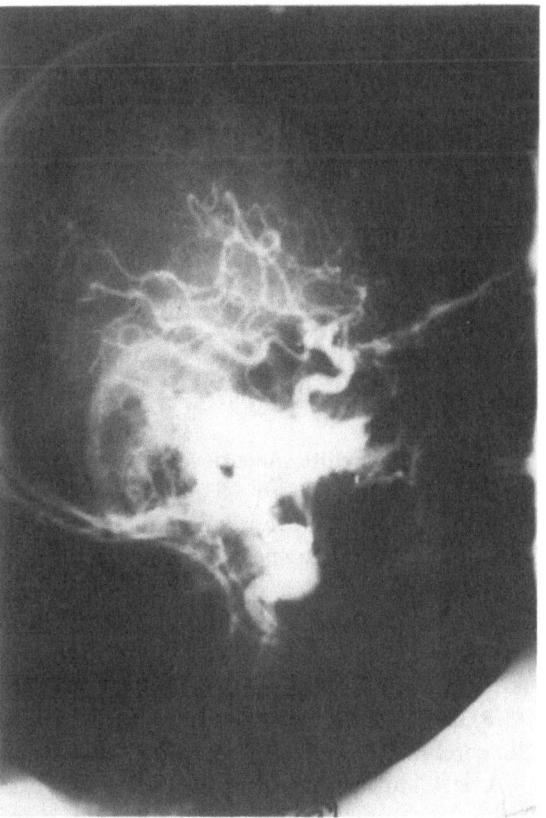

Fig. 38-5. Preoperative right lateral angiogram (case 4) demonstrating pseudoaneurysm of the right internal carotid artery at the level of C1–C2. The right posterior cerebral artery filled entirely from the right internal carotid artery.

Table 38-2. Mean arterial pressure measurements, case 4

Pressure	APCO$_2$	Unclamped	C.C. clamp +	(S$_1$) E.C. clamp +	(S$_2$) STA COMPR =	CGP
Before STA–MCA	30	120	90	40	—	—
	42	115	85	35	—	—
After STA–MCA	28	115	90	62	35	27
	40	115	90	65	33	32

would not be tolerated. A right superficial temporal–middle cerebral artery anastomosis was performed to augment the collateral circulation in the right hemisphere. After this was completed the stump pressure changes were measured once again and indicated that ligation would probably be tolerated. The contribution of CGP to ipsilateral internal carotid artery stump pressure was 27 mm Hg. A slight increase of CGP to 32 mm Hg was produced by relative hypercapnia.

A temporary Crutchfield clamp was placed around the internal carotid artery and postoperative arteriography confirmed that the anastomosis was patent (Figs. 38-6, 38-7). There was collateral filling of approximately four major branches of the middle cerebral artery with retrograde filling down the main middle cerebral artery.

Case 6—B.B.   Right Internal Carotid Stenosis, Left Middle Cerebral Stenosis

A 65-year-old white male developed right arm weakness lasting 10 to 15 minutes, approximately 3 weeks before admission. On examination there were no specific neurologic deficits although there was a decreased right carotid pulse. Transfemoral cerebral arteriography disclosed a high-grade stenosis of the right internal carotid artery at the bifurcation (Fig. 38-8) and a high-grade stenosis of the left middle cerebral artery at the genu (Fig. 38-9).

A left superficial temporal–middle cerebral artery anastomosis was performed and postoperative arteriography indicated a patent anastomosis (Fig. 38-10). Approximately 2 weeks later a right carotid endarterectomy was carried out, at which time stump pressure and col-

lateral graft pressure measurements were made above and below the stenotic lesion and following endarterectomy (Table 38-3).

A significant drop in pressure associated with external carotid clamping indicated relatively poor hemispheric collateral pressure. The contribution of collateral graft pressure to hemispheric collateral pressure cannot be assessed in the presence of a significant stenosis proximal to the bypass graft. The patient did well postoperatively with no further signs or symptoms of cerbrovascular insufficiency. He has been followed for 27 months.

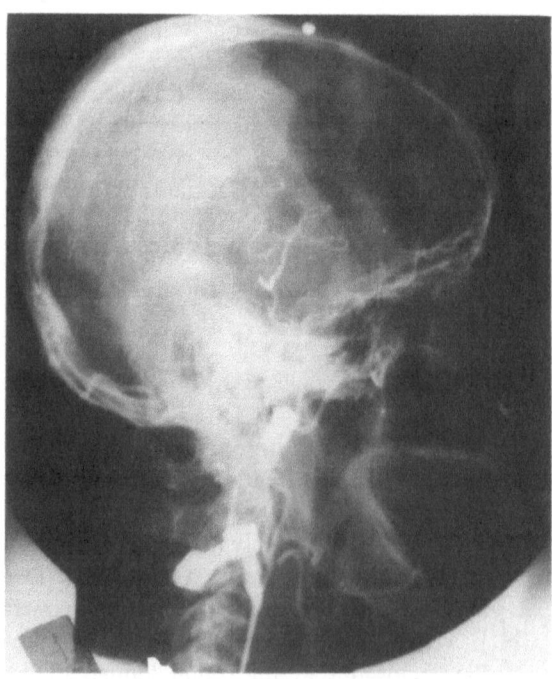

Fig. 38-6. Postoperative right lateral carotid angiogram demonstrating complete occlusion of the internal carotid artery with the Crutchfield clamp and patency of the bypass.

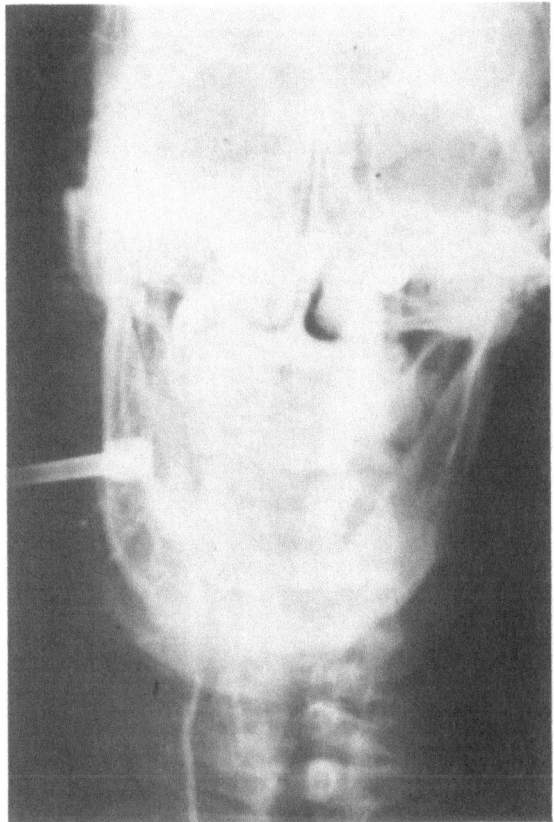

Fig. 38-7. Postoperative AP angiogram (case 4) showing complete occlusion of the right internal carotid artery by the Crutchfield clamp.

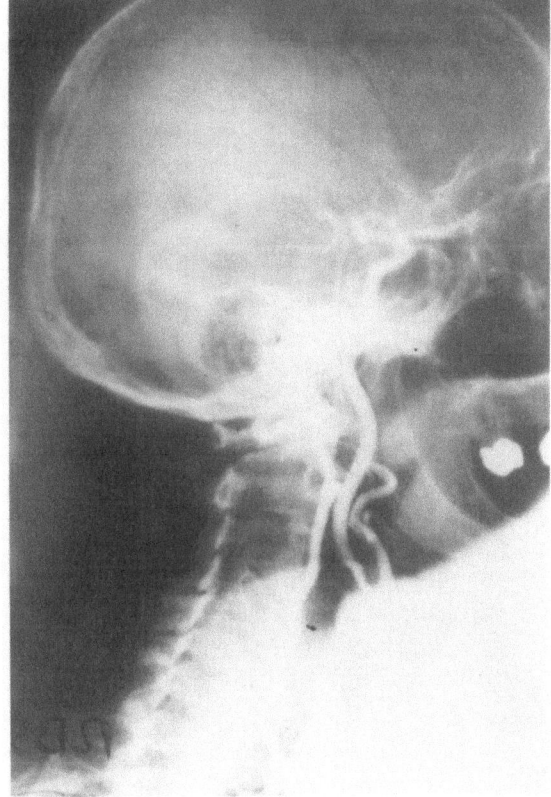

Fig. 38-8. Right lateral angiogram (case 6) showing stenosis of internal carotid artery. The carotid bifurcation is partly obscured.

Case 10—C.B.   Left Internal Carotid Occlusion, Right Internal Carotid Stenosis: Atretic Anterior Communicating Artery

A 57-year-old hypertensive female had recurrent transient episodes of difficulty in speech associated with a right hemiparesis. On examination the left carotid pulse was absent and there was decreased rapid alternating move-

ments in the right hand. RCBF (^{133}Xe) disclosed ischemic foci in both opercular regions. Angiography revealed a complete occlusion of the left internal carotid artery (Fig. 38-11). Furthermore the right-sided injection failed to fill the left anterior cerebral artery (Fig. 38-12).

A STA–MCA anastomosis was performed on the left side and patency of the bypass was verified 3 days after surgery (Fig. 38-13). Three

Table 38-3. Mean arterial pressure measurements, case 6 ($APCO_2 = 37$ mm Hg)

Pressure	Unclamped +	C.C. clamp +	(S$_1$) E.C. clamp +	(S$_2$) STA COMPR	= CGP
Common carotid (below lesion)	90	75	45	45	0
Internal carotid (above lesion)	90	60	47	47	0
After endarterectomy	90	82	55	55	0

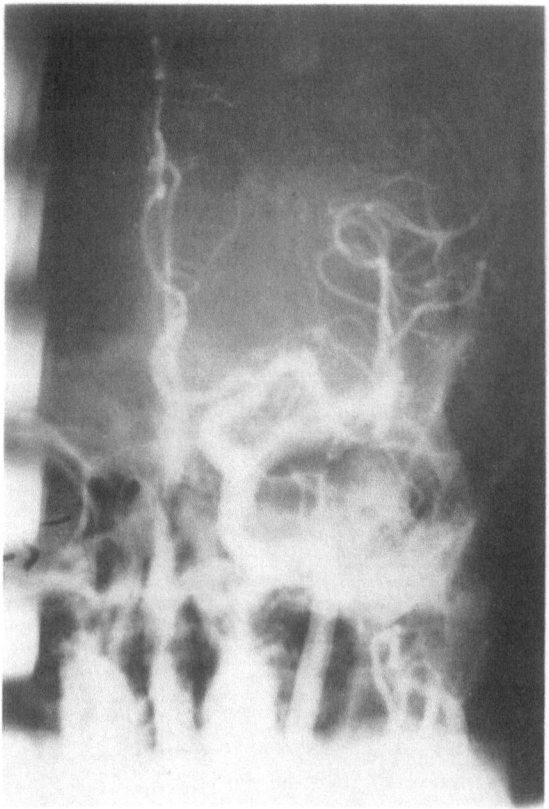

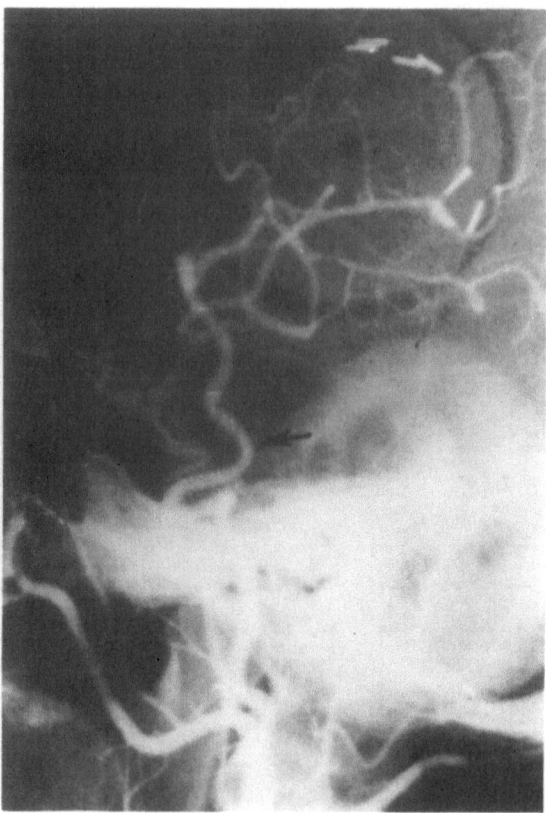

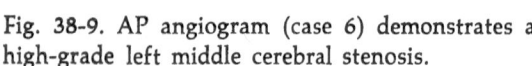

Fig. 38-9. AP angiogram (case 6) demonstrates a high-grade left middle cerebral stenosis.

Fig. 38-10. Postoperative left lateral angiogram (case 6) demonstrating filling of 3 or 4 branches of the MCA complex by the bypass.

weeks after the first surgical procedure a right carotid endarterectomy was planned. The stump pressure measurements (Table 38-4) indicated significant reversal of flow in the external carotid artery.

There was no significant contribution of the collateral graft pressure to collateral hemispheric perfusion pressure. Postoperative rCBF (^{133}Xe) showed a 40% increase in flow in the left opercular probe and a 25% increase in flow in the right opercular probe.

Discussion

The changes in collateral circulation produced by an STA–MCA bypass have been studied with conventional,[1] cine,[10] and fluorescence an-giography,[9] blood flow measurement,[11] Doppler sonography,[8] and oculoplethysmography.[5] Collateral graft pressure measurements provide a quantitative measurement of the function of the collateral circulation after the bypass procedure. In patients undergoing subsequent cervical carotid procedures there is an opportunity to assess the contribution of the STA graft to collateral hemisphere pressure by measuring the pressure in the internal carotid artery stump before and after percutaneous compression of a previously placed ipsilateral or contralateral STA graft (Table 38-5).

For the purposes of these measurements a graft may be classified as communicating or noncommunicating depending on whether a significant stenotic or atretic segment is interposed between the anastomosis and the point at which the stump pressure is measured. Five

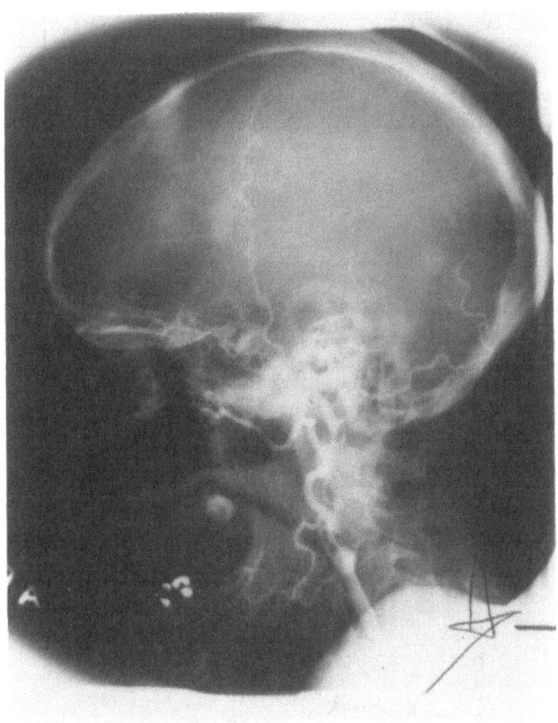

Fig. 38-11. Preoperative left lateral angiogram (case 10) showing complete occlusion of the internal carotid artery.

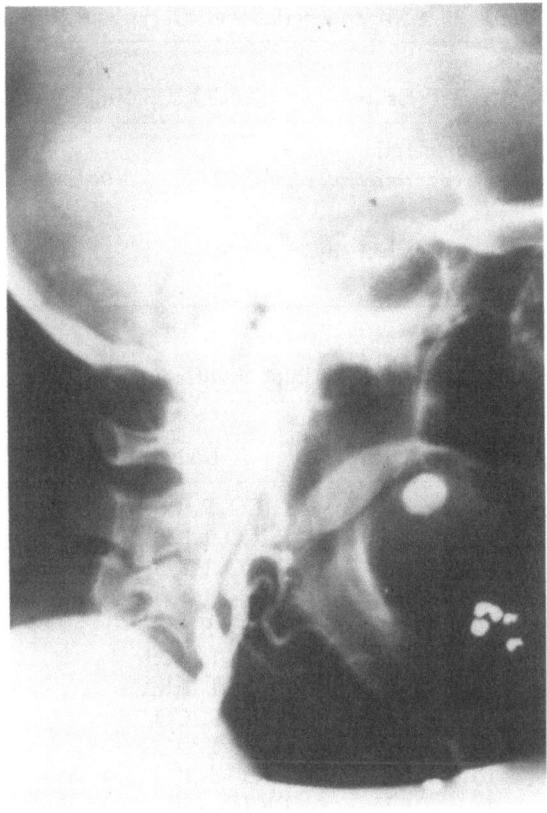

Fig. 38-12. Preoperative right lateral angiogram (case 10) showing a high-grade stenosis of the right internal carotid artery.

cases in this series were noncommunicating. In four the graft was placed for a stenosis of the middle cerebral artery. This stenosis produced a significant resistive element limiting the transmission of collateral pressure. In one case the anterior circle of Willis was atretic and this segment limited free transmission of collateral graft pressure.

In patients with bilateral internal carotid lesions where CGP could be measured, there was a correlation between this measurement and the degree of filling observed on the arteriogram. Reichman observed a similar correlation between the blood flow rate in the graft and the number of branches of the middle cerebral artery visualized through the anastomosis.[10]

Woodhall[14] measured the pressure in the ipsilateral middle cerebral and internal carotid arteries during occlusion of the cervical internal carotid arteries and found that the relative pressure reduction in these vessels and in the cervical internal carotid artery was similar.

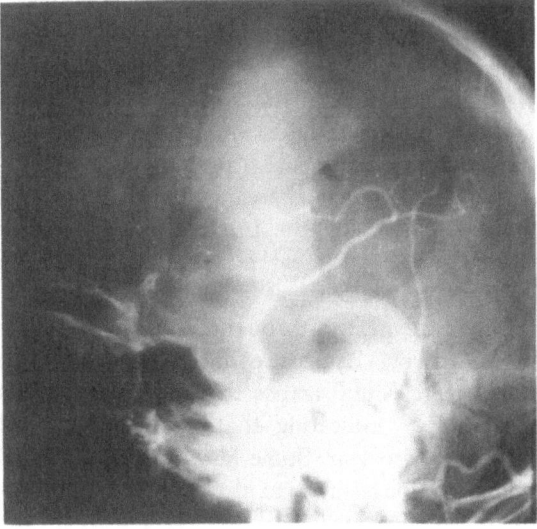

Fig. 38-13. Postoperative left lateral angiogram (case 10) showing the filling and reflux within the middle cerebral complex.

Table 38-4. Mean arterial pressure measurements, case 10

Pressure	APCO	Unclamped +	C.C. clamp +	(S₁) E.C. clamp +	(S₂) STA COMPR	= CGP
Common carotid						
Before endarterectomy	32	90	80	60	60	0
	40	84	75	62	62	0
After endarterectomy	34	92	75	70	70	0
	40	85	75	70	70	0

Table 38-5. Relationship of intraoperative stump pressure changes and arteriographic findings

Case	Patient	Lesion	Collateral graft pressure (mm Hg)	Stump pressure (mm Hg)	Branches filled
1	M.N.	L.ICO, R.ICS	12	51	3
2	H.P.	R.ICO, L.ICS	15	50	all
3	D.M.	R.ICO, L.ICS	23	71	all
4	R.C.	R. pseudoaneurysm	27	62	all
5	G.F.	L.ICO, RICS	0	60	4
6	B.B.	R.ICS, L.MCS	0	47	3
7	B.G.	R.ICS, L.I&MCS	0	49	2
8	I.H.	L.ICS, R.ICO	8	58	3
9	F.R.	R.ICS, L.MCO	0	55	4
10	C.B.	L.ICO, R.ICS	15	47	all
11	S.U.	RICO, LICS	11	70	2
12	C.S.	LICO, RI&MCS	0	47	4

Bakay and Sweet[2] also showed a concomitant percentage fall in the middle cerebral artery and in the cortical artery pressure after reducing the pressure in the ipsilateral or contralateral carotid artery in man and the macaque. This suggests that the internal carotid and middle cerebral arteries, along with their cortical branches, constitute a pressure reservoir or conducting system. If the arterial network, the bypass graft, and the internal carotid artery stump were an ideal conducting system, a change in pressure at either end should be freely transmitted throughout the entire system. However, pressure differences of up to 20% were found across this proximal arterial system,[12, 13] indicating that it is not an ideal pressure reservoir. Some loss of pressure head from a bypass graft to the point of measurement in the ipsilateral and certainly in the contralateral internal carotid artery is therefore predictable. The pressure in the STA segments was higher than that of the cortical artery in eight patients in this group in which these measurements were also made at the time of the bypass. STA pressure was also higher than the subsequently measured contralateral internal carotid artery pressure.

The intravascular flow pattern measured by rCBF and the direction of flow seen on angiography are directly dependent on intravascular standing pressure gradients. The collateral pressure in a high-pressure bed, however, may be lowered if a contribution from a lower-pressure efferent channel is temporarily eliminated, as is the case when the STA compression reduces pressure in the intermediary low-pressure bed. CGP was probably significantly lower than the graft pressure at the time of endarterectomy as well.

The ability of the STA graft to support collateral hemispheric pressure may be an important factor in planning the sequence of staged procedures for bilateral occlusive disease. The mortality rate for elective carotid endarterec-

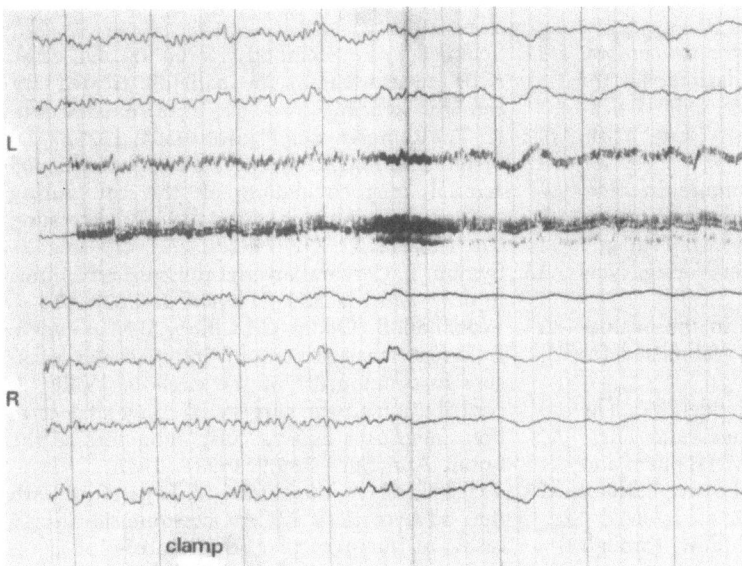

Fig. 38-14. Intraoperative EEG during reclamping for internal shunt removal in a patient with left internal carotid stenosis and right common carotid artery occlusion. Both hemispheres were dependent on the stenotic internal carotid artery. When this was clamped, the well-organized and symmetrical alpha rhythm gave way to severe degrees of slowing more on the right than the left. This is consistent with ischemic insufficiency and illustrates the stresses induced by carotid endarterectomy when there is contralateral occlusion.

tomy for unilateral internal carotid stenosis is approximately 4%. However, in the presence of a complete occlusion of the contralateral internal carotid artery the mortality rate may be as high as 22%.[4] This risk is related to a critical decrease in cerebral perfusion pressure of the most distal tissue during temporary carotid clamping or to fluctuations in systemic arterial blood pressure. The degree of ischemic stress in patients with ipsilateral internal carotid stenosis and contralateral occlusion can be appreciated by reference to Fig. 38-14. EEG slowing and a precipitous drop in internal carotid artery mean pressure is often produced by temporary clamping for placement and removal of an internal shunt during endarterectomy. The frequency of resulting neurologic deficits is enough to consider alternative strategies in the high-risk patient. Augmentation of the collateral circulation with STA–MCA anastomosis on the side of a complete internal carotid artery occlusion may offer significant immediate protection to this tissue at risk. Furthermore, these measurements of collateral graft pressure indicate that it appears to make a small but significant contribution to total cerebral hemispheric perfusion pressure. For this pressure to be widely transmitted, however, it is necessary that the conducting arterial system be in free communication from the point of anastomosis to the site of measurement in the contralateral internal carotid artery. If resistive elements are present either in the form of an atretic circle of Willis (case 10) or atherosclerotic narrowing of the proximal middle cerebral artery (cases 6, 7, 9, 12), the collateral graft pressure will only contribute to the perfusion pressure of a restricted region of brain.

References

1. Anderson, R.E., Reichman, O.H., Davis, D.O. Radiological evaluation of temporal artery–middle cerebral artery anastomosis. Radiology 113:73, 1974.
2. Bakay, L., Sweet, W.H. Cervical and intracranial intra-arterial pressure with and without vascular occlusion. Surg Gynecol Obstet 95: 67–75, 1952.
3. Bannister, C.M., Mundy, L.A., Mundy, J.A. Anastomosis of small arteries in growing animals. In Microneurosurgical Anastomosis for Cerebral Ischemia, G.M. Austin, editor, Charles C Thomas, Springfield, 1976.
4. Bauer, R.B., et al. Joint study of extracranial arterial occlusion. JAMA 208:509–518, 1969.
5. Carney, A.L. Ocular plethysmography and suction opthalmodynamometry in the diagnosis of carotid occlusive disease. In Microvascular Anastomosis for Cerebral Ischemia, J.M. Fein and

250 Jack M. Fein

O.H. Reichman, editors, Springer-Verlag, New York, 1978.

6. Fein, J.M. Oxidative metabolism in cerebral ischemia. In Microvascular Anastomosis for Cerebral Ischemia, J.M. Fein and O.H. Reichman, editors, Springer-Verlag, New York, 1978.

7. Fein, J.M. Contemporary techniques in cerebral revascularization. In Microvascular Anastomosis for Cerebral Ischemia, J.M. Fein and O.H. Reichman, editors, Springer-Verlag, New York, 1978.

8. Fein, J.M. Doppler sonography in the evaluation of the STA–MCA bypass (submitted for publication).

9. Murray, P.J., Yamamoto, L., Feindel, W. The watershed area following microvascular anastomosis. In Cerebral Function, Metabolism and Circulation, P. Ingvar and N.A. Larsen, editors, Munksgaard, Copenhagen, 1977.

10. Reichman, O.H. Estimation of flow through STA by-pass graft. In Microvascular Anastomosis for Cerebral Ischemia, J.M. Fein and

O.H. Reichman, editors, Springer-Verlag, New York, 1978.

11. Schmiedek, P., Steinhoff, H., Gratzl, O., et al. rCBF measurements in patients treated for cerebral ischemia by extra–intracranial vascular anastomosis. Eur Neurol 6:364, 1971.

12. Stromberg, D.D., Fox, J.R. Pressures in the pial arterial microcirculation of the cat during changes in systemic arterial blood pressure. Circ Res 31:229–239, 1972.

13. Symon, L. Cerebral arterial pressure recordings in dogs and Macaca. J Physiol 165:62, 1963.

14. Woodhall, B., Odom, G.L., Bloor, B.M., Golden, J. Direct measurement of intravascular pressure in components of the circle of Willis. A contribution to the surgery of congenital cerebral aneurysms and vascular anomalies of the brain. Ann Surg 135:911–921, 1952.

15. Yasargil, M.G., Yonekawa, Y. Experience with the STA–cortical MCA anastomosis in 46 cases. In Microvascular Anastomosis for Cerebral Ischemia, J.M. Fein and O.H. Reichman, editors, Springer-Verlag, New York, 1978.

39

Measurement of Intracranial Arterial Pressure in Patients Undergoing Extracranial to Intracranial Microsurgical Anastomosis for Cerebrovascular Ischemia

H. W. Stephens, Jr.

Arterial blood pressure was first measured in 1773 by Stephen Hales, the British clergyman who connected an 8-foot column of glass filled with blood to the artery of a mare, using a goose quill and a goose trachea as a cannula. This method was a direct invasive technique which demonstrated pulsatile blood flow, which in turn led to a better understanding of the physiology of blood flow.

The measurement of blood flow has become much more sophisticated now with the introduction of the electromagnetic flowmeter, ultrasonic Doppler, ultrasonic flowmeter, plethysmograph, impedence plethysmograph, and direct vascular cannulization using physiologic pressure transducers and digital recording systems.

Intra-arterial pressure measurements in the neck and brain were first reported by Bakay and Sweet in 1953.[1] These introductory investigations on the carotid arteries in the neck have been extended to studies of the cerebral vessels to better understand the effect of pressure changes after ligation of the carotid artery.

The introduction of microsurgical techniques in the treatment of ischemic cerebrovascular disease and the availability of cortical branches of the intracranial vessels, where both direct and indirect evaluations of cerebral blood flow can be made, has renewed interest in evaluation of intravascular pressure dynamics.

Clinical Material and Methods

Adequate data from both noninvasive and invasive studies were available in 27 patients, all of whom had cerebrovascular ischemic disease and were considered as candidates for extracranial–intracranial microvascular anastomosis. All patients had been evaluated by a neurologist interested in the study of TIAs, a vascular surgeon interested in the correction of occlusive vascular disease in the neck, and a neurosurgeon experienced in over 180 EC–IC procedures. Patients had either diagnosed TIAs, stroke in evolution, or signs of low cerebral perfusion syndrome. Selective 4-vessel angiography had established the vascular lesion(s) correlatable with the patient's clinical symptoms, and these were considered inaccessible to usual vascular surgical techniques, because of either total occlusion of the internal carotid artery or tandem lesions in inaccessible areas. Several of the patients had bilateral carotid lesions, such as total occlusion of one internal carotid artery, with a 75% or greater stenosis of the contralateral carotid artery. These patients underwent "staged" procedures; the initial procedure was the microvascular anastomosis on the side of the totally occluded vessel, followed later by carotid endarterectomy of the contralateral stenosed vessel.

At the time of surgery, all patients had controlled endotracheal ventilation with neuro-leptic anesthesia. Blood pressure was monitored peripherally with a radial artery cannula pre-calibrated and measured on a digital display. The apparatus used to measure intra-arterial pressures of the superficial temporal artery, cortical branches of the middle cerebral artery, posterior cerebral artery, and/or the vertebral-basilar arteries was a Hewlett-Packard strain-gauge transducer, precalibrated with a mano-meter, and recorded on a digital display and calibrated paper strips (Fig. 39-1). The cannula used to measure the intraluminal arterial pres-sures was a silicone catheter with an inner diameter of 1.5 to 2 mm coupled to the strain-gauge transducer.

With the patient in a stable state, the peri-pheral blood pressure was recorded from the radial artery, and simultaneous recording of the intraluminal pressure of the superficial temporal artery and the proximal and distal branches of the selected cortical arteries being used for the anastomosis. In double and triple shunts, the intra-arterial pressures were re-corded after completion, of the anastomosis for comparison of serial flow characteristics.

In several patients, measurements were made of the intraluminal arterial pressure, during transient reduction of the patient's systemic arterial pressure to record the effect on the intracranial blood pressures.

In patients with angiographically confirmed collateral circulation, intraluminal pressures were measured with and without digital occlu-sion of the collateral circulation to determine if reduction in cerebral perfusion pressures could be observed. In those patients having bilateral EC–IC anastomoses with established cross-circulation, digital pressure was applied to the functioning anastomosis and recordings made to measure the effect on the intra-arterial pressures. The significance of pulsatile blood flow was taken into consideration.

In selected cases the ophthalmic artery pres-sure measured by oculopneumoplethysmo-graphy (OPG-Gee) technique was compared to direct measurement of pressure in the ophthal-mic artery.

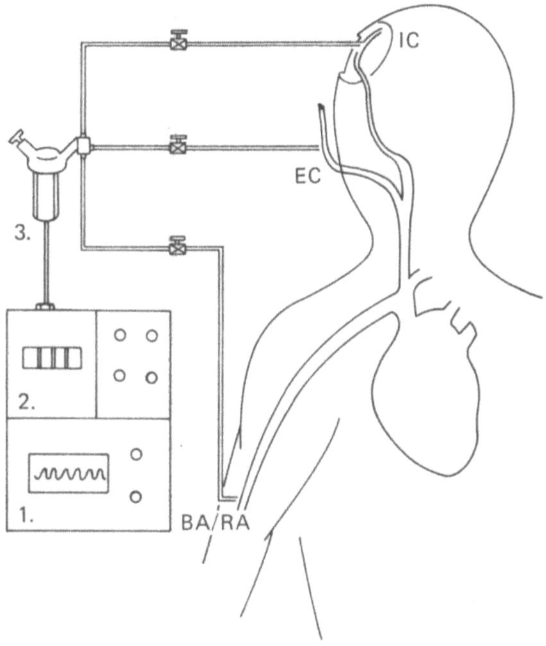

Fig. 39-1. Schematic plan. (1) Recorder, (2) digital read-out unit, (3) pressure transducer, (4) pressure transmission tubing. BA = brachial artery, and/or radial artery, extracranial artery, intracranial artery.

Results

The direct intra-arterial measurements have shown definite value in demonstrating phy-siologic changes in intraluminal pressure in each of our cases. In comparing the systemic pressure with that of the superficial temporal artery used as the donor vessel, a range from 12 to 16 mm Hg was found in most cases (aver-age drop of 35 mm Hg). The comparisons of the superficial temporal artery pressure to the pressure found in the proximal portion of the cortical branches of the middle cerebral artery showed a difference ranging from 38 to 80 mm Hg, with a mean difference of 45 mm Hg. This demonstrated a definite decrease in the intra-luminal perfusion pressure above the area of pathologic occlusion or stenosis. It also demon-strated the pressure difference we felt signifi-cant to justify the anastomosis and to maintain EC–IC flow until such time that intracranial col-lateral circulation could build up to a pressure that would equal that of the superficial temporal artery. This explains why some shunts convert from a "demanding" shunting system to a "passive" shunting system and possibly go on to occlusion when no longer required to perfuse an area of the brain which has reestablished adequate collateral circulation.

In several cases with total occlusion of the ipsilateral carotid artery and 75% or greater stenosis of the contralateral carotid artery, a definite drop in perfusion in both the proximal and distal branches of the cannulated middle cerebral artery could be demonstrated when digital pressure was applied to the stenosed vessel, thereby limiting crossover flow to the ischemic hemisphere and demonstrating the justification for carrying out prophylactic EC–IC anastomosis before doing a second "staged" operation on the stenosed internal carotid artery.

In those patients demonstrating an established collateral circulation on angiography, coming from the external carotid artery via the ophthalmic artery, measurements of the proximal and distal portions of the cortical branches of the middle cerebral artery demonstrated a precipitous drop in perfusion pressure when digital pressure was placed over the portion of the superficial temporal artery supplying collateral circulation to the ophthalmic artery, thereby demonstrating the importance of not using the previously established and functioning branch of the collateral circulation to the brain which might inadvertently be utilized as the anastomosing external carotid vessel instead of selecting another branch or branches of the external carotid artery. This also demonstrates the importance of considering endarterectomy of the external carotid artery on the side of a totally occluded internal carotid, when the tissue vessel supplies important collateral circulation to that hemisphere, and has been shown to be stenosed by angiography. This would prove to be an acceptable method of providing extra blood while establishing collateral pathways between the extracranial and intracranial arteries.

The importance of recognizing this collateral circulation and using it, is best demonstrated with a complex system of circular formations, one inside the other, as in the nine complex systems of angular ring formations discussed by Yasargil and Krayenbuhl.[5]

Serial measurements of cortical vascular pressures during multiple shunts have also been done, and have led us to conclude that double and triple EC–IC microanastomosis are of definite benefit in terms of both flow and pressure to the ischemic hemisphere.

A Comparison of Noninvasive Oculoplethysmography-Gee with Invasive Intraluminal Pressure Measurements

In 27 patients undergoing EC–IC anastomosis for cerebrovascular ischemia, a definite correlation has been demonstrated between the ophthalmic systolic pressure measured by the noninvasive modified OPG-Gee method and the intraluminal pressure of the middle cerebral artery in the proximity of the ophthalmic artery. All patients who demonstrated an elevated ophthalmic artery pressure by the noninvasive OPG-Gee method, also demonstrated a similar elevation of pressure with the invasive technique.

Of 19 patients who underwent EC–IC shunting, the procedure was bilateral in six, a total of 25 procedures; however, one of these procedures connected an occipital artery to a posterior cerebral artery, and in this latter circumstance the OPG-Gee measurement is felt to have no validity. Of the 24 EC–IC shunts evaluated preoperatively and postoperatively by the OPG-Gee technique, 17 of the 24 (71%) demonstrated improvement. The improvement was unilateral in 4 of the 17, definitely bilateral in 8, and possibly bilateral in 5.

A graph of the data on two of the EC–IC shunt patients can best demonstrate the difference between improvement with the EC–IC shunt in one patient, and how the shunt may not have contributed significantly to the clinical improvement of the second patient (Fig. 39-2). The patient labeled A, on the left side of the graph, underwent a bilateral EC–IC shunting procedure. Prior to the first procedure, the systemic blood pressure was 104 mm Hg; the ophthalmic systolic pressures were equal, at a level of 75 mm Hg. After the second procedure, with a systemic pressure of 130 mm Hg, oph-

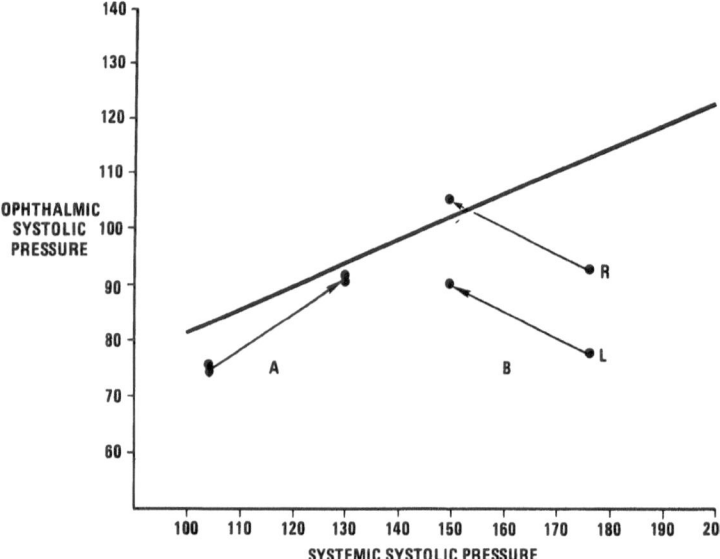

Fig. 39-2. Comparison of two patients undergoing EC–IC shunts showing changes in ophthalmic systolic pressure folling shunting procedures. Correlation of systemic (brachial) and ophthalmic systolic pressure in two patients (A on the left, B on the right) before and after EC–IC shunts. The respective arrows point from the preoperative to the postoperative data. Both patients were improved following shunting procedures.

thalmic systemic pressures remained equal and at a level of 91 mm Hg. Clinically, the patient was much improved; however, the increase in the ophthalmic systolic pressures is probably principally the result of the increase of the systemic systolic pressure. It is our feeling that, at best, the shunts have only slightly improved the physiologic status of this patient, and may have contributed in no way to his clinical improvement.

In contrast, the data for patient B on the right side of the graph relates to a single EC–IC shunt on the right side. The patient became symptomatic only when his antihypertensive regimen resulted in orthostatic hypotension: Angiography demonstrated bilateral internal carotid artery occlusion, and a significant left external carotid stenosis. Preoperatively, at a systemic systolic pressure of 176 mm Hg, the right and left ophthalmic systolic pressures were 93 and 78 mm Hg, respectively. After his right EC–IC shunt, he had a systemic systolic pressure of 150 mm Hg, and right and left ophthalmic pressures of 105 and 90 mm Hg, respectively. Thus, in spite of a 26-mm Hg fall in systemic systolic pressure, there has been an elevation of the ophthalmic pressure of 12 mm Hg. Note that the postoperative right ophthalmic systolic pressure is within normal limits. The patient remained asymptomatic although his antihypertensive regimen was continued.

We have thus demonstrated the importance of the noninvasive OPG-Gee technique for measuring ophthalmic systolic pressure, both preoperatively and postoperatively, which can give us a better understanding of the dynamics of blood pressure and cerebral perfusion in patients undergoing EC–IC revascularization procedures.

In several patients postoperatively demonstrating a drop in ophthalmic systolic pressure, the use of Lasix and Decadron was soon followed by clinical improvement and elevation of the ophthalmic artery pressure as measured with this noninvasive technique (OPG-Gee).

In several patients who had amaurosis fugax prior to an EC–IC shunt, the amaurosis fugax was stopped. This may be explained by the increase in ophthalmic pressure. In one documented case, with a lesion above the siphon, distal to the ophthalmic artery, the patient underwent a multiple shunting procedure to the ischemic hemisphere and continued to exhibit amaurosis fugax, but no cortical symptoms. No increase in ophthalmic pressure followed the procedure.

We also noted in another patient with preoperative retinal ischemia a definite improvement of vision after the EC–IC shunt, which we feel is definitely related to the increase in ophthalmic pressures secondary to the shunt.

In conclusion, we have had no operative mortality or morbidity in any of our patients who underwent direct cannulization of the cortical branches of the middle cerebral artery to evaluate intravascular pressures, but we did observe that the postoperative course did not appear to be as dramatic as that of those patients who did not undergo cannulization procedures.

In several cases, low leptomeningeal perfusion pressures down to 15 mm Hg were recorded and no postoperative deficits were found. It is recommended that those branches of the external carotid circulation which are supplying collateral blood via the ophthalmic artery not be used for EC–IC procedures, and that other branches of the external carotid circulation be used to better perfuse an ischemic hemisphere.

It is also suggested that multiple shunts be considered to such cortical branches as the angular, opercular, and frontal branches of the middle cerebral artery, since we have demonstrated definite pressure improvements with the multiple shunting techniques and have demonstrated the best pressure elevations with our triple shunts.

We feel that the noninvasive OPG-Gee technique is quite acceptable in selected cases and can be used both pre- and postoperatively to accurately reflect changes in intravascular pressure in ischemic cerebral hemispheres. This technique has not proven of value in stenotic lesions above the take-off of the ophthalmic artery from the internal carotid artery, and it does not appear to be applicable to shunting procedures in the posterior circulation.

The postoperative OPG studies have documented pressure improvement in patients undergoing EC–IC anastomoses and have shown 50% of these cases to have bilateral improvement in ophthalmic artery pressure.

There have also been cases where we have demonstrated preoperative orthostatic hypotension which has been relieved following EC–IC shunting. In several patients with longstanding history of migraine, the attacks ceased following the shunting procedure. In selected cases where a shunting procedure was performed distal to an occlusion, there has been improvement in neurologic status, and it has led us to believe that anastomosis into specific ischemic areas of the brain should prove to be beneficial.

Several patients who have undergone EC–IC

anastomosis to ischemic areas of the brain have demonstrated increase in brain volume on serial CT scanning of a previous ischemic area of the brain. We feel that this is secondary to the shunting procedure.

In several patients with field cuts secondary to ischemia of the posterior cerebral artery, we have demonstrated improvement in vision and regression of visual field cuts after increasing perfusion to this ischemic area of the brain.

The concept of a "demand shunt" that delivers adequate blood flow and perfusion to an ischemic area of the brain and a "passive shunt" that can go on to occlusion as collateral circulation develops to an ischemic area of the brain demonstrates why some shunts may function initially, and later become occluded, and why, in those cases without the ability to reestablish collateral circulation, the demand shunt goes on to increase in size and perfuse larger areas of ischemic brain.

In cases of vertebral-basilar insufficiency, where the noninvasive OPG-Gee method and other noninvasive techniques may not prove of value, direct intravascular measurements may prove to be the best way of evaluating increase in blood flow. In an especially challenging problem of a vertebral artery stenosis, the measurement of an adequate perfusion pressure from the occipital artery to the posterior inferior cerebellar artery enabled us to do an intracranial vertebral artery endarterectomy to remove the stenotic plaque and reestablish blood flow into the vertebral-basilar system, eliminating vertebral-basilar symptoms with no postoperative neurologic sequelae.

The cannulization of cortical and deep intracranial branches in ischemic cerebrovascular disease has given us an understanding of the pathophysiology of ischemic cerebrovascular disease and of why the patient is benefited by EC–IC microvascular anastomosis.

References

1. Bakay, L., Sweet, W.H. Intraarterial pressures in the neck and brain. Late changes after carotid closure. J Neurosurg 10:353–359, 1953.
2. Barr, P. Percutaneous puncture of the radial artery with a multi-purpose Teflon catheter for

indwelling use. Acta Physiol Scand 51:343–347, 1961.

3. Geddes, L.A. The Direct and Indirect Measurement of Blood Pressure. Yearbook Medical Publishers, Chicago, 1970.

4. Gee, W., Smith, C.A., Hinsen, C.E., Wylie, E.J. Ocularpneumoplethysmography in carotid artery disease. Med Instru 8: 4, 1974.

5. Krayenbuhl, H.A., Yasargil, M.G., Cerebral Angiography—Collateral Circulation. J.B. Lippincott, Philadelphia, 1968, pp. 129–142.

6. McDonald, D.A. Blood Flow in Arteries. London, Edward Arnold, 1960.

7. McDonald, P.T., Rich, N.M., Collins, G.J., Anderson, C.A., Kozloff, L. Doppler cerebrovascular examination, ocularplethysmography and ocular pneumoplethysmography. Arch Surg 113:1321–1349, 1978.

8. Symon, L., Ishikawa S., Meyer, J.S. Cerebral arterial pressure changes and development of leptomeningeal collateral circulation. Neurology 13:237–250, 1963.

9. Sweet, W.H., Sarnoff, S.J., Bakay, L.A. Clinical method for recording internal carotid pressure; significance of changes during carotid occlusion. Surg Gynecol Obstet 90:327–334, 1950.

10. Wright, R.L., Sweet, W.H. Carotid or vertebral occulsion in the treatment of intracranial aneurysms; value of early and late readings of carotid and retinal pressures. Clin Neurosurg 9:163–192, 1963.

VII
Clinical Aspects

40

High Cervical Carotidopathies

William A. Friedman and Albert L. Rhoton, Jr.

Extracranial vascular lesions account for 30 to 40% of cerebrovascular ischemic events.[16] Most of these lesions are located at the carotid bifurcation and are easily accessible, by well-established techniques, to surgical management.[27] Atherosclerosis is the etiology of greater than 90% of these lesions.[33] The disease primarily involves the intima and is found in a predominantly older age group (over 50 years).

A much smaller group of carotid lesions is found in the high cervical area. The etiology of high cervical carotidopathies includes dissection, arteriosclerosis, kinks and coils, fibromuscular dysplasia,[12] trauma,[4] and congenital malformations.[20] These lesions tend to occur in a younger age group.[18] Surgery in this area is technically much more difficult. Accordingly, patients with such lesions have been considered for extracranial–intracranial bypass procedures.

Very few cases of spontaneous, cervical carotid, dissecting aneurysms have been reported. The following paper concerns four patients with this disease, referred for possible EC–IC bypass. The case reports and a review of the literature are presented. The natural history of this disease process is discussed, particularly as it pertains to EC–IC bypass surgery.

Case Reports

Case 1

This 52-year-old female experienced an episode of amaurosis fugax (OS) and transient agraphia in January 1977. She was hospitalized and underwent transfemoral cerebral angiography. This revealed severe stenosis of the left high cervical and petrous carotid artery, consistent with spontaneous dissection (Fig. 40-1). The patient underwent anticoagulation. With the exception of one further TIA, she remained well. She was referred, in September 1977, for possible EC–IC bypass. Physical examination was normal except for a left Horner's syndrome. Follow-up angiography was within normal limits (Fig. 40-2). The anticoagulants were stopped and the patient has remained asymptomatic.

Case 2

This 46-year-old female complained of generalized headache and intermittent diplopia for one week. Subsequently, on 8 February 1978, she experienced the sudden onset of aphasia and right hemiplegia. Transfemoral cerebral an-

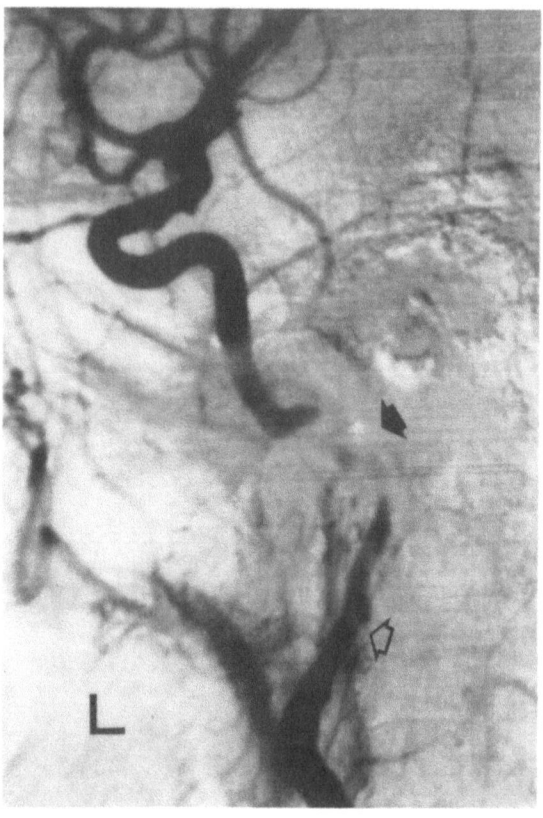

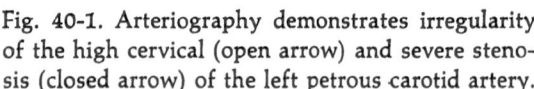

Fig. 40-1. Arteriography demonstrates irregularity of the high cervical (open arrow) and severe stenosis (closed arrow) of the left petrous carotid artery.

giography revealed tapering and severe stenosis of the left high cervical carotid, consistent with dissection (Figs. 40-3, 40-4). The left middle cerebral artery and anterior cerebral artery filled well on a right carotid injection (Fig. 40-5). During March, she was referred for possible EC–IC bypass. Physical examination revealed marked receptive dysphasia and moderate right hemiparesis. Follow-up angiography was within normal limits (Fig. 40-6).

Case 3

This 59-year-old female experienced two transient episodes of amaurosis fugax (OS) and right upper extremity paresis in September 1977. Transfemoral cerebral angiography revealed high-grade stenosis of the left internal carotid artery, consistent with dissection (Figs. 40-7, 40-8). Evidence of small-vessel emboliza-

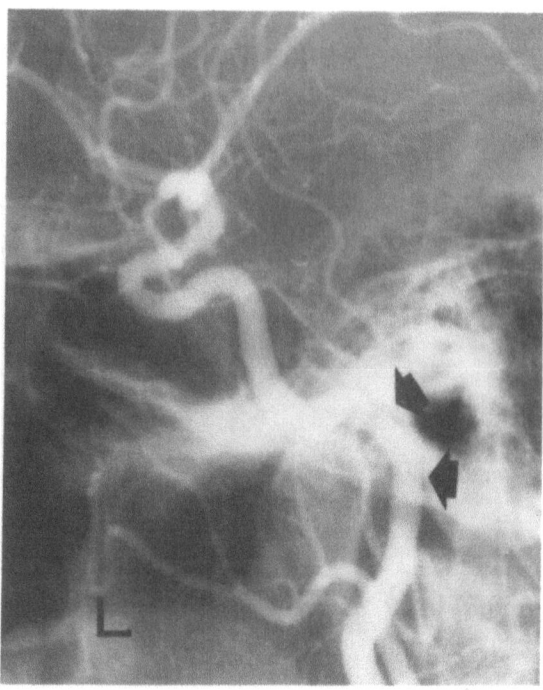

Fig. 40-2. Follow-up arteriography demonstrates recanalization (closed arrows).

tion was seen (Fig. 40-9). She was heparinized and referred for further evaluation. At the University of Florida Medical Center she was placed on coumadin and treated as an outpatient. She was readmitted in December. Physical examination was unremarkable; follow-up angiography was within normal limits (Fig. 40-10). The anticoagulants were discontinued and the patient has remained asymptomatic.

Case 4

This 45-year-old female complained of multiple episodes of amaurosis fugax (OS) associated with left-sided headache. She also noted episodes of right arm dysesthesia. Physical examination disclosed a left carotid bruit. Transfemoral cerebral angiography revealed a filling defect in the left internal carotid artery at the level of Cl (Fig. 40-11). She was placed on coumadin and followed for 3 months. Physical examination was within normal limits (no bruit), and follow-up angiography was unremarkable (Fig. 40-12). Our neuroradiologic

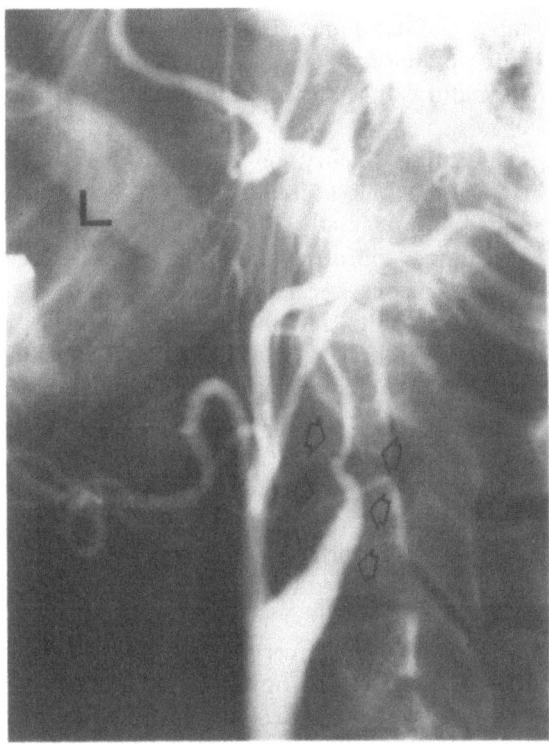

Fig. 40-3. Arteriography demonstrates tapering and stenosis (open arrows) of the left internal carotid artery, above the bifurcation.

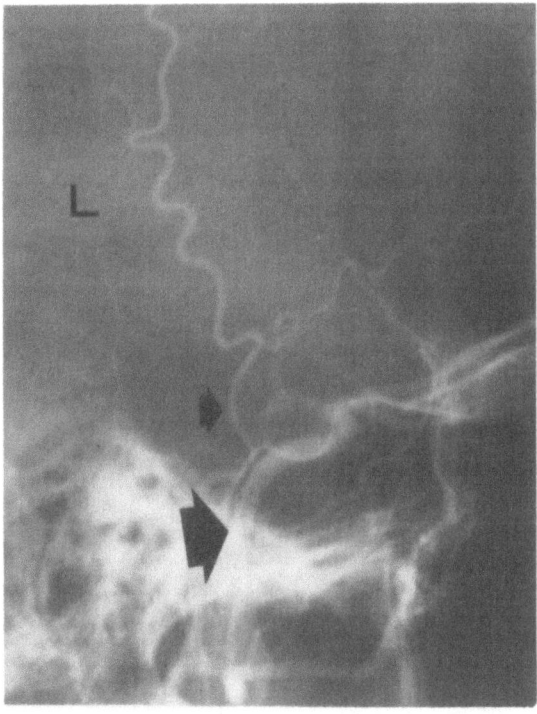

Fig. 40-4. The intracavernous carotid artery (large arrow) is visualized at the same time as the prominent superficial temporal artery (small arrow). This indicates extremely slow flow in the internal carotid.

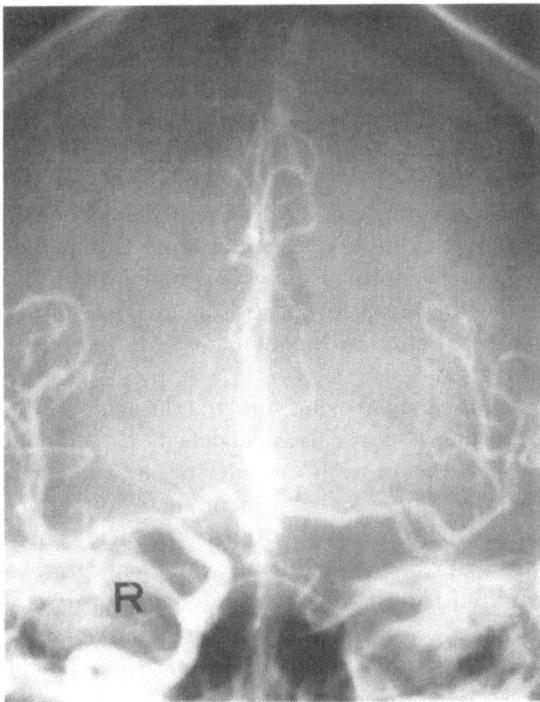

Fig. 40-5. Arteriography demonstrates good collateral flow from the right internal carotid to the left hemisphere.

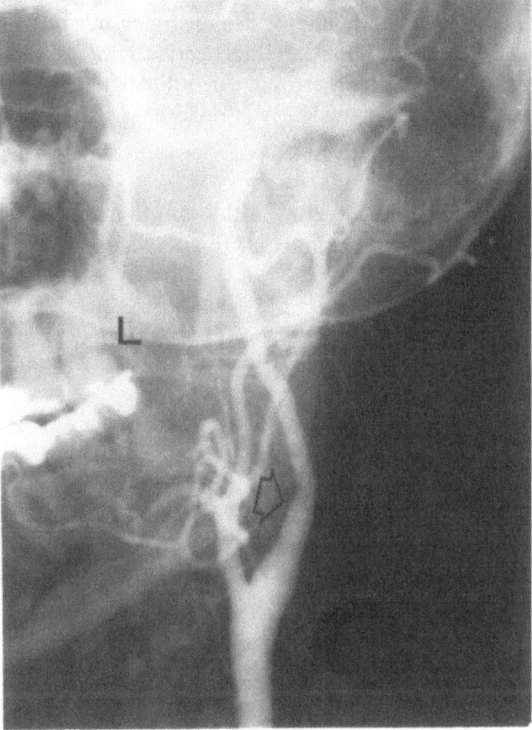

Fig. 40-6. Follow-up arteriography demonstrates recanalization (open arrow).

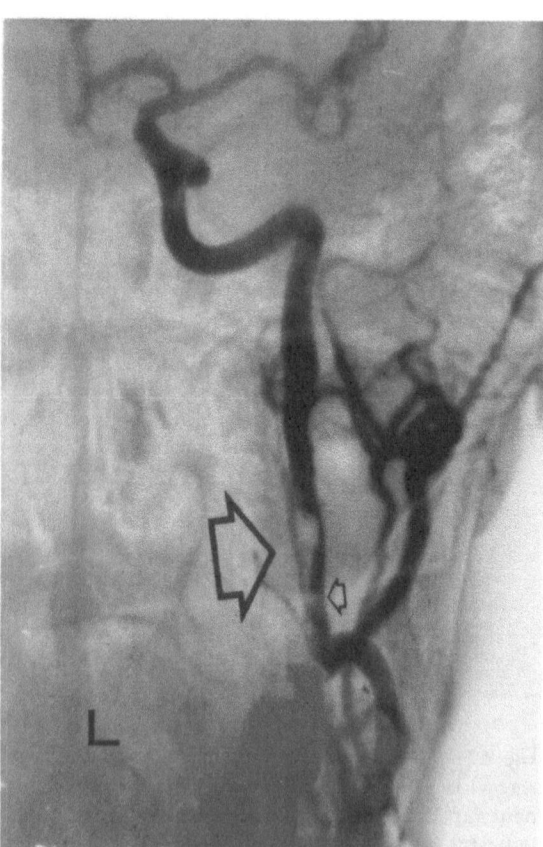

Fig. 40-7. Arteriography demonstrates irregularity and stenosis of the left high cervical internal carotid artery (large arrow). An intimal flap is visualized (small arrow).

interpretation of the initial angiogram could not exclude fibromuscular dysplasia or catheter spasm.

Discussion

The large majority of dissecting aneurysms occur in the aorta.[32] Degenerative disease of the media has been implicated in this lesion, though the etiology of the degenerative process remains unknown.[14, 29] Gore felt that the pathophysiology of the lesion was as follows (Fig. 40-13): The primary event is an intramural hemorrhage. This dissects through the media, enlarging the vessel wall and reducing the caliber of the true lumen. If the hemorrhage ruptures through the intima, into the true lumen, a false lumen is established. Recanalization of the true or false lumen may occur.[15] The natural mortality of the process is 75 to 90%.[7]

Dissecting aneurysms occur in peripheral arteries much less frequently.[10, 32] When described intracranially, the clinical course has been almost uniformly fatal.[3, 8, 24, 26] One case of spontaneous recanalization has been reported.[31] Wisoff[30] felt that it was a prominent cause of cerebral arterial thrombosis in children. On pathologic examination, the plane of dissection is usually subintimal rather than intramedial. This suggests a pathophysiology different from that of aortic dissection.

Cervical carotid dissecting aneurysms have rarely been reported. Most commonly they have been associated with traumatic percutaneous angiography.[9, 25] They have also been described as a result of cervical trauma.[22] "Spontaneous" dissection, however, has been reported in only thirteen cases prior to this paper; these are summarized in Table 40-1. The average age of presentation was 45 (range 31 to 70). There were nine males and eight females. The lesions were left sided (10), right sided (4), bilateral (2), or unspecified (1). Clinical presentation included TIAs (6), asymptomatic bruit (1), seizures (1), and completed stroke (9). Of those with stroke, six experienced prodromal symptoms—amaurosis in 2, headache in 2, hemiparetic spells in 2. Treatment included surgery (5), anticoagulants (3), and supportive measures only (9). The outcome is shown in Table 40-2. All of those with pathologically confirmed dissection had intramedial hemorrhage, as in aortic lesions. The role of distant trauma in "spontaneous" dissections is uncertain.

Of the patients who survived the acute insult, only one had progressive deficit. He did not receive the possible benefits of anticoagulant therapy. The remainder maintained a stable or slowly improving neurologic picture. These survivors are the patients who may later be referred for possible EC–IC bypass surgery.

Three of our patients exhibited angiographic features clearly consistent with spontaneous dissection.[23] Case 4 had clinical and angiographic findings consistent with, but not diagnostic of, this lesion. All four of our patients experienced complete angiographic resolution.

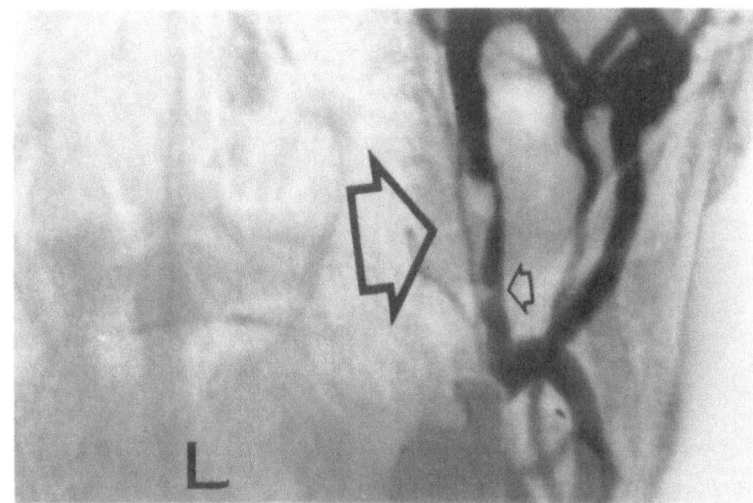

Fig. 40-8. Magnification view of the area of dissection.

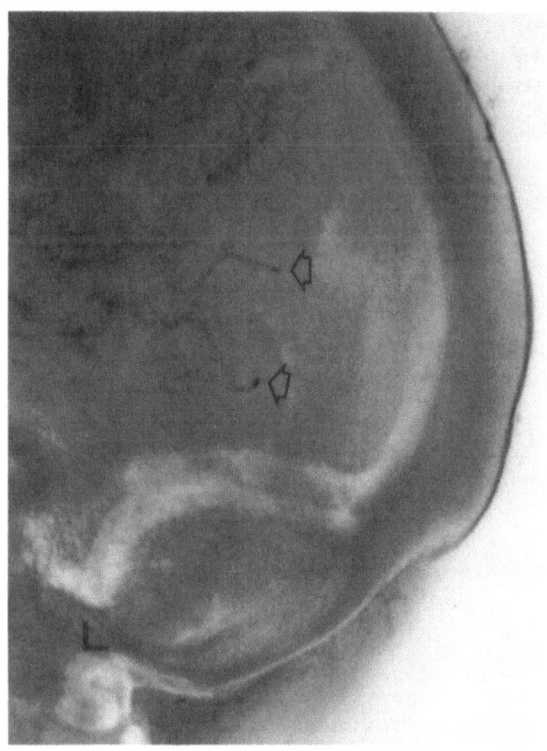

Fig. 40-9. Left carotid arteriogram demonstrates emboli in distal middle cerebral artery branches (open arrows).

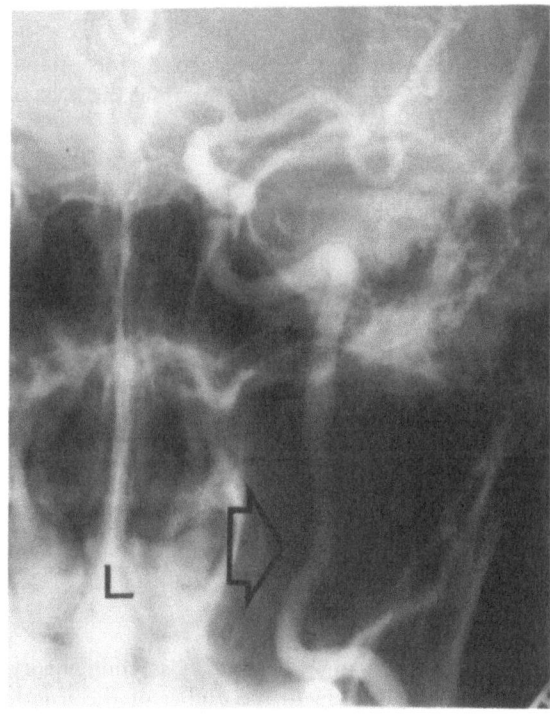

Fig. 40-10. Follow-up arteriography demonstrates recanalization (open arrow).

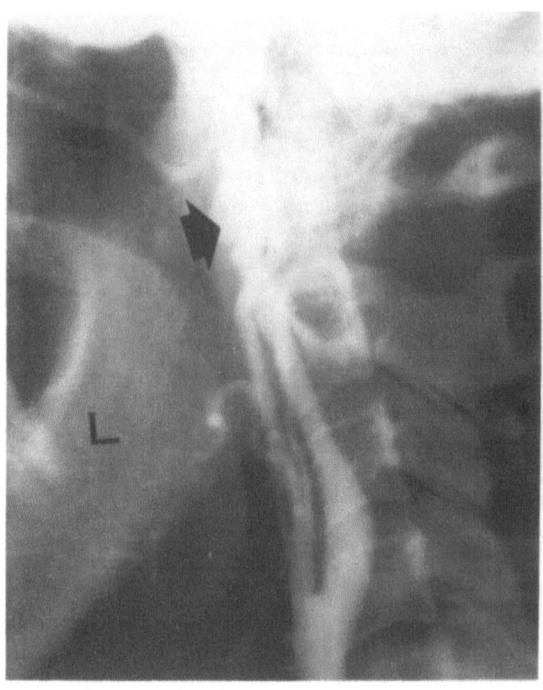

Fig. 40-11. Arteriography demonstrates focal steno-sis of the left internal carotid artery at the level of C1 (closed arrow).

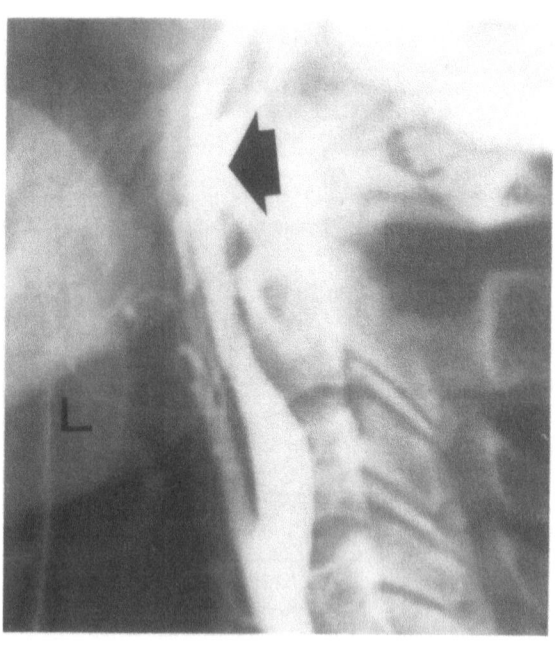

Fig. 40-12. Repeated arteriography demonstrates resolution of the lesion (closed arrow).

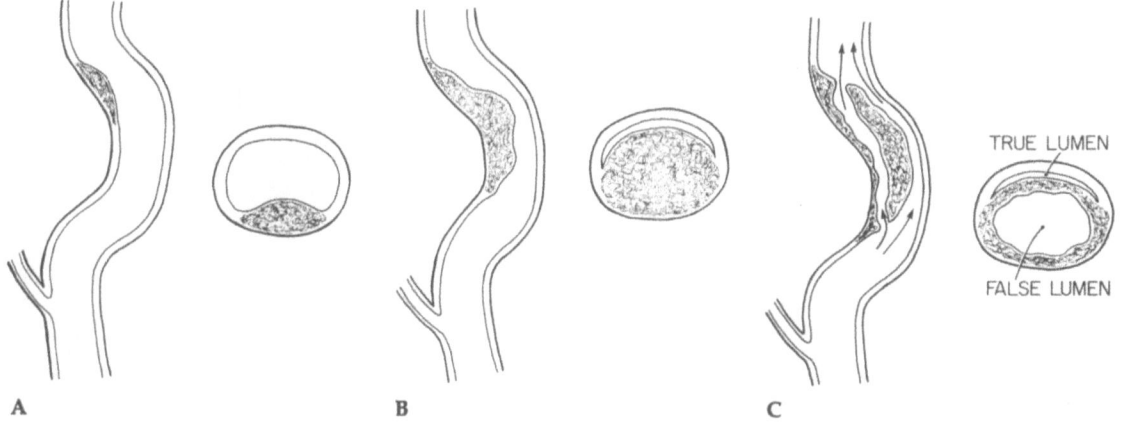

Fig. 40-13. The pathogenesis of a dissecting aneurysm. A. Spontaneous intramural hemorrhage. B. Enlarg-ing hemorrhage reduces the caliber of the true lumen. C. Intimal reentry and recanalization leads to the formation of a false lumen.

Table 40-1. Summary of clinical cases

Case	Author	Age	Sex	Side	Symptoms & signs	Therapy	Outcome
1	Jentzer[19]	31	Female	Bilateral	Amaurosis (OS) Headache Exophthalmos	Left ICA ligation	Death, 8 years later 2° R. ICA aneurysm
2	Anderson[2]	41	Male	Left	Right hemiplegia Coma	Supportive	Death
3	Hardin[17]	51	Male	Left	Bruit (AS)	Fenestration & graft	Decreased bruit Left IX, X paresis
4	Brice[6]	40	Female	Left	Right hemiplegia Aphasia	Supportive	Death
5	Brice[6]	35	Male	Right	Amaurosis (OD) Left hemiplegia Coma	Supportive	Death
6	Brice[6]	38	Female	Left	Headache Right hemiplegia Coma	Supportive	Death
7	Bostrom[5]	53	Male	Right	Transient left hemiparesis Left hemiplegia Coma	Refused	Repeat angiograph shows progression Death
8	Bostrom[5]	70	Male	Right	Seizures	Supportive	Death (cardiac disease)
9	Thapedi[28]	35	Male	Left	Coma	Supportive	Death
10	Lloyd[21]	38	Female	Bilateral	Transient left hemiparesis Left hemiparesis	Recanalization	Stable
11	Ojemann[23]	41	Male	Left	Amaurosis (OS) Right hemiplegia Aphasia	Vein graft	Slow improvement
12	Wylie[33]	38	Male	—	Transient hemiparesis	Supportive	Repeat angiograph shows occlusion
13	Wylie[33]	48	Male	Right	Transient left hemiparesis	Vein graft	Stable
14	Friedman	52	Female	Left	Amaurosis (OS) Transient agraphia	Anticoagulants	Stable with angiographic resolution
15	Friedman	46	Female	Left	Headache Diplopia Right hemiplegia Aphasia	Supportive	Stable with angiographic resolution
16	Friedman	59	Female	Left	Amaurosis (OS) Transient right arm paresis	Anticoagulants	Stable with angiographic resolution
17	Friedman	45	Female	Left	Amaurosis (OS) Left carotid bruit	Anticoagulants	Stable with angiographic resolution

Table 40-2. Results of treatment

	Death	Stable
Surgery		5
Anticoagulation		3
Supportive care	7	2
	7	10

This phenomenon of recanalization is well documented.[1, 11, 13] The frequency of the process is unknown. It may be that good collateral flow (as in case 2) could predispose toward successful recanalization.[13] The same factor certainly contributes toward surviving the initial ischemic event. Thus, our four surviving patients may have been predisposed to recanalize.

It appears that the natural history of those patients who survive a cervical carotid dissection is one of stability or improvement. In addition, they may be strongly predisposed toward recanalization of the involved vessel. These factors suggest prudence on the part of the consulting microvascular surgeon. A trial of medical therapy and follow-up arteriography may be indicated prior to EC–IC bypass surgery.

Summary

Four patients with cervical carotid dissecting aneurysms were referred for possible EC–IC bypass. Repeated angiography revealed complete resolution of the vascular lesion in all cases. A review of the literature suggests that the patients with this lesion who survive to see a consulting microvascular surgeon may be predisposed toward a stable clinical course and recanalization. A trial of medical therapy and follow-up angiography may be indicated before EC–IC bypass surgery.

References

1. Allcock, J.M. Occlusion of the middle cerebral artery: Serial angiography as a guide to conservative therapy. J Neurosurg 27:353, 1967.

2. Anderson, R.M., Schechter, M.M. A case of spontaneous dissecting aneurysm of the internal carotid artery. J. Neurol Neurosurg Psychiatry 22:195, 1959.

3. Bigelow, N.H. Intracranial dissecting aneurysm. Arch Pathol 60:271, 1955.

4. Boldrey, E., Maass, L., Miller, E. The role of atlantoid compression in the etiology of internal carotid thrombosis. J Neurosurg 13:127, 1956.

5. Bostrom, K., Liliequist, B. Primary dissecting aneurysm of the extracranial part of the internal carotid and vertebral arteries. Neurology 17:179, 1967.

6. Brice, J.G., Crompton, M.R. Spontaneous dissecting aneurysms of the cervical internal carotid artery. Br Med J 2:790, 1964.

7. DeBakey, M.E., Cooley, D.A., Creech, O. Surgical consideration of dissecting aneurysm of the aorta. Ann Surg 142:586, 1955.

8. Dratz, H.M., Woodhall, B. Traumatic dissecting aneurysm of the left internal carotid, anterior cerebral and middle cerebral arteries. J Neuropathol Exp Neurol 6:286, 1947.

9. Fleming, J.F.R., Park, A.M. Dissecting aneurysms of the carotid artery following arteriography. Neurology 9:1, 1959.

10. Foord, A.G., Lewis, R.D. Primary dissecting aneurysms of peripheral and pulmonary arteries. Arch Pathol 68:87, 1959.

11. Fox, J.L. Cerebral arterial revascularization: The value of repeated angiography in selection of patients for operation. Neurosurgery 2:205, 1978.

12. Galligioni, F., Iraci, G., Marin, G. Fibromuscular hyperplasia of the extracranial internal carotid artery. J. Neurosurg 34:647, 1971.

13. Gannon, W.E., Chait, A. Occlusion of the middle cerebral artery with recanalization. Am J Roentgengol 88:24, 1962.

14. Gore, I., Seiwert, V. Dissecting aneurysm of the aorta. Arch Pathol 53:121, 1952.

15. Gore, I. Pathogenesis of dissecting aneurysm of the aorta. Arch Pathol 53:142, 1952.

16. Gurdjian, E.S., Lindner, D.W., Hardy, W.G., et al. Completed stroke due to occlusive cerebrovascular disease. Neurology 11:724, 1961.

17. Hardin, C.A., Snodgrass, R.G. Dissecting aneurysm of the internal carotid artery treated by fenestration and graft. Surgery 55:207, 1964.

18. Hymphrey, J.G., Newton, F.H. Internal carotid occlusion in young adults. Brain 83:565, 1960.

19. Jentzer, A. Dissecting aneurysm of the left internal carotid artery. Angiology 5:232, 1954.

20. Lerner, M.A., Braham, J. High cervical carotidopathies. Clin Radiol 22:296, 1971.

21. Lloyd, J., Bahnson, H.T. Bilateral dissecting aneurysms of the internal carotid arteries. Am J Surg 122:549, 1971.

22. Northcroft, G.B., Morgan, A.D. A fatal case of traumatic thrombosis of the internal carotid artery. Br J Surg 32:105, 1944.

23. Ojemann, R.G., Fisher, C.M., Rich, J.C. Spontaneous dissecting aneurysm of the internal carotid artery. Stroke 3:434, 1972.

24. Sinclair, W. Dissecting aneurysm of the middle cerebral artery with migraine syndrome. Am J Pathol 29:1083, 1953.

25. Sirois, J., Lapointe, H., Cote, P.E. Unusual local complication of percutaneous cerebral angiography. J Neurosurg 11:112, 1954.

26. Spudis, E.V., Schanyj, M., Alexander, E., et al. Dissecting aneurysms in the neck and head. Neurology 12:867, 1962.

27. Taveras, J.M., Wood, E.H. Occlusive and stenotic lesions. In Diagnostic Neuroradiology, 2nd ed, Vol 2, Williams & Wilkins Co, Baltimore, 1976, pp 857–911.

28. Thapedi, I., Asherhurst, E.M., Rozdilsky, B. Spontaneous dissecting aneurysm of the internal carotid artery in the neck. Arch Neurol 23:549, 1970.

29. Tyson, M.D. Dissecting aneurysms. Am J Pathol 7:851, 1931.

30. Wisoff, H.S., Rothballer, A.B. Cerebral arterial thrombosis in children. Arch Neurol 4:258, 1961.

31. Wolman, L. Cerebral dissecting aneurysms. Brain 82:276, 1959.

32. Wychulis, A.R., Kincaid, O.W., Wallace, R.B. Primary dissecting aneurysms of peripheral arteries. Mayo Clin Proc 44:804, 1969.

33. Wylie, E.J., Ehrenfeld, W.H. Extracranial Occlusive Cerebrovascular Disease, W.B. Saunders Co, Philadelphia, 1970.

41

Extra–Intracranial Arterial Bypass Surgery for Cerebral Ischemia in Patients with Normal Cerebral Angiograms

P. Schmiedek, V. Olteanu-Nerbe, O. Gratzl, D. Leaschem, and F. Marguth

The indications for extra–intracranial bypass surgery have been fairly well established over the past few years.[2, 7, 8] Next to the neurologic symptoms, the radiologic criteria are considered to be of decisive importance for the selection of appropriate candidates for this operation. Accordingly, the procedure has been recommended only for those patients with a recognizable lesion, either stenotic or occlusive, within the surgically inaccessible portion of the internal carotid artery. It is well known, however, that a considerable number of patients with symptoms or signs of cerebral ischemia have negative cerebral angiograms. The common explanation for this is either that in a previously occluded cerebral artery spontaneous recanalization took place before angiography was performed or, on the other hand, that the lesion is located distally within the vascular territory and therefore is not visible on normal angiograms.[4, 7] It should be emphasized that this is not a benign condition. Marshall and Wilkinson reported on a series of 68 patients with TIAs and normal angiograms and found an incidence of subsequent TIAs and strokes in these patients similar to that in those with positive angiographic findings.[5] These patients are probably in an even worse position than those in whom an etiologically related lesion can be found and treated. These considerations have led us to evaluate the possible role of extra–intracranial bypass surgery in the management of patients with symptoms of cerebral ischemia and normal angiograms. Our preliminary experience as well as the rationale for this procedure in this particular group of patients will be presented in this report.

Clinical Material (Table 41–1)

Ten patients were included in this study: six women and four men who ranged in age from 32 to 60 years, with a mean of 48 years. All of them were admitted to the hospital because of a history of symptoms of neurologic deficits attributable to cerebral ischemia. One 60-year-old lady had a completed stroke on the left side with marked residual weakness of the leg. Five patients exhibited prolonged reversible ischemic neurologic deficits (PRINDs). All of the latter exhibited minor neurologic defects when they were examined initially. Four patients had histories of previous TIAs. Only those patients have been included here, with a postoperative follow-up period of at least 12 months.

Preoperative Studies (Table 41–2)

Cerebral angiography was performed in all cases. In nine patients no radiologic abnormalities could be demonstrated. In one patient a recanalized middle cerebral artery occlusion

Table 41-1. Clinical presentation

Patient no.		Age	Sex	History	Type of CVD
1	M.H.	44	F	4 episodes of left hemiparesis	TIA
2	E.H.	54	M	3 episodes of left hemiparesis	TIA
3	H.J.	32	F	Multiple episodes of numbness of right hand	TIA
4	K.S.	60	F	Left hemiparesis with incomplete recovery	CS
5	S.R.	28	F	Left hemiparesis	TIA
6	S.L.	65	F	Left hemiparesis	PRIND
7	S.J.	54	F	Right hemiparesis	PRIND
8	B.F.	48	M	Right hemiparesis with aphasia	PRIND
9	S.R.	39	M	Multiple episodes of numbness of left side	PRIND
10	H.R.	54	M	2 episodes of right hemiparesis with aphasia	PRIND

Table 41-2. Summary of angiographic, CT and rCBF findings

Patient no.	Angiography	CT	rCBF
1	MCA–O, recanalized	Normal	FR
2	Normal	Normal	RFR
3	Normal	Normal	FR
4	Normal	Normal	RFR
5	Normal	Normal	FR
6	Normal	Small infarct	FR
7	Normal	Normal	FR
8	Normal	Normal	FR
9	Normal	Normal	FR
10	Normal	Small infarct	RFR

was noted 3 weeks following the initial study. A later review of her x-rays, however, revealed that there was still a relatively slow antero-grade filling of the middle cerebral vasculature at the postrecanalized stage. Therefore this pa-tient does not entirely fulfill the criteria for in-clusion in this study. Except for two cases who had some evidence of cerebral infarction, the CT scan was reported as normal. In all patients measurement of rCBF, using the intra-arterial xenon-133 injection method with 16 regional scintillation detectors, was performed over the appropriate hemisphere.[8] Without exception, positive findings were obtained in all patients. Seven patients had only minor focal abnor-malities of rCBF (FR) which, however, were considered to be of pathologic significance in spite of a normal flow within the nonfocal re-gions. Three patients had a relative focal re-duction of CBF, which is defined as a circum-scribed disturbance of CBF associated with a generalized decrease of the hemispheric flow outside of the focus. There were no patients with more severe changes of CBF, such as mod-erate or severe general reduction of rCBF.

From our earlier experience with rCBF studies in the selection of patients for extra–intracranial bypass surgery, it has become evi-dent that patients with focal changes of rCBF (FR and RFR) would be the best candidates for bypass surgery. Although all of our earlier cases had additional angiographically demon-strable lesions, it was thought that the patients of this group, who all had convincing clinical manifestations of cerebral ischemia and proven abnormalities on CBF studies, could eventually benefit from bypass surgery as well. The ten patients were subsequently operated on.

Results (Table 41–3)

No operative morbidity or mortality was encountered in this group and all patients are still alive. The postoperative follow-up period ranged from 12 to 29 months, with a mean of 19 months. Patients were readmitted to the hospital at regular intervals during the postoperative course. According to the most recent neurologic examination, the clinical condition was reported to be as follows: Seven patients were found to be asymptomatic, including all patients with preoperative history of TIAs. None of them had experienced an episode of TIA since he had been operated on. Three patients of the PRIND group had also become asymptomatic meanwhile. Two other patients with a PRIND reported a considerable improvement of symptoms during the postoperative period; however, they still had minor residual neurologic deficits. Essentially unchanged was the condition of the only patient of this series who had had a completed stroke preoperatively.

Graft patency (Table 41-4) was evaluated postoperatively at various times, with different techniques or a combination of them. Most often the Doppler technique was employed. The Doppler method revealed evidence of a functioning bypass during the early postoperative period, usually on the seventh postoperative day, in all cases. When the study was repeated several months later, the result suggested an occlusion of the bypass in two cases

Table 41-3. Clinical results

Patient no.	Follow-up period (months)	Clinical result
1	29	No further TIAs, asymptomatic
2	27	No further TIAs, asymptomatic
3	22	No further TIAs, asymptomatic
4	20	Unchanged, weakness of left side
5	18	No further TIAs, asymptomatic
6	17	Complete recovery of left hemiparesis, asymptomatic
7	16	1 episode of weakness of right hand for 10 min
8	15	Complete recovery of right hemiparesis, asymptomatic
9	14	Episodes of numbness reduced
10	12	Complete recovery of right hemiparesis, asymptomatic

Table 41-4. Evaluation of bypass function

Patient no.	Doppler Early	Doppler Late	Angiography	rCBF
1	+	+	Bypass patent, MCA–O	Normalized
2	+	+	Bypass patent	Normalized (extern. study)
3	+	+	Not done	Not done
4	+	–	Bypass occluded	Not done
5	+	+	Bypass patent	Not done
6	+	+	Not done	Not done
7	+	+	Bypass patent	Normal
8	+	+	Bypass patent	Normal
9	+	+	Bypass patent	Unchanged, FR
10	+	–	Not done	Not done

with positive findings in the remaining eight patients.

Late postoperative control angiography was performed in seven patients. Patency of the bypass could be demonstrated in six patients. Using the grading system of Ausman[1] to describe the angiographic quality, two patients had grade-2 filling, the remainder grade-1 filling. An occlusion of the bypass was found in the completed stroke case.

In five patients postoperative rCBF studies could be obtained. In one instance the isotope was injected into the external carotid artery. In the other four patients an identical approach was used in both the pre- and postoperative situation, thereby allowing a direct comparison of results. A completely normal CBF was found in two patients postoperatively; evidence for an increase of CBF over the preoperative study was seen twice, and one patient had identical results pre- and postoperatively.

Case Reports

Case 1 (Fig. 41–1)

As mentioned earlier, this 44-year-old woman, with a history of four previous transient ischemic episodes involving her left side, had a middle cerebral artery occlusion on her initial right angiogram. Three weeks later the study was repeated and at this time revealed an anterograde filling of the middle cerebral artery territory. However, a phase difference of contrast filling was noticed, with slower filling of the middle cerebral artery. The rCBF study which was performed during the postrecanalized stage showed a focal reduction of flow values, corresponding to the middle cerebral artery. She was operated on and had an uneventful postoperative course. When she was seen again, 29 months later, she was asymptomatic and had not had any further TIAs. Control angiography showed a good functioning bypass with filling of the middle cerebral artery tree. An additional selective internal carotid study demonstrated again a complete occlusion of the right middle cerebral artery. On her rCBF study only minor flow abnormalities could be seen.

Case 2 (Fig. 41–2)

This 54-year-old patient had three episodes of transient left hemiparesis before he was admitted to the hospital. The decision to operate on him was based on the result of the rCBF study, which showed a relative focal reduction of CBF. During the 27 months of his postoperative follow-up period, he remained asymptomatic. The late postoperative control angiogram showed a good functioning bypass. The rCBF study was performed at the same time. However, because of injection of the isotope into the external route, the result could be interpreted only as suggestive of a normalization of flow values.

Case 8 (Fig. 41–3)

This 48-year-old man had a right-sided hemiparesis with aphasia 7 months before he was admitted to the hospital. His neurologic symptoms had completely resolved over a couple of days and he was asymptomatic when he was seen in the hospital. Cerebral angiography and CT scan were both within normal limits. The rCBF study showed a small focus with ischemic values. The patient was operated on and remained asymptomatic during the postoperative period. Control angiography done 15 months later showed a functioning bypass, which, however, according to present standards, would have been considered to be of only poor quality. A comparison of pre- and postoperative rCBF results revealed a normal hemispheric blood flow on his postoperative study.

Discussion

The rationale for extra–intracranial bypass surgery in the treatment of cerebral ischemia is to increase the collateral blood supply to an ischemic brain region, secondary to a hemodynamically effective obstruction of the conducting cerebral arteries. Accordingly, it can be expected that the quality of the bypass, and at the same time the volume of blood which is supplied via the anastomosis, are directly proportional to the extra–intracranial pressure

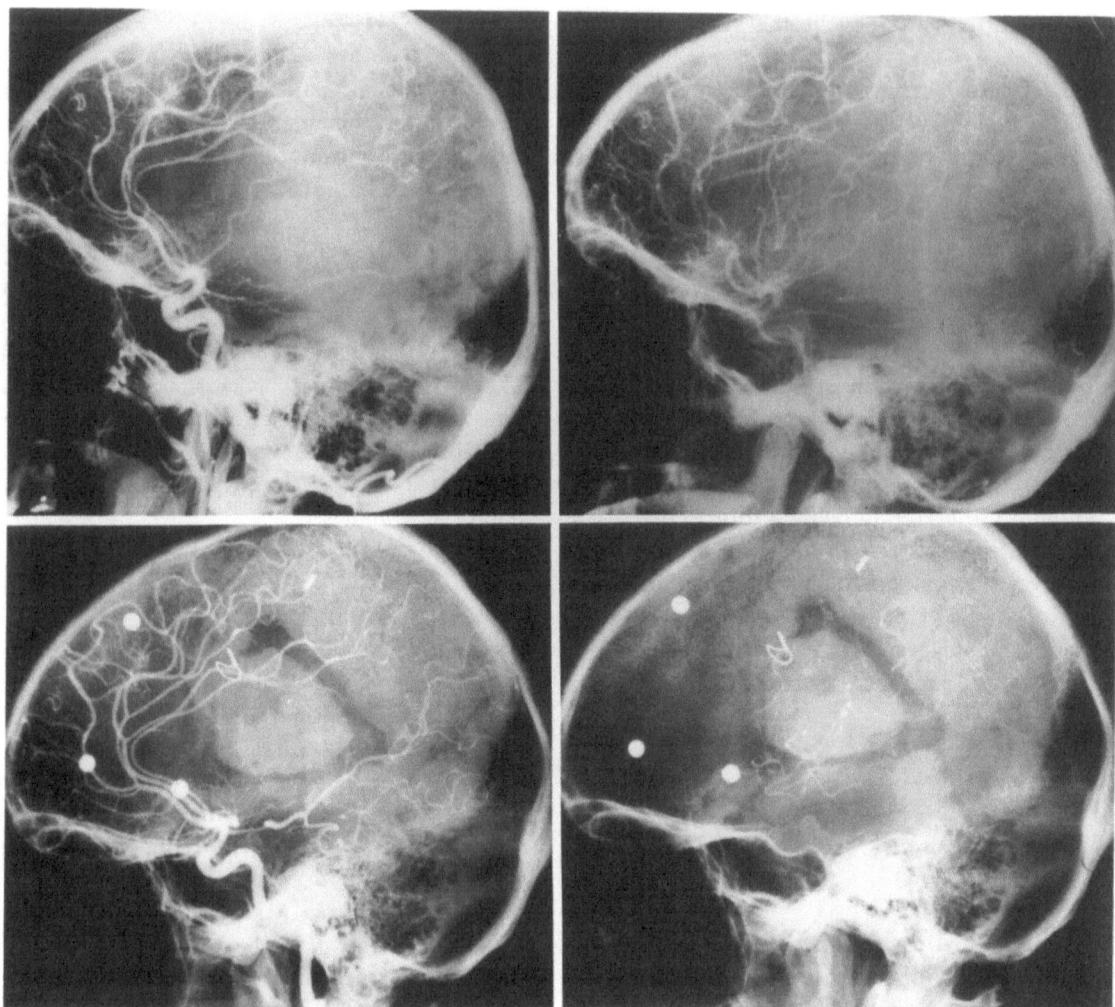

Fig. 41-1. (L) carotid angiograms of a 44-year-old woman. Left middle cerebral artery occlusion shown in upper left. Upper right shows collateral filling of middle cerebral branches. Bottom postoperative control angiograms 29 months after bypass; showing filling of middle cerebral tree with external carotid injection on (R) and persistent failure of middle cerebral filling with internal carotid injection on left.

gradient between the two vascular territories. Theoretically, this pressure gradient should be highest when middle cerebral artery occlusion is due to a lack of sufficient natural collateral channels. An occlusion of the internal carotid artery will probably also result in a rise of this pressure gradient depending, however, on the compensatory capacity of the circle of Willis. Finally, a third situation can be speculated on, namely, an unobstructed flow within the cerebral arteries, which obviously will prevent the development of a considerable extra–intracranial pressure gradient. The results of this study are not entirely in support of this concept, at least with regard to the last point, because it could be demonstrated that a well-functioning bypass can be seen in a patient despite an angiographically normal cerebral vasculature. In fact, this could mean an extension of our present criteria for the selection of patients who may benefit from an extra–intracranial bypass procedure. Although the data from this study are as yet inconclusive, we think that it is justified to operate on a patient with symptoms of cerebral ischemia, even in the absence of an appropriate vascular lesion,

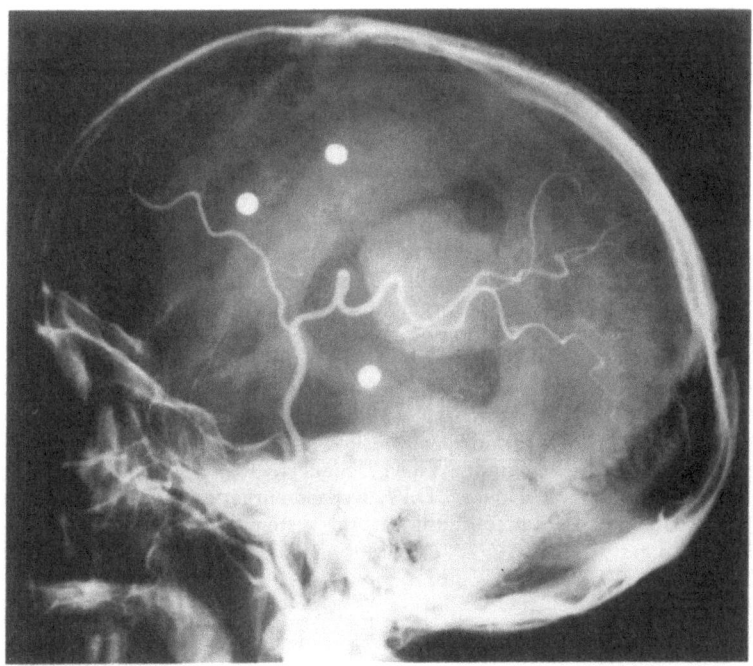

Fig. 41-2. Postoperative angiogram in 54-year-old man 27 months following bypass.

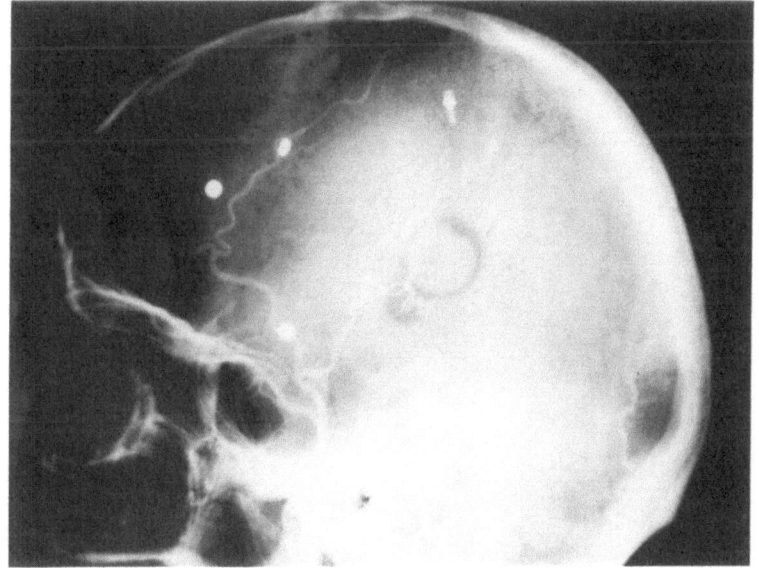

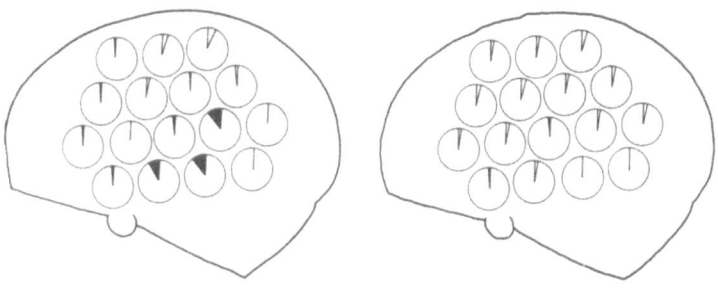

Fig. 41-3. A. Postoperative angiogram in 48-year-old man showing minimal flow across anastomosis. B. Preoperative rCBF study showing area of relative ischemia. C. Postoperative rCBF study showing normalization of hemispheric flow.

provided his symptoms are definitely attributable to an insufficient blood supply to the brain.

References

1. Ausman, J.I., Latchaw, R.E., Lee, M.C., Ramirez-Lassepas, M. Results of multiple angiographic studies on cerebral revascularization patients. In P. Schmiedek, O. Gratzl, and R. Spetzler, editors, Microsurgery for Stroke, Springer-Verlag, New York, 1977, p 222.
2. Gratzl, O., Schmiedek, P., Spetzler, R., Steinhoff, H., Marguth, F. Clinical experience with extra–intracranial arterial anastomosis in 65 cases. J. Neurosurg 44:313, 1976.
3. Høedt-Rasmussen, K., Sveinsdottir, E., Lassen, N.A. Regional cerebral blood flow in man determined by intra-arterial injection of radioactive inert gas. Circ Res 18:237, 1966.
4. Irino, T., Taneda, M., Minami, T. Angiographic manifestations in postrecanalized cerebral infarction. Neurology 27:471, 1977.
5. Marshall, J., Wilkinson, I.M.S. The prognosis of carotid transient ischemic attacks in patients with normal angiograms. Brain 94:395, 1971.
6. Schmiedek, P., Gratzl, O., Spetzler, R. (editors). Microsurgery for Stroke, Springer-Verlag, New York, 1977.
7. Sindermann, F., Dichgans, J., Bergleiter, R. Occlusion of the middle cerebral artery and its branches: angiographic and clinical results. Brain 92:607, 1969.
8. Sundt, Th.M., Siekert, R.G., Piepgras, D.G., Houser, D.W. Bypass surgery for vascular disease of the carotid system. Mayo Clin Proc 51:677, 1976.

42

Revascularization in the Acute Stage of the MCA Occlusion

Yasuhiro Yonekawa, Hajime Handa, Mitsumasa Terano,
and Tetsuaki Teraura

Thromboembolectomy of the middle cerebral artery (MCA) was successfully performed by Welch in 1954 and a considerable number of patients underwent this procedure thereafter, with or without refinement of microsurgical techniques.[2, 9, 15, 17, 18] The procedure lags, however, somewhat behind the superficial temporal artery–middle cerebral artery (STA–MCA) bypass pioneered by Yasargil and Donaghy in 1967.[17] The purpose of this report is to present our experience with thromboembolectomy of the MCA in the acute stage on two cases and to reappraise the procedure.

Case Reports

Case 1. T.F.

This 65-year-old female suffered from exophthalmos on the left side. Angiographic study revealed a giant aneurysm of the left internal carotid artery (ICA) at the cavernous portion. Although carotid ligation was thought to be the treatment of choice, collateral circulation to the left cerebral hemisphere was displayed to be insufficient by the Matas test as well as by angiographic study. The STA–MCA bypass was therefore performed prior to the carotid ligation. The bypass was revealed, however, by follow-up angiography to have occluded. A gradual occlusion of the cervical ICA with Crutchfield clamp was later performed.

On 12 October 1977 the clamp was closed completely but was reopened 5 minutes later, as signs of ischemia developed. The patient became suddenly unconscious and soon drowsy, aphasic, and hemiplegic on the right side. A MCA embolism was diagnosed, and thrombus formed at the site of the cervical ICA distal to the Crutchfield clamp was considered to have detached when the clamp was reopened. Angiography disclosed a complete occlusion of the left MCA (Fig. 42-1). Hypotension was carefully avoided by giving Reomacrodex 500 ml IV, which acts also as antisludging agent.

Operation. Complete revascularization was accomplished 8 hours after the onset of embolization (Fig. 42-2). A pterional approach to the left MCA was performed by rongeuring the sphenoid ridge. The MCA was dissected by opening the sylvian fissure with microsurgical technique. The brain was neither edematous nor anemic. The dislodged embolus was observed at the MCA bifurcation. The relatively hard dark-red embolus was taken out through a small arteriotomy (3 mm in length), by milking and sucking. The lumen was rinsed with heparin-saline and the arteriotomy was closed by interrupted microsutures of 8-0 monofilament. A complete revascularization was thus achieved.

Course. Postoperative course was uneventful. No specific anticoagulant therapy was used ex-

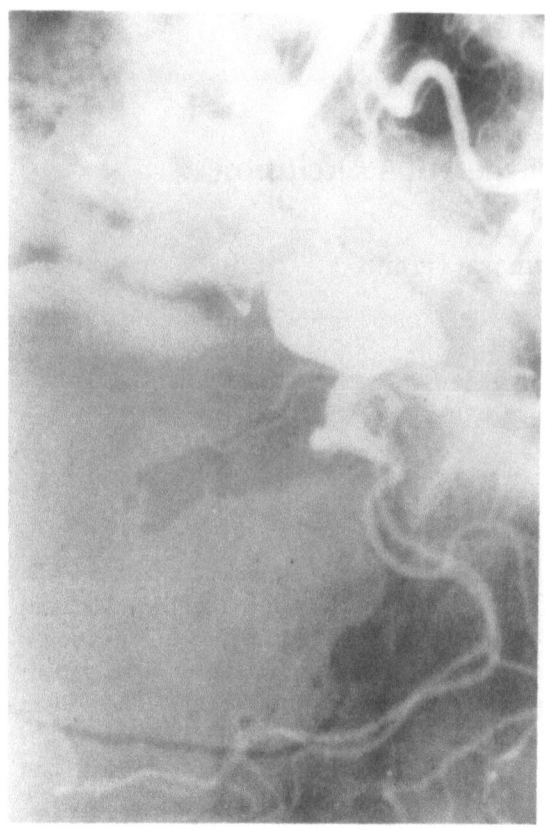

Fig. 42-1. Complete occlusion of the MCA is shown. Giant aneurysm and previous craniotomy for the STA–MCA bypass are also observed. Only lateral view was done.

cept Rheomacrodex and acetylsalicylic acid (ASA). Consciousness disturbance almost cleared up on the first postoperative day. Hemiparesis and aphasia improved rapidly. Urinary incontinence remained about 2 weeks. Postoperative CT scan on the fifth postoperative day revealed low density at the site of operation and the left subcortical area (Fig. 42-3). A small high-density area was also observed, which would indicate small hematoma or hemorrhagic infarction. Follow-up CT scan 3 weeks postoperatively revealed patchy low-density areas in the left hemisphere (Fig. 42-4). Follow-up angiography 1½ months after the operation revealed a complete vascularization of the MCA territory, with no stenotic lesion at the sutured site (Fig. 42-5). At the time of angiography the patient was almost free of abnormal neurologic findings except for exophthalmos and a very slight right hemiparesis.

Case 2. T.N.

This 61-year-old male became suddenly hemiplegic and drowsy on 26 February 1978. Angiographic study revealed a complete occlusion of the right MCA just distal to the origin of the posterior temporal branch (Fig. 42-6). No cardiac disorder was observed and MCA thrombosis was thus diagnosed.

Operation. Complete revascularization was achieved in 18 hours after the onset of thrombosis (Fig. 42-7). The MCA was dissected by the approach described above. It was filled with a hard yellow-white thrombus from the middle part of the M1 to bifurcation. The lenticulostriate arteries were fully involved. Milking out of the thrombus through a small arteriotomy was impossible. Thromboendarterectomy was performed through an arteriotomy 1.5 cm in length, as illustrated in Fig. 42-7. After the lumen was rinsed with heparin-saline, the arteriotomy was closed by continuous sutures of 8-0 monofilament. Perfusion of the MCA territory was thus reestablished.

Course. No special anticoagulant therapy was given except Rheomacrodex and ASA. Postoperative course was uneventful but neurologic deficits remained unchanged in spite of the complete reperfusion of the right MCA territory, as was ascertained by follow-up angiography (Fig. 42-8).

Discussion

Patency rate of the revascularized MCA of reported cases has been relatively low: occlusion in one of Welch's two cases and in both of Jacobson's cases.[9, 15] As Crawford et al. have already mentioned,[3] endarterectomy of arteries of this small size (2 to 3 mm in diameter) usually complicates lumen constriction, which would be partly avoided by technical refinement using microsurgery.[9, 17] In the case of embolectomy in the acute stage as in Chou's case or our first case, endarterectomy is not necessary and neat closure of arteriotomy with microsurgical technique would promise a long-lasting patency of the MCA.[2]

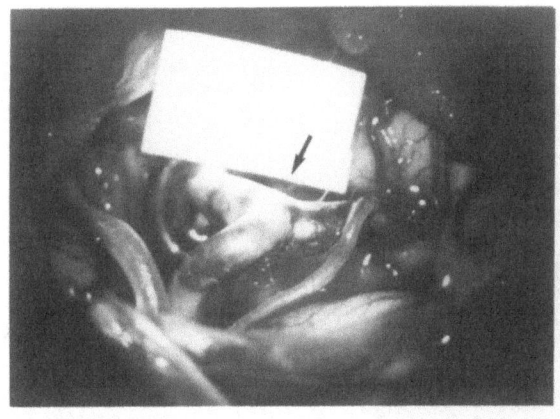
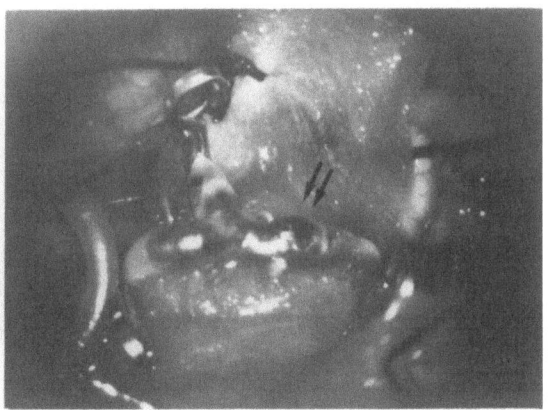

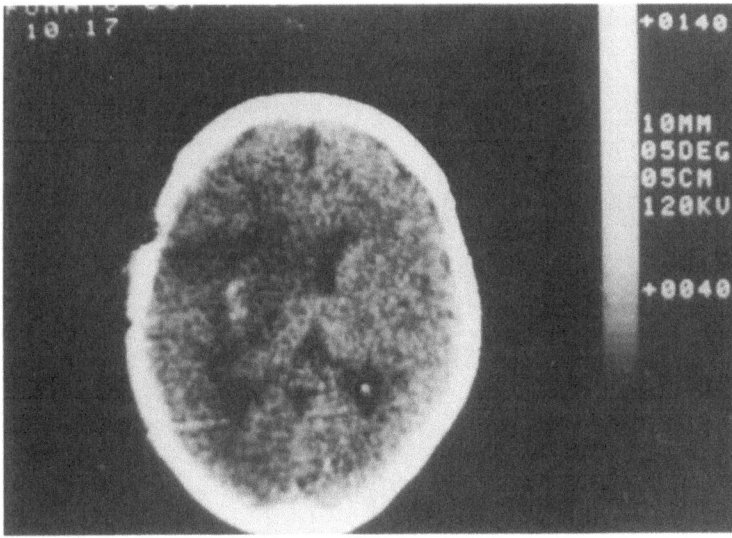

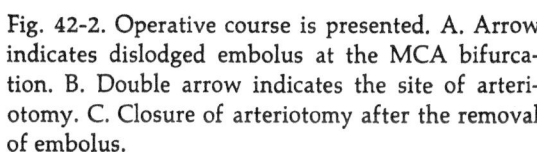

Fig. 42-2. Operative course is presented. A. Arrow indicates dislodged embolus at the MCA bifurcation. B. Double arrow indicates the site of arteriotomy. C. Closure of arteriotomy after the removal of embolus.

Fig. 42-3. CT scan on the fifth postoperative day indicates low density at the site of operation and subcortical area and also small high-density area, which may be small hematoma or hemorrhagic infarction.

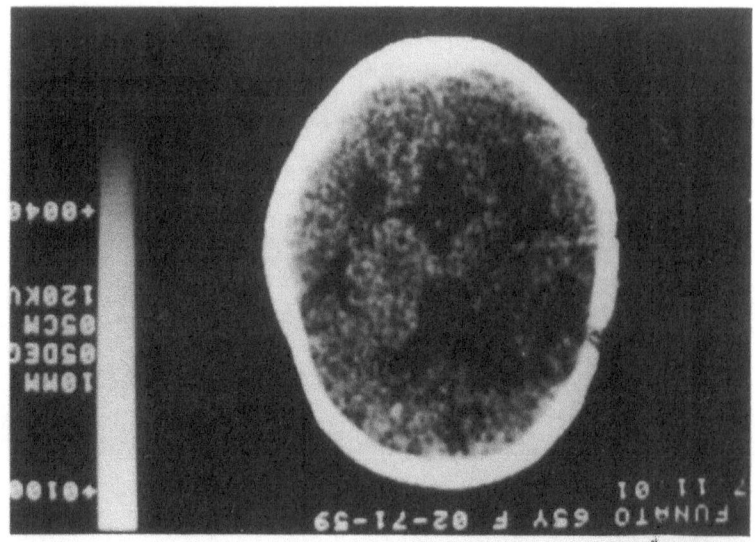

Fig. 42-4. CT scan 3 weeks later indicates patchy low-density area in the left hemisphere.

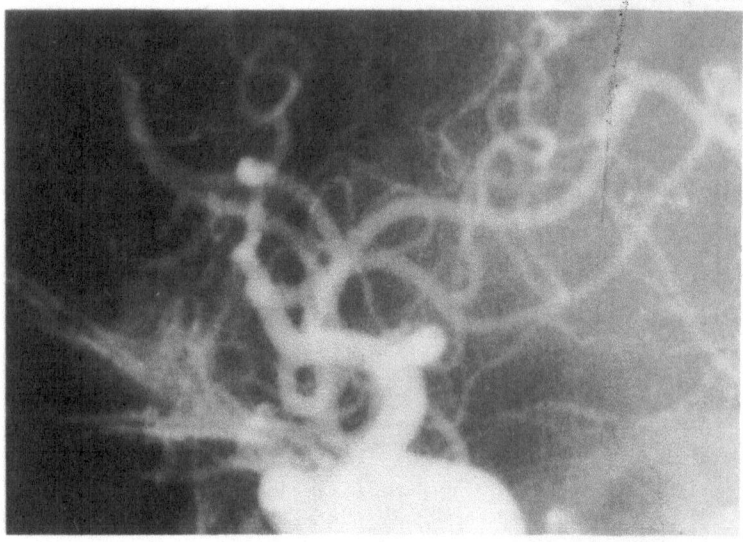

A

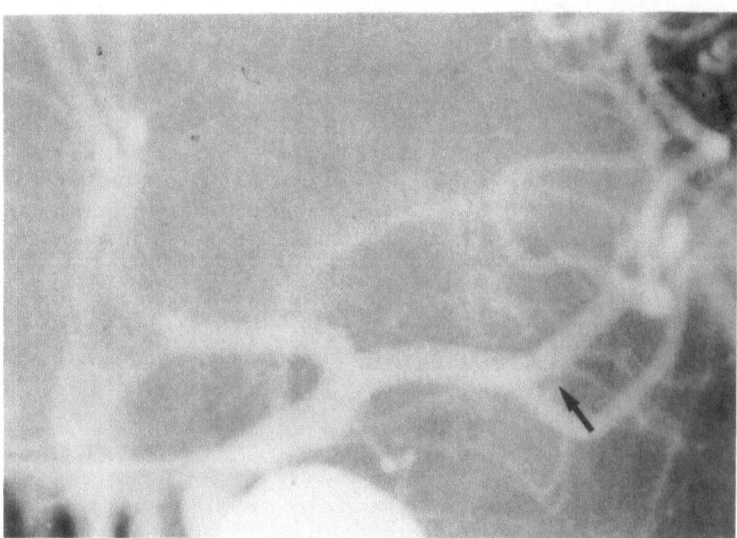

B

Fig. 42-5. Follow-up angiography 1½ months after the operation reveals complete reperfusion in the MCA territory. A. Lateral view. B. AP view. Arrow indicates site of microsutures.

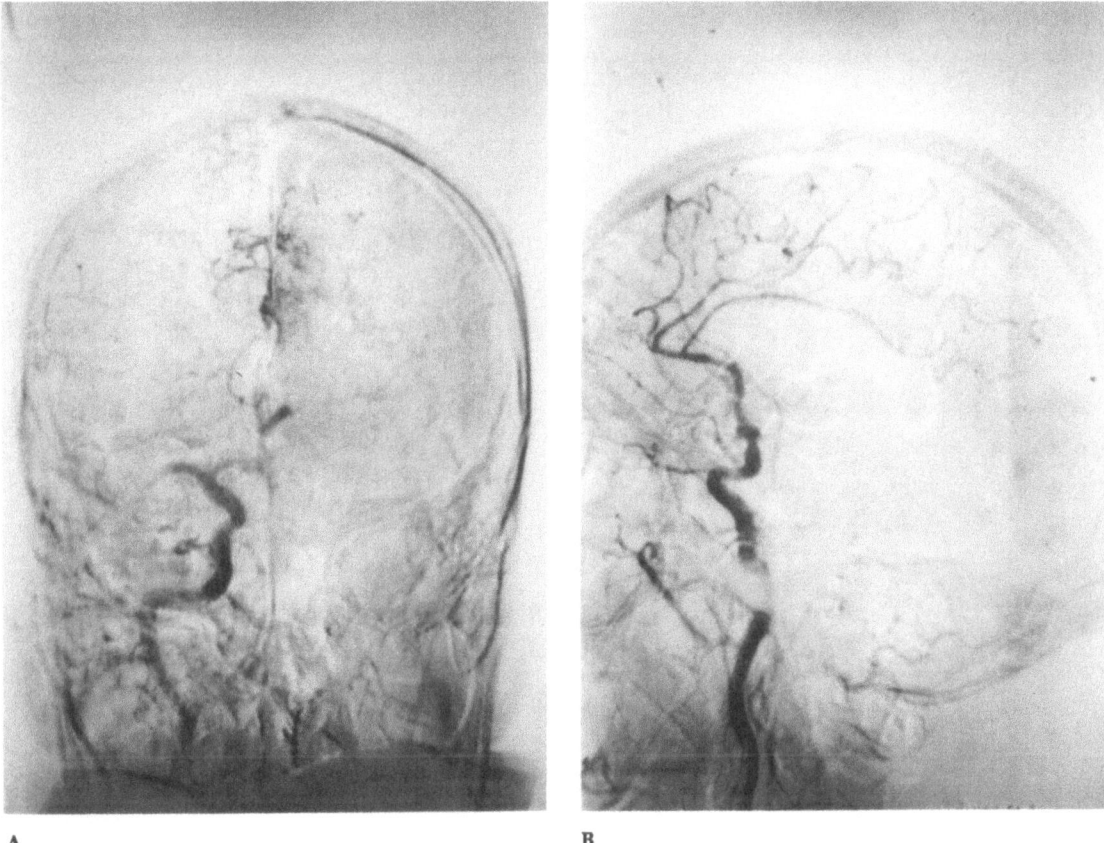

A   B

Fig. 42-6. Complete occlusion of the MCA just distal to the posterior temporal branch. A. AP view. B. Lateral view.

It has been reported that the brain can tolerate absolute ischemia for a considerable time experimentally, e.g., one hour according to Hossman et al.[7] MCA occlusion causes no absolute ischemia and collateral circulation as in leptomeningeal anastomosis would modify further development of infarction. Experimental ischemia from the MCA occlusion has been reported to be largely reversible if flow is restored in 3 to 6 hours.[14] Irreversible neuronal changes are considered to take place thereafter.[12, 13] The interval might be lengthened by hyperosmolar agents[11] or other known treatment such as induced hypertension, hypothermia, hyperbaric oxygen chamber, antisludging agent, etc. The shortest interval from the vascular accident to the embolectomy was 40 min in a case of Yasargil's series.[17] Nine hours elapsed in Chou's case[2] and 8 hours in our first case. The latter two cases had angiographically verified reperfusion and fair functional recovery. The lack of functional recovery of our second case is attributed to unduly long ischemic intervals (18 hours) and to involvement of the perforating arteries, which will also determine functional prognosis after a revascularization procedure. CT scan, SEP,[8] or other new methods of examination such as positron-emission CT would bring much more information concerning the functional prognosis.

Good results of acute revascularization by the STA–MCA bypass have been experimentally and clinically documented.[4, 5, 6] The advantages of direct MCA thromboembolectomy in the acute stage to the STA–MCA bypass would be: (1) larger blood flow through the direct MCA revascularization, and (2) faster revascularization (may be an hour faster). The disadvantages would be: (1) operative intervention of greater magnitude, and (2) technical difficulty because of the depth of operative fields.

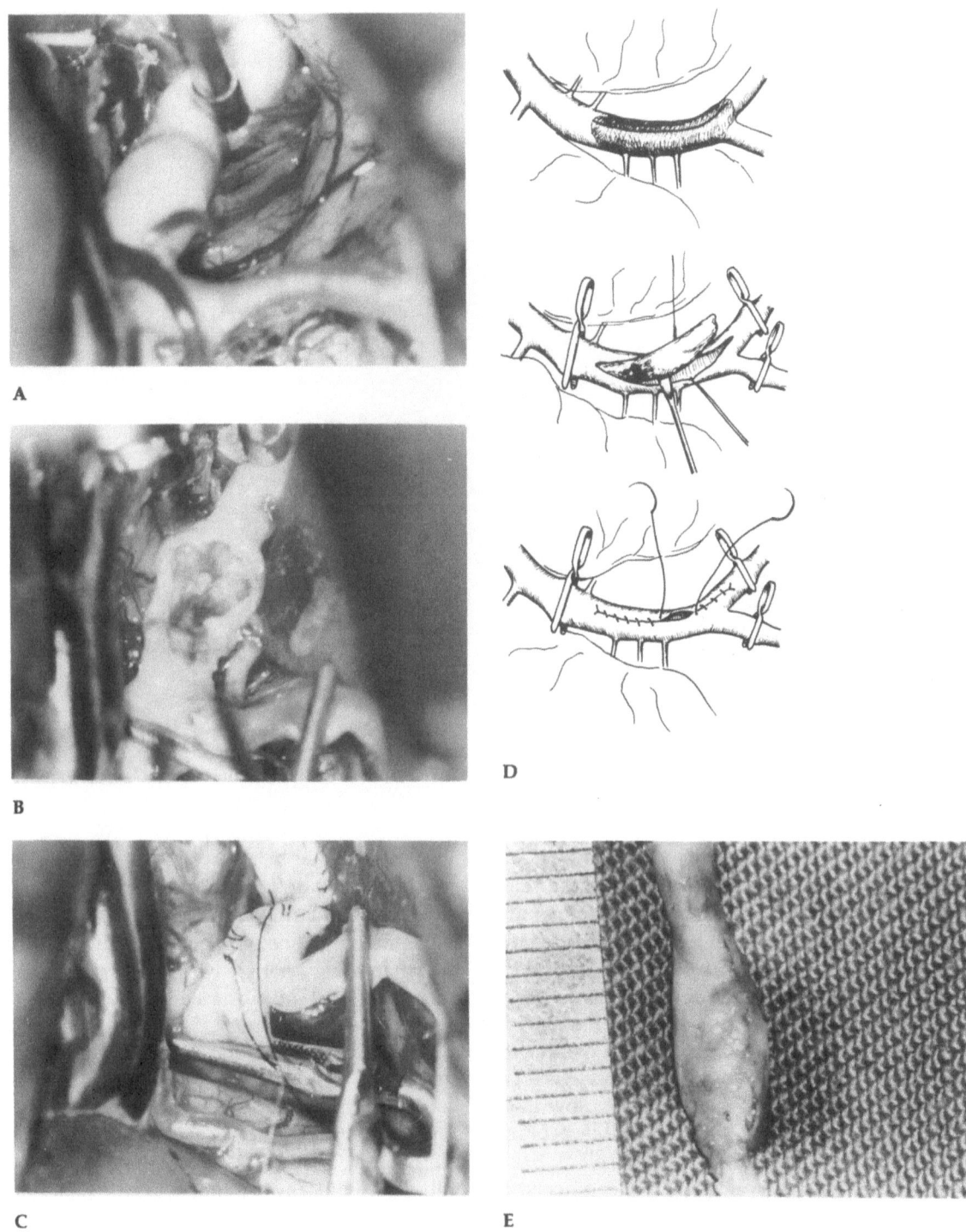

Fig. 42-7. Operative course. A. The MCA is fully thrombosed. B. Arteriotomy and removal of thrombus. C. Closure of the arteriotomy with continuous sutures. D. Schematic representation of thromboembolectomy. E. Removed thrombus.

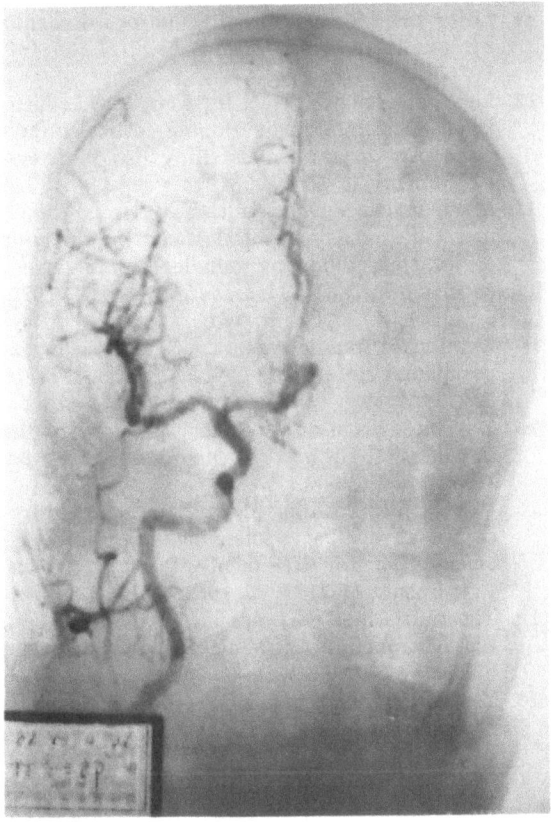 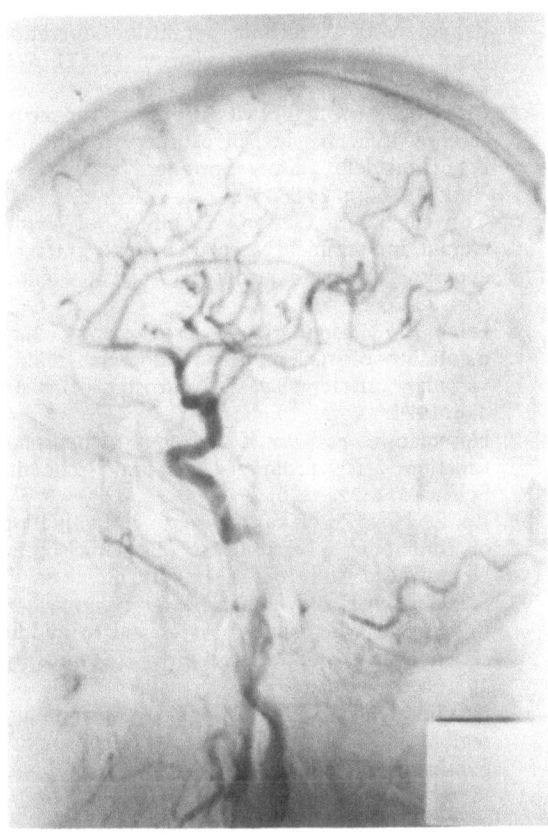

A   B

Fig. 42-8. Postoperative angiography reveals complete revascularization.

Revascularization in the acute stage has been contraindicated for fear of hemorrhagic infarction.[1, 16] In none of the cases in which the MCA thromboembolectomy was performed within 48 hours was hemorrhagic infarction reported. It has been shown experimentally that hemorrhagic infarction occurs rarely or on a small scale, if at all, in such acute revascularization.[10]

In conclusion, thromboembolectomy of the MCA, especially embolectomy in the acute stage, should be considered into account seriously in selected cases, with the expectation of good functional recovery.

Summary

Two cases of revascularization in the acute stage of the middle cerebral artery have been presented. A 65-year-old female was submitted to MCA embolectomy 8 hours from onset of MCA embolism as a complication of the use of a Crutchfield clamp. A 61-year-old male underwent thromboembolectomy in 18 hours from onset of MCA thrombosis. Follow-up angiography revealed patent MCA in both cases. Functional recovery was observed in the former case and not in the latter. Clinical aspects and theoretical background of this procedure have been briefly reviewed.

References

1. Blaisdell, W.F., Clauss, R.H., Galbraith, J.G., et al. Joint study of extracranial arterial occlusion. IV. A review of surgical considerations. JAMA 209:1889–1895, 1969.
2. Chou, S.N. Embolectomy of middle cerebral artery. Report of a case. J Neurosurg 20:161–163, 1963.
3. Crawford, E.S., Beall, A.C., Ellis, P.R. Jr., De-

Bakey, M.E. A technic permitting operation upon small arteries. Surg Forum 10:671–675, 1960.

4. Crowell, R.M. STA–MCA bypass for acute cerebral ischemia. In Microsurgery for Stroke, P. Schmiedek, editor, Springer-Verlag, New York, 1976, pp 244–250.

5. Crowell, R.M., Olsson, Y. Effects of extracranial intracranial vascular bypass graft on experimental acute stroke in dogs. J Neurosurg 38:26–31, 1973.

6. Fein, J.M., Molinari, G. Experimental augmentation of regional blood flow by microvascular anastomosis. J Neurosurg 41:421–426, 1974.

7. Hossman, K.A., Sato, K. Recovery of neuronal function after prolonged cerebral ischemia. Science 168:375–376, 1970.

8. Ito, Z., Hen, R., Nakajima, K., et al. Evaluation of functional reversibility of ischemic brain. Neurol Med Chir 16:121–129, 1976.

9. Jacobson, J.H., Wallman, L.J., Schumacher, G.A., et al. Microsurgery as an aid to middle cerebral artery endarterectomy. J Neurosurg 19:108–115, 1962.

10. Kamijo, Y., Garcia, J.H., Cooper, J. Temporary regional ischemia in the cat. J Neuropathol Exp Neurol 36:338–349, 1977.

11. Little, J.R. Modification of acute focal ischemia by treatment with mannitol. Stroke 9:4–9, 1978.

12. Little, J.R., Sundt, T.M. Jr., Kerr, F.W.L. Neuronal alterations in developing cortical infarction. An experimental study in monkeys. J Neurosurg 39:186–198, 1974.

13. MacDonald, V.D., Sundt, T.M. Jr., Winkelmann, R.K. Histochemical studies in the zone of ischemia following middle cerebral artery occlusion in cats. J Neurosurg 37:45–54, 1972.

14. Sundt, T.M. Jr., Grant, W.C., Garcia, J.H. Restoration of middle cerebral artery flow in experimental infarction. J Neurosurg 31:311–322, 1969.

15. Welch, K. Excision of occlusive lesions of the middle cerebral artery. J Neurosurg 13:73–80, 1956.

16. Wylie, E.J., Hein, M.F., Adams, J.E. Intracranial hemorrhage following surgical revascularization for treatment of acute strokes. J Neurosurg 21:212–215, 1964.

17. Yasargil, M.G., Krayenbühl, H.G., Jacobson, J.H. Microneurosurgical arterial reconstruction. Surgery 67:221–233, 1970.

18. Zlotnik, E.I. Thromboembolectomy of the middle cerebral artery. Case report. J Neurosurg 42:723–725, 1975.

43

Cerebral Microvascular Surgery in Completed Stroke

Michael J. Jerva and Nicola Pintozzi

The use of microvascular surgical techniques in the management of transient ischemic attacks has been well known since 1967 when the elegant work of Yasargil[4] and Donaghy[1] was published. The use of cerebral bypass procedures in patients who have sustained a completed stroke is much less established. It is a generally accepted principle, however, that revascularization procedures are considered to be ineffective when attempting to improve a sustained neurologic deficit of a moderate to severe degree.[3] Whether the procedure will be of benefit to this type of patient remains unsettled, and possibly will continue to be unsettled in light of the restrictions placed on microvascular surgeons with the anticipated international multicenter cooperative study of EC–IC bypass surgery. The current study is intended to eliminate patients who have aphasia, dementia, and loss of ambulation from being included as candidates for an extracranial–intracranial bypass procedure.

The prospective study has created somewhat of a dilemma. Experienced microvascular surgeons are available to carry out EC–IC bypass procedures. Because of the limitations of the prospective study, it will be impossible for all patients who have sustained moderate to severe sustained neurologic deficit to receive the benefits of the procedure. The critical feature is that this study and others like it will be given the credit for assessing the value of an operation which has as its rationale the improvement of cerebral blood flow to a symptomatic area of cerebral circulation.

This presentation reviews two patients who would have been excluded from having an EC–IC bypass on the basis of the prospective criteria. Although carefully selected, both of these patients have had a marked improvement in neurologic status which has been sustained over a long period of time.

Case Reports

F.M. (Hospital #160524)

A 63-year-old male experienced the sudden onset of a left homonymous hemianopia and hemiplegia on 16 April, 1976. He was treated with intensive physical therapy until 1 June, 1976, when it became apparent that no improvement had taken place. At that time he remained in a wheelchair with the previously mentioned hemiplegia and was totally dependent for all his needs upon those around him.

Cerebral angiography was performed on 2 June, 1976, revealing a right internal carotid artery occlusion. Superficial temporal–middle cerebral artery anastomosis was performed on 14 June, 1976. Ten days after surgery he returned to physical medicine for further treatment.

On follow-up examination on 8 August, 1976, the patient was living independently, did not wear a brace for his extremities but occasionally would use a cane for support. By August 1978 he was driving his own car and living a totally independent existence.

Comment. In this instance a STA–MCA bypass procedure did not seem to be advisable because of the sustained severe neurologic deficit. On the other hand, the family and the family physician on repeated occasions requested that the patient have the operative procedure in the slim hope that he would benefit from it. Because of the constant urging of all concerned, the patient underwent surgery.

P.P. (Hospital #290646)

A 66-year-old male awoke on 20 January 1978, complaining of numbness in the right calf and ankle. This progressed to a right hemiplegia, mental confusion, slurred speech, and a short attention span. In spite of intensive efforts at physical medicine and rehabilitation, the patient showed no improvement whatsoever by 20 February, 1978.

A computerized tomographic brain examination revealed two left cerebral hemisphere infarctions, one along the anterior margin of the frontal lobe and the other medially along the parietal lobe. Cerebral angiography revealed complete occlusion of the left callosomarginal artery, diffuse cerebrovascular arteriosclerosis, and stenosis of the middle cerebral complex. A superficial temporal–middle cerebral artery anastomosis was performed on 28 February, 1978.

This patient returned to physical medicine and rehabilitation on 7 March, 1978, and was discharged on 21 April, 1978, walking independently and performing independent activities of daily living.

Comment. The rationale behind this procedure was exactly the same as that in the previous patient. He had not improved at all in a sustained period of time. The family and the family physician urged the operation be performed since it was apparent to them that he

would remain a total burden upon his family and society.

Discussion

The fundamental indication for EC–IC bypass procedures is disabling transient ischemic cerebral attacks which cannot be adequately controlled by medical management.[2] There are other goals for the bypass which might also be considered. Whether or not life can actually be prolonged as a result of this procedure is undetermined. Improvement in the survival rate in patients with stenosis or occlusion of the major cerebral arteries seems to be an acceptable goal. Severe disease of the cerebral vessels, in whom medical management alone carries a high risk, unquestionably is a more serious consideration. Repeated strokes in areas of low perfusion from diffuse cerebrovascular arteriosclerosis and in whom medical management with anticoagulation or platelet suppression therapy is of no benefit may derive stabilization of their condition with an EC–IC bypass. Maintaining a low operative mortality and a high graft patency rate should always be considered essential.

Excluded from consideration of EC–IC bypass would be those patients who have totally inoperable cerebral vessels or severe complicating diseases such as metastatic carcinoma, severe hypertension, and so on.

While the above seem to be acceptable medical goals for cerebral bypass procedures, there are also social goals which should be taken into consideration. Patients should be returned to productive life so that they may resume their previous occupations or in some way support their families or themselves. Therefore, a social spin-off of a cerebral bypass procedure is the dignity of an independent life-style.

Assessing the therapeutic value of an operative procedure can be difficult. Clinical experience is an acceptable method. Relief of the signs and symptoms is a reasonable approach to evaluating an operation. Unfortunately, all of these techniques require the analysis through the "retrospectroscope." For this reason, a study should take into consideration the retrospective analysis of patients and their response, follow-up evaluations at repeated intervals, and a combined effort among neurologists and neurologic surgeons to determine the efficacy of the EC–IC procedure. Different treatment modalities must be considered to expand the study of transient ischemic cerebral attacks. It is indeed possible that more rather than fewer patients will benefit from surgical operations of this sort.

The objectives of this study should be to delay the recurrence of transient ischemic attacks or multiple strokes, to prolong the disease-free intervals, and ultimately to improve the survival rate. It is important to recall that cerebrovascular arteriosclerosis is an incurable disease.

No matter what the response, certain considerations must be made. The disease-host relationship is established at the onset of the disease and has a significant bearing on its natural history. Since cerebrovascular arteriosclerosis itself is an incurable disease, all treatments are palliative in the sense that they are trying to control the march of the disease process. Lastly, patients with cerebral atherothrombotic disease may be living for an extended period of time asymptomatically with the incurable disease. Interruption of this symbiotic relationship may be inadvisable. All claims which are made should be carefully analyzed to take these matters into consideration.

Summary

The objectives of cerebral bypass surgery are to obtain lasting relief from intractable transient ischemic attacks and, possibly, to improve cerebral function.

There is no certainty whatsoever whether a life will be saved or prolonged by EC–IC bypass. The quality of life should be improved, thereby lessening the burden on family and society.

Because of the nature of the involvement of family and family physician in the treatment of various diseases, it will be these individuals who will influence our approach to the treatment modality. Strict adherence to criteria may have to be abandoned from time to time.

References

1. Donaghy, R.M.P. Neurologic surgery. Surg Gynecol Obstet 134:269–271, 1972.
2. Millikan, C.H. Cerebral circulation. JAMA 239: 1313–1315, 1978.
3. Samson, D.S., Boone, S. Extracranial–intracranial (EC–IC) arterial bypass: Past performance and current concepts. Neurosurgery 3:79–86, 1978.
4. Yasargil, M.G. Anastomosis between the superficial temporal artery and a branch of the middle cerebral artery. In Microsurgery Applied to Neurosurgery, M.G. Yasargil, editor, Charles C Thomas, Springfield, 1976, pp 359–367.

44

Extra–Intracranial Anastomosis Operation Associated with Hyperbaric Oxygenation in the Treatment of Completed Stroke

K.-H. Holbach and H. Wassmann

A completed stroke (CS) is most frequently due to an occlusive vascular lesion resulting in cerebral hypoxia, ischemia, or a combination of these.[3] Whether in such poststroke states the neurologic disorder is due to reversible or irreversible neuronal alterations cannot be predicted. In case the neurons have lost their function but are still alive, it appears reasonable to assume that improving the oxygenation of the brain tissue either by increasing the oxygen concentration in the arterial blood or by increasing the cerebral blood supply may result in an improvement of the neurologic deficit.

Material and Methods

A total of 112 patients (90 males, 22 females, mean age 50.3 years) with CS was studied. These patients had persisting neurologic deficits caused by internal carotid occlusion in 99 cases and by middle cerebral artery occlusion in 13. They were considered suitable to undergo extra–intracranial arterial bypass surgery if necessary. Among these patients were 26 with mild neurologic deficit who had EC–IC surgery and 86 with severe neurologic deficit who were randomly assigned to a surgical or a medical treatment group. Each of the 112 patients underwent hyperbaric (HO) treatment before either surgical or medical treatment was performed. The average duration of time between the CS and the first HO treatment was 3 months. The HO therapy consisted of a series of 15 single sessions given daily. These were performed under spontaneous respiration of oxygen at a pressure of 1.5 atm and a period of exposure of 40 min.

Neurologic and EEG analytic examinations were carried out on each patient before beginning HO treatment, during its course, and at the conclusion of the treatment. EEGs also were recorded and analyzed from the hyperbaric chamber before the pressure phase under spontaneous respiration of air, during the respiration of air and subsequently of oxygen at 1.5 atm and 15 min after the change from oxygen to air respiration at normal ambient pressure (1.0 atm). Long-term follow-up neurologic and EEG analytic assessment was done in all patients during a period ranging from $1/2$ to $3\frac{1}{2}$ years. The EEG analysis system previously described[2] enables us to obtain values for the local electrical brain activity in the form of electrical power equivalent (EPE).

We tried to quantify the motor deficits by applying six grades of severity (6 = normal physical strength, 5 = slight paresis, 4 = active movement of extremities against moderate resistance, 3 = active movement of extremities against gravity, 2 = active movement of extremity upon exclusion of gravity, 1 = visible contraction without any effect of mobility, 0 = paralysis) which were separately assessed in arm, hand, and leg. The aphasic disturbances by applying four grades of severity (4 = undisturbed, 3 = slight dysphasia, 2 = moderate dysphasia, 1 = severe dysphasia, 0 = total aphasia). The latter were previously determined by others.[1]

Results

First, a typical case is presented to demonstrate the procedure of this study. A 54-year-old man suddenly developed aphasia and right hemiparesis in December 1974. Before admission to our clinic in March 1975 he was under intensive medical management. At this time we found that he had a spastic right hemiparesis and motor dysphasia (Table 44-1). Angiography revealed an occlusion of the left internal carotid artery with moderate retrograde filling of the ophthalmic artery feeding some suprasylvian arteries and a stenosis of the right internal carotid artery. HO therapy was begun subsequent to angiography, i.e., after the neurologic deficit had already persisted for 3½ months.

The EEG analysis, performed immediately before and during the first HO session, showed a lower alpha- and beta-wave activity over the affected left hemisphere than over the contralateral side (Fig. 44-1). Thirty minutes after the change from breathing air to oxygen at 1.5 atm there was a bilateral increase of the alphawave activity, in particular over the left side of the brain, and also a minor increase of the betawave activity. At the conclusion of this HO

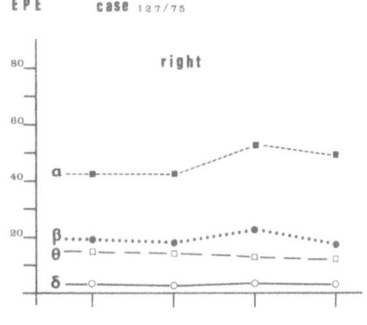

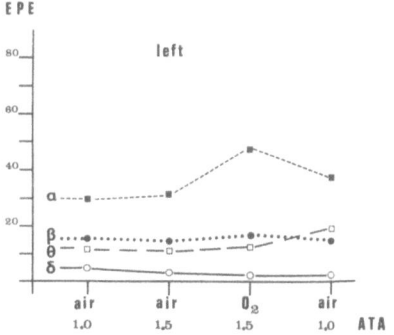

Fig. 44-1. EEG analyses before and during hyperbaric oxygenation session. EPE = electrical power equivalent value. ATA = atmospheres absolute.

session, i.e., after the change from breathing oxygen to air at 1.0 atm (normal ambient pressure), the improvement of the EEG receded almost completely. After the conclusion of the HO therapy consisting of a series of 15 single sessions, there was a considerable increase of

Table 44-1. Changes in neurologic findings: Neurologic follow-up

	Right extremities				Left extremities		
	Hand	Arm	Leg	Speech	Hand	Arm	Leg
December 1974: Completed stroke on left							
March 1975 Pre HO	2	3	4	2	6	6	6
Post HO	3	3	4	3	6	6	6
6 weeks post EC–IC	4	4	5	3	6	6	6
6 months post EC–IC	4	4	5	3	6	6	6
December 1975: Completed stroke on right							
January 1976 Pre HO	4	4	5	2	0	0	2
Post HO	4	4	5	2	2	2	3
6 weeks post EC–IC	4	4	5	3	3	3	4
6 months post EC–IC	4	4	5	3	3	3	4
February 1978	4	4	5	3	3	4	4
June 1978	4	4	5	3	3	4	4

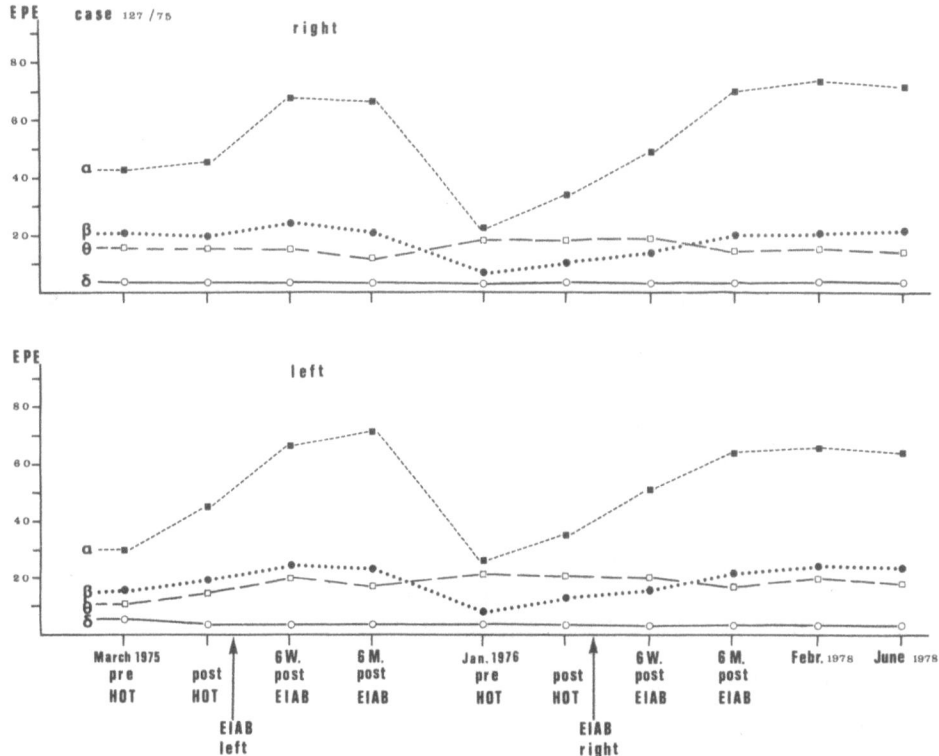

Fig. 44-2. Follow-up EEG analyses. EPE = electrical power equivalent values.

the alpha-wave activity over the left affected hemisphere (Fig. 44-2). At this time, the neurologic examination revealed an increase of motor function in the right hand and an improvement of the speech disorder.

Subsequently EC–IC surgery was carried out on the left side. Two days after the operation angiography revealed a patent anastomosis irrigating most of the middle cerebral territory.

EEG analyses performed 6 weeks and 6 months following operation showed a distinct increase of the alpha-wave activity over the affected left side as well as over the contralateral side of the brain. Also, the beta- and frequent theta-wave activity showed slight increases. At the same time, the neurologic examination revealed further recovery of the right hemiparesis.

After this satisfactory clinical course we suggested the removal of the stenosis in the right internal carotid artery. The patient, however, did not agree to this surgical procedure.

The postoperative neurologic status per-

sisted until December 1975. At this time, the patient abruptly developed a left hemiplegia and a renewed speech disorder. One month later he was admitted to our clinic demonstrating only little change in the severe left neurologic deficit. Angiography revealed an occlusion of the right internal carotid artery.

Follow-up EEG analyses indicated a distinct bilateral reduction of the alpha- and beta-wave activity. This was more pronounced over the right—at this time the mainly affected hemisphere—than over the contralateral side, which was perfused by the bypass.

Again HO therapy was given. At the conclusion of this treatment, i.e., after 15 sessions, we found an improvement of the left neurologic deficit and a bilateral increase of the alpha- and beta-wave activity. Subsequently a right EC–IC bypass was carried out. Following operation the speech disorder, the impaired motor functions, and the reduced mental activity improved. Finally the patient became able to walk on his own and to take care of himself. The postoperative follow-up EEG analyses showed further improvement which was maintained.

The last postoperative angiography, done 3½ years after the left and 2½ years after the right EC–IC surgery, revealed that the left bypass was filling the territory of the left middle cerebral artery and that the right bypass was irrigating the complete right hemisphere and also the territory of the left anterior cerebral artery, i.e., both cerebral hemispheres of this patients were completely perfused by the extra–intracranial anastomoses (Fig. 44-3).

All in all, we treated and observed 112 patients with CS and obtained the following results (Table 44-2).

Under the respiration of oxygen at 1.5 atm, 84% of the patients with mild neurologic deficit, 55% of the surgically treated patients, and 47% of the medically treated patients with severe neurologic deficit showed improvement in the EEG.

After the conclusion of the HO therapy, i.e., after a series of 15 single sessions, EEG analysis and neurologic examinations revealed improvements in 67% of the patients with mild neurologic deficit in both parameters, in the surgically treated group of patients with severe neurologic deficit, 58% in EEG and 56% in neurologic status, and in the corresponding

medically treated group, 59% in EEG and 55% in neurologic status.

The long-term follow-up examinations revealed an improvement of the patients with mild neurologic deficits, 83% in EEG and 87% in neurologic status. An improvement of the surgically treated patients with severe neurologic deficit was seen in 61% in EEG and in 59% in neurologic status and in the corresponding group of the medically treated patients in 30% in both parameters.

While the percentage of improved patients with severe neurologic deficits was significantly higher in the surgically treated group, the percentage of unimproved patients and deaths was significantly higher in the medically treated group.

During the long-term postoperative follow-up we found that the percentage of improved patients with mild neurologic deficit was significantly higher than the percentage of improved patients with severe neurologic deficit.

Furthermore, we have assessed the relationship between the effects of HO and EC–IC surgery on impaired neurologic functions:

1) Changes in EEG recorded under the respiration of oxygen at 1.5 atm corresponded to those seen after EC–IC surgery in 95% of the patients with mild neurologic deficit and in

Table 44-2. Results of HO and EC–IC bypass on EEG and neurologic status in complete stroke (CS) with mild and severe neurologic deficit

		Under O₂ respiration at 1.5 atm	After conclusion of HO therapy		Follow-up results after ½ to 3½ yr	
		EEG	EEG	N S	EEG	N S
C S	Improved	84%	67%	67%	83%	87%
Mild N D	Unchanged	16%	33%	33%	13%	9%
(N = 26 pat.)	Worsened	—	—	—	4%	4%
	Died	—	—	—	—	—
C S	Improved	55%	58%	56%	61%	59%
Severe N D	Unchanged	45%	42%	44%	33%	35%
With EC–IC	Worsened	—	—	—	4%	4%
(N = 46 pat.)	Died	—	—	—	2%	2%
C S	Improved	47%	59%	55%	30%	30%
Severe N D	Unchanged	53%	41%	45%	30%	28%
Without surgery	Worsened	—	—	—	23%	25%
(N = 40 pat.)	Died	—	—	—	17%	17%

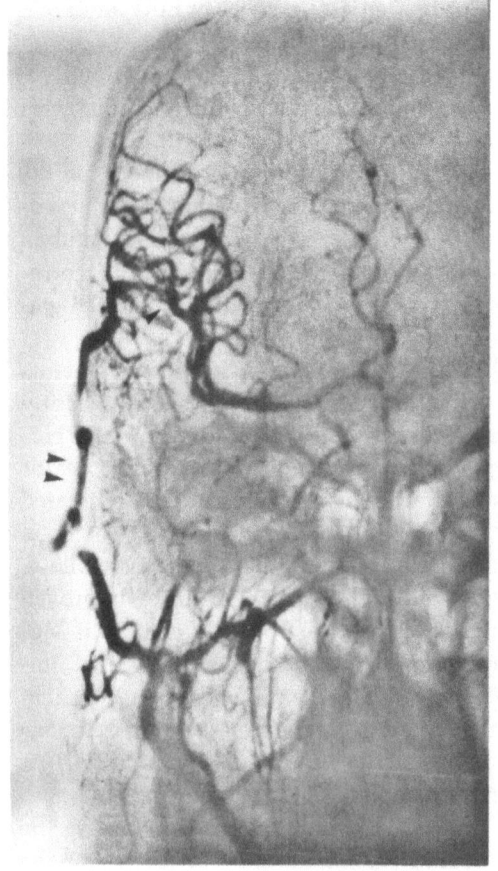

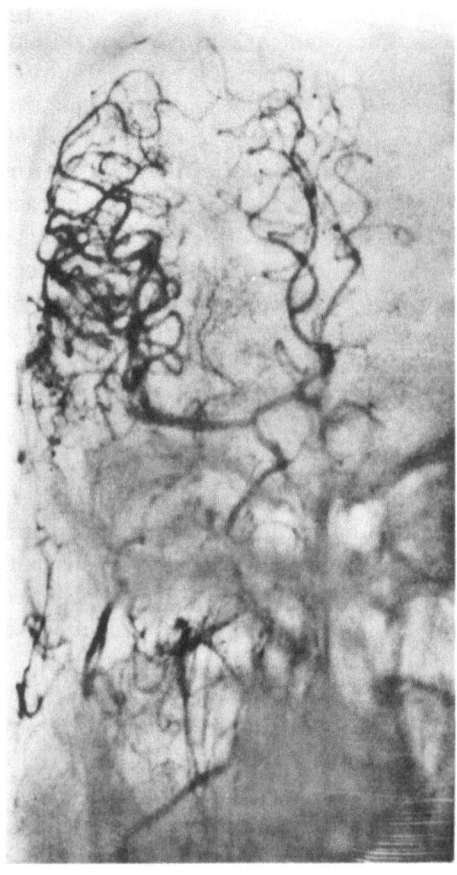

A

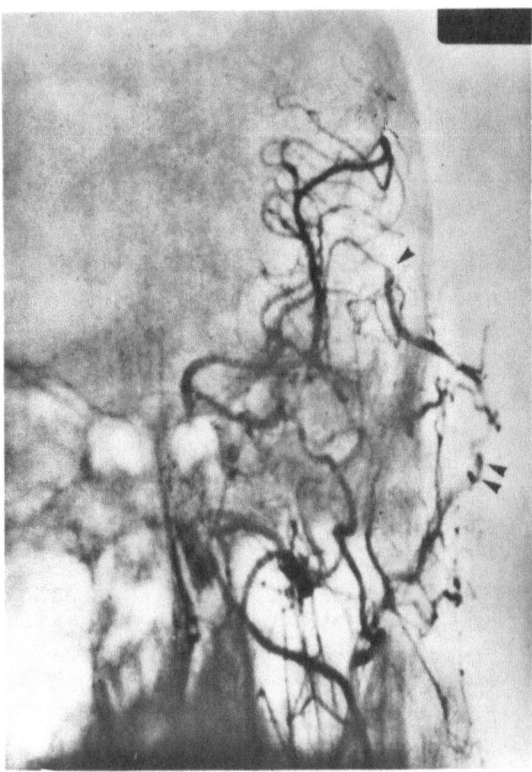

B

Fig. 44-3. Postoperative right and left carotid angiography.

87% of the patients with severe neurologic deficit.

2) Changes in EEG registered after the conclusion of the HO therapy corresponded to those seen after EC–IC surgery in 92% of the patients with mild and in 94% of the patients with severe neurologic deficit.

3) Changes in neurologic status found after the conclusion of the HO therapy corresponded to those observed after EC–IC surgery in 83% of the patients with mild and in 91% of the patients with severe neurologic deficit.

Consequently, practically all the patients with a favorable electroencephalographic and/or neurologic response to HO show a positive response to EC–IC surgery, while the patients where HO treatment is considered to be ineffective show no or little change in impaired neuronal functions subsequent to EC–IC surgery.

These findings made in complete stroke patients indicate:

1) HO treatment can improve hypoxic ischemic alterations of the brain.

2) Subsequent EC–IC surgery can result in additional improvement of neurologic deficit and in maintaining the level of improved neuronal function.

3) The evaluation of the effect of HO treatment on hypoxic ischemic alterations of the brain, particularly by EEG interval-amplitude analysis, can be helpful in differentiating between reversible and irreversible poststroke changes. Consequently, response to HO treatment may be used as a criterion for the prognosis of the cerebrovascular lesion and also for selection of patients for EC–IC surgery.

References

1. Herrschaft, H., Kunze, U. Relationship between rCBF-changes and restitution of neurological and electroencephalographic disturbances in patients with focal ischemia. In Proceedings of the 8th International Salzburg Conference on Cerebral Vascular Disease, J.S. Meyer, H. Lechner, and M. Reivich, editors, Excerpta Medica, Amsterdam-Oxford, 1977, pp 88–94.
2. Holbach, K.-H., Wassmann, H., Hohelüchter, K.L. Reversibility of the chronic post-stroke state. Stroke 7:296–300, 1976.
3. Ingvar, D.H. The pathophysiology of stroke related to findings in EEG and to measurements of regional cerebral blood flow. In Stroke, A. Engel, and T. Larsson, editors, Thule Int Sympos, Nordiska Bokhandelns Förlag, Stockholm, 1967.

45

Extra–Intracranial Arterial Bypass Surgery in Patients with Bilateral Internal Carotid Artery Occlusions

V. Olteanu-Nerbe, P. Schmiedek, O. Gratzl, and F. Marguth

Immediate mortality[6, 8, 9] and morbidity[2, 4] from cerebral infarction following internal carotid artery occlusion (ICAO) are known to be high. The natural history, however, is extremely variable,[3, 4, 8, 12] depending among other things on the availability of collateral circulation to the ischemic carotid system.[7] Since endarterectomy of chronic carotid occlusions is not feasible,[3] surgical therapy of carotid thrombosis consists in reestablishing the circulation by an extra–intracranial arterial bypass.[1, 13] Yasargil operated upon the first patient presenting bilateral internal carotid artery occlusions (ICAOs) with additional thrombosis of one vertebral artery and reestablished the carotid circulation by using a superficial temporal artery–middle cerebral artery anastomosis (STA–MCA anastomosis).[1, 13]

The incidence of bilateral ICAOs in several series reported varies from 1.5 to 2.5%.[11] In our total series of 250 operated cases, however, it was 4.5%.

Continuing our previous studies,[5, 10] it is the purpose of this report to evaluate the long-term results after STA–MCA bypass surgery in patients with bilateral ICAOs.

Clinical Material

Between February 1973 and July 1977 a group of 12 consecutive patients with angiographically proven bilateral internal carotid artery oc-clusions were treated by STA–MCA anastomosis. There were 10 males and 2 females, ranging in age from 39 to 66 years. The mean age was 50.8 years.

Nine patients (Table 45-1) had a history of bilateral symptoms of cerebral ischemia, whereas three patients had only unilateral symptoms. From the group with unilateral symptoms, two had a history of transient ischemic attacks (TIAs), one of prolonged reversible ischemic neurologic deficits (PRINDs) and one of mild completed stroke (CS). From those cases with bilateral cerebral ischemia, two had a history of bilateral TIAs and six patients had completed stroke (CS) of one hemisphere and an additional history of contralateral TIAs. One patient had a bilateral mild completed stroke (CS).

Two patients had an additional history of amaurosis fugax (Table 45-2) and another two of vertebral-basilar transient ischemic attacks. Seizures were reported in one patient. Finally, in one case mild dementia was noted.

Methods

Four-vessel angiography was performed before surgery in all cases. In addition to bilateral ICAOs, the following angiographic findings were demonstrated: external carotid artery stenosis in one case and a stenotic lesion within the vertebral-basilar system in four cases.

Table 45-1. Clinical presentation

Type of CVD	No. cases
Unilateral	3
TIAs	1
PRIND	1
CS (mild)	1
Bilateral	9
TIAs	1
TIAs and PRIND	1
TIAs and CS (mild)	5
TIAs and CS (severe)	1
CS (mild)	1

Table 45-2. Symptoms related to numbers of brain hemispheres

Clinical symptoms	No.*
Transient ischemic attacks (TIAs)	
Retinal	2
Cerebral	9
Vertebral-basilar	2
Prolonged reversible ischemic neurologic deficit (PRIND)	2
Completed stroke (CS)	
Mild or moderate neurologic deficit	7
Severe neurologic deficit	1
Seizures	1
Dementia	1

*Related to number of brain hemispheres.

Table 45-3. Computer tomographic findings

Computerized tomography	No. cases
Brain infarct	9
Unilateral	7
Middle cerebral artery territory	4
Middle and anterior cerebral artery territory	2
Middle and posterior cerebral artery territory	1
Bilateral	2
Middle cerebral artery territory	1
Middle and anterior cerebral artery territory	1
Brain atrophy	6

Preoperative computer tomographic (CT) studies (Table 45-3) were performed in ten cases. Unilateral cerebral infarction was appar-ent in seven cases, bilateral infarction in two. Infarction areas were mostly seen within the middle cerebral artery territory; in addition, however, they were found within the anterior and posterior cerebral artery distribution.

Brain atrophy of varying degree was detected in six patients (one case shown in Fig. 45-1). Bilateral STA–MCA anastomosis was performed in eight patients. A unilateral STA–MCA bypass was performed in those three cases with one-sided symptoms and in one case with bilateral symptoms who, however, had a completed stroke (CS) of one hemisphere.

Results

There was no operative morbidity or mortality. One patient, however, died during the early postoperative period from acute septicemia. Graft patency rate, as evaluated by angiography and/or Doppler sonographic studies, was 100%.

None of those cases with preoperative carotid TIAs suffered any further TIAs (Table 45-4). Vertebral-basilar TIAs disappeared in one patient; in this case bilateral follow-up angiography demonstrated an excellent filling of the MCA tree, including the right anterior cerebral artery via the superficial temporal arteries (Fig. 45-2). In patients who exhibited preoperative amaurosis fugax no further attacks occurred during the follow-up period.

Both patients with preoperative PRINDs became asymptomatic following bypass surgery (Table 45-4). In the group of eight patients with mild completed stroke (CS) there was an improvement of neurologic deficit in seven cases (Table 45-4). In one case, however, the improvement was minimal and additionally

Table 45-4. Clinical results

Type of CVD	No.	Asymptomatic	Improved	Death
TIAs	10	10		
PRIND	2	2		
CS	8		7	1*

*Death on ninth postoperative day of acute septicemia.

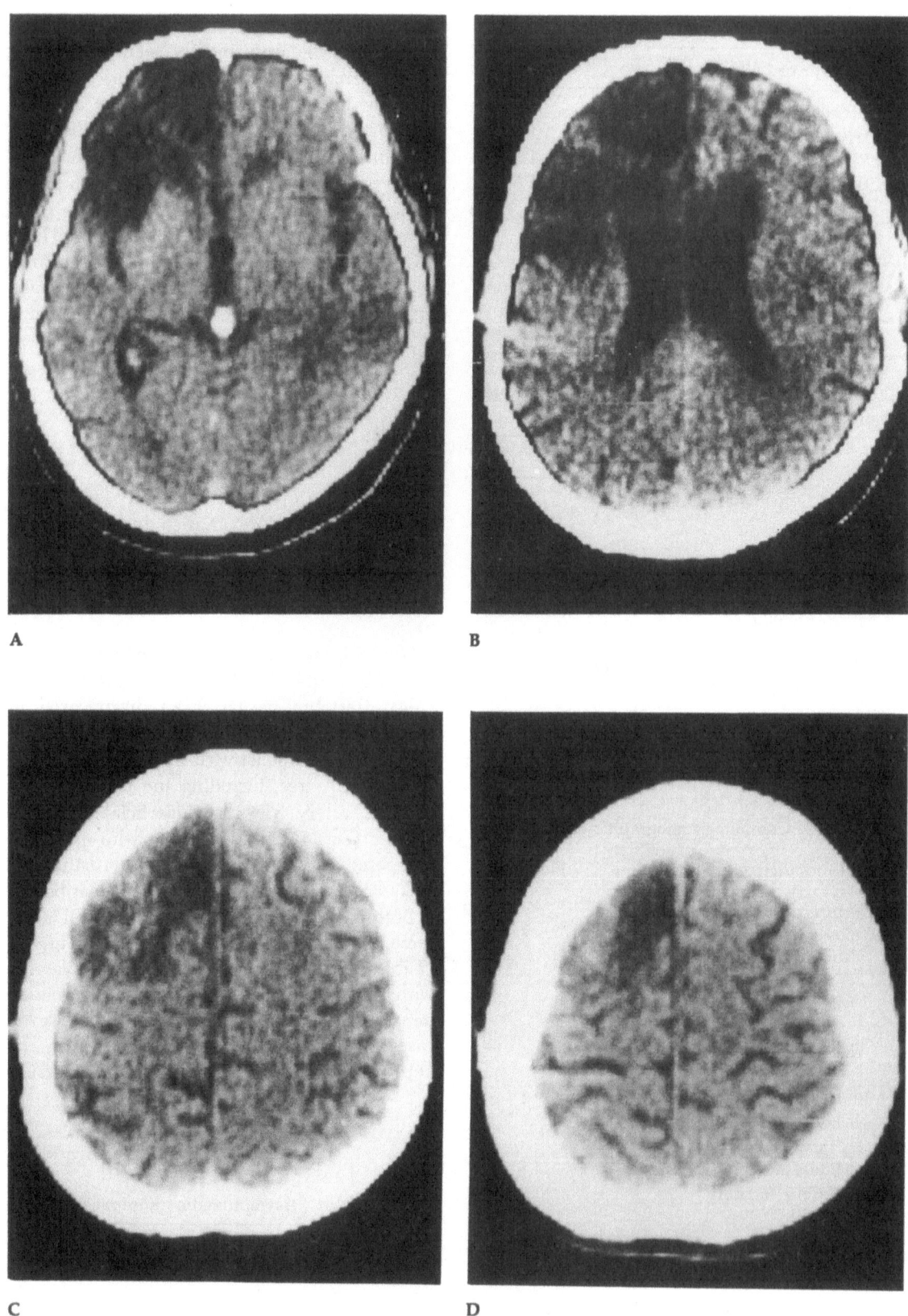

A

B

C

D

Fig. 45-1. CT in a 57-year-old man showing generalized brain atrophy.

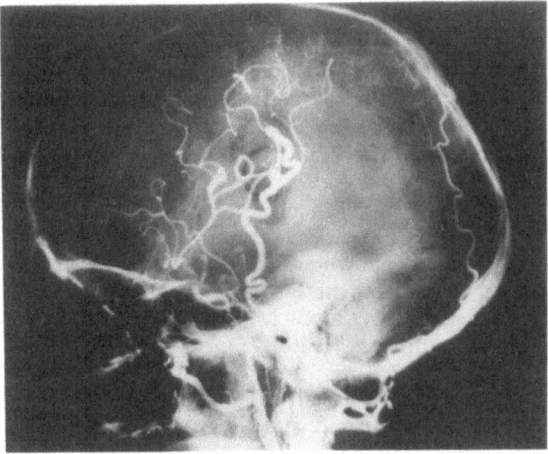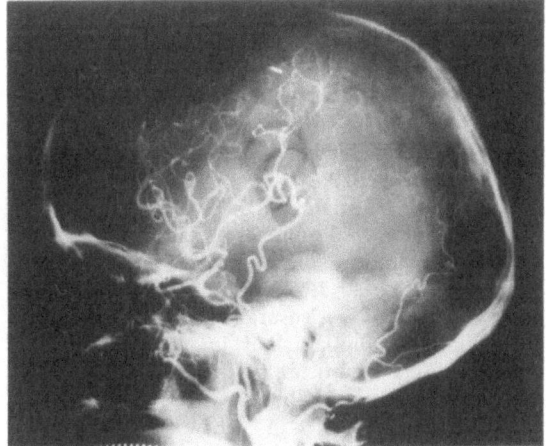

Fig. 45-2. Postoperative angiograms 1 year after bilateral EC–IC bypass in a 46-year-old patient with carotid and vertebral-basilar TIAs. Excellent filling bypasses.

mental disturbance remained unchanged. No occurrence of new strokes during the follow-up period was noted, either in the bilaterally or in the unilaterally operated patients.

Discussion

Our material represents a biased series of patients who, because of a sufficient natural collateral circulation, remained alive after bilateral occlusion of the internal carotid arteries (ICAs). The natural collateral blood supply obviously was not sufficient to prevent permanent neurologic deficits which were found in 75% of our cases, while the remaining 25% had transient symptoms of carotid and/or vertebral-basilar insufficiency. Moreover, in 50% of cases generalized brain atrophy, probably a result of chronic cerebral ischemia, could be detected by CT studies.

Long-term follow-up angiographic studies demonstrated in all performed anastomoses an excellent filling of the middle cerebral artery tree via the superficial temporal arteries. As a result of the improvement of the cerebral circulation 90% of patients had a clinical outcome judged to be good or excellent, without occurrence of any further TIAs or improvement of mild neurologic deficits.

Postoperative improvement of hemodynamics within the circle of Willis may even result

in normalization of those vertebral-basilar TIAs, which are considered to be caused by a carotid steal phenomenon.

Clinical and CT follow-up studies revealed also that reappearance of new strokes and even the continuing process of cerebral atrophy seem to be arrested.

We conclude from these data that patients with bilateral internal carotid artery occlusions (BICAOs) clinically exhibiting transient ischemic attacks (TIAs), prolonged reversible ischemic deficits (PRINDs), and/or mild completed strokes (CS) are probably some of the most ideal candidates for the STA–MCA bypass procedure.

References

1. Donaghy, R.M.P., Yasargil, M.G. Microvascular Surgery, Report of First Conference, October 6–7, 1966. C.V. Mosby, St. Louis, 1967.
2. Dyken, M.L., Klatto, E., et al. Complete occlusion of common or internal carotid arteries. Clinical significance. Arch Neurol 30:343–346, 1974.
3. Fields, W.S., Maslenicov, V., et al. Joint study of extracranial arterial occlusion. Progress report of prognosis following surgery or nonsurgical treatment for transient cerebral ischemic attacks and cervical carotid artery lesions. JAMA 211:1992–2003, 1970.
4. Fisher, C.M. The natural history of carotid occlusion. In Microneurosurgical Anastomoses

for Cerebral Ischemia, G.M. Austin, editor, Charles C Thomas, Springfield, 1976.

5. Gratzl, O., Schmiedek, P., et al. Long-term clinical results following extra–intracranial arterial bypass surgery. In Microsurgery for Stroke, P. Schmiedek, editor, Springer-Verlag, New York, 1977.

6. Grillo, P., Patterson, R.H. Occlusion of the carotid artery: Prognosis (natural history) and the possibilities of surgical revascularization. Stroke 6:17–20, 1975.

7. Krayenbühl, H., Yasargil, M.G. Der cerebrale kollaterale Blutkreislauf im angiographischen Bild. Acta Neurochir (Wien) 6:30–80, 1958.

8. Matsumoto, N., Whisnant, J.P., et al. Natural history of stroke in Rochester, Minnesota, 1955 through 1969: an extension of a previous study, 1945 through 1954. Stroke 4:20–29, 1973.

9. McDowell, F.H., Pates, J., et al. The natural history of internal carotid and vertebro-basilar artery occlusion. Neurology 11:153–157, 1961.

10. Olteanu-Nerbe, V., Schmiedek, P., et al. Late followup studies in a selected group of patients with extra–intracranial arterial bypass. In Microsurgery for Stroke, P. Schmiedek, editor, Springer-Verlag, New York, 1977.

11. Peerless, S.J., Chater, N.L., et al. Multiple-vessel occlusions in cerebrovascular disease—a further followup of the effects of microvascular bypass on the quality of life and the incidence of stroke. In Microsurgery for Stroke, P. Schmiedek, editor, Springer-Verlag, New York, 1977.

12. Whisnant, J.P., Matsumoto, N., et al. Transient cerebral ischemic attacks in a community—Rochester, Minnesota, 1955 through 1969. Mayo Clin Proc 48:194–198, 1973.

13. Yasargil, M.G. Microsurgery Applied to Neurosurgery. Georg Thieme, Stuttgart, 1969.

46

The Surgical Management of Bilateral Carotid Artery Occlusive Disease

Stephen C. Boone

Fifty percent of our patients undergoing EC–IC bypass surgery have been found to have bilateral carotid artery occlusive disease. The purpose of this paper is to analyze this small number of patients to see if a logical sequence of surgical therapy can be arrived at. A similar series of patients was reported by Moran et al.[4] It was their recommendation that in patients with a symptomatic unilateral carotid occlusion and a contralateral carotid stenosis a STA–MCA bypass should be done first on the occluded side. Then a prophylactic carotid endarterectomy could be performed on the other side. Some surgeons might disagree with this sequence by arguing that a carotid endarterectomy done first might alleviate the symptoms on the occluded side, via collateral flow through the anterior communicating artery. If this were the case, then only one operation would be necessary, i.e., the ischemic symptoms on the occluded side would be alleviated and the brain on the stenotic side would be prophylactically protected. This paper attempts to describe a logical means of making the decision as to which operations should be done and in what sequence, by estimating the amount of collateral blood flow to the hemisphere of the occluded carotid artery. The type of surgery will depend on whether the vascular lesions are accessible or inaccessible to the standard extracranial endarterectomy. Therefore, carotid artery occlusions and stenotic lesions above the angle of the jaw would be considered inaccessible. In the joint study on extracranial arterial occlusion, 39.3% of patients with symptoms of cerebrovascular ischemia were found to have inaccessible lesions.[3] The great majority of this group (84%) had a combination of accessible and inaccessible lesions.

Subjects and Methods

From 1975 to 1977, twenty-six patients have undergone EC–IC bypass. Thirteen of these were done for unilateral disease and thirteen for bilateral carotid occlusive disease. The patients with bilateral carotid artery disease can be divided into three groups: (1) bilateral carotid artery occlusion—3, (2) unilateral carotid artery occlusion and contralateral carotid stenosis—9, (3) bilateral carotid artery stenosis—1 (Table 46-1).

The management of patients in groups (1) and (3) i.e., those with bilateral carotid artery occlusions or bilateral carotid artery stenosis,

Table 46-1. Bilateral carotid artery occlusive lesions

Lesion	Number
Bilateral carotid occlusion	3
Unilateral carotid occlusion ⎫ Contralateral carotid stenosis ⎭	9
Bilateral carotid stenosis	1
Total	13

is fairly straightforward. The symptomatic side is treated first by either an endarterectomy or an EC–IC bypass, depending on its accessibility. If this first operation results in the resolution of symptoms bilaterally, then the decision may be not to do the other side. If a 50% or greater carotid stenosis is found accessible on the asymptomatic side, then an endarterectomy is performed as a prophylactic measure. However, an inaccessible lesion on the asymptomatic side is currently not felt to be an indication for an EC–IC bypass.

The difficult but challenging group of patients to manage are those with unilateral carotid occlusion and contralateral carotid stenosis because, unlike the other two groups, surgery of the symptomatic side in this group is not always done first. The evaluation of collateral blood flow is very important in these patients. Nine of our cases exhibited this combination. Five of the patients were symptomatic on the side of the occlusion while only one was symptomatic on the stenotic side. Three patients were symptomatic on both sides. The key questions in the surgical management of these cases are: (1) What surgical procedures should be done? (2) Which side should be done first? (3) Is it necessary to operate on both sides? If the patient is symptomatic only on the side of the stenotic lesion, then only this side should be operated on. If the patient is symptomatic on the occluded side, then adequacy of collateral flow to the occluded side helps determine the side to be done first.

If there is good collateral flow to the occluded side, we have chosen to perform an endarterectomy on the stenotic side if it is an accessible lesion below the angle of the jaw. The collateral flow is determined angiographically and in the vascular laboratory using the OPG-Gee. The presence of a well-functioning anterior communicating artery angiographically suggests that a carotid endarterectomy will increase the flow to both hemispheres. The OPG-Gee basically measures the stump pressure of the occluded internal carotid artery. If the pressure is greater than 60 mm Hg on the occluded side, it is felt that collateral flow is adequate and that an endarterectomy on the stenotic side would further increase flow.

If the collateral flow is poor as witnessed by nonfunctioning anterior communicating artery or by a stump pressure of less than 60 mm Hg as measured by the OPG-Gee, it is felt that the hemisphere on the side of the occluded carotid is at an increased risk of infarction during the endarterectomy. For this reason, it is proposed to perform an EC–IC first on the occluded side.

It may not be necessary to operate on both sides. In cases with good collateral to the occluded side, a carotid endarterectomy on the stenotic side may prevent any further TIAs. If symptoms persist on the occluded side, after the endarterectomy, however, then an EC–IC bypass will be needed on the occluded side.

Three patients in this group of unilateral carotid occlusion and contralateral carotid stenosis will be presented who required three different operative approaches. The first is symptomatic on the stenotic side. The second is symptomatic on the occluded side, but has good collateral flow to that side. The third is also symptomatic on the occluded side but has poor collateral flow to that side. It is hoped that the discussion of these patients will illustrate our method of surgical management.

Case Reports

Case 1

This patient is the only one who was symptomatic on the stenotic side. She is a 47-year-old right-handed white female with an 8-month history of TIAs involving the left face and arm. In the week prior to admission these TIAs had been occurring with increasing frequency and severity. Past history revealed a one-day episode of dysphasia ten years previously. During arteriography, she developed a left-sided paresis, although she remained alert. Her blood pressure was 126/82. She was not a smoker. Laboratory evaluation revealed a type IV hyperlipidemia. Her arch study revealed an occlusion of the left internal carotid. A right lateral carotid arteriogram revealed stenosis of approximately 80% of the right internal carotid artery in the siphon. A right AP common carotid arteriogram showed the stenotic siphon lesion and the absence of crossover via the anterior communicating artery (Fig. 46-1). A left

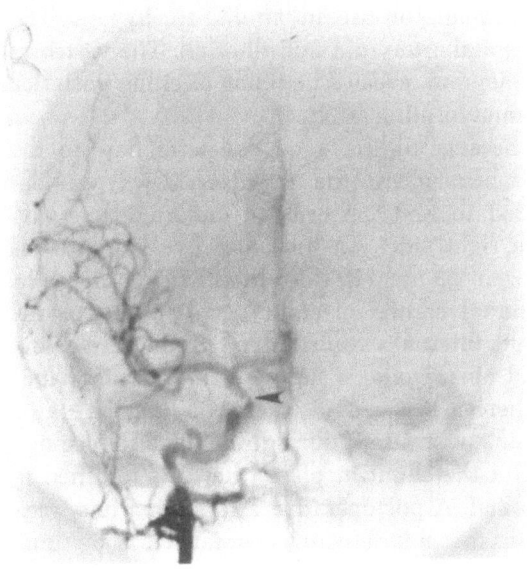

Fig. 46-1. Case 1. Right carotid arteriogram showing an 80% stenosis of the carotid artery in the siphon and the absence of anterior communicating artery collateral flow to the occluded left side.

lateral common carotid arteriogram revealed an occlusion of the left carotid artery in the siphon with marked narrowing proximal to the occlusion (Fig. 46-2). The left vertebral arteriograms revealed excellent collateral filling of the anterior circulation, via both posterior communicating arteries.

It was decided to perform only a right STA–MCA bypass since only her right hemisphere was symptomatic. The operation was done as an emergency since her TIAs were becoming more frequent and more severe. Her postoperative right carotid arteriogram confirms the patency of the anastomosis, with the right STA increasing in size from 1.2 mm to 1.8 mm (Fig. 46-3). The patient has been asymptomatic since surgery. Her left hemiparesis cleared within 24 hours. No surgery was contemplated for the left side since it was asymptomatic and angiographically she had excellent collateral to the left hemisphere.

Case 2

This patient had good collateral flow to the symptomatic occluded side. He is a 58-year-old right-handed white male, who had one 2-hour

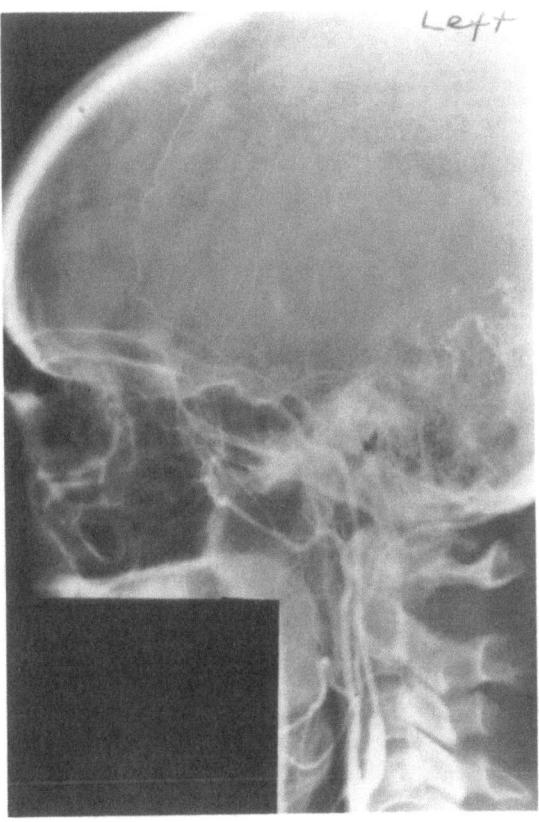

Fig. 46-2. Case 1. Left carotid arteriogram showing occlusion of the left carotid artery in the siphon with marked proximal narrowing.

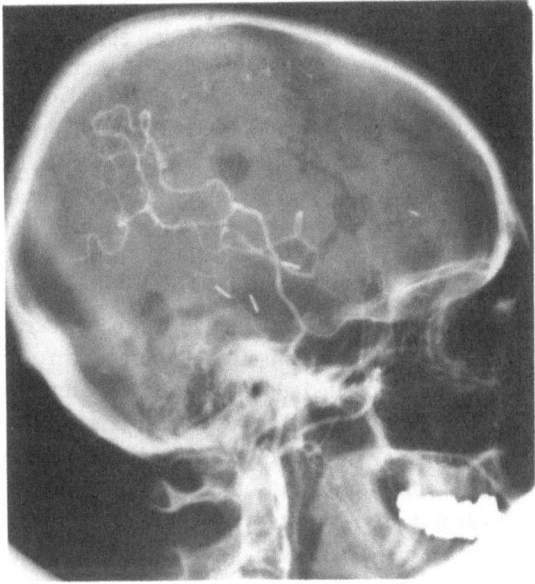

Fig. 46-3. Case 1. Postoperative right carotid arteriogram confirming patency of the right STA–MCA bypass.

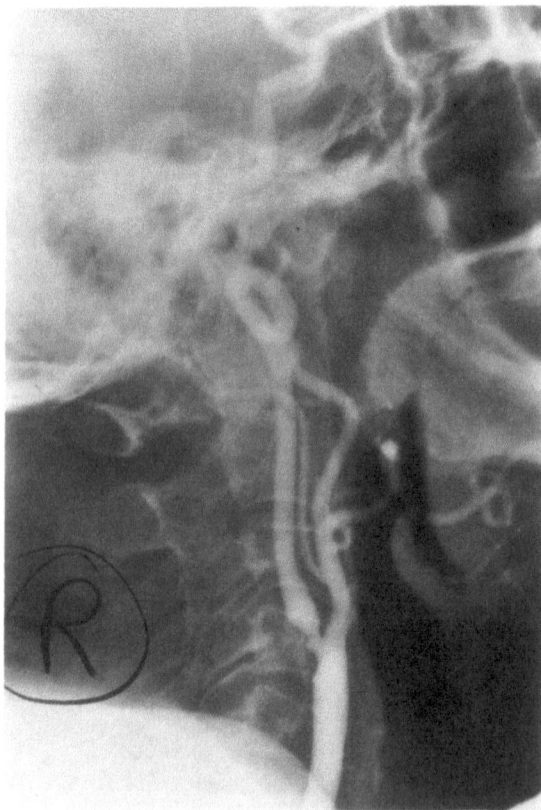

Fig. 46-4. Case 2. Right carotid arteriogram revealing an 80% stenosis of the origin of the internal carotid artery.

too small for use in an EC–IC bypass. The occipital artery did not fill at all. The vertebral angiogram revealed no filling of either posterior communicating arteries.

Because of the good collateral flow to the left hemisphere (the occluded side), it was decided to first perform an endarterectomy on the right side. An intraoperative stump pressure of 25 mm Hg was obtained from the right internal carotid artery. Test occlusion of the right internal carotid artery produced slowing and then voltage suppression in both hemispheres. Because of these findings, a Javid shunt was used during the endarterectomy. With the shunt in place, the EEG returned to normal. A postoperative arteriogram one week after the endarterectomy revealed it to be functioning well.

Although improved, the patient was still symptomatic with intermittent episodes of lightheadedness and near loss of consciousness. It was, therefore, decided to try to further increase the flow to the left hemisphere by performing an EC–IC bypass. A left external carotid endarterectomy was performed in hopes of

episode of aphasia and three brief episodes of loss of consciousness. He was a heavy smoker. Neurologic examination revealed a blood pressure of 102/60 and a harsh right carotid bruit. His laboratory values were normal except for increased platelet aggregation. His dynamic brain scan revealed decreased flow on the left side. The OPG-Gee revealed a left stump pressure of 80 mm Hg. His arch study suggested a right carotid stenosis and a left internal carotid artery occlusion. His right common carotid arteriogram revealed a significant 80% stenosis at the origin of the internal carotid (Fig. 46-4). The right AP view demonstrated a functional anterior communicating artery (Fig. 46-5). His left carotid arteriogram revealed a complete occlusion of the left internal carotid artery at its origin and an approximate 30 to 40% narrowing point of the left external carotid artery (Fig. 46-6). The left superficial temporal artery was found to be 0.7 mm in diameter and thus

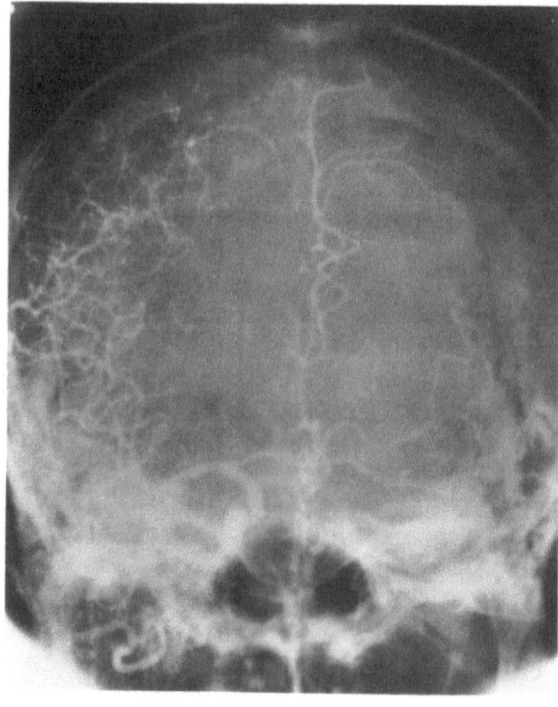

Fig. 46-5. Case 2. Right carotid arteriogram revealing some crossover to the left hemisphere by the anterior communicating artery.

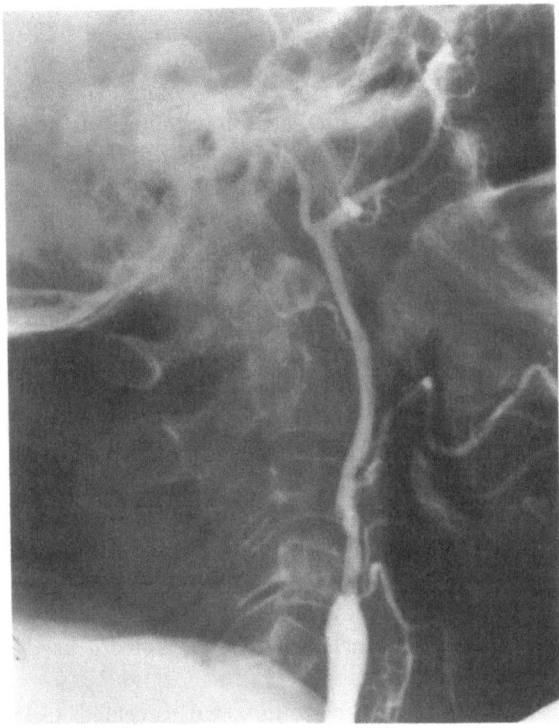

Fig. 46-6. Case 2. Left carotid arteriogram showing complete occlusion of the internal carotid artery and a 30 to 40% stenosis of the external carotid artery.

increasing the size of the left STA. The arteriogram after this procedure revealed a good result, with the plaque being gone and the occipital artery now filling. The left superficial temporal artery was also seen to have increased in size from 0.7 mm to 1.2 mm. With this increase in size of the STA, the bypass was performed. The postoperative angiogram revealed excellent function of the bypass (Fig. 46-7). The diameter of the superficial temporal artery had increased from 1.2 mm to 2.4 mm. Clinically, the patient has had no further ischemic attacks following completion of these three surgical procedures.

In summarizing this case, it was decided to do the right carotid endarterectomy first for the following reasons: (1) The presence of a functional anterior communicating artery and a left carotid stump pressure of 80 mm Hg suggested that collateral to the left hemisphere was good. (2) It was felt that the right carotid endarterectomy might increase the flow to the left hemisphere and thus stop the TIAs. Therefore,

only one surgical procedure would have been necessary. (3) It was felt that with an 80% stenosis an endarterectomy would have to be performed even though the right hemisphere was not specifically symptomatic. (4) Since the left STA was too small without performing a left external endarterectomy, it was felt unwise to proceed with these two operative procedures with an 80% stenosis on the opposite side. When the patient remained symptomatic following his right endarterectomy, it was then decided to go ahead with the left STA–MCA bypass. In order to do the bypass, a left external carotid artery endarterectomy had to be done.

Case 3

This patient had poor collateral flow to the symptomatic occluded side. He is a 49-year-old hypertensive right-handed white male who had had five bouts of right amaurosis fugax within the last 5 months. Past history revealed a 24-hour episode of left hand and face weakness in 1967. His physical examination was normal. Laboratory examinations revealed a type IV hyperlipidemia. The static and flow brain scans were normal. The CT scan suggested some atrophy in the right sylvian area. His arch study

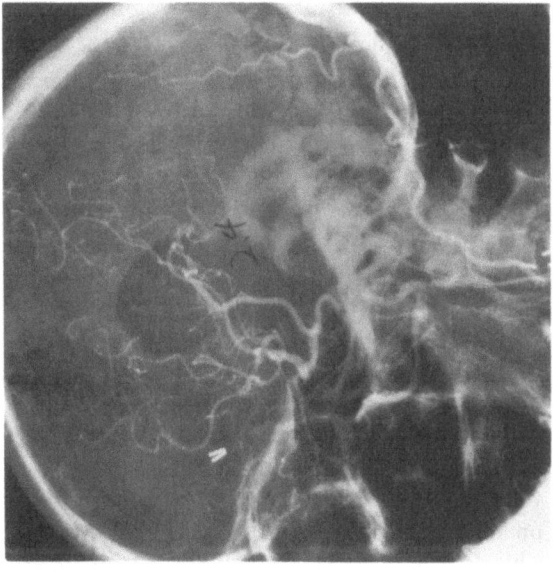

Fig. 46-7. Case 2. Postoperative left carotid arteriogram showing a well-functioning STA–MCA bypass with the STA measuring 2.4 mm in diameter.

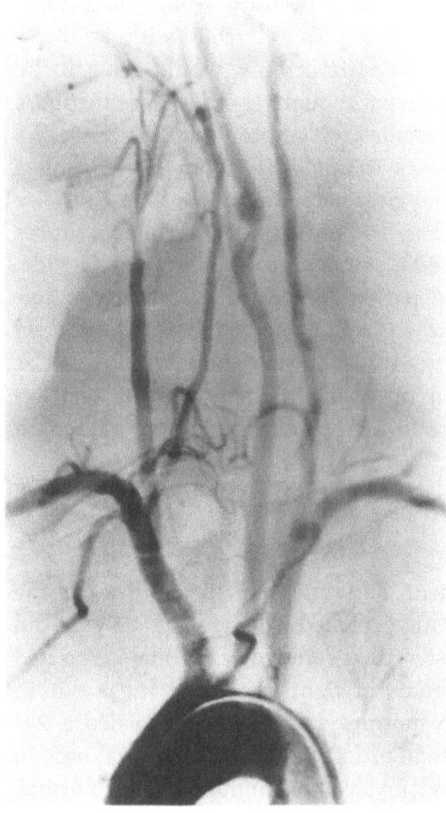

Fig. 46-8. Case 3. Arch study revealing a right internal carotid artery occlusion at its origin and a 50% stenosis of the left internal carotid artery and its origin.

It was decided that the patient should have both a right STA–MCA bypass and a left carotid endarterectomy for two reasons: (1) Both procedures would increase blood supply to the ischemic right hemisphere. (2) The left carotid stenosis was 50% and, therefore, it was felt that an endarterectomy should be done as prophylactic protection for the left hemisphere.

It was decided to do the right STA–MCA first because: (1) The right side was the symptomatic hemisphere. (2) Even though both the anterior and posterior communicating arteries were seen to function, the OPG-Gee was less than 60 mm Hg on the right, suggesting inadequate collateral flow. (3) Since the collateral flow was judged to be low it was felt that the occlusion of the left internal carotid during the endarterectomy might lead to right cerebral infarction if it was not protected by a functioning bypass. Both branches of the STA were used in the EC–IC bypass.

The postoperative angiogram revealed excellent flow through both of these branches of the superficial temporal artery with enlargement from 1.3 mm to 1.6 mm and 1.2 mm to 1.5 mm (Fig. 46-9). The postoperative course was complicated by some superficial necrosis of the wound edge which healed in 2 weeks and was probably caused by the use of both branches of the STA. Two weeks later the left

revealed a right internal carotid artery occlusion and a 50% stenosis of the left internal carotid artery at its origin (Fig. 46-8). The neck view of the right common carotid arteriogram revealed an occlusion at the origin of the internal carotid and the absence of significant disease of the external carotid artery. Cranial views of the right common carotid arteriogram revealed an excellent superficial temporal artery with a large anterior and posterior branch. No other lesions were found on complete cerebral angiography except the 50% stenosis at the origin of the left internal carotid artery. His anterior and posterior communicating arteries were both seen to function but the OPC-Gee on the occluded side was less than 60 mm Hg. This low stump pressure suggested an inadequate collateral flow to the right side even though the anterior communicating artery was patent.

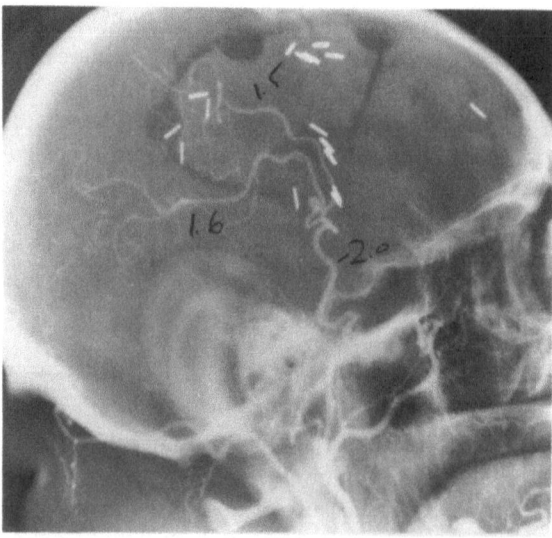

Fig. 46-9. Case 3. Postoperative right carotid arteriogram revealing excellent flow through both branches of the STA.

carotid endarterectomy was done without diffi-culty. Since the completion of these two opera-tive procedures, the patient has remained neurologically intact and has had no further TIAs.

Patient Characteristics

Table 46-2 presents the patient characteristics found in our thirteen cases. The mean age was 50. There were eight males and five females. Eleven were white and two were black. Risk factors found in these thirteen patients are pre-sented in Table 46-3. Twelve of the thirteen patients were heavy smokers. Eight had type IV hyperlipidemia, five had adult onset diabetes mellitus, and three had hypertension. The re-sults of surgery are summarized in Table 46-4. There were no deaths. There were two cases of superficial necrosis of the edge of the scalp flap and there were two RINDs postoperatively that took 4 and 7 days to clear. Ninety-four percent of the bypasses were open postoperatively and all of the endarterectomies were patent. It was felt that all patients had some clinical improve-ment. Four patients had mild improvement with cessation of the TIAs but no change in neuro-logic deficit. Nine patients had a moderate im-provement manifested by the absence of TIAs and improvement neurologically.

Table 46-2. Patients with bilateral carotid occlusive disease

Number	13
Mean age	50
Males	8
Females	5
White	11
Black	2

Table 46-3. Risk factors in patients with bilateral carotid occlusive disease

	Patients
Total	13
Heavy smoking	12
Type IV hyperlipidemia	8
Diabetes mellitus	5
Hypertension	3

Discussion

Patients with bilateral carotid occlusive disease are obviously more at risk than are those with only unilateral disease. Bilateral carotid occlu-sions can be treated surgically only by an EC–IC bypass. Patients with unilateral carotid ar-terial occlusion and contralateral stenosis can be treated surgically with an EC–IC bypass, a carotid endarterectomy, or both. Fields and Lemak[2] reported that 43% of patients in this category either died or had a stroke as the result of surgical intervention. Analysis of this high morbidity and mortality revealed that most of the deaths occurred in patients in whom opening of an occluded internal carotid had been attempted, or in patients operated on during the acute phase of a stroke. Thompson and Talkington[6] and Patterson[5] in separate series reported no increased morbidity or mor-tality when endarterectomies are performed in this group of patients. In the Walter Reed series of patients[1] with unilateral carotid arterial oc-clusion and contralateral carotid stenosis, 21 patients were having TIAs. Twenty of these 21 were relieved of their symptoms by carotid endarterectomy. When the endarterectomy does not relieve the symptoms, then an EC–IC should be performed on the occluded side. Al-though there were no deaths in the Walter Reed series, there was an 11% stroke rate. It is felt that this stroke rate could be lowered by the careful evaluation of collateral flow to the side of the occluded carotid artery. If col-

Table 46-4. Clinical results in patients with bilateral carotid occlusive disease

	Number	Percent
Mortality	0	0
Morbidity		
A. Minimal scalp necrosis	2	15
B. Postop. neurologic deficit		
1. TIA	0	0
2. RIND	2	15
3. Infarct	0	0
Patency of EC–IC	16/17	94
Patency of endarterectomy	8/8	100
Clinical improvement	13	100
A. Mild	4	30
B. Moderate	9	70

lateral flow is poor, then an EC–IC bypass should probably precede the endarterectomy. The zero percent mortality and infarct rate in the present study would support this conclusion.

References

1. Andersen, C.A., Rich, N.M., Colins, G.J., Mc-Donald, P.T., Boone, S.C. Unilateral internal carotid arterial occlusion: Special considerations. Stroke 8:699–671, 1977.

2. Fields, W.S., Lemak, N.A. Joint study of extracranial arterial occlusion. X. Internal carotid occlusion. JAMA 235:2734–2738, 1976.

3. Hass, W.K., Fields, W.S., North, R.R., Kricheff, I.I., Chase, N.E., Bauer, R.B. Joint study of extracranial arterial occlusion. JAMA 203:961–968, 1968.

4. Moran, J.M., Reichman, O.H., Baker, W.H. Staged intracranial and extracranial revascularization. Arch Surg 112:1424–1428, 1977.

5. Patterson, R. H. Risk of carotid surgery with occlusion of the contralateral carotid artery. Arch Neurol 30:188–189, 1974.

6. Thompson, J.E., Talkington, C.M. Carotid endarterectomy. Ann Surg 184:1–15, 1976.

47

Indications for Surgery in Patients with Several Cerebrovascular Lesions

L. M. Auer and F. Heppner

This study covers patients with TIA (transient ischemic attacks), PRIND (persistent reversible ischemic neurologic deficit), or minor CS (completed stroke) who were considered for EC–IC bypass surgery (extracranial–intracranial arterial bypass) and/or TEA (thrombendarterectomy). In a series of 53 patients with cerebrovascular insufficiency we found 14 suffering from more than one cerebrovascular lesion. The main point of interest was to learn more about priorities when two or more operative procedures become disputable in one patient. Another question of equal interest was the limits regarding age of patient and number of operable lesions. A problem much discussed in recent years is the value of EC–IC bypass in patients with carotid stenosis at one bifurcation and internal carotid artery (ICA) occlusion on the contralateral side (SO patients).[2, 3, 6, 7, 14, 15, 18, 20, 23, 26, 28] ICA stenosis and aneurysm in the same patient have been treated following differing priorities with varying success.[1, 16, 17, 24, 25, 27]

Selection of Patients and Diagnostic Procedures

This study covers 11 men and 3 women (Table 47-1). The mean age at the time of operation was 52 years (range 16 to 67 years). Seven patients exhibited TIAs or PRIND, and seven a completed stroke. All stroke patients had an infarcted area on CT scan (5 recent infarctions,

2 old infarctions); one patient suffered from visual disturbance and had a pituitary adenoma.

Two TIA patients also showed small infarctions in the middle cerebral artery (MCA) area; two had occipital infarction combined with visual disturbance.

Four-vessel angiography was performed in all patients: Six had ICA occlusion on one side and stenosis at the bifurcation of the other side (SO patients). Three of them have persistent neurologic deficit, three had come with TIAs.

Neurologic symptoms occurred on the occluded side in five, on the stenosed side in one. One patient had ipsilateral extra- and intracranial stenosis of an ICA and 90% stenosis of both vertebral arteries. One patient suffered ICA bifurcation stenosis on both sides. The patient with tumor of the sella region had stenosis of both his supraclinoidal portions and the left infraclinoidal portion of ICA. One patient had multiple stenoses of the intracranial ICA and the MCA trunk and arterior cerebral artery (ACA) of the right side, one had an MCA trunk stenosis. One patient had bilateral ICA occlusion. Two patients had an aneurysm of the ICA; one of them additionally had stenosis of the contralateral carotid bifurcation, the other ipsilateral ICA occlusion.

The mean follow-up period was 11 months, the range from 2 to 26 months.

For selection of patients suffering from CS we tried additionally EEG analysis and neuro-

Table 47-1. Description of 14 patients with multiple cerebrovascular lesions

Patients	Age	Neurological symptoms					Lesions							Operations					Follow-up				Follow-up time in months
		Visual defect	TIA	PRIND	CS	Asympt.	ICAS	ICAO	MCAS	MCAO	Pituit. tumor	ICA aneurysm	VAS	EC–IC	TEA	Tu	Aneurysm	PICA	Asympt.	Idem	Pejus	Melius	
M	63				R		R	L						1	2					X			4
M	61		L				L	R						1	2				X				6
M	67	X	R				L								2X				X				4
M	61	X	R				LR						LR	1	2			3	X		X		4
M	60				L		L	R						1	2					X			8
M	46				R		R	L						1	2					X			6
M	54	X			R		L					X			X					X			6
F	16				L		R		R					1								X	18
M	60		R				L	R						1	2				X				23
M	51		L				L	R						1	2				X				26
F	43	L	L					R				R		2			1		X				2
M	46		L						R					–	–					X			—
M	52		L					LR												X			—
F	53						L					R							X				12

Abbreviations: Male (M); female (F); internal carotid artery stenosis (ICAS); internal carotid artery occlusion (ICAO); middle cerebral artery stenosis (MCAS); middle cerebral artery occlusion (MCAO); vertebral artery stenosis (VAS); extracranial-intracranial arterial bypass (EC–IC); thrombendarterectomy (TEA); intracranial tumor (Tu); occipital artery–posterior inferior cerebellar artery anastomosis (PICA); patient free of symptoms (Asympt.); neurological symptoms unchanged (Idem); Deterioration (Pejus); Improvement (Melius).

logic control during hyperbaric oxygenation, as reported elsewhere.[4, 21]

Operative Procedures

In SO patients and intracranially stenosed ICA, EC–IC bypass was performed first, regardless of the side of neurologic deficit. The skin incision for bypass was made right over the STA in nine cases; in two cases a skin flap was made around the vessel. While scalp necrosis occurred in both flap patients, we have never seen necrosis since we have incised the skin along the STA. Control angiography showed all bypasses to be patent.

In patients with brain infarction, operation was not performed until 6 weeks after the stroke. CT controls were made to determine healing of an infarcted area. Nevertheless, TEA after EC–IC bypass is performed using an internal shunt. In one patient, the ICA aneurysm was clipped one week prior to TEA. The patient with bilateral carotid stenosis had both carotids operated on by TEA.

The pituitary adenoma of the patient with intracranial ICA stenosis was operated on by the transsphenoidal approach after EC–IC bypass.

In the girl with ipsilateral intracranial ICA, MCA, and ACA stenoses, an EC–IC bypass was done on this side.

Special procedures will be described in the case history.

Results

Two patients—one with MCA stenosis, the other with bilateral ICA occlusion—suffered massive infarction while waiting for the operation; one died 2 weeks later.

None of the operated patients have yet died. Patients with TIAs or PRIND are free of previous symptoms from the brain regions fed by the MCA; one case of unaffected and progressive insufficiency of posterior circulation will be described in detail in a case history. Four of the operated CS patients remained unchanged; the fifth improved markedly the day after bypass. None deteriorated neurologically, none suffered reinfarction. Some interesting cases are described and illustrated in the following:

Case 1 (F.J.)

A 61-year-old man had suffered several attacks of TIAs on the left side days before admission to the hospital. Ten years before, a PRIND had occurred. Labile hypertonus was known for many years. On admission, the patient had no neurologic deficit; CT scan showed an old small infarct in the right basal ganglia. Angiography detected ICA occlusion on the right, stenosis at the bifurcation of the left side (Fig. 47-1 A, B). As a first step, we performed EC–IC bypass on the right side, followed by TEA on the left side one week later. The patient recovered quickly, and remained free of symptoms. Control angiography 4 months later confirmed the left ICA open, the right bypass patent; the STA had enlarged to almost double its original diameter and filled the angular, posterior parietal, temporal branches and trunk of the MCA (Fig. 47-1 C, E). Six months after the operations, the patient is—objectively and subjectively—free of symptoms.

· Case 2 (L.R.)

A 60-year-old man came to the hospital a few hours after his second attack of brief right hemiparesis; the first TIA had been about 10 minutes, the next a few seconds. CT scan was normal; angiography revealed right ICA occlusion and left stenosis (Fig. 47-2 A, B). One week after EC–IC bypass on the right, TEA was performed on the left side. The patient had been free of any symptoms for 2 days after the second intervention when TIAs recurred on the right side according to left stenosis pre-

operatively. Control angiography showed the bypass to be patent, but there was again stenosis at the left bifurcation (Fig. 47-2C). TEA was repeated immediately and the patient remained free of symptoms during a follow-up period of 23 months.

Case 3 (H.J.)

A 46-year-old man wanted to be operated on for amelioration of his 2-year-old faint right hemiparesis. CT showed the typical old infarction in the region of the basal ganglia, angiography left ICA occlusion and right stenosis (Fig. 47-3 A, B). After left EC–IC we performed right TEA; the patient remained neurologically unchanged. On control angiography after 4 weeks the bypass was open, yet the right common carotid turned out to be occluded from the aortic arch onward (Fig. 47-3 C, D). Five months later the patient was neurologically still more or less unchanged, neurologic deficit improving very faintly.

Case 4 (N.W.)

A 65-year-old man with a history of hypertension and heart infarction had suffered a series of short hemiparesis attacks on the right side, one immediately prior to admission to the hospital. On admission, the patient had irregular defects of the visual field on both sides, no other neurologic defect. CT scan revealed recent bilateral occipital infarction, angiography left-sided 50% ICA stenosis at the bifurcation and 80% stenosis at the siphon as well as bilateral 90% vertebral artery stenosis about 2 cm before the origin of the basilar artery (Fig. 47-4 A–E). Since his general condition was very good, we decided to perform left EC–IC after 6 weeks, left TEA 1 week later. Three months after these two operations, no further TIAs had occurred but the visual defects were unchanged, the patient was suffering first signs of brain stem ischemia, and collateral circulation to the posterior circulation was very poor. We therefore decided, as a third step, to perform an occipital artery–posterior inferior cerebellar artery anastomosis. Although TIAs no longer occurred, the defects of the visual

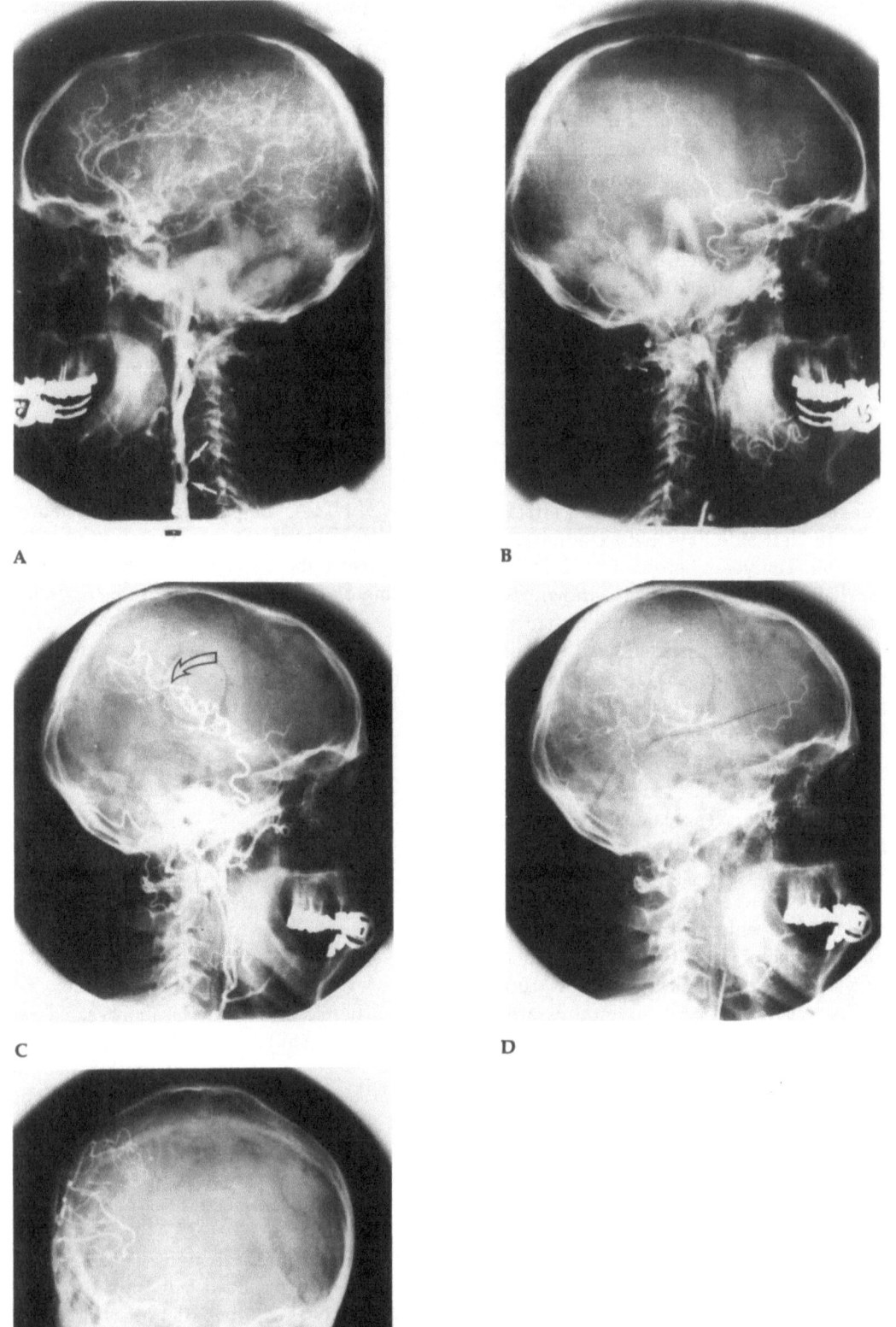

A

B

C

D

E

Fig. 47-1. Carotid angiography from a 61-year-old
man (case 1), suffering from TIAs. A. Left carotid
bifurcation stenosis. B. Right ICA occlusion, control angiography after 4 months. C–E. Markedly
enlarged STA leading to a patent anastomosis and
filling several branches of the MCA peripherally
as well as the MCA trunk retrogradely.

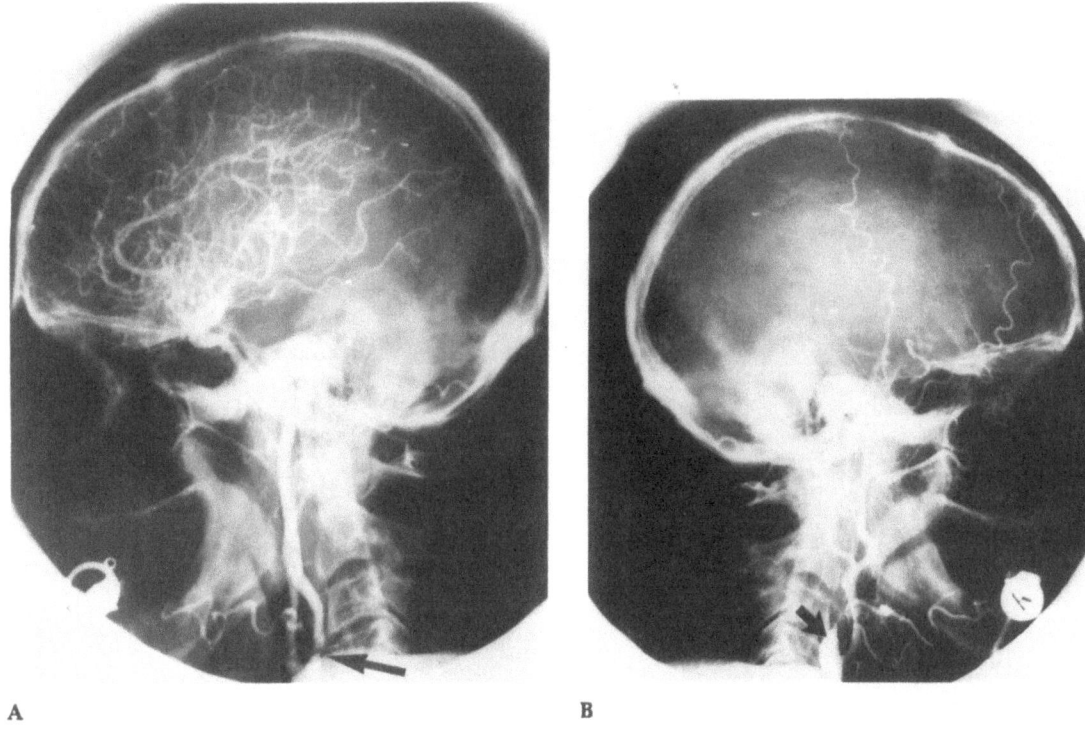

A   B

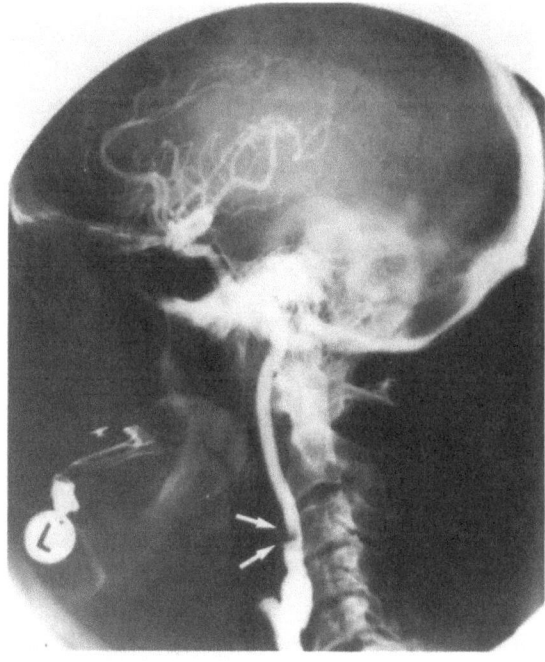

C

Fig. 47-2. Bilateral carotid angiogram of a 60-year-old man (case 2) suffering from TIAs. A. Left ICA stenosis at the bifurcation. B. Right ICA occlusion, control angiography few days after bypass and TEA with the patient suffering again from TIAs on the right side. C. The anastomosis is patent.

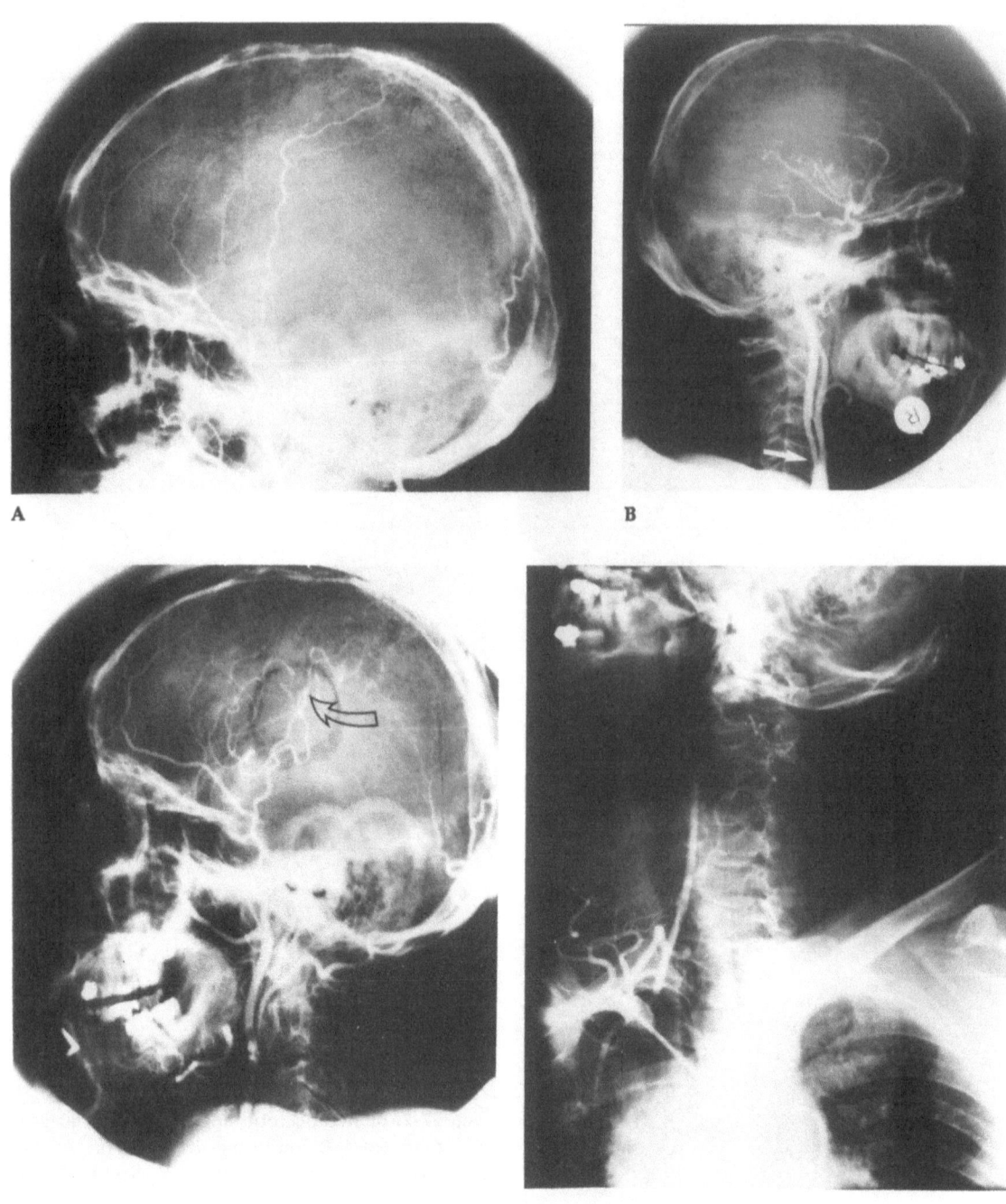

A

B

C

D

Fig. 47-3. Bilateral carotid angiogram of a 46-year-old man (case 3) with 2-year-old CS. A. Left ICA occlusion. B. Right ICA stenosis at the bifurcation, control angiography 4 weeks after bypass and TEA. C. Patent bypass on the left side. D. Common carotid artery occlusion after TEA on the right side.

field remained the same; brain stem symptoms had even progressed 3 months after the third operation, control angiography showing the progressive nature of arteriosclerosis and the patent anastomoses (Fig. 47-4 F–H).

Case 5 (W.I.)

A 43-year-old woman had been operated on for aneurysm of the right internal carotid artery (Fig. 47-5A). The intervention was complicated by longitudinal rupture of ICA distal to the aneurysm; the vessel had to be clipped. Next day, the patient had dozens of short attacks of left hemiparesis. Control angiography confirmed intracranial occlusion of the right ICA (Fig. 47-5B), the aneurysm being clipped. Symptoms turned to a PRIND on the third day; CT scan was normal. We decided to perform right EC–IC bypass when the patient could hardly move arm and fingers and had marked facial nerve palsy. Four hours after operation, she was happy to show almost normal function of her left arm and hand; facial nerve palsy was normalized the day thereafter. Control angiography showed the anastomosis to be patent (Fig. 47-5C). After a week, the patient was free of symptoms.

Discussion

The most frequent incidence of multiple cerebrovascular lesions is stenosis or occlusion of both carotid arteries. Thus, the situation of stenosis at one carotid bifurcation and occlusion of the contralateral carotid (SO patients) has been discussed in a number of recent papers; thus far, considerably differing suggestions have been made. From a joint study, Fields and Lemak[15] drew the conclusion that medical therapy showed better effects than surgical therapy. In contrast to this opinion, it has been proposed to do surgery for both lesions, namely EC–IC bypass for the occluded side and TEA at the side of stenosis; these authors suggested that the bypass be performed prior to TEA.[3] There is also an opinion between these two extremes, as published by Andersen et al.,[2] who advised doing only TEA in most SO patients irrespective of the side of neurologic symptoms and/or cerebral lesions. To this conclusion, an exception, to also do a bypass on the occluded side, should be made in patients with poor collateral circulation and those who remain symptomatic after TEA. The TEA complication rate of that study ran up to 11%: two thirds of those 11% had symptoms on the side of previous stenosis, one third on the occluded side. The TEA complication rate fits well with other communications, such as that

of Denck on 700 cases with 11% failure in patients with TIA and those free of symptoms.[9] Samson et al. reported a 29% post-TEA stroke incidence[26] in a group of patients who refused to have the bypass. Stroke incidence after TEA in 228 cases of Easton and Sherman was 14%.[12] Collins et al. reported on the incidence of stroke in 509 patients after TEA; they found postoperative stroke in 2%—all of these 10 cases, however, suffering from contralateral carotid stenosis or occlusion.[8]

Our own experience includes two cases of complication that after TEA ended up without persistent neurologic deficit. One patient became symptomatic due to the complication. The other remained unchanged; we had performed EC–IC bypass prior to TEA. The question of causalities is undoubtedly of great interest in such a case. However, it appears preferable to perform preliminary bypass in all of these cases, to remain uncertain about the pathophysiologic background but to have a lower complication rate than 11% (1 patient in our material).

A further argument for EC–IC in the SO group is the observation in the present study and others[2] that most cases suffer from neurologic symptoms referred to the occluded side.

Comparing data with medically treated patients, the latter appear to be at a disadvantage[15] when certain principles for indication to surgery are considered; among these are not to operate on a recent stroke nor on a stroke in evolution. There may be an indication for anticoagulant therapy in patients without a history of hypertension[19] worth a comprehensive prospective study. Arteriosclerotic patients lacking hypertension are in the minority, however, and anticoagulant therapy might numerically remain a possibility for patients whose angiograms do not show an operable cerebrovascular lesion. Following a study of Eisenberg et al.,[13] this probability is around 10% for patients with amaurosis fugax and TIA. Platelet aggregation therapy alone was shown from a series of 178 patients to have no significantly different results from placebo therapy.[16] It should, therefore, be stressed that bypass is a prophylactic measure with an extremely low risk for patients with TIA, PRIND, or minor stroke, such therapy showing the lowest rate of stroke in the follow-up period of all other

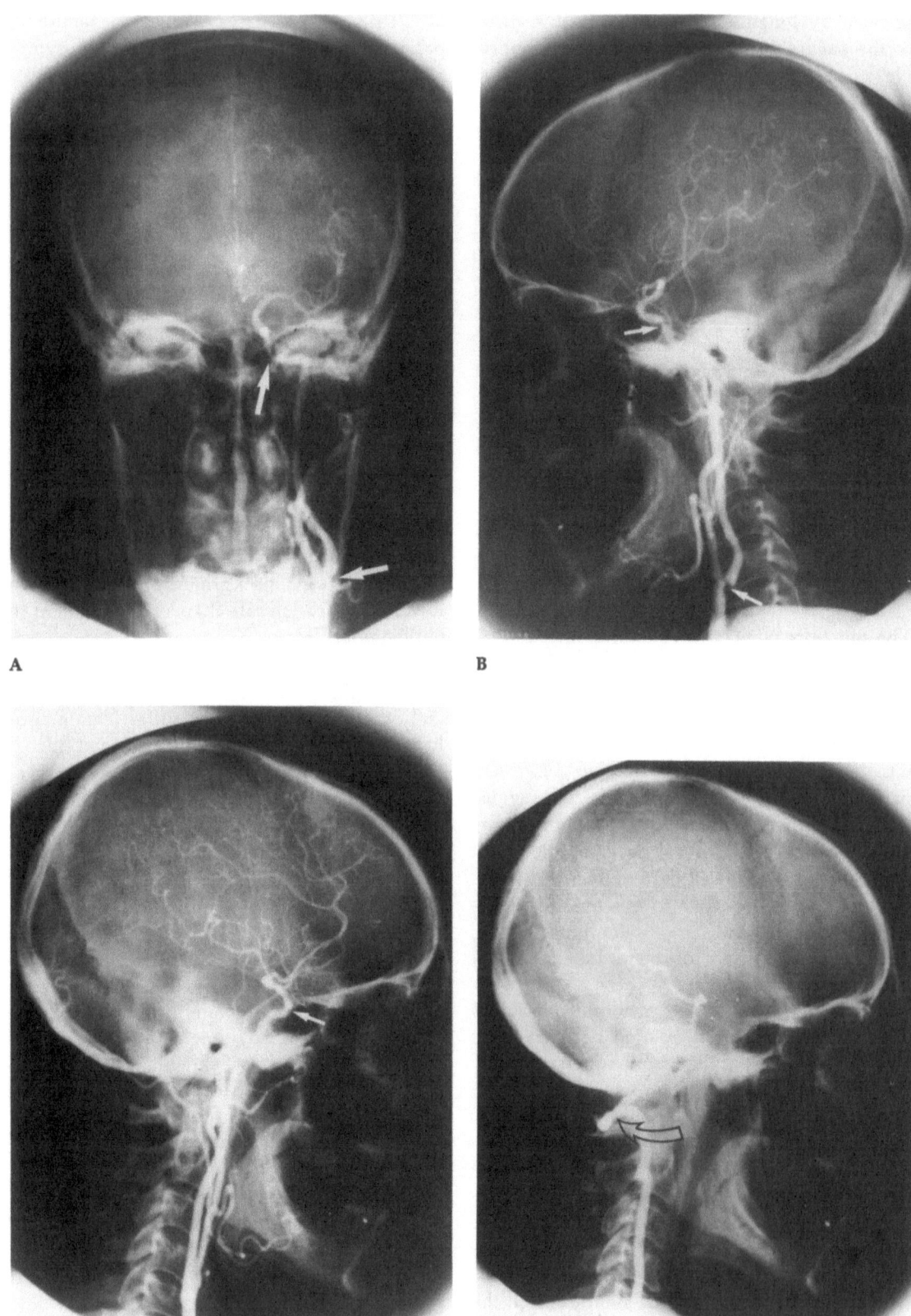

A

B

C

D

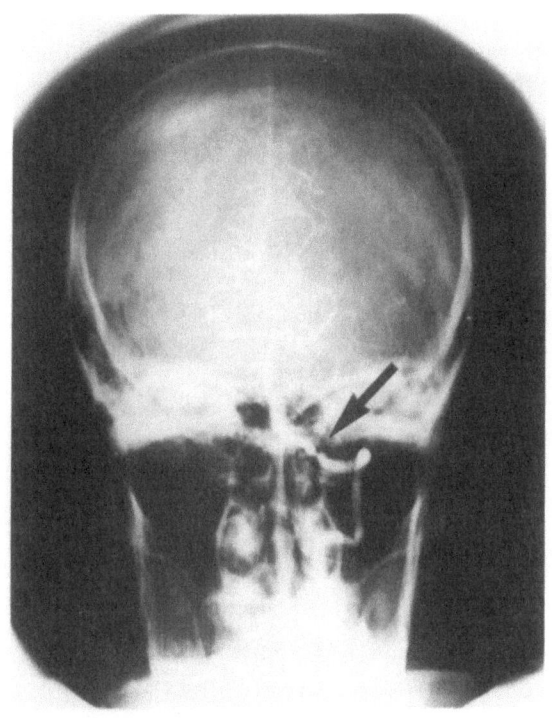

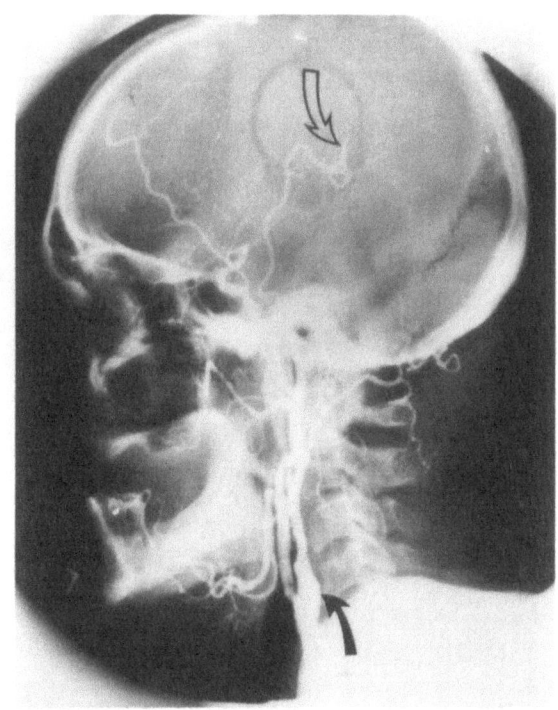

E

F

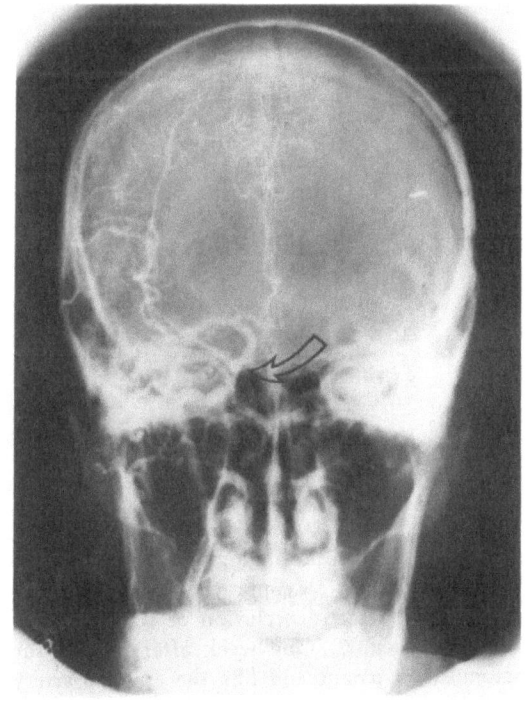

Fig. 47-4. Four-vessel angiograms of a 65-year-old man (case 4). A, B. AP and lateral view of left carotid showing 50% stenosis at the bifurcation and 80% stenosis at the siphon. D, E. Bilateral vertebral artery 90% stenosis above the arch of C1. Control angiography 5 months after first angiography and 3 months after bypass, TEA, and occipital artery–PICA anastomosis. F. Left carotid bifurcation is widely open, bypass is patent, left occipital artery–PICA anastomosis patent but filling posterior circulation very poorly. G. Increasing multiple stenoses at right siphon.

G

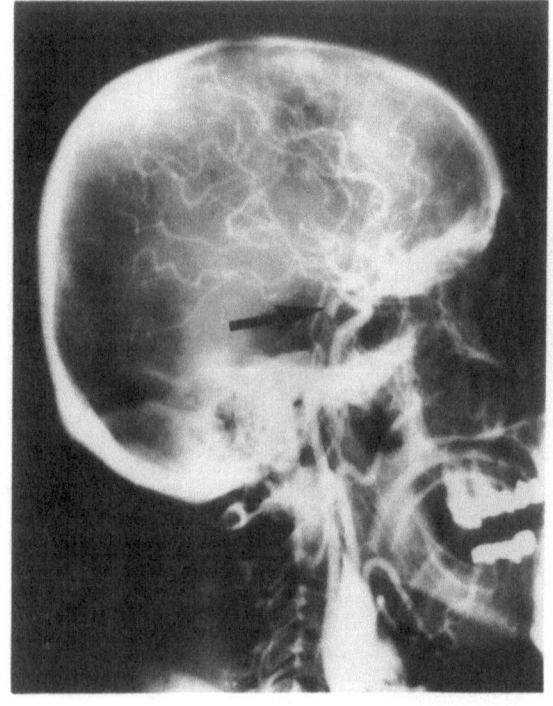

A

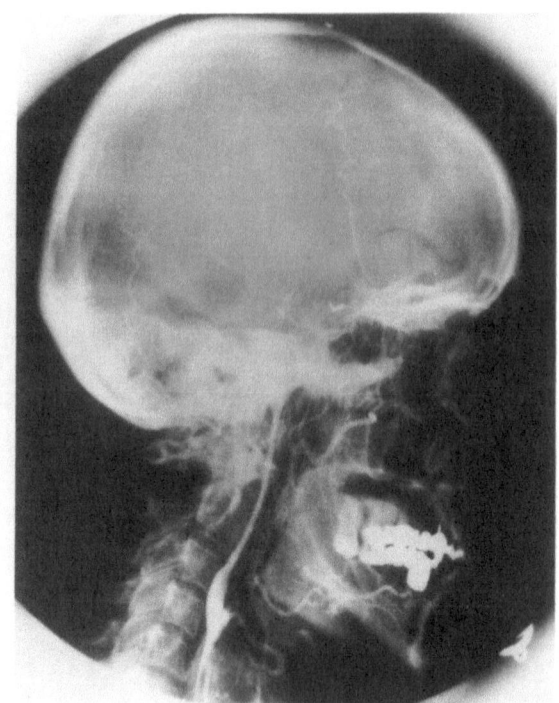

B

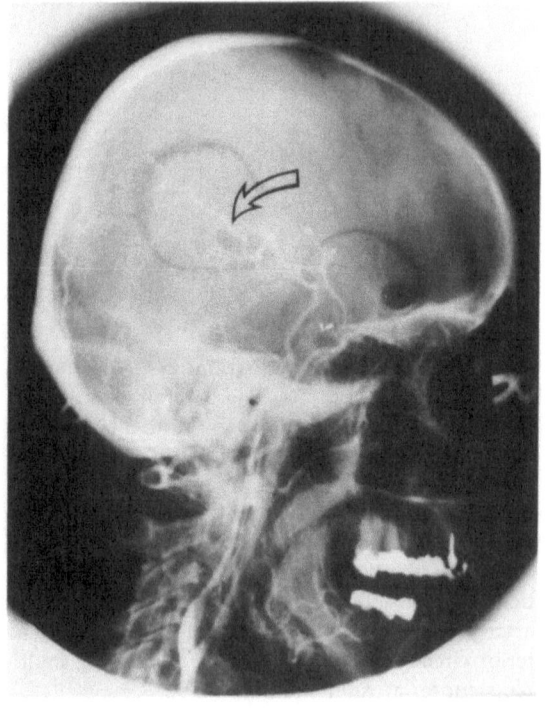

C

Fig. 47-5. Right carotid angiograms of a 43-year-old woman (case 5). A. Supraclinoidal ICA aneurysm. B. Postoperative occlusion of ICA with the STA being open. C. One week after bypass the anastomosis is patent and fills the angular artery as well as the MCA trunk retrogradely.

types of therapy combinations. The decision to try therapy with as much as possible prophylactic effect can almost be called a compulsory one. The patients are suffering from insufficient collateral circulation; otherwise they would not have become symptomatic. It appears not adequate to decide only from an angiogram whether collateral circulation is sufficient or not and to determine from such a postulation whether EC–IC bypass should be performed after TEA, as proposed by other authors.[2]

The other cases presented in this paper are rare events that show the beneficial effect of bypass performed at equally low risk. Again, the idea of prophylaxis should dominate considerations.

Cases of coincidental carotid stenosis and intracranial aneurysm have been presented and discussed in a number of papers.[1, 10, 17, 24, 25, 27] They outline a possibly crucial situation where it is difficult to decide which operation to perform first; doing aneurysm surgery first in a patient with symptomatic carotid stenosis may mean an increased risk for ischemic lesions. Performing TEA as the initial step may lead to rupture of the aneurysm, caused by increase of flow and peak pressure. In summary, however, the risk of operating on the aneurysm first may be the minor risk regarding the patient's survival chances.

Discussing operative procedures in patients with atherosclerosis generally, we have always to be aware of operating into an unaffected florid process as seen in one of our patients (case 4). It appears difficult to predict the nature of a process; we do not know whether a stenosing and surgically inaccessible plaque forms microemboli or not,[11] thus questioning any bypass procedure a priori. The excellent results in patients with mild neurologic deficit and adequate general condition, however, indicate such processes to be rare.

Mild completed strokes are worth operating on even when follow-up studies show that most of the patients do not improve after operation but remain neurologically unchanged. Comparing these results with those during conservative therapy and recurrence of stroke, the better results in operated patients are unquestionable.[4, 5, 20 ,22]

Conclusions

Multiple cerebrovascular lesions are worth being operated on with more than one intervention; the same criteria should be applied for selection of candidates as discussed for any cerebrovascular surgery in patients with cerebral ischemia. Thus, operative interventions are indicated in patients with TIAs, PRINDs and mild CS, when their biological ages are adequate.

EC–IC bypass surgery should be considered as a prophylactic rather than a therapeutic measure in patients with multiple lesions. Therefore, it can always be performed as the first operation, followed by TEA or tumor extirpation.

EC–IC bypass surgery can drastically and acutely ameliorate neurologic deficit irrespective of presence or absence of ischemic infarction.

Control angiography is indicated in all patients who remain or become symptomatic after surgery; there might be an operable complication.

References

1. Adams, H.P. Carotid stenosis and coexisting intracranial aneurysm. Arch Neurol 34:515–516, 1977.
2. Andersen, Ch.A., et al. Unilateral internal carotid arterial occlusion: special considerations. Stroke 8:669–671, 1977.
3. Anderson, R.E., Reichman, O.H., Davis, D.O. Radiological evaluation of temporal artery–middle cerebral artery anastomosis. Radiology 113:73–79, 1974.
4. Auer, L., Oberbauer, R., Lanner, G. Zur neurochirurgischen Behandlung des Schlaganfalls. Proc Ost Chir Kongreß 1978, in press.
5. Auer, L., Oberbauer, R. Carotid angiography findings before and after extra–intracranial arterial bypass operation. Seara Med Neurocir Brasil 7:43–62, 1978.
6. Chater, N. Surgical results and measurements of intraoperative flow in microneurosurgical anastomosis. In Microneurosurgical Anastomosis for Cerebral Ischemia, G.M. Austin, editor, Charles C Thomas, Springfield, 1976, pp 295–304.
7. Clark, E., Harrison, C.V. Bilateral carotid artery occlusion. Neurology 6:705–712, 1956.
8. Collins, G.J., et al. Stroke after carotid endarterectomy. Stroke 8:14, 1977.
9. Denck, H. Chirurgische Schlaganfallprophylaxe. Pro Med Nov 14–21, 1976.

10. Denton, I.C., Gutman, L. Surgical treatment of symptomatic carotid stenosis and asymptomatic ipsilateral intracranial aneurysm. J Neurosurg 38:662–665, 1973.

11. Donaghy, P. Pitfalls in extracranial–intracranial blood flow diversion. In Microneurosurgical Anastomoses for Cerebral Ischemia, G. M. Austin, editor, Charles C Thomas, Springfield, 1976, pp 305–307.

12. Easton, J.D., Sherman, D.G. Stroke and mortality rate in carotid endarterectomy: 228 consecutive operations. Stroke 8:565–568, 1977.

13. Eisenberg, R.L., et al. Relationship of transient ischemic attacks and angiographically demonstrable lesions of carotid artery. Stroke 8:483–486, 1977.

14. Fields, W.S., Edwards, W.H., Crawford, E.S. Bilateral carotid artery thrombosis. Arch Neurol 4:369–375, 1961.

15. Fields, W.S., Lemak, N.A. Joint study of extracranial arterial occlusion. X. Internal carotid artery occlusion. JAMA 235:2734–2738, 1976.

16. Fields, W.S., et al. Controlled trial of aspirin in cerebral ischemia. Stroke 8:301–314, 1977.

17. Fields, W.S., Weibel, J. Coincidental internal carotid stenosis and intracranial saccular aneurysm. Trans Am Neurol Assoc 95:237–238, 1970.

18. Fisher, C. M. Senile dementia—A new explanation of its causation. Can Med Assoc J 65:1–7, 1951.

19. Gallhofer, B., Ladurner, G. Lechner, H. Prognosis of prophylactic anticoagulant treatment in ischemic stroke. Neurology, in Druck, 1978.

20. Gratzl, O., Schmiedek, P., Steinhoff, H., Enzenbach, R. Microneurosurgical anastomoses for cerebral ischemia in 39 patients—clinical results, angiography and regional cerebral blood flow. In Microneurosurgical Anastomoses for Cerebral Ischemia, G.M. Austin, editor, Charles C Thomas, Springfield, 1976, pp 308–319.

21. Holbach, H.K., et al. Differentiation between reversible and irreversible post-stroke changes in brain tissue: its relevance for cerebrovascular surgery. Surg Neurol 7:325–331, 1977.

22. Koos, W.T., Kletter, G. Experiences with extra–intracranial arterial bypass in patients with completed stroke.

23. Peerless, S.J., Chater, N.L., Ferguson, G.F. Multiple vessel occlusion in cerebrovascular disease—a further follow-up of the effects of microvascular bypass on the quality of life and the incidence of stroke. In Microsurgery for Stroke, P. Schmiedek, editor, Springer-Verlag, New York, 1978, pp 251–259.

24. Pool, L.J., Potts, D.G. Aneurysms and Arteriovenous Anomalies of the Brain: Diagnosis and Treatment. Harper & Row, New York, 1965.

25. Portnoy, H.D., Avellanosa, A. Carotid aneurysm and contralateral carotid stenosis with successful surgical treatment of both lesions. J Neurosurg 32:476–482, 1970.

26. Sampson, D., Watts, C., Clark, K. Cerebral revascularization for transient ischemic attacks. Neurology, in press.

27. Shoumaker, R.D., Avant, W.S., Cohen, G.H. Coincidental multiple asymptomatic intracranial aneurysm and symptomatic carotid stenosis. Stroke 7:504–506, 1976.

28. Wortzmann, G., Barnett, H., Lougheed, W. Bilateral carotid artery occlusion. Can Med Assoc J 99:1186–1192, 1968.

48

Further Experience with Occipital Artery–Caudal Loop–PICA Anastomosis for Vertebrobasilar Insufficiency

G. Khodadad

The rationale for the consideration of an occipital artery–caudal loop–posterior inferior cerebellar artery (OA–caudal loop–PICA) anastomosis, the patient selection, and the surgical techniques have been previously described.[1-7] In this report, after a general summary of the patients who underwent this procedure, four patients who either showed postoperative neurologic deficits or died will be discussed.

To date, twenty patients have been operated upon, and nineteen anastomoses are completed. In one patient, the anastomosis was not done because of the patient's repeated transient apnea during the surgical procedure. This patient will be discussed in detail in this report.

Of twenty patients, there were nineteen males and one female. The youngest patient was a diabetic man 26 years of age,[1] and the oldest a man of 71. Of the entire group, nineteen patients showed symptoms and signs of vertebrobasilar insufficiency and the remaining patient was thought to be brain-stem stroke prone. All the patients had arteriographic evidence of impaired blood flow in the vertebrobasilar system. Most had either complete occlusion of both vertebral arteries or complete occlusion of one vertebral and severe stenosis of the other vertebral artery. None of the angiograms demonstrated sufficient collateral flow through the posterior communicating arteries to the vertebrobasilar system.

Of twenty patients, three died. The remaining seventeen were discharged home either improved or unchanged, except for one patient who had a moderate degree of cerebellar ataxia. This patient will also be discussed in this report. The longest follow-up period is 3 years and the shortest 1 month.

A total of eleven patients had postoperative angiograms; of these, eight showed a patent anastomosis at the first angiogram 1 to 3 weeks postoperatively. Two patients showed patent occipital artery without visualization of the cerebellar artery on the first angiograms. Angiograms done months later in these two patients, however, showed a patent anastomosis and filling of the posterior inferior cerebellar artery. The angiograms of the remaining patient did not show the anastomosed occipital artery.

The three patients who died and the one who developed ataxia postoperatively will be discussed below.

Description of Patients

Case 1

This was a 62-year-old diabetic, hypertensive, and heavy-smoking black man with a past history of myocardial infarction and prostate surgery who started having difficulties in remembering recent events and in writing about 6 months prior to his admission. Subsequently, within a couple of months he developed slurred speech, episodes of blurred vision, and dizziness lasting for a few minutes. Later he noted difficulties in walking and in hearing, and also started having drop attacks.

On admission, the patient's blood pressure was 164/70, pulse 64, and respiration 18 per minute. The general physical and neurologic examination was within normal limits except for slurred speech, bilateral diminished hearing, left upgoing toes, and right equivocal upgoing toes.

Cerebral angiograms revealed the following:

Almost complete occlusion of the right vertebral artery. Very severe atherosclerotic changes of a small left vertebral artery which supplied basically the ipsilateral posterior inferior cerebrellar artery.

Moderate irregularity of the right cavernous and supraclinoid carotid artery.

Filling of the tip of the basilar artery, right posterior cerebral artery, and both superior cerebellar arteries through the right posterior communicating artery.

Sixty-seventy percent narrowing of the left cavernous carotid artery.

Bilateral intracranial occlusive small vessel disease.

Moderately large lateral ventricles.

On the basis of the history, clinical picture, and neurologic and angiographic findings, the diagnosis of vertebrobasilar insufficiency was made. Under general anesthesia, in the prone position, and with controlled respiration, the patient underwent a right OA–caudal loop–PICA anastomosis. Throughout the operation, his blood pressure was not very stable. The systolic pressure ranged from 180 to 140 with one episode as high as 200, and two episodes as low as 105 and 115, each lasting for 5 minutes. The diastolic pressure ranged from 110 to 80. It should be mentioned, however, that the diastolic pressure was not measured during the two periods that the systolic pressure dropped. The pulse rate throughout the operation ranged between 60 and 100. Immediately following the operation, the patient was able to be roused and his pupils were equal and reactive to light. Several hours later, however, he suffered cardiac and respiratory arrest and died on the first postoperative day.

The postmortem examination, in addition to diffuse severe cerebral atherosclerosis, old myocardial infarcts, acute ischemic encephalopathy, and a 1-cm organizing infarct in the pons, showed acute myocardial infarcts in both the anterior and posterior walls of the left ventricle. Postmortem angiograms of the anastomosed arteries showed a patent anastomosis. It was reported that "At autopsy the immediate cause of death was acute myocardial infarction."

Case 2

This was a 46-year-old obese and known hypertensive black man with a history of multiple strokes. Five years previously, he had two strokes, 2 months apart. The first one produced weakness of the left side of the body. The second one caused both weakness of the left side of the body and slurred speech. Four months before his admission to the hospital he developed both further weakness of the left side and further slurred speech. Subsequently, he developed both weakness of the right arm and right side of the face.

On admission, his blood pressure was 160/100, pulse 72, and respiration 28 per minute. The general physical examination was within normal limits. The neurologic examination showed the following:

Slurred speech.

Left hemiplegic gait.

Right central facial palsy.

Diminished strength in the left arm and leg.

Bilateral increased deep tendon reflexes.

Bilateral upgoing toes.

Diminished pain sensation on the left side of the face.

Intact cerebellar function.

Cerebral angiograms revealed:

Complete occlusion of the right vertebral artery.

Fifty percent stenosis of the distal left vertebral artery.

Atherosclerotic changes of the basilar artery.

Irregularities of both cavernous carotid arteries.

With the diagnosis of multiple and bilateral brain-stem strokes, the patient underwent a right OA–caudal loop–PICA anastomosis under general anesthesia, in the prone position, and with controlled respiration. Throughout the operation there were three periods of drop of blood pressure as follows:

First period—1.5 hours after the induction of anesthesia, the blood pressure dropped from a starting value of 120/80 to 85/35 and lasted 10 minutes.

Second period—2 hours after the induction, the blood pressure dropped to 90/50 and lasted 15 minutes.

Third period—3 hours after the induction, the blood pressure dropped to 75/35–30 and lasted 30 minutes.

The cerebellum or brain stem was not exposed during the first 3.3 hours of the operation. During the entire operation, the pulse rate for the most part ranged from 80 to 100 per minute, except on two occasions when it increased to 110 and 120; both were associated with elevation of the blood pressure.

The postoperative course was stormy. The patient was restless and had a great amount of pulmonary secretion. He developed a left lower lobe pneumonia, partial right upper lobe collapse, and fever, and require a tracheostomy. He gradually recovered and was discharged 21 days after his operation. No postoperative angiograms were done.

On discharge, the patient was neurologically worse than at the time of admission, and in addition to his original objective neurologic findings he showed a cerebellar gait and diplopia.

Case 3

This was a 52-year-old known hypertensive, heavy-drinking, black man who was transferred from another hospital with a possible diagnosis of subdural hematoma. There was a history of a questionable stroke 3 years previously and a recent fall. Two days before his admission, he was seen having difficulties in walking and subsequently he became drowsy.

On admission, his blood pressure was 200/100, pulse 100, and respiration 22 per minute. The general physical examination was within normal limits. The neurologic examination showed:

Drowsiness.

Severe dysarthria.

Orientation to person, but not to place or time.

Left central facial palsy.

Deviation of the tongue to the left.

Deviation of the uvula to the right.

Nystagmus in all directions.

Disconjugate gaze with both eyes deviated downward.

Weakness of the left arm and leg.

Bilateral hyperactive deep tendon reflexes.

Bilateral upgoing toes.

Questionable diminished pain sensation of the right arm and leg.

Right carotid bruit.

Cerebral angiograms showed:

Complete occlusion of the right vertebral artery.

Complete occlusion of the origin of the left vertebral artery. Distally this artery was patent and received its supply retrograde from the anterior spinal artery.

Ninety-five percent occlusion of the right cervical carotid bifurcation.

Irregularities of the right petrous, cavernous, and supraclinoid carotid artery with 50% occlusion.

Irregularity of the left carotid artery.

Diffuse irregularity of the left middle cerebral artery.

Extremely slow cerebral circulation.

Following the angiogram, he became drowsier.

The diagnosis of bilateral brain-stem stroke was made, and the patient first underwent a right carotid endarterectomy. He tolerated this procedure well, and a postoperative angiogram several days later showed a well-repaired and patent carotid artery. Neurologically, however, the patient did not show any significant improvement, and in fact his drowsiness became worse; at times he became comatose when his blood pressure dropped 20 to 30 degrees. Since he was not getting better, it was decided to perform a right OA–caudal loop–PICA anastomosis. This procedure was done under general anesthesia, in the sitting position, with controlled respiration, 17 days following the right carotid endarterectomy.

Throughout the operation, there were two periods of drop in blood pressure. The first period occurred 30 minutes after the induction. The blood pressure dropped from the starting values of 160/100 to 100/60 and lasted 15 minutes. The second developed 1 hour and 10 minutes after the induction. The pressure dropped to 105/50 and lasted also for 15 minutes.

During the entire operation the pulse rate remained relatively stable, and ranged between 70 and 90 per minute. Postoperatively the patient moved all four extremities, but the right pupil was fixed to light. Later that evening, he had a grand mal seizure which lasted 5 minutes. One day postoperatively he no longer responded to painful stimulation and his blood pressure started dropping. Medical treatment was continued unsuccessfully, and the patient finally died 5 days after the operation.

Postmortem examination revealed generalized atherosclerotic vascular disease with marked involvement of the vertebrobasilar system, severe acute ischemic encephalopathy with superimposed respirator brain, thrombosis of occasional cortical vessels of the brain, and a recent superior sagittal sinus thrombosis.

No antemortem or postmortem cerebral angiography was performed. The anastomosed right occipital and right posterior inferior cerebellar arteries, however, were sectioned and examined histologically. It was found that the lumina of both the donor and the recipient arteries were patent. The final note of the prosector stated that the patient had died as the result of a brain-stem stroke.

Case 4

This was a 50-year-old, obese, diabetic, hypertensive white man with a past history of two myocardial infarctions at the age of 39 who started having frontal headaches and transient attacks of dizziness 3 months before his admission. The headaches were associated with "a draining type of sensation" in the front of the head.

The attacks of dizziness, aside from being associated with nausea and vomiting, were at times so severe that the patient had to lie on the ground. Subsequently, he experienced transient attacks of tinnitus in both ears and paresthesia on the right side of his lips, face, arm, and hand. About a month prior to his admission, he lost his vision in the right field and developed a vertical diplopia.

On admission to a local hospital in Washington, D.C., his blood pressure was 120/80, pulse 80, and respiration 14 per minute. The general physical examination was within normal limits and the neurologic examination showed a right homonymous hemianopia.

A CT scan revealed a left occipital infarct, and the cerebral angiograms (Figs. 48-1 to 48-3) showed:

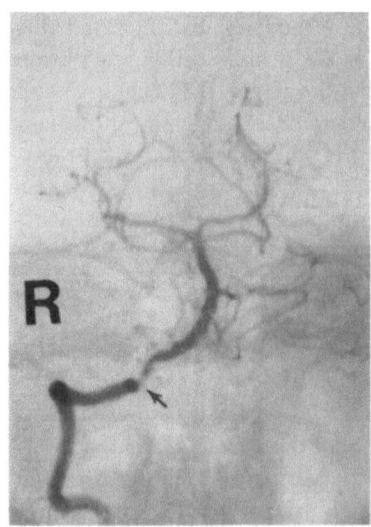
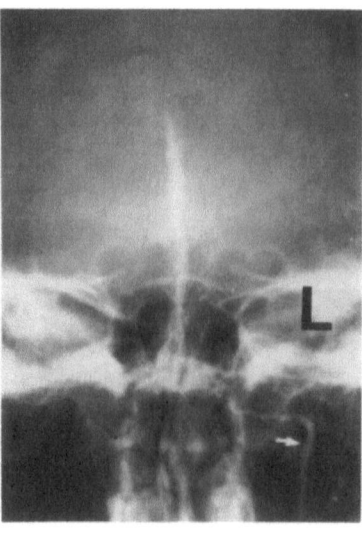

Fig. 48-1. Case 4. R and L show the anteroposterior views of the left and right vertebral angiograms. The black arrow points to the site of the severe narrowing and the white arrow to the hypoplastic vertebral artery with no filling of the basilar artery.

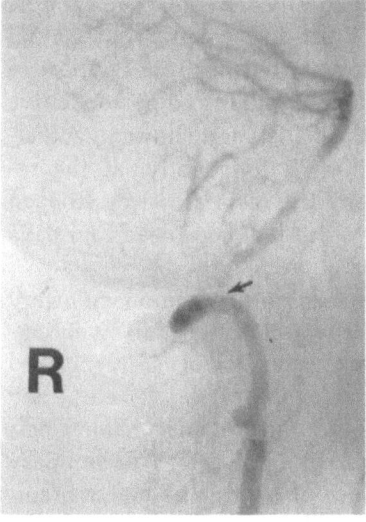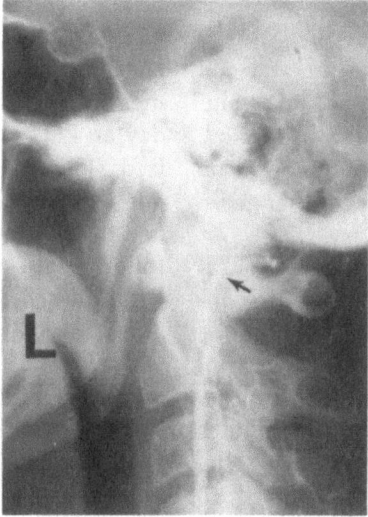

Fig. 48-2. Case 4. R and L show the lateral view of the corresponding right and left angiograms seen in Fig. 48-1. The arrow on R again shows the site of the narrowing and the arrow on L the hypoplastic vertebral artery.

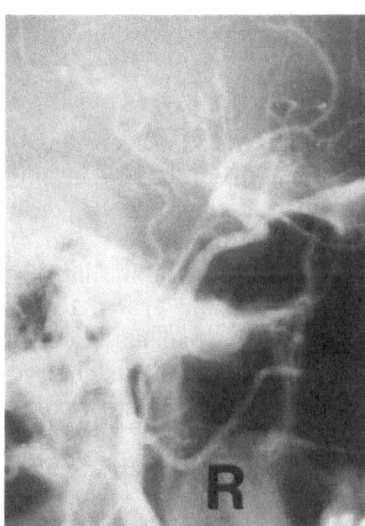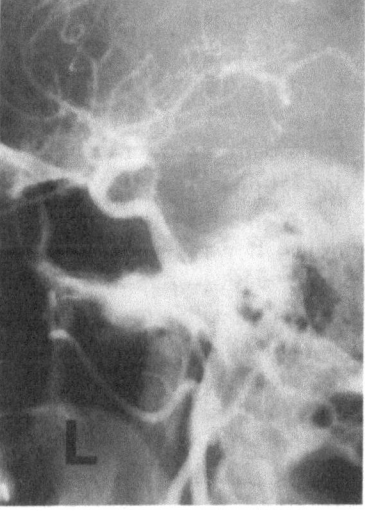

Fig. 48-3. Case 4. R and L show the lateral views of the right and left carotid angiograms. No significant posterior communicating arteries are seen.

Severely stenotic (95% or more) right vertebral artery.

Complete occlusion of the left vertebral artery.

No radiologically recognizable posterior communicating arteries.

Widely patent bilateral carotid arteries.

Following the angiography his neurologic condition became worse and he developed:

Diminished hearing in the right ear.

Ataxia of the right arm and leg.

Transient dysarthria.

Nystagmus in looking to the right side.

After the angiography, the diagnosis of ver-

tebrobasilar insufficiency was confirmed, and anticoagulant and steroid therapy was begun. Shortly afterward, the patient was transferred by air to Cincinnati. While in the air, he had two episodes of loss of consciousness, each one lasting a few minutes. On admission, the neurologic examination showed:

Orientation to persons, place and time.

Dysarthria.

Conjugate deviation of the eyes to the left.

Inability to conjugate the eyes to the left beyond the midline.

Right homonymous hemianopia.

Slight left facial weakness.

Right hemihypesthesia.

Ataxia of the right arm and leg.

Later on the day of admission, he was put in a sitting position for 30 minutes and evaluated neurologically during and after this period. He tolerated this position well and showed no further neurologic abnormality or change in level of consciousness.

On the following day, under general anesthesia, in the sitting position and with controlled respiration, a right OA–caudal loop–PICA anastomosis was attempted, but was not completed because of four episodes of apnea.

The first occurred 1 hour and 15 minutes after the induction of anesthesia, during the dissection of the occipital artery. It lasted 10 minutes and was associated with a bradycardia of 60 (the starting pulse was 80), and a drop of blood pressure to 90 systolic (the starting systolic pressure was 130). The diastolic pressure was not recorded throughout the operation. During the entire period of apnea, the patient's respiration was controlled.

The second apneic episode developed 40 minutes later (2 hours and 5 minutes following the induction), still during dissection of the occipital artery, and lasted 40 minutes. It was not associated with any change of blood pressure or pulse. Again, during the period of apnea, the patient's respiration was controlled.

The third episode occurred 30 minutes after the second one (3 hours and 15 minutes following the induction) during the elevation of the right cerebellar tonsil. It lasted only 5 minutes and was not associated with any pulse or blood pressure changes. It was during this episode that a small bubble of air was noted in one of the cortical cerebellar veins.

The fourth respiratory difficulty developed when the left PICA was temporarily clamped for 2 minutes. The patient's respiration did not stop, but dropped from 20 to 10 per minute; it was 20 minutes before it returned to the earlier rate.

Because of these intermittent failures of respiration, it was decided to discontinue the operation.

Immediately following the operation, the patient moved all his extremities to painful stimulation and squeezed hand at request. He had, however, shallow respirations and had to be assisted mechanically. The next morning he was no longer breathing spontaneously, and his blood pressure started to drop. Supportive measures continued. On the third postoperative day an EEG was obtained and showed generalized slow activities. Subsequently, at the request of his family the respirator was stopped and the patient was pronounced dead four days following the operation.

At autopsy, in addition to "coronary artery atherosclerosis, severe, 3 vessel (narrowing 65-90%)," and focal myocardial scar, marked atherosclerotic narrowing of the vertebral and basilar arteries and diffuse encephalomalacia were found. It was the prosector's preliminary note that the cause of death was major brainstem and/or cerebral infarction.

Discussion

All four patients had moderate to severe symptoms and signs of the vertebrobasilar insufficiency. All of them had at least one stroke in the past. At least in three (cases 1, 2, and 4) this stroke was due to the vertebrobasilar disease. Two patients (cases 1 and 4) had 1 or 2 myocardial infarctions. Two patients (cases 1 and 4) were also diabetic. All patients showed angiographic evidence of severe atherosclerotic occlusive vertebrobasilar disease. CT scan in one patient (case 4) showed a left occipital infarct.

The first two patients were operated upon in the prone position and the other two patients in the sitting position. General anesthesia with sodium pentothal and oral endotracheal tube was used. Throughout the operation, the blood pressure of all the patients was monitored by an intra-arterial radial catheter. Both Doppler and right atrial catheter were used for the detection of possible air embolism. Other supportive measures such as elastic bandages for legs and an abdominal binder in the sitting position were applied. No EEG monitoring was done.

The first patient, although he did not have a very stable blood pressure during the operation in the prone position, was rousable immediately following the procedure and was recovering from the anesthesia when he had a massive anterior and posterior myocardial infarction and died.

This patient had a myocardial infarction in the past and died of another one shortly after the operation. Regardless of whether or not the operation had a major role in the production of the infarction, the practical point is that postoperative anticoagulant or at least platelet-inhibiting medications might have been of value.

The second patient had three episodes of drop of blood pressure, lasting 10 to 30 minutes with diastolic pressure as low as 35. Following a long, stormy postoperative period he survived but had additional neurologic signs of brain-stem and cerebellar dysfunction. It seems reasonable to consider the episodes of hypotension during the operation as the cause of the patient's neurologic worsening. Fortunately, at least the surgery was done in the prone position. In the sitting position, it is probable that the patient would not have survived the procedure or would have had much more severe neurologic deficits.

Since arterial hypertension is relatively common among stroke patients and at times is very difficult to regulate, the surgeon must treat any hypotensive episode quickly and effectively. In addition and most importantly, these procedures should not be done in the sitting position.

The third patient also had two episodes of hypotension, each lasting 15 minutes, with a diastolic pressure of 50 to 60. Postoperatively the patient's right pupil was fixed to light and he eventually died of a brain-stem stroke. This patient was very much sicker both pre- and postoperatively than the second patient, but another unfortunate factor was that the operation was done in the sitting position which probably intensified the effect of hypotension on the brain stem. Certainly, he would have had much better chance to fight the hypotensive periods in the prone or a similar position than in the sitting position.

The fourth patient had episodes of apnea which were probably caused by the impairment of brain-stem circulation. The first episode was associated with a bradycardia and a drop of systolic pressure to 90, lasting 10 minutes. The diastolic pressure was not recorded. A small air bubble was also seen in one of cortical cerebellar veins during this episode of apnea. There was, however, no other objective or clinical evidence of air embolism. No anastomosis was performed and the patient died following the procedure because of a brain-stem infarction.

Unfortunately, this patient's operation was also done in the sitting position, and he was not protected against cerebral ischemia. He was the only patient whose respiration was not controlled during the operation and thus the episodes of apnea and further brain-stem ischemia were recognized. If the procedure had been done under controlled respiration, most probably it would have been continued and the anastomosis completed. In that case the cause of problems and bad results would not have been as clear as it is now. Again a position different from the sitting and a better control of blood pressure might have been of significant value.

Detailed analysis of these four cases calls for certain modifications and considerations in surgical techniques and postoperative care of patients who undergo an OA–caudal loop–PICA anastomosis or similar operations.

The sitting position should be avoided. The sitting position is convenient for the surgeon, but dangerous for the patient. The surgeon sits straight and parallel to major anatomic landmarks, which makes the exposure easier and wider, there are less bleeding and swelling, the cerebrospinal fluid (CSF) does not puddle in the tonsillar region as it does in the prone position. These are technical advantages, but the great danger is an irreversible brain-stem ischemia especially in hypertensive patients with unstable and hard-to-control blood pressure.

The prone position, although it is protective when there is a fall of blood pressure and also alleviates the problem of air embolism, has the disadvantages of venous stasis, swelling of the brain, and puddling of the CSF in the area where the anastomosis is being performed.

The last patient in our series of twenty was operated upon in a lateral and slightly prone position with the head and neck flexed and slightly above the chest level. The bleeding, venous stasis, and swelling were not of any problem and a good exposure of the tonsillar region was obtained. Although a lumbar spinal needle was inserted preoperatively to drain the CSF during the operation, it was not used since the operative field was free of CSF. Both the operation and postoperative course went smoothly and the patient felt that his neurologic condition had improved.

This "lateral-semiprone" position appears to be superior to either the sitting or prone position and we plan to use it in future operations.

Aside from the surgical position, careful control of the blood pressure and rapid correction of any hypotensive episodes are of absolute importance. The value of any method, such as EEG, possibly spontaneous respiration or others, by which the brain-stem function could be monitored cannot be sufficiently emphasized.

The major cause of mortality and morbidity of the OA–caudal loop–PICA anastomosis is further impairment of the blood flow to the brain stem. Measures can be taken both to avoid and to treat this major complication. Patients with previous history of myocardial infarction or occlusive coronary artery disease should also receive appropriate therapy immediately following operation.

References

1. Ausman, J.I., Nicoloff, D.M., Chou, S.N. Posterior fossa revascularization: Anastomosis of vertebral artery to PICA with interposed radial artery graft. Surg Neurol 9:281–286, 1978.
2. Khodadad, G. Arteriosclerotic occlusive disease of the vertebrobasilar system in young adults and its surgical consideration. Neurochir 45: 147–154, 1978.
3. Khodadad, G. Brain stem strokes and microvascular anastomosis. Reprinted from International Congress Series No. 433, Neurological Surgery, R. Correa, editor, Proceedings of the Sixth International Congress of Neurological Surgery, São Paulo, June 19–25, 1977.
4. Khodadad, G. Occipital artery–posterior inferior cerebellar artery anastomosis. Surg Neurol 5: 225–227, 1976.
5. Khodadad, G., McLaurin, R. L. Syndromes of vertebrobasilar insufficiency and their possible surgical treatment. J Fam Pract 6:1185–1190, 1978.
6. Khodadad, G., et al. Possible prevention of brain stem stroke by microvascular anastomosis in vertebrobasilar system. Stroke 8:316–321, 1977.
7. Sundt, T.M., Piepgras, D.G. Occipital to posterior inferior cerebellar artery bypass surgery. J Neurosurg 48:916–928, 1978.

49

New Approaches in Cerebral Revascularization

James I. Ausman and Norman L. Chater

With the development of microvascular surgery and improved angiographic techniques the interest of neurologists and neurosurgeons in cerebral vascular disease has increased. These advances have confronted us with patients having complicated vascular lesions requiring innovative surgical approaches. In this paper we will discuss our approach to three such problems.

Case Reports

Case 1[1]

During the 6 years prior to admission this 50-year-old man suffered two transient ischemic attacks. Cerebral angiography performed after the second event revealed a left vertebral artery occlusion. In December of 1976, 3 months before his admission to the University of Minnesota Hospital, the patient experienced a brain-stem infarction consisting of numbness on the left side of his face, dysmetria, nausea, vomiting, left Horner's sign, and weakness of both lower extremities. On cerebral angiography, at that time, an occlusion of the left vertebral artery above Cl and of the right vertebral artery beyond the right posterior inferior cerebellar artery (PICA) was seen. No posterior communicating vessels were visualized. The patient was placed on coumadin and improved

clinically, maintaining only a residual broad-based gait. Upon admission in March of 1977, follow-up angiography was unchanged. Neurologic examination was as described.

Because it was our belief this patient, now 50 years old, would be at increased risk for further brain-stem vascular ischemic events[8] and because of the severely compromised posterior fossa, revascularization procedure was planned.

Because we were reluctant to temporarily occlude the only vessel in his posterior fossa, the right PICA, it was decided to open the posterior fossa bilaterally and search for a suitable vessel and then use a radial artery graft connecting the distal end of the open portion of the left vertebral artery to any appropriate vessel on the cerebellum which could be found. Because this flexibility in approach was necessary, the occipital artery could not be used since it was not certain which vessel in the posterior fossa and which side would be eventually utilized for the procedure. It was decided to use a radial artery graft.

Bilateral radial artery angiograms were normal, indicating that there was no disease in these vessels.

The patient was brought to surgery for a radial artery graft to be connected between the left vertebral artery and the right PICA. After exploration of the posterior fossa, the right PICA was the only vessel which was found. After lightening the anesthesia and observing the patient neurologically with the right PICA temporarily occluded for a period of 8 minutes during surgery, it was decided this vessel could be utilized.

Postoperatively the patient has had no further ischemic events and is no longer taking anticoagulant therapy.

At 6 months and 1 year postoperatively follow-up angiography revealed the radial artery graft to be patent with excellent filling of the posterior fossa vascular structures demonstrated on angiography.

Case 2[2]

This 58-year-old man was referred for evaluation of multiple episodes of amaurosis fugax in the left eye. The patient was developing severe pain in the left eye and changes consistent with ischemic retinopathy. Angiography 4 months previously had indicated occlusion of the right internal carotid artery, left internal, and left common carotid arteries, with no superficial temporal artery visualized.

The patient was neurologically negative. Repeated cerebral angiography at our institution revealed the findings described above; however, on injection of the left vertebral artery collateral filling of the left external carotid artery could be seen, with faint visualization of the origin of the superficial temporal artery.

To stop the amaurosis fugax in the left eye and possibly to prevent further ischemic retinopathy in that eye, reconstruction of the circulation to the left cerebral hemisphere was planned. A saphenous vein graft from the left subclavian artery to the left external carotid artery was performed. Follow-up angiography revealed a patent graft with filling of the left external carotid artery and demonstration of the left superficial temporal artery. Then a left STA–MCA bypass procedure was performed. Angiography after the bypass operation revealed the entire graft and bypass circulation to the patent with filling of the intracranial circulation in the left hemisphere. The patient's ischemic retinopathy stabilized and his headaches disappeared, although the vision in his left eye did not improve. A subsequent transient ischemic spell in his right cerebral hemisphere, even while receiving aspirin therapy, was treated by a right STA–MCA bypass pro-

cedure. Subsequently, the patient is asymptomatic.

Case 3

This 63-year-old man experienced multiple attacks of vertebral basilar insufficiency and was referred for further evaluation. Angiography revealed severe stenosis of the midportion of the basilar artery above the take-off of both anterior inferior cerebellar arteries and below both superior cerebellar arteries. The right posterior communicating artery was occluded and a faint visualization of the left posterior communicating artery between the left carotid circulation and the tip of the basilar artery could be seen.

The patient was placed on intravenous heparin therapy after angiography while an approach to his problem was considered. Three days later, he experienced another brain-stem ischemic event consisting of internuclear ophthalmoplegia, left hemiparesis, left Horner's syndrome, and transient loss of consciousness.

It was felt that this patient needed additional collateral filling to the tip of his basilar artery beyond the stenotic region and a revascularization procedure was planned. It was decided to avoid the risks of the sitting position because of the compromised posterior fossa circulation; thus, in the supine position a long segment of the patient's right superficial temporal artery was dissected, the right temporal lobe was elevated, a hole was made in the tentorium, and an anastomosis between the right superficial temporal artery and the superior cerebellar artery (SCA) was accomplished.

Postoperatively the patient experienced a mild ischemic infarction to the upper midbrain from which he gradually recovered over a 6-month period. Follow-up angiography revealed only visualization of the superficial temporal artery as it approached the posterior fossa structures with no filling of the posterior fossa vasculature. Subsequent angiography on two additional occasions one year following operation revealed partial resolution of the stenotic lesion in the midbasilar artery and much better demonstration of both posterior cerebral arteries on the vertebral artery angiographic study. The superior cerebellar arteries were visualized only in the later angiographic phases, suggesting that these vessels were filling either late or by collateral flow from other channels. This suggested a stenosis of the origin of both superior cerebellar arteries. Although the filling of the posterior fossa vasculature could not be demonstrated angiographically, the superficial temporal artery was angiographically patent and was filling; it was probable that there was patency of the anastomosis although filling of the posterior fossa circulation was probably meager. There are two reasons why there was an insignificant amount of intracranial filling: (1) The small caliber of the superior cerebellar artery, slightly less than 1 mm in diameter, may not have enlarged. (2) The poor runoff to the basilar artery secondary to stenosis of the origins of the superior cerebellar arteries may have prevented filling of the basilar tip. However, this approach would seem to offer an alternative providing circulation to the basilar tip.

Conclusion

Three unusual cases of complicated cerebral vascular occlusive disease are presented and the innovative approaches to treatment of these problems are briefly discussed.

References

1. Ausman, J.I., Nicoloff, D.M., Chou, S.N. Posterior fossa revascularization: Anastomosis of vertebral artery to PICA with interposed radial artery graft. Surg Neurol 9:281–286, 1978.
2. Ausman, J.I. Cerebral revascularization: Extracranial–intracranial bypass procedures for cerebrovascular disease. In Vascular Surgery, J.S. Najarian and J.P. Delaney, editors, Symposia Specialists, Miami, 1978, pp 343–357.
3. Cartilage, N.F., Whisnant, J.P., Elveback, L.R. Carotid and vertebral-basilar transient cerebral ischemic attacks. Mayo Clin Proc 52:117–120, 1977.

50

Failure of EC–IC Bypass to Alter Ischemia

M. Peter Heilbrun

Retrospective studies to date suggest that EC–IC bypass has a definite role in preventing progression to severe completed stroke in patients with transient ischemic attacks, prolonged reversible ischemic deficits, and some cases of mild completed strokes.[1,2,3] A prospective random study is in progress to analyze this role further.

In a group of 54 patients evaluated from September 1973 to December 1977, EC–IC bypass was performed in three patients in an attempt to alter a state of progressive or severe cerebral infarction, and in two patients to alter ischemia associated with combined vascular and brain parenchymal lesions. Bypass failed in all five cases. Three cases will be described in detail to elucidate the variables encountered in dealing with progressing cerebral infarction.

Case Reports

Case 1 (J.X.)

This 46-year-old white male 3 weeks before admission fell and as a result sustained a fracture of his posterior malleous. At the time, he struck his head but was not unconscious. He was asymptomatic until the day of admission. While sitting in a chair, he suddenly lost the ability to speak, appeared to complain of pain below the cast, then headache, following which he collapsed with right-sided weakness.

The past history was not remarkable.

Examination 45 minutes after onset showed a well-developed, well-nourished white male with normal blood pressure and pulse. No nuchal rigidity was present. Neurologic examination showed a patient who was intermittently stuporous and agitated with global aphasia, dense right central facial palsy, and a spastic right hemiplegia.

Hospital Course. Initial CBC, electrolyte findings, urinalysis, and skull and chest radiographs were normal. Immediate cerebral angiography showed complete occlusion of the left internal carotid artery 5 mm above the anterior clinoid. The right carotid injection showed no significant collateral circulation to the left hemisphere except for minimal flow from anterior cerebral leptomeningeal branches. After discussion with the family about the alternative therapies of supportive care, anticoagulation, intracranial embolectomy, and revascularization, the patient was taken to surgery where a left extracranial–intracranial bypass was performed. At the time of surgery, the cortex initially was noted to be pale; the cortical vessels were not full, although there was circulation through the recipient cortical vessel. The anastomosis was completed and open 11 hours and 45 minutes after the onset of the stroke. At this point there was increased filling of the cortical vessels; it was also noted that by this time there was moderate swelling of the left hemisphere. No hemorrhage occurred after the anastomosis was opened.

Postoperatively the patient was maintained on controlled respiration and dexamethasone. Over the next 24 hours he progressively deteriorated and lapsed into coma. During this period there was good pulsation of the donor artery and the flap. The patient died on the second postoperative day. No autopsy was performed, but a postmortem CT scan showed massive left hemisphere swelling with decreased density and no evidence of hemorrhagic infarction.

Comment. This case illustrates failure of revascularization to provide substantial increased circulation, even when completed early in the face of severe neurologic deficit associated with early decreased level of consciousness. In our experience, sudden occlusion of the major vascular supply to a hemisphere without evidence of direct collateral to the ipsilateral middle cerebral is generally associated with massive infarction and death.

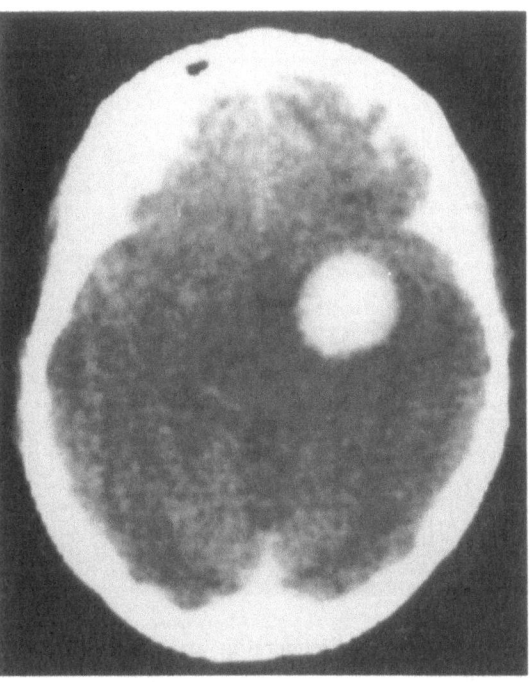

Fig. 50-1. Case 2. Preoperative CT scan demonstrating right giant aneurysm.

Case 2 (L.McC.)

This 34-year-old white female for one year preceding admission had intermittent occipital and right frontal headache and episodes of olfactory hallucinations, followed by flushing, nausea, and generalized weakness. Neurologic examination was normal. EEG showed minor temporal sharp activity with nasopharyngeal leads. A CT scan showed a giant aneurysm filling the right temporal fossa (Fig. 50-1).

Hospital Course. Angiography demonstrated a giant aneurysm arising from the distal right internal carotid just proximal to the anterior and middle cerebral bifurcation (Fig. 50-2). A left carotid injection with cross compression of the right common carotid showed excellent crossing, filling the right middle cerebral without any filling of the aneurysm (Fig. 50-3). In view of the excellent collateral circulation it was elected to treat the aneurysm with progressive occlusion of the right internal artery with a clamp. To avoid sequelae of embolization from the thrombosing internal carotid, the patient was placed on heparin during the occlusion. At the time of placement of the clamp, the internal carotid stump pressure was noted to be 36 mm Hg, so it was concluded that occlusion should be gradual.

The clamp was tightened over a period of 3 days during which the patient was noted to have slight headache and occasional premature ventricular contractions. On the fourth postoperative day, the patient was alert without headache or neurologic deficit. The heparin was discontinued. That evening she complained of progressively severe headaches and appeared slightly lethargic with mild left central facial palsy and arm drift, but no nuchal rigidity. The patient was placed on dexamethasone. The following morning the headache was improved but the right hemisphere deficit was worse. The blood pressure was 100 to 110 systolic. A CT scan was performed which showed thrombosis of the posterior one third of the aneurysm (Fig. 50-4). Angiography showed partial occlusion of the right middle cerebral (Fig. 50-5). The first series was performed with a blood pressure of 106/85, at which time the patient was lethargic. Using phenylephrine the blood pressure was raised to 140 to 150 over 95 to 98. The patient became more alert but showed no change in her left arm drift, and a second injection showed faster angiographic circulation

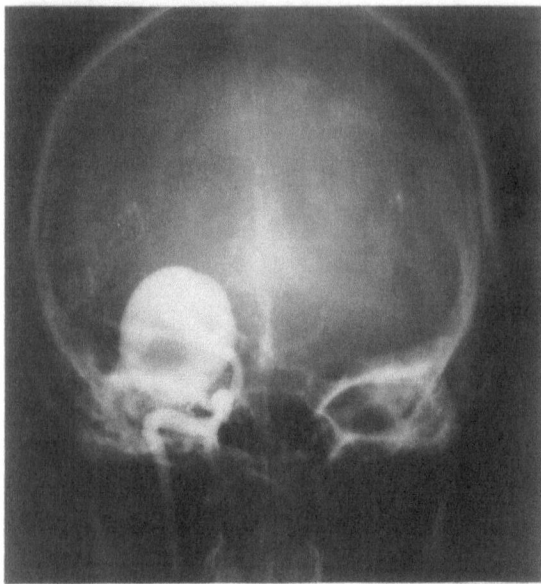

Fig. 50-2. Case 2. Preoperative angiogram demonstrating right internal carotid giant aneurysm.

time but no change in the occlusion. The patient was maintained on the phenylephrine and heparin for 2 days without significant improvement in her focal left-sided weakness. On the sixth postoperative day a STA–MCA anastomosis was performed. At surgery, before clamping of the recipient cortical vessel, an embolus was noted to pass rapidly through the vessel. Over a period of 7 days the patient's neurologic deficit cleared. She had good pulsation of the superficial temporal artery. Before discharge, a CT scan showed that the thrombosis had completely cleared from the aneurysm (Fig. 50-6).

Subsequent Course. It was elected to restudy the patient within 3 months. Her posthospital course was characterized by marked emotional lability with bouts of euphoria and depression. No further seizures occurred. Two days preceding readmission for further studies, her husband reported that, while lying on a sofa waiting to go out for lunch with friends, she suddenly let out a loud gasp and died immediately. Autopsy showed massive rupture of the aneurysm.

Comment. This case illustrates the spectrum of problems that can occur in treating giant aneurysms. Initial studies suggested that carotid occlusion alone should be sufficient. The internal carotid rather than the common carotid was clamped so that the superficial temporal would be available to treat ischemic complications if they occurred. Heparin was utilized to counteract complications of thrombosis and embolization. The patient not only did well until the heparin was discontinued but the aneurysm also showed evidence of partial thrombosis. Once embolization occurred in the absence of heparin, the associated ischemic neurologic deficit was partially improved with elevation of the systemic pressure and completely relieved by bypass. However, the presence of the bypass was also associated with lysis of the thrombus within the aneurysm. Thus, no treatment was accomplished.

During the interval before further studies could be accomplished to see how the aneurysm could be isolated from it superficial temporal feeders, it ruptured.

It would have to be concluded that, if bypass is to be utilized as an adjunct in the treatment of giant aneurysms, if technically possible all potential arterial feeders to the aneurysm should be trapped.

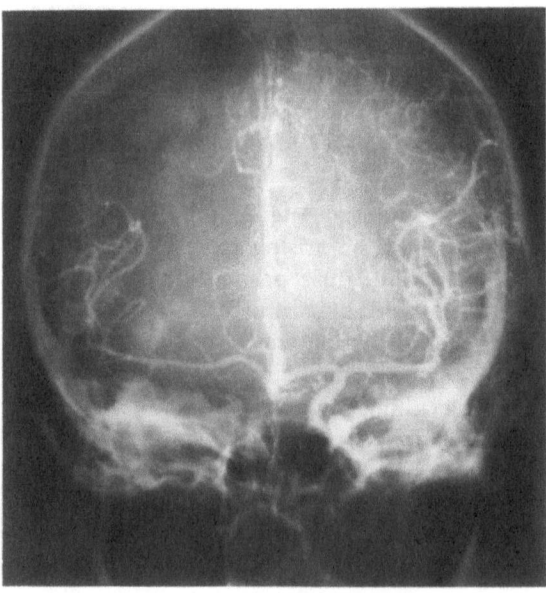

Fig. 50-3. Case 2. Preoperative angiogram demonstrating right middle cerebral filling with cross compression of the right common carotid.

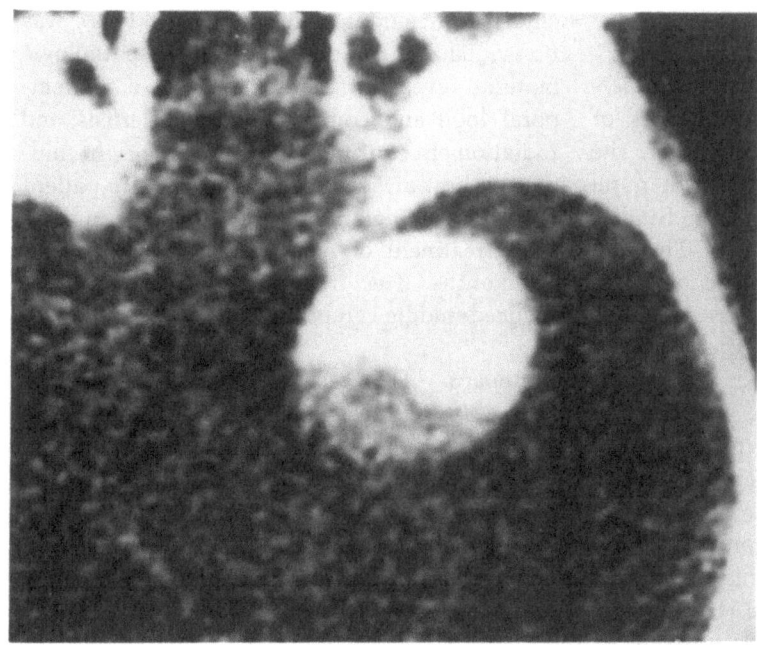

Fig. 50-4. Case 2. Postoperative CT scan demonstrating thrombosis of the posterior portion of the aneurysm.

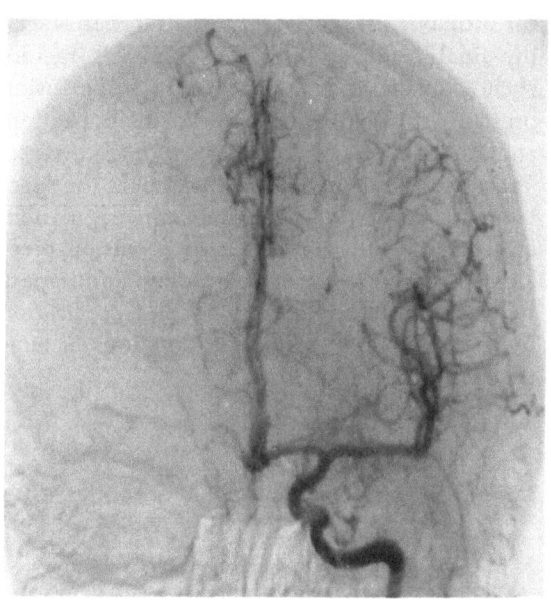

Fig. 50-5. Case 2. Postoperative angiogram demonstrating partial occlusion of the right middle cerebral artery.

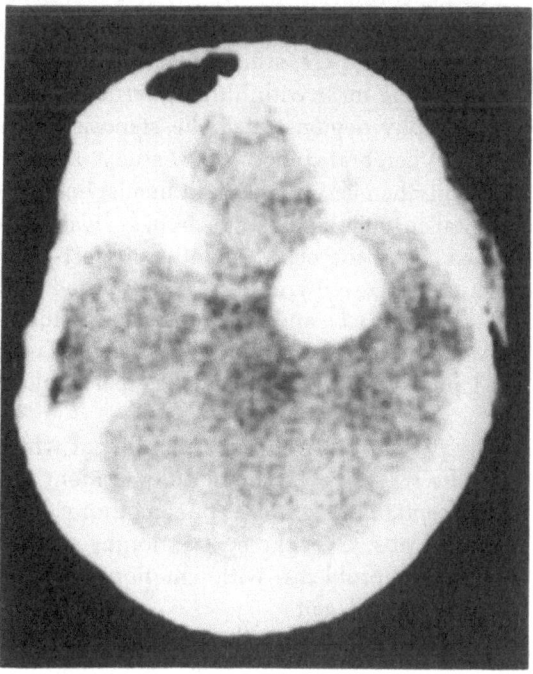

Fig. 50-6. Case 2. Second postoperative CT scan demonstrating partial occlusion of the right middle cerebral artery.

Case 3 (C.S.)

This 58-year-old white female exhibited personality change and intermittent episodes of left hemiparesis. Eighteen months earlier, she had developed enlargement of the right pupil and drooping of the right eyelid. Studies showed evidence of a pituitary tumor. Through a supratentorial approach a large adenoma was removed, leaving a portion which surrounded the right internal carotid and invaded the cavernous sinus. Postoperatively, her third nerve palsy resolved and she received a course of radiation therapy. Five months later she developed emotional lability and intermittent left-sided weaknesses which initially were felt to be seizures and were partially controlled with medication. The episodes continued at a rate of one per month. Seven months later angiography showed a long segment of stenosis of the right middle cerebral.

Examination on admission showed a female appearing chronically ill with marked emotional lability, slight weakness of the left side, and a wide-based gait. CT scan showed evidence of an enhancing mass within the cavernous sinus. Angiography demonstrated the stenosis and a regional cerebral blood flow study showed marked ischemia over the right hemisphere. An occipital-to-middle cerebral bypass was performed. Over the next 3 months, no left-sided weakness occurred and her gait improved. She was readmitted and postoperative studies showed a well-functioning anastomosis with focal improvement in regional cerebral blood flow.

The patient did well for 7 months, at which time she was involved in an auto accident and was hospitalized with a pneumothorax and fractured ribs. Over the next 5 months she had progressive problems with emotional lability and wide-based gait.

A repeated CT scan showed an increase in the parasellar enhancing mass. The patient was readmitted. Clinical examination at that time suggested marked bilateral frontal lobe disease and repeated angiography showed a functioning bypass but, now, occlusion of the left middle cerebral artery.

Although the outlook was poor, it was elected to explore the sellar area. Only necrotic temporal lobe was found with a fibrotic occluded right middle cerebral artery. There was no evidence of tumor. Review of the pathologic material revealed radiation necrosis of the temporal lobe and combined atherosclerosis and radiation effect of the segment of the right middle cerebral artery. Postoperatively the patient progressively deteriorated and died 30 months after treatment of her pituitary adenoma and 13 months after treatment of her radiation-induced middle cerebral stenosis.

Comment. This case illustrates that the bypass appeared to relieve the focal symptoms related to the right middle cerebral stenosis; however, the unrelenting progressive diffuse deficit associated with radiation effects to both frontal lobes, the temporal lobe, and both middle cerebral arteries could not be halted.

Conclusion

These cases point out that EC–IC bypass, as carotid endarterectomy, works best if utilized for prophylaxis. Once cerebral infarction starts, the final result is related to multiple factors such as available collateral channels, perfusion pressures, thrombogenesis and embolization, and associated brain parenchymal disease. Treatment regimens which encompass the spectrum of proper oxygenation, anticoagulation, antiedema agents, elevation of perfusion pressure, thrombectomy, embolectomy, and bypass require careful serial analysis and application to the pathologic processes that are encountered.

References

1. Chater, N., Popp, J. Microsurgical vascular bypass for occlusive cerebral vascular disease: Review of 100 cases. Surg Neurol 6:115–118, 1976.
2. Gratzl, O., Schmiedek, P., Spetzler, R., Steinhoff, H., Marguth, F. Clinical experience wtih extra–intracranial arterial anastomosis in 65 cases. J Neurosurg 44:313–324, 1976.
3. Sundt, T.M.Jr., Siekert, R.G., Piepgras, D.G., Sharbrough, F.W., Houser, O.W. Bypass surgery for vascular disease of the carotid system. Mayo Clin Proc 51:677–692, 1976.

51

Hemorrhagic Infarction after Microsurgical Cerebral Revascularization

Roberto C. Heros and Paul N. Nelson

Since the early days of carotid surgery, clinicians have feared that acute revascularization of ischemic brain may result in hemorrhagic infarction. We have recently encountered such a complication after an extracranial–intracranial (EC–IC) bypass graft. Only two similar cases have been reported in the literature.[22, 28]

This study was performed to determine the incidence of hemorrhagic infarction after EC–IC bypass surgery and to attempt to define the clinical setting of such complication and specific factors that may contribute to its development. With these aims we reviewed the literature and surveyed a number of surgeons known to have an interest in microsurgical revascularization.

Case Report

A 66-year-old hypertensive male had two reversible episodes of right hemiparesis and expressive aphasia lasting for several days each in 1975. He did well until December 1977, when he had a similar episode which left him with mild residual expressive aphasia. He was treated with heparin. Two weeks later heparin was stopped in preparation for angiography. Six hours later he had a left hemispheric transient ischemic attack (TIA). Angiography showed complete occlusion of the left cervical internal carotid artery (ICA) with reconstituted supracavernous ICA which, on retrospective

study, seemed to lodge an irregular plaque with a small intraluminal thrombus (Fig. 51-1). He was entered in the cooperative EC–IC study and randomized for surgery. Heparin, which was restarted after angiography, was stopped the night before surgery. The patient awoke with a severe right hemiparesis and global aphasia, and the operation was cancelled. A CT scan showed a small low-density area in the left hemisphere (Fig. 51-2).

Anticoagulation was resumed and he made a good recovery over the next several weeks. Some fluctuation in his deficit, at times postural, led us to suspect that, although repeated embolism was largely responsible for his ischemic episodes, hemodynamic factors may also be playing a role. He was rehospitalized, coumadin was stopped, and heparin was restarted until the time of surgery.

A left superficial temporal-to-middle cerebral (STA–MCA) bypass graft was performed on 3 March, 1978, 8 weeks after his last stroke. There were no unusual technical problems at surgery. The systolic pressure ranged between 140 and 160 except for a 15-min period of pressures around 100 early during the operation. Clamping time was about 35 minutes. Upon arrival at the recovery room the blood pressure was 240/120 but his neurologic status was unchanged from the preoperative state. Over the next 40 hours he was stable neurologically and, indeed, our neurologic consultant felt that he was somewhat improved over his

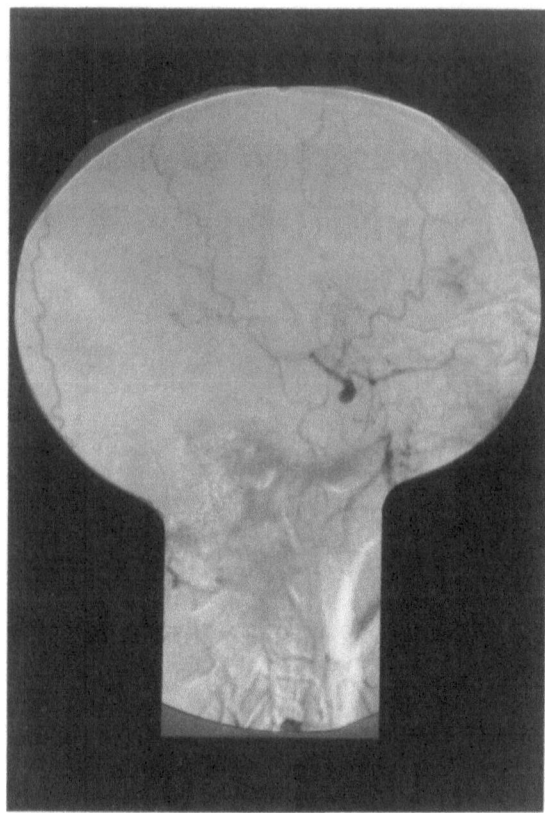

Fig. 51-1. Preoperative left common carotid angiogram. Note the irregular plaque with probable intraluminal thrombus in the supracavernous segment of the ICA.

preoperative status. Considerable difficulty was experienced controlling the blood pressure first with nitroglycerin and later with nitroprusside.

The second postoperative day he developed significant worsening of his aphasia and some drowsiness. A CT scan showed a hemorrhagic area (Fig. 51-3). Reoperation, undertaken to rule out an extracerebral hematoma, disclosed a swollen brain with obvious hemorrhagic infarction. The anastomosis was patent. Since then he has recovered to almost the preoperative status but still has considerable difficulty expressing himself. In addition he has had some focal seizures involving the right upper extremity. A follow-up angiogram has shown fair segmental filling of the MCA through the anastomosis. The STA is smaller, throughout its length, than in the preoperative angiogram (Figs. 51-4, 51-5).

Case Analysis

The relationship of each of this patient's recent ischemic events to the discontinuation of anticoagulants strongly suggests that the basic problem was one of repeated embolism. The retrospective recognition of a probable intraluminal thrombus in the supracavernous segment of the left ICA makes this the most likely site of origin of the emboli. Technical factors are not likely to have played a major role in the production of his subsequent deficit, since he was at least unchanged and possibly slightly improved the first postoperative day. For the same reason it is unlikely, though not impossible, that the hemorrhagic infarction occurred at the time of surgery or immediately postoperatively. If the only significant factor had been reperfusion of an ischemic area, the problem would have been most likely to have developed immediately after reperfusion—although it is possible that vasospasm may have

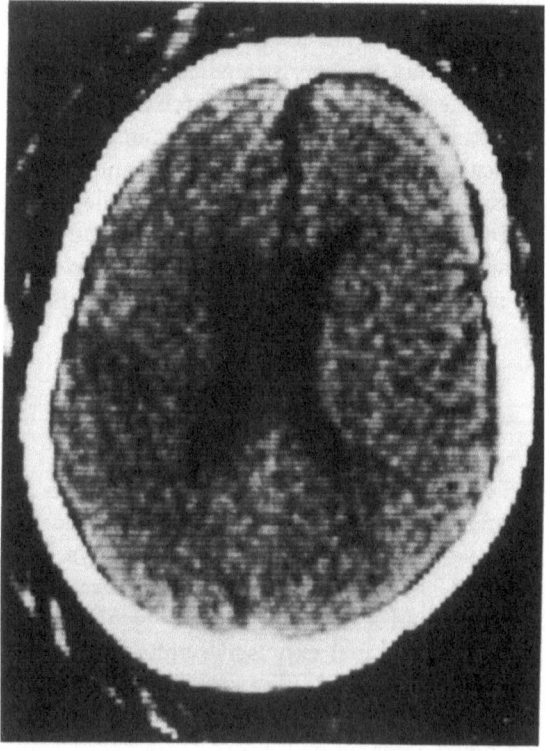

Fig. 51-2. Preoperative CT scan. Note small low-density area in the left posterior frontal-parietal region indicative of a bland infarct.

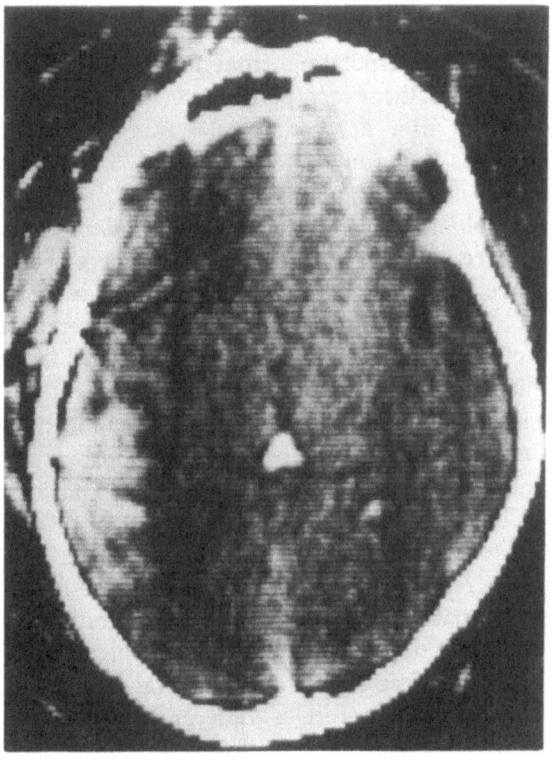

Fig. 51-3. CT scan 48 hours after surgery. Note high-density area indicative of hemorrhagic infarction.

not have been considered a candidate for STA–MCA; instead, he should have been treated with long-term anticoagulation. In addition we should have been much more strict in controlling the postoperative blood pressure, especially during the critical period of transportation from the operating table to the recovery room.

Summary of Other Cases

We have restricted our analysis to cases in which a hemorrhagic infarction or gross intracerebral hemorrhage occurred postoperatively in the general area potentially "revascularized," namely, the middle cerebral territory, since all the cases collected involved anastomosis to a middle cerebral branch. Thus we have excluded

maintained the flow through the anastomosis at a low level initially. We feel that it is more likely that this patient experienced further embolism into his middle cerebral territory postoperatively since anticoagulants were not restarted after surgery. In addition it appears quite likely that the postoperative hypertension contributed significantly to the hemorrhagic nature of his infarct.

The role played by the anastomosis itself remains unclear to us. Although the anastomosis is patent in the follow-up angiogram, the flow through it does not appear to be great at this time. It is possible that it was higher initially and decreased with time as a result of lesser demand from the grossly infarcted tissue, but whether this actually occurred remains speculative. It is of interest in this regard that the STA is smaller throughout its length in the follow-up angiogram, which is the first time we have observed this phenomenon.

In retrospect we feel that this patient should

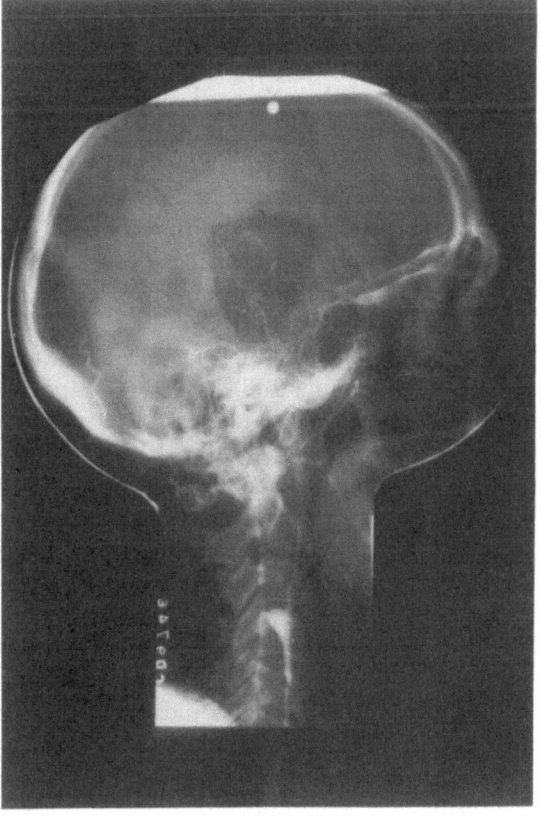

Fig. 51-4. Left common carotid angiogram 4 months after surgery; early arterial phase. Note small STA starting to fill some MCA branches.

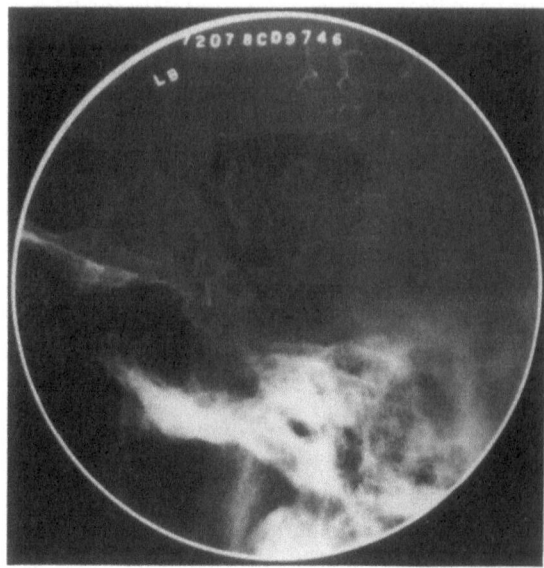

Fig. 51-5. Later arterial phase of postoperative angiogram showing fair segmental filling of MCA arterial territory.

two cases of postoperative cerebellar hemorrhage reported by Yasargil and Yonekawa which were clearly related to postoperative hypertension.[34] Even though the subject of this review is "hemorrhagic infarction" we are including intracerebral hemorrhages occurring in relation to the anastomosis because in most cases this differentiation could not be made clinically and only two cases came to autopsy.

Table 51-1 summarizes the salient features of each case. Cases 1 and 2 have been reported in the literature.[22, 28] Summaries of cases 3 through 8 were obtained through the kindness of the surgeon involved in each case. Forty surgeons were contacted and 32 replies were obtained. From these replies and from other series in the literature that allude specifically to complications,[2, 4, 10, 15, 18, 22, 24, 28, 29, 34] a total of about 1600 cases of EC–IC bypass operations were collected. The exact number is not known because several respondents did not recall the total number of cases personally performed or gave only an approximate number. An effort was made to ascertain the total number of cases performed after a recent stroke. Many respondents, however, did not have these specific figures and some operations were performed for "TIAs with residual deficit" or "slowly

progressive deficit" which would be hard to classify. Interpolating from the several series in which the exact percentage of cases performed after a recent stroke was known, it appears that roughly about 10 to 25% of the cases might be in this category. In most, the neurologic deficit was minimal to moderate and apparently very few patients with severe deficit have been operated upon. Thus, the nine cases of hemorrhagic infarction or intracerebral hemorrhage we have collected out of this large number of operations represents an overall incidence of about 0.5% for this complication. In cases with a recent stroke the approximate incidence appears to be between 2% and 5%.

The ages of the cases collected range from 43 to 70 years and there were six males and three females. All the anastomoses were found to be patent either by direct inspection at reoperation or by angiography or Doppler sonography. In case 5 the distal occipital artery was small, and therefore a vein graft was interposed between the proximal occipital artery and a cortical middle cerebral branch. The rest of the operations were STA–MCA bypass grafts. In case 2, in addition to an STA–MCA graft an embolectomy was performed in an angular branch, and this may have contributed to the subsequent hemorrhagic infarction.[22] In case 5 the patient deteriorated several days postoperatively and generalized spasm of the middle cerebral artery was found angiographically. This was treated with hypertensive agents which may have contributed to the subsequent hemorrhage.

Perhaps the most striking finding is that in all seven instances in which this question was answered specifically the patient experienced significant postoperative hypertension prior to clinical deterioration. In the other two cases no information about the postoperative blood pressure was obtained.

Discussion

The first clinical reports of hemorrhagic infarction after surgical revascularization appeared soon after the development of carotid surgery.[3, 14, 23, 31] Many of these early cases occurred after thromboendarterectomy of com-

Table 51-1. Clinical summary

Case	Hx of ↑ BP[a]	Angiography[b]	Recent stroke	Postop ↑ BP[c]	Complication	Day P OP[d]	Result	Comment
1[e]	No	R ICA L ICA	No	Yes	Frontal hemorrhage	0	Mild hemiparesis	Hematoma not directly under graft
2[f]	Yes	R ICA L ICA	Mild 2 weeks	Yes	Hemorrhage + hem. infarct	1	Died	Embolectomy of cortical branch
3	Yes	R ICA L ICA	Moderate 10 weeks	Yes	Large F–P hemorrhage	2	Died	
4	?	L ICA	No	?	Hem. infarct	1	Moderate hemiparesis	Hypotension intra-op
5	Yes	L ICA R ICA(s)	No	Yes	Massive hemorrhage	14	Died	MCA spasm Rx with ↑ BP
6	Yes	?	Moderate 8 weeks	Yes	F–T deep hemorrhage	1	Hemiplegia aphasia	
7	?	R MCA(s)	No	Yes	Hemorrhage + hem. infarct	0	Died	
8	?	L I–C ICA(s) R ICA	Moderate "recent"	?	Hemorrhage + hem. infarct	4	Hemiplegia	
9[g]	Yes	L ICA	Moderate 8 weeks	Yes	Hem. infarct	2	Moderate aphasia	Probable embolism from I–C ICA

[a] History of hypertension preoperatively.
[b] Preoperative angiographic findings: ICA = cervical internal carotid occlusion; I–C ICA = intracranial internal carotid occlusion; (s) = stenosis.
[c] Significant elevation of the blood pressure postoperatively.
[d] Postoperative day in which the complication became clinically apparent.
[e] Sundt's case.[28]
[f] Reichman's case.[22]
[g] Present case.

pletely occluded carotids soon after the occurrence of a severe neurologic deficit. An analysis of these reports, however, reveals that in some instances the gross pathologic description resembled more a typical hypertensive hemorrhage than a true hemorrhagic infarction. No mention is made in any of these early reports of the postoperative blood pressure. Wylie later admitted that postoperative hypertension was common after carotid endarterectomy and may have played a significant role in some of his early fatalities from brain hemorrhage.[32] It is also clear from the early reports that, although most patients did have a recent completed stroke or a stroke in evolution, some did not and were operated upon because of TIAs. These ischemic episodes were sometimes referable to the opposite hemisphere or to the posterior circulation. An additional mechanism that may have been responsible for some of the hemorrhagic infarctions reported is cerebral embolism from dissection around the carotid plaque, as recently suggested by Sundt.[27] It is well known that cerebral embolism commonly leads to hemorrhagic infarction and in fact the latter may be quite rare in cerebral ischemia from nonembolic occlusions.[12] In summary, we agree with Fisher's opinion that there is no substantial evidence for the claim that reestablishment of cervical carotid flow can convert a pale infarct into a hemorrhagic one[13] unless complicated by postoperative hypertension or intraoperative embolism. Several large endarterectomy series reinforce this conclusion.[8, 21, 27, 30]

Direct restoration of flow in the middle cerebral artery, however, would logically appear more likely to result in hemorrhagic infarction. In this case the occlusion is closer to the area of ischemia and distal to the circle of Willis with consequent less opportunity for collateralization. In other words, middle cerebral occlusion with subsequent reestablishment of flow closely resembles the usual mechanism of spontaneous hemorrhagic infarction.[12] Thus it is not surprising that experimentally hemorrhagic infarction can be produced by reestablishing flow after about 6 hours of temporary occlusion of the middle cerebral artery by a clip[5] or artificial embolus.[11] At least three clinical cases of hemorrhagic infarction after acute middle cerebral embolectomy have been reported.[26, 33]

Anastomosis of a relatively small extracranial artery to a cortical cerebral artery is quite different, from a hemodynamic point of view, from restitution of either carotid or middle cerebral flow. Blood flow through such anastomosis averages roughly 28 to 35 ml/min acutely[1, 24, 25] as opposed to an average flow of about 120 ml/min for the middle cerebral artery and about 250 ml/min for the internal carotid artery.[7, 16, 20, 24] In spite of this relatively small flow, at least in one study, STA–MCA grafts performed 4 and 24 hours after MCA occlusion in dogs resulted in a high incidence of hemorrhagic infarction.[9] An earlier report had indicated that when the anastomosis was completed by about 2 hours after MCA ligation the incidence of hemorrhagic infarction was less in the animals with anastomosis than in the control animals with MCA ligation.[6]

We attempted to define the period of time after a stroke during which an EC–IC bypass operation would carry a high risk of resulting in hemorrhagic infarction. Some of the experimental evidence just alluded to suggests that if revascularization is accomplished before 6 hours after occlusion the incidence of hemorrhagic infarction is lower than when revascularization is delayed beyond this period.[6, 9, 11] Crowell collected twelve clinical cases of EC–IC bypasses performed 4 hours to 4 days after acute ischemia. No patient developed a hemorrhagic infarction but three patients who were obtunded and had panhemispheric deficits prior to surgery continued to deteriorate and died from progressive cerebral edema and herniation.[7] Pathologic evidence suggests that, after cerebral arterial occlusion, progressive brain

softening becomes maximal at one week and progressive healing occurs during the following 8 weeks.[17, 19] It is likely that after this period of time revascularization should be safe. Indeed, the cases in the present series that developed hemorrhagic infarction after a stroke did so between 2 and 8 weeks after the stroke. Of course some patients developed hemorrhagic infarction who did not have a previous stroke. Therefore, no definite statement can be made from the data available, but it appears likely that an EC–IC bypass procedure performed on a patient who has had a stroke more than 2 months previously carries no significantly higher risk of hemorrhagic infarction than if done on patients without a recent stroke.

Conclusions

The overall incidence of postoperative hemorrhagic infarction after EC–IC bypass grafts is probably less than 1%. The incidence in cases operated on after a completed stroke is probably no higher than 5%.

Postoperative hypertension preceded clinical deterioration in the majority of the cases of hemorrhagic infarction collected here. Therefore it is likely that strict control of the blood pressure postoperatively could prevent many of these complications.

An analysis of our case suggests that, at least in this particular patient, postoperative cerebral embolism, complicated by postoperative hypertension, may have been responsible for the hemorrhagic infarct. It is possible that treatment with anticoagulants instead of surgery may avoid such complication in patients with suspected recurrent cerebral embolism. Confirmation of this assumption, however, must await the result of a well-controlled cooperative study.

Acknowledgment

We are grateful to Dr. O.M. Reinmuth, Chief of Neurology at the University of Pittsburgh, for his invaluable assistance in managing this patient and for his helpful comments about the subject of this paper.

References

1. Austin, G., Laffin, D., Hayward, W. Cerebral blood flow in patients undergoing microanastomosis for modification or prevention of stroke. Ann Clin Lab Sci 5:229–235, 1975.
2. Austin, G., Hayward, W., Laffin, D. Modification of cerebral ischemia by microsurgical intracranial anastomosis. In Microneurosurgical Anastomoses for Cerebral Ischemia, G.M. Austin, editor, Charles C Thomas, Springfield, 1976, pp 281–294.
3. Bruetman, M.E., Fields, W.S., Crawford, E.S., De Bakey, M.E. Cerebral hemorrhage as a complication of surgery in carotid artery occlusion. Trans Am Neurol Assoc 88:52–55, 1963.
4. Chater, N., Popp, J. Microsurgical vascular bypass for occlusive cerebrovascular disease: review of 100 cases. Surg Neurol 6:115–118, 1976.
5. Crowell, R.M., Olsson, Y., Klatzo, I., Ommaya, A. Temporary occlusion of the middle cerebral artery in the monkey: clinical and pathological observations. Stroke 1:439–448, 1970.
6. Crowell, R.M., Olsson, Y. Effect of extracranial–intracranial vascular bypass graft on experimental acute stroke in dogs. J Neurosurg 38:26–31, 1973.
7. Crowell, R.M. STA–MCA bypass for acute focal cerebral ischemia. In Microsurgery for Stroke, P. Schmiedek, editor, Springer-Verlag, New York, 1977, pp 244–250.
8. De Bakey, M.E., Crawford, E.S., Cooley, D.A., Morris, G.C., Garrett, H.E., Fields, W.S. Cerebral arterial insufficiency: one to eleven year results following arterial reconstructive operation. Ann Surg 161:921–945, 1965.
9. Diaz, F.G., Ausman, J.I., Mastri, A. The value of cerebral revascularization after acute ischemic infarction. Abstract. Neurosurgery 2:158, 1978.
10. Donaghy, P. Evaluation of extracranial–intracranial blood flow diversion. In Microneurosurgical Anastomoses for Cerebral Ischemia, G. M. Austin, editor, Charles C Thomas, Springfield, 1976, pp 256–274.
11. Dujovny, M., Osgood, C.P., Barrionuevo, P., Hellstrom, R., Maroon, J. Experimental middle cerebral artery microsurgical embolectomy. Acta Neurochir 35:91–96, 1976.
12. Fisher, C.M., Adams, R.D. Observations of brain embolism with special reference to the mechanism of hemorrhagic infarction. J Neurosurg Exp Neurol 10:92–94, 1951.
13. Fisher, C.M. The natural history of carotid occlusion. In Microneurosurgical Anastomoses for Cerebral Ischemia, G.M. Austin, editor, Charles C Thomas, Springfield, 1976, pp 194–201.
14. Gonzales, L.I., Carson, M.L. Cerebral hemorrhage following successful endarterectomy of the internal carotid artery. Surg Gynecol Obstet 122:773–777, 1966.
15. Gratzl, O., Schmiedek, P., Spetzler, R., Steinhoff, H., Marguth, F. Clinical experience with extra–intracranial arterial anastomosis in 65 cases. J Neurosurg 44:313–324, 1976.
16. Hardesty, M.H., Roberts, B., Toole, J.P., Royster, H.P. Studies on carotid artery flow. Surgery 49:251–256, 1961.
17. Harvey, J., Rasmussen, T. Occlusion of middle cerebral artery; experimental study. Arch Neurol Psychiatry 66:20, 1951.
18. Merei, T.F., Bodosi, M. Microsurgical anastomosis for cerebral ischemia in ninety patients. In Microsurgery for Stroke, P. Schmiedek, editor, Springer-Verlag, New York, 1977, pp 264–270.
19. Meyer, J.S. Importance of ischemic damage to small vessels in experimental cerebral infarction. J Neuropathol 17:571, 1958.
20. Nornes, H., Wikeby, P. Cerebral arterial blood flow and aneurysm surgery. Part I: Local arterial flow dynamics. J Neurosurg 47:810–818, 1977.
21. Ojemann, R.G., Crowell, R.M., Roberson, G. H., Fisher, C.M. Surgical treatment of extracranial carotid occlusive disease. Clin Neurosurg 22:214–263, 1975.
22. Reichman, O.H. Complications of cerebral revascularization. Clin Neurosurg 23:318–335, 1976.
23. Rob, C.G. Operation for acute completed stroke due to thrombosis of the internal carotid artery. Surgery 65:862–865, 1969.
24. Samson, D.S., Boone, S. Extracranial–intracranial (EC–IC) arterial bypass: past performance and current concepts. Neurosurgery 3:79–85, 1978.
25. Spetzler, R., Chater, N. Microvascular bypass surgery. Part 2: Physiological studies. J Neurosurg 45:508–513, 1976.
26. Sundt, T.M., Nofzinger, J.D. Clip-grafts for aneurysm and small vessel surgery. J Neurosurg 27:477–489, 1967.
27. Sundt, T.M., Sandok, B.A., Whisnant, J.P.: Carotid endarterectomy. Complications and preoperative assessment of risk. Mayo Clin Proc 50:301–306, 1975.
28. Sundt, T.M., Siekert, R.H., Piepgras, D.G., Sharbrough, F.M., Houser, O.W. Bypass surgery for vascular disease of the carotid system. Mayo Clin Proc 51:677–692, 1976.
29. Tew, J.M. Reconstructive intracranial vascular surgery for prevention of stroke. Clin Neurosurg 22:264–280, 1975.
30. Thompson, J.E., Austin, D.J., Patman, R.D. Carotid endarterectomy for cerebrovascular insufficiency. Ann Surg 172:663–679, 1970.
31. Wylie, E.J., Hein, M.F., Adams, J.E. Intracranial hemorrhage following surgical revascularization for treatment of acute strokes. J Neurosurg 21:212–215, 1964.

32. Wylie, E.J. Discussion of paper by Thompson, J.E., Austin, D.J., Patman, R.D. endarterectomy of the totally occluded carotid artery for stroke. Arch Surg 95:791–801, 1967.

33. Yasargil, M.G. Diagnosis and indications for operations in cerebrovascular occlusive disease. In Microsurgery Applied to Neurosurgery, M. G. Yasargil, Verlag-Stuttgart Academic Press, New York, pp 95–118.

34. Yasargil, M.G., Yonekawa, Y. Results of microsurgical extra–intracranial arterial bypass in the treatment of cerebral ischemia. Neurosurgery 1:22–24, 1977.

52

Extracranial–Intracranial Anastomosis in Cerebrovascular Disease

D. Shaw

The development of microvascular techniques has made possible the revascularization of parts of the cerebrum by direct surgical approach. The operation of extracranial–intracranial (EC–IC) anastomosis has been performed frequently throughout the world but we are aware of only three reported cases in Britain. During the past year eleven such operations have been performed in Newcastle without preoperative or postoperative mortality and with little morbidity. These cases are described and possible indications for the operation are briefly discussed.

Patients and Methods

The clinical details of the eleven patients are shown in Table 52-1. Ten had suffered episodes of transient cerebral ischemia in either the retinal or cerebral circulation and seven had mild residual deficit. One patient had no history of transient ischemic attacks but had suffered a right hemisphere stroke. Eight patients had complete occlusion of one or both internal carotid arteries, two had stenosis of the internal carotid artery which was inaccessible to carotid endarterectomy, and one had a large inoperable aneurysm of the left middle cerebral artery which was associated with transient ischemic attacks in the territory of that artery.

All operations were carried out according to the standard technique. A suitable branch of the superficial temporal artery is isolated and,

through a small craniectomy, is anastomosed end to side to a branch of the middle cerebral artery on the surface of the brain. The vessels used are of the order of 1 to 2 mm in diameter, necessitating the use of an operating microscope.

Results

Of the eleven patients, nine have had postoperative angiograms after a period of 6 to 24 weeks, and in all the anastomoses were patent. Two patients suffered postoperative deep vein thrombosis; one developed a small pulmonary embolus but there were no other complications, and no patient suffered an increase in neurologic deficit as a result of vascular manipulation at the time of the operation.

One patient died of a myocardial infarction 8 months after operation; at autopsy the anastomosis was shown to be patent.

The three patients who had transient ischemic attacks without residual deficit still have no abnormal neurologic signs after 15, 8, and 6 months. Of those who originally had deficits, two have recovered completely and the others have shown improvement.

Discussion

Newcastle experience has simply confirmed the feasibility of EC–IC anastomosis between

Table 52-1. Extracranial–intracranial arterial anastomosis

Patient	Age	Sex	Symptoms	Angiography	Result	Outcome	Check angiography anastomosis
R.L.	62	M	Left hemisphere TIAs and stroke	Large aneurysm of left middle cerebral artery	Improved with persisting dysphasia	Alive after 15 months	Refused
R.M.	65	M	Left hemisphere TIAs	Stenosis of intra-cranial portion of left internal carotid artery	No deficit	Alive after 15 months	Patent
F.E.	65	M	Right hemisphere TIAs and stroke	Occlusion right ICA	No deficit	Alive after 15 months	Patent
D.G.	65	F	Bilateral hemi-sphere TIAs and left hemisphere stroke	Occlusion left ICA Stenosis right ICA	Persisting dysphasia Deep vein thrombosis	Death after 8 months from myo-cardial infarct	Patent
J.M.	63	M	Bilateral hemi-sphere TIAs and left stroke, confusion	Bilateral occlu-sion ICA	Improved but residual dysphasia	Alive after 10 months	Patent
D.G.	43	F	Left hemisphere TIAs and stroke, confusion	Occlusion left ICA Stenosis right ICA	Marked improvement Dysphasia and right hemi-paresis	Alive after 10 months	Patent
E.D.	53	F	Right hemisphere TIAs	Occlusion right ICA	No deficit	Alive after 8 months	Patent
L.G.	56	M	Right hemisphere TIAs and stroke	Occlusion right ICA	Persisting left hemiparesis	Alive after 6 months	Patent
F.R.	59	M	Right amaurosis fugax	Right carotid siphon and bifurcation stenosis	No deficit	Alive after 6 months	Patent
B.M.	65	M	Left hemisphere TIAs, confusion	Occlusion right ICA Stenosis left ICA	No deficit, improved mental state	Alive after 4 months	Patent
J.B.	56	M	Right hemisphere stroke	Occlusion right ICA	Mild left hemiparesis	Alive after 2 months	Not yet done

branches of the superficial temporal artery and middle cerebral artery. The operation, which is relatively safe, appears to help some patients with cerebrovascular disease, but the extent of the benefit achieved and the precise indications for its performance remain uncertain. It has a rational basis for patients with occlusion or inoperable stenosis of the carotid artery who are suffering from ischemic symptoms in appropriate territory. It is less logical to perform an anastomosis on patients with completed strokes due to lesions distal to stenosis or oc-clusions, but the possibility exists that terri-tories of the brain may suffer prolonged ische-mia without infarction and, in this circum-stance, infarction might be prevented by an-astomosis. A third group are patients with dif-fuse disease and without focal symptoms; the rationale for operation in these cases seems dubious.

The indications for this operation are thus yet to be defined. While all eleven patients in our series showed improvement, we cannot assess what their progress might have been if managed conservatively. Like many others who have perfromed this operation, we are not in a position to draw any firm conclusions about its efficacy. Furthermore, it is not entirely without hazard; nor is the preliminary arteriography which is a prerequisite.

How then is the future role of this operation to be established? We are reminded of the aphorism of the late Lord Cohen that the feasibility of an operation is not necessarily an indication for its performance. There is a danger that a procedure which is technically success-ful may become part of established therapeutic practice without proper evaluation. The story of carotid endarterectomy is a case in point. We are optimistic about the future of the anastomotic procedure but are convinced of the need for its careful monitoring. As participants, we look forward to the outcome of the cooperative study of EC–IC arterial anastomosis which is directed by Dr. Henry Barnett of London, Ontario, and funded by the National Institutes of Health and which involves 32 centers in North America and Europe.

53

Results in 51 Patients with EC–IC Bypass: Technical and Clinical Considerations

R. Deruty, J. Lecuire, P. Bret, and J. Capdeville

During the past 6 years, we have operated on 51 patients with EC–IC bypass, performing a total of 60 bypasses.

The purpose of this paper is to review our material and our results, to discuss some technical aspects, and to emphasize some clinical problems.

Material and Methods

Fifty-one patients were operated on from 1972 to 1978. Every patient suffered from cerebral ischemia; none of them was operated on prior to other surgery (aneurysm or tumor surgery).

Clinically, 17 patients had suffered with transient or reversible ischemia; they were asymptomatic at the time of surgery. Thirty-three patients had suffered with stroke and still presented a deficit—either mild in most cases, or complete palsy in other cases. One patient was admitted with a stroke in evolution and had a severe hemiplegia at the time of surgery.

No patient was operated on in emergency. Most were operated on within 3 months after the ischemic accident; in four patients, surgery was carried out after a long delay, 1 year or more after the onset of stroke.

The superficial temporal artery was used in 47 patients; in the other four, the bypass was performed with the occipital artery. In 42 patients, one bypass was performed; in the other nine, two bypasses were carried out, using both branches of the STA, during the same operation. Thus 60 bypasses were achieved.

As far as cortical arteries are concerned, we used: a temporal or the angular artery in 38 cases, and a parietal or a fronto-opercular artery in 22 cases.

To assess the bypass patency, we tried to perform an angiographic control in each case within 15 days after surgery. This was possible in 47 patients. In the other four, patency was assessed either by Doppler examination or by the pulse of STA at the site of the craniectomy. In fourteen patients, a second angiographic control was performed one year later.

Results

Patency Rate

Forty-seven patients underwent an early angiographic control and thus 56 anastomoses were angiographically studied; 41 were patent. Of the other four, patency was presumed in two cases by means of Doppler examination or pulse palpation. Thus the early patency rate is 43 out of 60 anastomoses.

A second angiographic control was performed later in 14 patients, checking 18 bypasses. Of the latter, 4 bypasses, not visualized on the first angiography, happened to be patent on the second one.[3] No patent bypass happened to be occluded on the second angiography.

In the cases of double bypass (9 patients), both anastomoses were patent in 6 cases; one anastomosis was occluded in 3 cases.

The definitive patency rate, evaluated after one year, is 46 bypasses out of 60 (76.6%); on 51 patients, 41 (80.3%) have at least one patent bypass.

Clinical Results

Mortality-Morbidity. One patient died after surgery (intratemporal hematoma); one patient was impaired (acute subdural hematoma). Minor and transient complications occurred in 5 patients (4 transient aphasia, 1 chronic subdural hematoma).

Functional Results. Seventeen patients were asymptomatic at the time of surgery; 2 presented a further recurrence of ischemia, due to the same pathology in 1 of them. Thirty-four patients out of 51 were operated on with a deficit; 16 improved after surgery. Such an improvement was presumably related to surgery in 7 of them; for the other 9, the same improvement probably would have occurred without surgery.

Discussion

As do many people, we think that the main questions raised by this surgery are not about the technical procedure. The most questionable problems concern the clinical results and the actual effectiveness of the procedure.

Several questions are to be asked, which we will try to answer with the help of our limited experience.

First Question

What is the effectiveness of the bypass surgery for the prevention of cerebral ischemia? Is a bypass of real value to prevent the recurrence of TIAs or to prevent the onset of a stroke? This is the major question, since patients with transient or reversible ischemic attacks are considered the best candidates for this surgery.

There is some support for effectiveness, angiographic as well as hemodynamic and clinical. For example, in some of our cases we could demonstrate on angiography that the bypass is able to act as a communicating artery (Fig. 53-1). On the lateral view of this angiograph, the bypass was patent, located on a temporal or angular artery. No fronto-opercular artery was supplied through the bypass. During the same angiography a digital compression of the contralateral carotid artery was performed, and at this time the fronto-opercular arteries became supplied through the bypass. So, in this case, the bypass spontaneously did not fill the complete territory of MCA. Should the contralateral carotid artery be occluded, however, then the bypass could possibly supply some additional arteries.

Clinically, one cannot say with certainty whether such an additional blood supply would be able to prevent ischemic damage. For instance, in a patient with bilateral stenosis of the siphon, a bypass was performed on the right side. A good patency was obtained, as shown on the angiographic control 15 days after surgery (Fig. 53-2). Meanwhile, however, a complete thrombosis of the affected carotid artery was demonstrated as a result of the bypass surgery. The patient was doing well immediately after surgery, but another reversible ischemic attack occurred 3 weeks later; at this time, the CBF value was unchanged when compared with the preoperative values.

Second Question

What is the effectiveness of the bypass surgery for the treatment of a stroke? Is a bypass of any value to improve a patient with hemiplegia?

The answer to this question is really difficult, for the natural history of stroke is well known. Everybody knows that a spontaneous improvement may occur during the months following the stroke. When the improvement occurs early and dramatically after the bypass surgery (as it occurred in 7 of our cases), such an improvement can possibly be connected to the bypass. This is not a certainty, however, but only a presumption. For a lot of people, the bypass surgery is not indicated in cases of stroke with

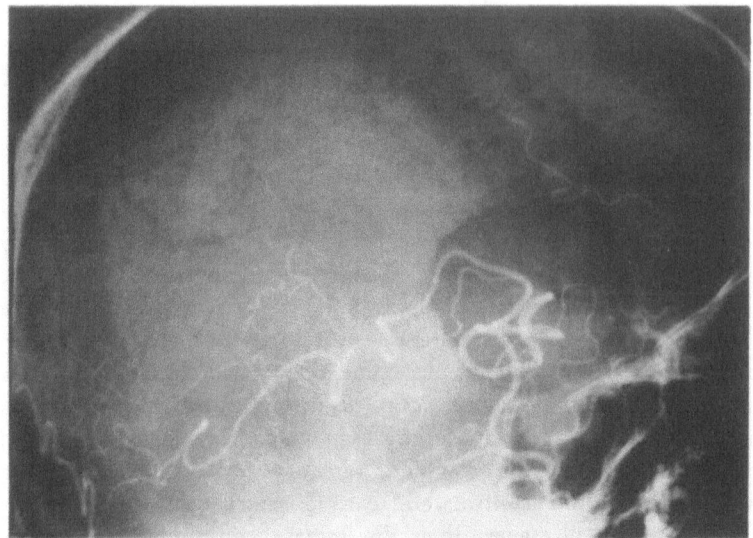

A

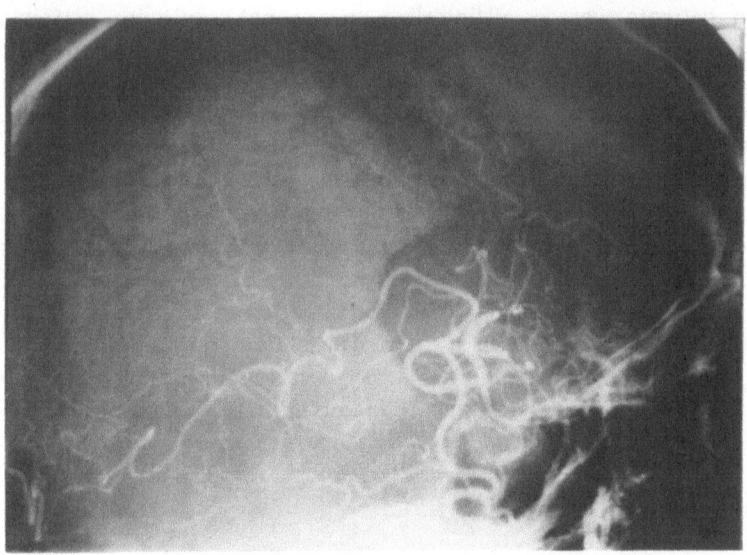

B

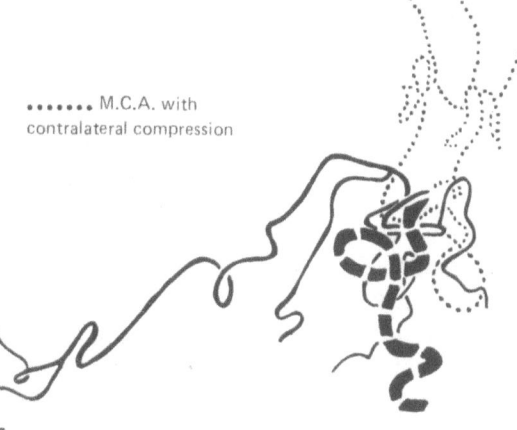

•••••• M.C.A. with
contralateral compression

C

Fig. 53-1. Possible extension of a temporal bypass.
A. Simple angiography. Note the lack of fronto-
opercular arteries. B. Angiography with compression of the contralateral angiography. Note the filling of fronto-opercular arteries. C. Drawing of
Fig. 53-1B.

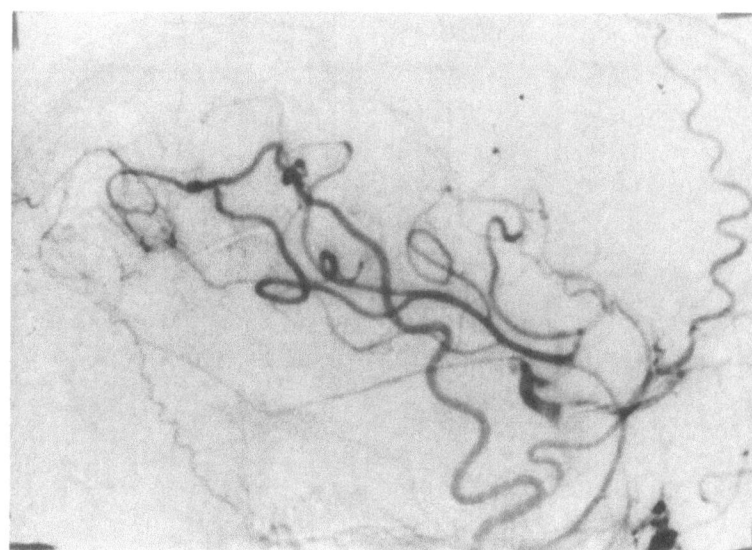

Fig. 53-2. Bypass in a case of siphon stenosis. Note the complete obliteration of the siphon 15 days after surgery.

severe deficit; we think that in some patients a bypass may help the recovery.

Third Question

Is the location of the bypass of any importance for the result or, on the contrary, is either cerebral artery able to ensure the same result, provided the bypass is patent?

It is striking that in most cases a bypass performed on a temporal cerebral artery spontaneously does not supply the fronto-opercular arteries, at least at the beginning. During the following months or years, the bypass usually enlarges and extends[1, 2] and may act as a communicating artery, as we have previously noticed. Thus, in case of transient ischemia, the choice of the cerebral artery may not be of great importance since the bypass works as a spare supply when needed.

In case of stroke, the answer may be different. The choice of the brain artery can possibly be of value. In our series, the improvement of patients seems to have been better in case of frontal or parietal bypass (Fig. 53-3) (of the 7 patients who presumably were improved by surgery, 5 had a bypass supplying the fronto-opercular arteries).

Furthermore, the next question raised by this statement is: Is a double bypass more useful than a single bypass in a patient with stroke? Despite a very small number of pa-

tients, good results seem to have been obtained in cases of double bypasses (Figs. 53-4, 53-5), especially when performed on frontal or parietal arteries (3 improvements out of 5).

Last Question

What is the place of bypass surgery in case of bilateral ischemic lesions: occlusion of one side and contralateral stenosis?

This is a rather frequent condition. In this condition, the cerebral blood flow may have low values in both hemispheres, and the hypothesis of an intracranial steal may arise. In such cases, we would perform a bypass on the side of the occluded carotid artery, whether the patient has a deficit or not. As shown on the CBF measurements, this bypass may be of some use in saving the blood flow coming from the stenotic carotid artery; furthermore, it may allow a safer treatment of this stenotic carotid artery.

Conclusion

Bypass surgery is nowadays routine. There are some arguments for its efficacy as protective surgery in case of transient or reversible ischemia. Its efficacy in case of stroke with hemiplegia is not so well acknowledged. In our opinion, the bypass surgery may be of some

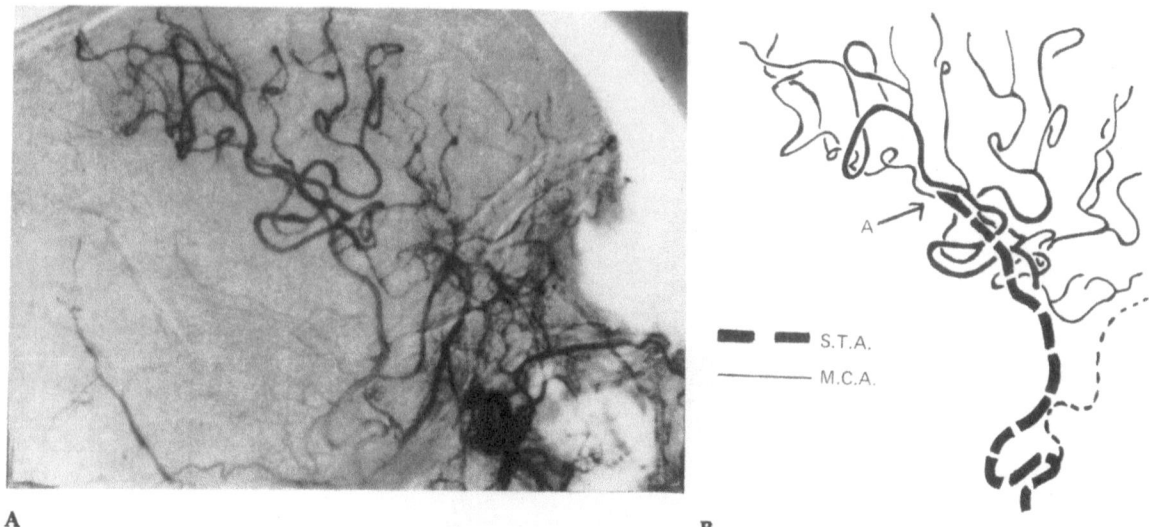

A   B

Fig. 53-3. A. Example of frontal bypass. B. Drawing of Fig. 53-3A.

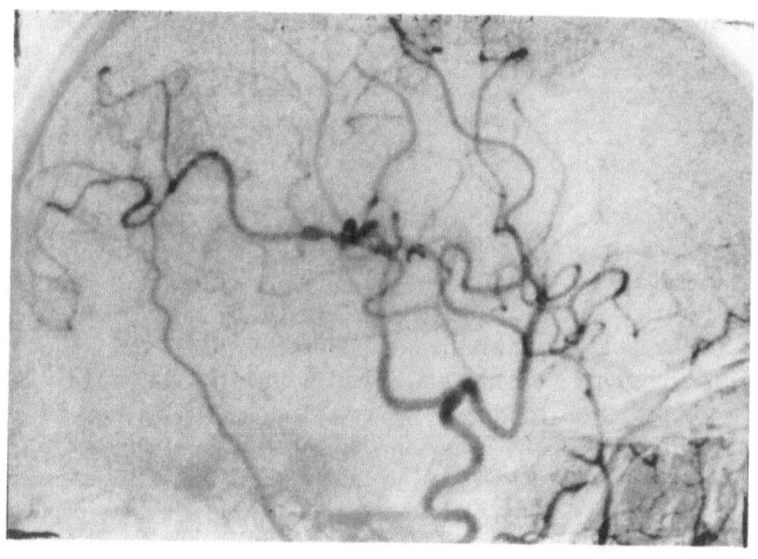

A

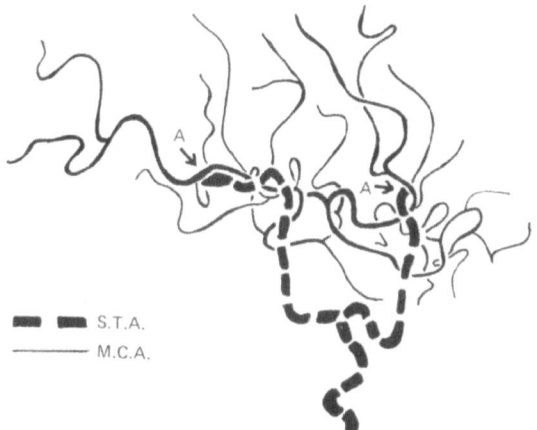

B

Fig. 53-4. A. Example of double bypass (frontal bypass and angular bypass). B. Drawing of Fig. 53-4A.

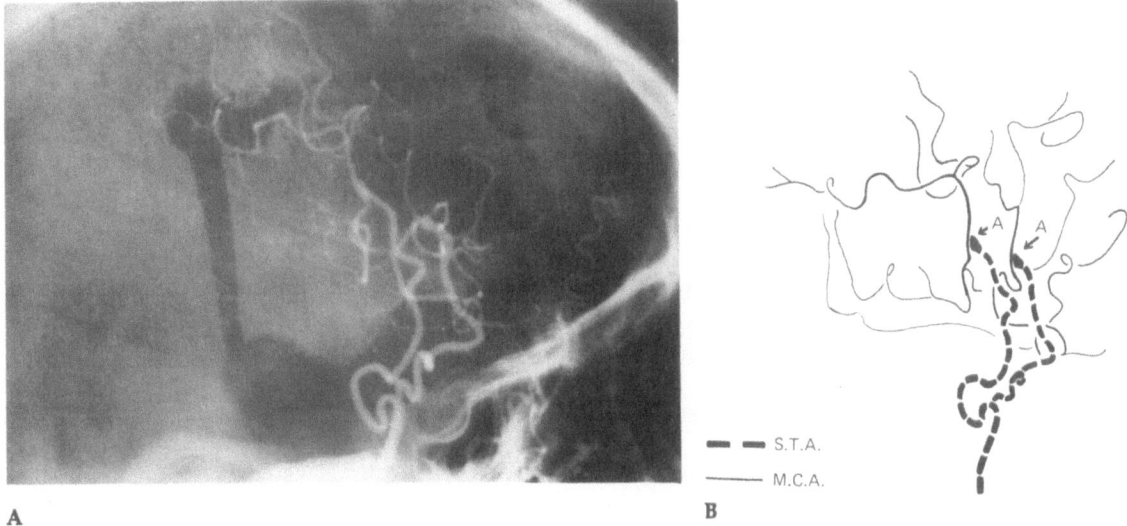

Fig. 53-5. A. Example of double frontal bypass. B. Drawing of Fig. 53-5A.

benefit for patients with hemiplegia; in such cases, the choice of the cortical artery could possibly be of some importance.

References

1. Anderson, R.E., Reichman, O.H., Davis, D.O. Radiological evaluation of temporal artery–middle cerebral artery anastomosis. Radiology 113:73–79, 1974.

2. Deruty, R., Duquesnel, J., Lecuire, J., Dechaume, J.P., Bret, P. L'anastomose extra–intracrânienne: correlations radio-cliniques. Neurochirurgie 22: 469–476, 1976.

3. Khodadad, G. Transient post-operative occlusion of the superficial temporal–middle cerebral artery branch anastomosis: spasm, swelling or thrombosis. Surg Neurol 3:341–345, 1975.

54

Microneurosurgical Arterial Bypass for Cerebral Ischemia: The San Francisco Experience

H. Maximilian Mehdorn, William F. Hoffman, and Norman L. Chater

At the last Symposium on Extracranial–Intracranial Anastomoses for Cerebral Ischemia in 1976,[16] our group presented our experience in a series of 140 patients[6] harboring vascular lesions that were otherwise inoperable or inaccessible. We would like—as Dr. Chater has put it—to "pause again and reflect on what has been factually accomplished, what is encouraging at the present time, and what are the problem areas awaiting solutions."

As microsurgical techniques have become more and more widespread, the extracranial-intracranial (EC–IC) bypass procedure has been applied with increasing frequency. At the present time, our series has increased to more than 200 patients operated on by N.L.C. Our attention will be focused on those 172 patients who have been followed for an average of 29.5 months, with a minimum of 6 months. These patients had reversible ischemic neurologic deficits due to atherosclerotic lesions in the area of the internal carotid artery; included are two patients who had fibromuscular hyperplasia and one who had vasculitis.

Indications

The indications for the EC–IC bypass that have been listed previously[6] remain essentially unchanged (Table 54-1). However, we have tried to evaluate the usefulness of surgical therapy as compared to the best available medical treatment—mainly aspirin. Since the cooperative study on EC–IC anastomoses was initiated only as of July 1977,[7] considerable time will elapse before its results become available. Therefore, a careful comparison of our series with those reported in the literature will be useful in giving a preliminary idea about the benefits and risks of this operative procedure.

Patient Population

The demographic breakdown of our series shows a male to female ratio of 137:35 (4:1), with an age range of 22 to 81 years. The average age is 59 years for the men, and 51 years for the women.

Table 54-1. Clinical presentation—Indications for EIAB (N = 172)

TIA	116*	
Stroke	55	
mild		15
moderate		17
severe		10
progressive		13
Prophylactic	1	
Seizures	3	

*18 patients with previous completed stroke and now having TIAs; 2 had previous stroke on opposite side.

The associated diseases and risk factors were hypertension and manifestation of atherosclerotic disease in other parts of the body, such as heart disease and peripheral vascular disease. This is the typical disease pattern encountered in all series of patients with cerebrovascular disease, both medical and surgical.

Table 54-2 compares the associated diseases in our patients with those in a series of patients undergoing carotid endarterectomy[15] and those in two series that studied the natural history of TIAs[1, 3] A similar pattern of associated diseases has been found in the Canadian cooperative study of aspirin and sulfinpyrazone in threatened stroke.[4]

Localization of Vascular Lesions

Except for palpation and auscultation of the cervical vessels, noninvasive diagnostic techniques were not used frequently in our series, but angiography was essential in obtaining precise localization of the suspected stenosis or occlusion. Unilateral internal carotid artery occlusion and multiple-vessel occlusion were responsible for cerebral ischemia in 114 of 172 patients; other lesions included unilateral internal carotid artery stenosis, bilateral carotid artery occlusion, and middle cerebral artery stenosis (Table 54-3).

Operation

The patients were operated on by N.L.C. using a modification of Yasargil's technique, described elsewhere.[13, 19]

Analysis of Results

TIA

A familiar difficulty in the analysis of TIA data is that there is no uniform opinion about the natural history of TIAs. In order to evaluate the risks and benefits of this surgical procedure, we compared our patients' results to those found in series of patients who progressed through a natural history of the disease, and to those in series of patients who underwent medical treatment. In these series, of the patients who experienced TIAs, 62%[2] to 76%[11] became free of TIAs; however, the latter series consisted of "chronic patients,"[18] and is not representative of our own patients. In our series of 114 patients who had TIAs, 85% had no further TIAs after EC–IC bypass surgery had been performed, and 12.3% had a marked reduction of TIA recurrence after operation (Fig. 54-1). The risk of subsequent stroke after TIA is estimated at approximately 30%[17] as compared to 5.3% in our series (Fig. 54-2). The

Table 54-2. Coexisting risk factors (in % of patients) and associated diseases in different series

Risk factors	N = 172 (present series)	N = 49[15]	N = 79[3]	N = 367[1]
Hypertension	61	31	63	63
Heart disease	40	51	41	54 (ECG)
angina	15			
post MI	14	30	32	
arrhythmia	11		3	
other (not specified)			6	
Peripheral vascular disease	20	51	11	9
Diabetes mellitus	18	14	6	2.7 men
				3.8 women
History of peptic ulcer	19		20	
Hyperlipidemia	7			
Hypercholesterolemia	3.5			

Table 54-3. Angiographic presentation (N = 172)

BICO	13	
UICO	70	(2 with fibromuscular hyperplasia)
UICS	23	
high cervical	3	
siphon	19	
supraclinoidal	1	
MCAO	8	
MCAS	13	
MVO	44	(1 with vasculitis)
CCO	1	

BICO = bilateral internal carotid artery occlusion; UICO = unilateral internal carotid artery occlusion; UICS = unilateral internal carotid artery stenosis; MCAO = middle cerebral artery occlusion; MCAS = middle cerebral artery stenosis; MVO = multiple vessel occlusion; CCO = common carotid occlusion.

mortality rate for patients following a natural course after TIAs is 14.1%.[2] This must be compared to a 3.5% mortality in our series, which includes the operative mortality occurring to one month after surgery (2.6%), and the death of one patient occurring at a later date as a result of massive gastrointestinal bleeding (Fig. 54-3).

Since it is thought that aspirin is the best available medical for TIAs,[9] we compared our surgically achieved results to those reported in the American aspirin (AITIA) study.[8] Although TIA recurrence is slightly higher in surgically treated patients, the difference is not statistically significant. The difference between the effects of aspirin and the EC–IC bypass with respect to cerebral or retinal infarction or death is more impressive: 14.8% in the AITIA study, as compared to 3.6% (Figs. 54-4, 54-5).

Stroke

Thus far, we have considered only the effect of therapy on TIAs. Now, we will give a brief look at the data available for patients who had suffered a stroke. Of 55 patients who were operated on for stroke, 45 (81.8%) improved, as compared to 66% of patients whose course followed a natural history[2] (Fig. 54-6). The mortality rate for untreated patients is 25.6% after a single stroke and 49.2% after multiple

strokes.[2] In our group of 55 patients who had suffered a stroke, 7.3% died during an average follow-up time of 29.5 months. This figure includes the operative mortality of 3.6% (Fig. 54-7). The data concerning stroke recurrence vary from 20% recurrence within 5 years[12] to 53% within 2 years.[10] Therefore, it is difficult to say whether or not the smaller stroke recurrence rate of 7.3% in our series is significantly different (Fig. 54-8). To our knowledge, no reliable data are available concerning stroke recurrence under medical therapy.

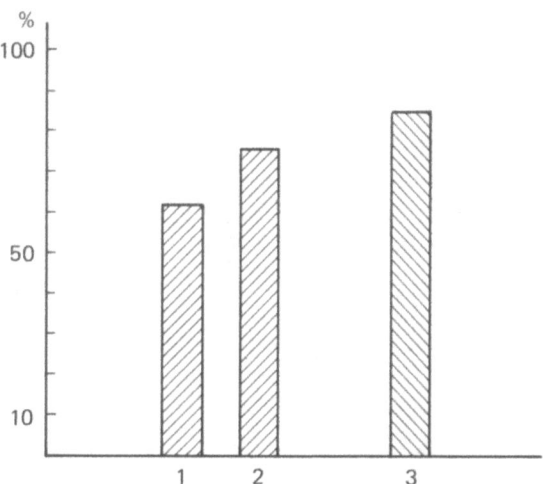

Fig. 54-1. Patients having experienced TIA who became free of TIA. (1) Natural history: follow-up 36 months.[2] (2) Natural history: follow-up 12 months.[11] (3) After EIAB: follow-up 29.5 months (our series; N = 114).

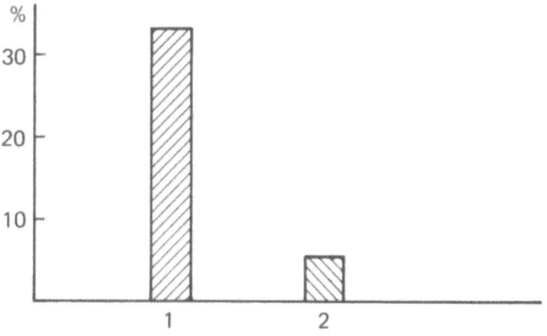

Fig. 54-2. Development of stroke after TIA. (1) Natural history.[17] (2) After EIAB (our series; N = 114).

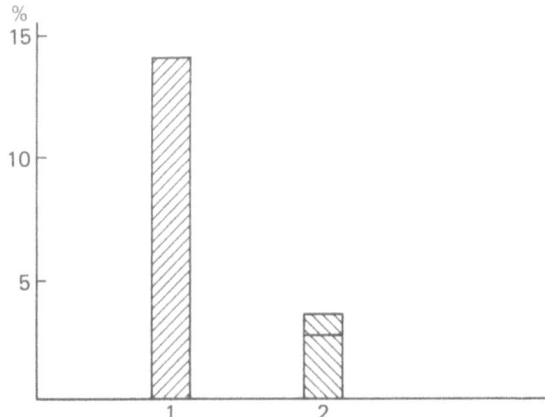

Fig. 54-3. Mortality in patients with TIA. (1) Natural history.[2] (2) After EIAB (our series; N = 114).

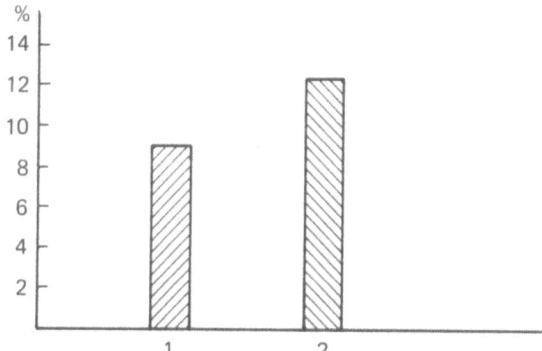

Fig. 54-4. TIA frequency under therapy. (1) Aspirin (N = 88).[8] (2) EIAB (our series; N = 112).

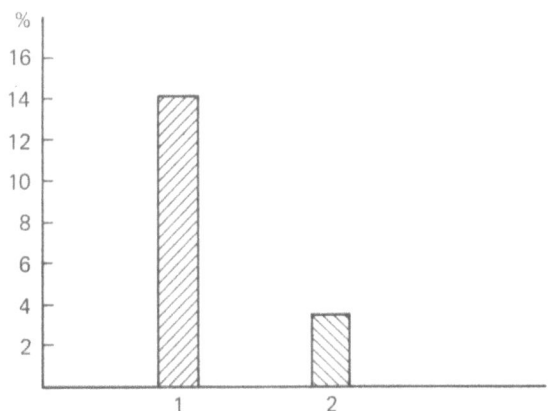

Fig. 54-5. Patients reaching "endpoints" under therapy. (1) Aspirin (N = 88).[8] (2) EIAB (our series; N = 112).

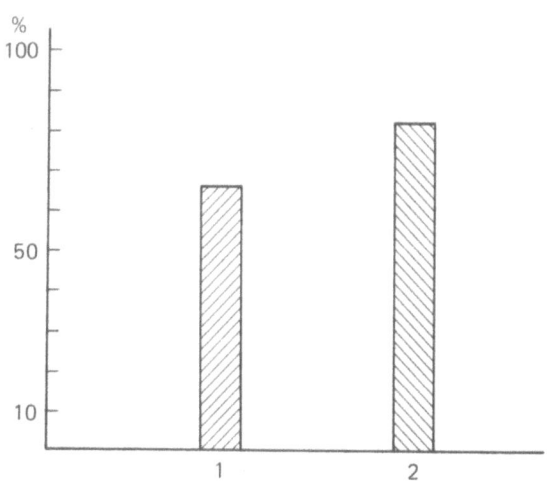

Fig. 54-6. Improvement after stroke. (1) Natural history.[2] (2) After EIAB (our series; N = 55).

Stroke in Evolution

In our series, 13 patients were operated on for stroke in evolution; 11 of them (83%) improved postoperatively; one survived with his deficit stabilized; and one, a 75-year-old patient, died of massive gastrointestinal bleeding 2 weeks after surgery (mortality rate, 7.6%). These data must be compared to those available from the control group in Meyer's series, in which improvement was seen in 58% of patients, and a mortality rate of 11% was found[14] (Fig. 54-9). In Carter's series of selected patients treated with anticoagulants, improvement was noted in 41% of patients; the mortality rate was 5%.[5] In Meyer's series, however, the mortality rate for treated patients was 35%, and improvement was noted in

43%. It is probably safe to say that the EC–IC bypass procedure is more effective than medical therapy in treating patients who have stroke in evolution. It also appears that the EC–IC procedure involves the same or a smaller risk than medical therapy.

Discussion

After this evaluation of the effect of the EC–IC bypass on cerebral ischemia, we conclude with

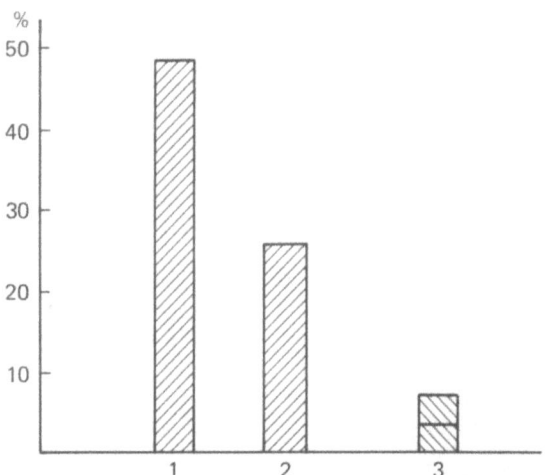

Fig. 54-7. Mortality after stroke. (1) Natural history after multiple strokes.[2] (2) Natural history after a single stroke.[2] (3) After EIAB (our series; N = 55).

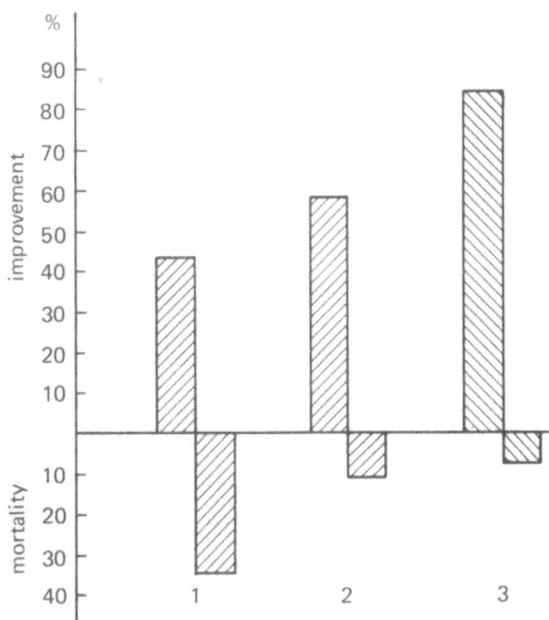

Fig. 54-9. Stroke in evolution. (1) Thrombolytic therapy.[14] (2) Natural history.[14] (3) After EIAB (our series; N = 13).

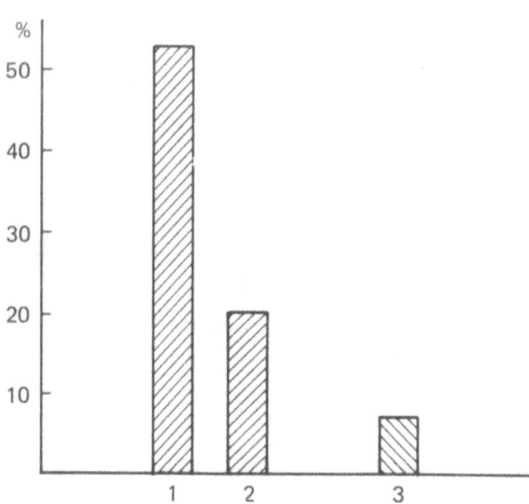

Fig. 54-8. Recurrence of stroke. (1) Natural history within 2 years.[10] (2) Natural history within 5 years.[12] (3) After EIAB within 29.5 months (our series; N = 55).

a brief look at the complications of this operation. If the long listing in Table 54-4 is somewhat overwhelming, it is because it includes all the complications that occurred during the early phase of our series. Variations of the preoperative care and diagnostic evaluation, modification of the details of the surgical procedure, a decrease in our operating time to 2.5 to 3

hours (including the time required for occlusion of the cortical vessel), and variations of the postoperative care all reduced the risk of the surgical procedure and the operative mortality remarkably, to the point that only one operative death occurred in our last 100 cases. Despite the complications we have encountered, the overall success of this operation has led us to perform the EC–IC bypass more willingly in patients who are considered high risks.

After analyzing those patients in our series who died after the EC–IC bypass operation, those who suffered cerebral infarction, and those who continued to have TIAs, we feel that it may be beneficial to:

1) Perform a bilateral bypass in a greater number of cases for patients who have generalized low-perfusion syndrome.

2) Use low doses of heparin intraoperatively and postoperatively in patients who have high-grade stenosis of the cerebral vessels.

3) Use aspirin in treating patients who experience TIAs after the bypass.

The experience gained from our series leads us to suggest that:

1) The EC–IC bypass is more effective than

Table 54-4. Temporary complications (N = 172)

Transient neurologic dysfunction	35	
Cerebral edema	2	
Seizures	5	
Subdural hematoma	5	(2 requiring operation; no sequelae)
Subdural hygroma	2	(2 requiring operation; no sequelae)
Subgaleal fluid collection	2	
Scalp ischemia (no surgery required)	4	
Stitch abscess	1	
Hypertensive crisis	2	
Pulmonary emboli	1	
Pulmonary edema	1	
UTI	10	
Aspiration pneumonia	1	
Cardiac arrhythmia	3	
Hepatitis	1	
Pancreatitis	1	
Bronchitis	2	
Gastritis	1	
Unexplained hypotension	1	
Myocardial infarction	1	

medical treatment in preventing the development of permanent neurologic deficit after a series of TIAs.

2) The EC–IC bypass is more effective than medical therapy in the treatment of stroke, although statistical evaluation is difficult.

3) The EC–IC bypass is more effective than medical therapy in the treatment of stroke in evolution.

4) The risks involved in the EC–IC bypass are comparable to those of aspirin therapy.

5) The EC–IC bypass is as effective as aspirin in preventing the recurrence of TIAs, although this will not be its major application. At a later date, it will be interesting to compare the results of our series with those of the ongoing cooperative EC–IC bypass study, and to evaluate further the efficacy of EC–IC bypass surgery.

References

1. Acheson, E.J. Factors affecting the natural history of "focal cerebral vascular disease." Q J Med 40:25, 1971.

2. Acheson, E.J., Hutchinson, E.C. The natural history of focal cerebral vascular disease. Q J Med 40:157, 1971.

3. Baker, R.N. Prospective study of transient ischemic attacks. In Seventh Princeton Conference on Cerebrovascular Disease, J. Moossy, and R. Janeway, editors, Grune and Stratton, New York, 1970, pp 166–169.

4. Canadian Cooperative Study Group. A randomized trial of aspirin and sulfinpyrazone in threatened stroke. N Engl J Med (in press).

5. Carter, A.B. Progressing stroke. Anticoagulant therapy. In Cerebral Vascular Diseases (Transactions of the Third Conference of the American Neurological Association and the American Heart Association), H.C. Millikan, R.G. Siekert, and J.P. Whisnant, editors, Grune and Stratton, New York, 1961, pp 151–156.

6. Chater, N.L., Weinstein, P.R., Spetzler, R.F. Microvascular bypass for cerebral ischemia—An overview, 1966–1976. In Microsurgery for Stroke, P. Schmiedek, editor, Springer-Verlag, New York, 1977, pp 79–88.

7. Cooperative Study of Extracranial/Intracranial Arterial Anastomosis Research Protocol, 1977.

8. Fields, W.S., Lemak, N.A., Frankowski, R.F., Hardy, R.J. Controlled trial of aspirin in cerebral ischemia. Stroke 83:301, 1977.

9. Genton, E., Barnett, H.J.M., Field, W.S., Gent, M., Hoak, J.C. XIV. Cerebral ischemia: The role of thrombosis and of antithrombotic therapy, Study group on antithrombotic therapy. Stroke 8:150, 1977.

10. Hutchinson, E.C., Acheson, E.J. Strokes. Natural History, Pathology and Treatment. W.B. Saunders, Philadelphia, 1975.

11. Marshall, J. The natural history of transient ischemic cerebrovascular attacks. Q J Med 33:309, 1964.

12. Matsumoto, N., Whisnant, J.P., Kurland, L.T., Okazaki, H. Natural history of stroke in Rochester, Minnesota, 1955–1969. An extension of a previous study, 1945–1954. Stroke 4:20, 1973.

13. Mehdorn, H.M., Hoffman, W.F., Chater, N.L. Microvascular neurosurgical arterial bypass for cerebral ischemia: A decade of development. World J Surg (in press).

14. Meyer, J.S., Gilroy, J., Barnhart, M.E. Therapeutic thrombolysis in cerebral thromboembolism: Randomized evaluation of intravenous streptokinase. In Cerebrovascular Diseases, Fourth Princeton Conference, P.R. Siekert, and J.P. Whisnant, editors, Grune and Stratton, New York, 1965, pp 200–213.

15. Moore, W.S., Hall, A.D. Importance of emboli from carotid bifurcation in pathogenesis of cerebral ischemic attacks. Arch Surg 101: 708, 1970.

16. Schmiedek, P. (ed.) Microsurgery for Stroke, Springer-Verlag, New York, 1977.

17. Toole, J.F. Management of transient ischemic attacks. In Cerebrovascular Diseases, 10th Princeton Conference, P. Scheinberg, editor, Raven Press, New York, 1976, pp 23–30.

18. Toole, J.F. Management of TIA's and acute cerebral infarction. Adv Neurol 16:71–80, 1977.

19. Yasargil, M.G. Microsurgery Applied to Neurosurgery, Academic Press, New York, 1969, pp 95–119.

55

STA–MCA Anastomosis: Further Analysis of Long-Term Results— A Neurologist's View

Myoung C. Lee, James I. Ausman, Fernando G. Diaz, Arthur C. Klassen, and Richard E. Latchaw

The superficial temporal artery (STA) to middle cerebral artery (MCA) anastomosis is being widely used in increasing numbers for patients with ischemic occlusive cerebrovascular disease in whom carotid endarterectomy is not technically feasible. The definite beneficial value of this procedure is yet to be determined, although information to date has been generally supportive.[4, 5, 7, 10] The results of multinational, multicenter cooperative study of STA–MCA anastomosis will not be available for several years. The purpose of this report is to update the long-term clinical results in our continuing follow-up study of the STA–MCA anastomosis of our first 40 patients with cerebral ischemia or infarction in the internal carotid artery distribution.

Materials and Methods

The study method, clinical protocols, and perioperative complications were in part previously described.[5] An independent neurologist examined and recorded the patients' pre- and postoperative medical and neurologic histories and objective neurologic findings. Of 32 men and 8 women with a median age of 56 years (range 27 to 71 years), 6 were diagnosed as having transient ischemic attacks (TIA), 22 as having had mild cerebral infarction with or without prior history of TIA or prolonged reversible ischemic neurologic deficit (PRIND)

but with mild neurologic deficits at the time of inclusion for the study, and 12 as having had moderately severe cerebral infarctions (Table 55-1). Two of six patients with TIAs exhibited amaurosis fugax as the only manifestation of cerebrovascular disease. Patients with severe neurologic deficits such as severe global aphasia and/or dementia, depressed sensorium, or complete paralysis with inability to ambulate even with assistance were excluded from the study.

The angiographic abnormalities in decreasing order of occurrence in these patients were (Table 55-2): unilateral internal carotid artery occlusion, 60%; bilateral internal carotid artery occlusion, 23%; multiple artery occlusions in internal carotid artery distribution, 10%; inoperable internal artery (ICA) or MCA stenosis or occlusion, 7%. There was no correlation between the types and severities of ischemic cerebrovascular disease and those of angiographic abnormalities.

Coexistent risk factors for cerebrovascular disease were quite common (Table 55-3). Although significant, these risk factors were not judged to be contraindications for the STA–MCA procedure. The median time between the patients' last ischemic episodes and their STA–MCA procedures was 2 months, ranging from 2 weeks to 40 months (Table 55-4). Neurologic deficits were thus considered stable for the time of the procedures. In three patients whose waiting period before the procedures was greater than 6 months (range, 10 to 40 months), the angiographic findings revealed the presence

Table 55-1. Clinical diagnosis and age distribution

Clinical diagnosis	Patients no.	Median age (years)	Age range (years)
TIA*	6	50	29–65
Mild cerebral infarction with/without TIAs or PRINDs**	22	57	33–71
Moderate to moderately severe cerebral infarction with/without TIAs or PRINDs	12	55	38–69
Total	40	56	29–71

*Transient ischemic attack.
**Prolonged reversible ischemic neurologic deficit.

Table 55-2. Clinical diagnosis vs. preoperative angiographic abnormalities

Angiographic abnormalities	Clinical diagnosis (No. patients)			
	TIA	Mild cerebral infarction	Moderate to moderately severe cerebral infarction	Total
Internal carotid artery occlusion(s)				
Unilateral	3	13	12	24 (60%)
Bilateral	1	6	2	9 (23%)
Inoperable ICA or MCA stenosis or occlusion(s)	1	2	—	3 (7%)
Multiple artery occlusions	1	1	2	4 (10%)
Total	6	22	12	40 (100%)

ICA = internal carotid artery; MCA = middle cerebral artery.

Table 55-3. Frequency of significant cerebrovascular risk factors

Risk factors	Frequency
Smoking	32 (80%)
Hypertension	23 (58%)
Obesity	11 (28%)
Myocardial infarction	10 (25%)
Hyperlipidemia	7 (18%)
Peripheral vascular disease	6 (15%)
Diabetes mellitus	4 (10%)

of bilateral ICA occlusions with inadequate angiographic evidence of collateralization. In another patient whose waiting period was unclear, angiographic findings were consistent with moyamoya disease with multiple arterial occlusions.

Results

The procedure was performed by the same surgeon in all cases. There was no operative mortality. Perioperative complication rate was minimal; one patient developed chest pain diagnosed as mild subendocardial infarction, which cleared. One patient developed subdural hematoma 48 hours after operation, which was evacuated with no residual deficit. Transient atrial fibrillation developed 10 hours after operation in one patient. The median duration of follow-up for all patients was 22 months, ranging from 2 to 42 months (Table 55-5).

Considering the episodes of amaurosis fugax, TIAs in these patients before and after surgery revealed a striking reduction in the frequency of recurrent episodes (Table 55-6). Preoperatively, nine patients had one ischemic episode,

Table 55-4. Time between last event and bypass

Time (months)	Diagnosis TIA	Mild stroke	Moderate stroke	Total
< 1	3 (50%)	4 (18%)	— —	7 (17.5%)
1–2	1 (17%)	10 (45%)	7 (58%)	18 (45.0%)
3–6	1 (17%)	7 (32%)	3 (25%)	11 (27.5%)
> 6	1 (17%)	1 (5%)	1 (8%)	3 (7.5%)
Unknown	— —	— —	1 (8%)	1 (2.5%)
Total	6 (100%)	22 (100%)	12 (100%)	40 (100%)
Median	0.75	1.5	2	2
Range	0.25–10	0.25–11	1–40	0.25–40

Table 55-5. Duration of follow-up—all patients

Duration of follow-up (months)	Clinical diagnosis TIA	Mild stroke	Moderate stroke	Total
≤ 6	— —	2 (9%)	— —	2 (5.0%)
7–12	1 (17%)	2 (9%)	4 (33%)	7 (17.5%)
13–24	1 (17%)	11 (50%)	3 (25%)	15 (37.5%)
25–36	4 (67%)	6 (27%)	2 (17%)	12 (30.0%)
37–42	— —	1 (5%)	3 (25%)	4 (10.0%)
Total	6 (100%)	22 (100%)	12 (100%)	40 (100%)
Median	27	21	21	21.5
Range	8–35	2–41	8–42	2–42

Table 55-6. Frequency of pre- and postoperative ischemia and/or infarction

	Postoperative None	One	Total
1	9	0	9
2–3	15	1*	16
4–5	4	1**	5
> 5	8	2***	10
Total	36	4	40

*TIA.
**PRIND.
***One amaurosis fugax; one amaurosis.

21 patients up to 5, and ten patients more than 5 such episodes. During the follow-up period for up to 42 months, four experienced ischemic events: one TIA, one PRIND, one amaurosis fugax, and one amaurosis. TIA occurred in the form of expressive aphasia approximately 3 months after the procedure in a patient with prior history of multiple TIAs superimposed on one moderately severe completed cerebral infarction. PRIND occurred in a patient who also had multiple TIAs and one episode of mild completed infarction approximately 10 months after the procedure. A single episode of amaurosis fugax and amaurosis occurred within 2 months after the operation in both patients who had multiple episodes of amaurosis fugax prior to the operation. No patient suffered from recurrent cerebral infarction with persistent focal deficit during the entire follow-up period. Thirty-six patients remained episode free.

Our neurologic findings during the follow-up examinations were graded from 0 to 5, 5 indicating total disability (being unable to walk even with assistance) (Table 55-7). Neurologic examinations in all patients remained unchanged or improved. All six patients with TIA

Table 55-7. Objective neurologic deficit before and after STA–MCA anastomosis (no. patients)

Clinical diagnosis	Preoperative	Postoperative		
		Worse	No change	Improved
Mild cerebral infarction	22	—	8	14
Moderate to moderately severe cerebral infarction	12	—	5	7
Total	34	0	13	21

Table 55-8. Deaths during follow-up period

Name	Type of cerebrovascular disease	Time after operation	Age of death	Cause of death	Significant medical diseases prior to operation
L.H.	Mild cerebral infarction	30 months	47	Acute MI*	MI
J.D.	TIA	18 months	55	Respiratory failure	Chronic obstructive pulmonary disease
E.E.	Moderate cerebral infarction	11 months	57	Probable MI	MI, peripheral vascular disease
G.H.	Mild cerebral infarction	5 months	58	Acute MI	Pulmonary emphysema, peripheral vascular disease
F.C.	Moderate cerebral infarction	27 months	59	Acute MI	MI, hypertension
H.L.	Mild cerebral infarction	18 months	67	Acute MI	MI, hypertension, peripheral vascular disease

*MI = myocardial infarction.

remained normal. In twenty-two patients with mild cerebral infarction, neurologic findings were improved in fourteen and unchanged in eight. In twelve patients with moderately severe cerebral infarctions, neurologic findings were improved in seven and unchanged in five.

Postoperative angiograms were obtained in 38 of 40 patients with 97% patency of the anastomosis. A reference is made to the detailed discussion by Doctors Latchaw and Ausman elsewhere in this volume.

There were six deaths during the follow-up period, five of which were attributed to acute myocardial infarction (Table 55-8). In four of these five patients, there was prior history of myocardial infarction. Another patient died from chronic obstructive pulmonary disease. With the exception of one patient who developed amaurosis 2 months after surgery, the neurologic status of these patients was stable at the time of their deaths.

Comments

In this well-defined patient population with cerebral ischemia or infarction in the internal carotid artery distribution who had undergone STA–MCA anastomosis and were followed up to 3½ years, no patient developed recurrent completed cerebral infarction. There was also a striking reduction in the frequency of recurrent TIAs and there was an objective clinical neurologic improvement in most of the patients who had had neurologic deficits prior to the operation. Previous studies on the natural history of TIAs and cerebral infarction have shown the incidence of completed cerebral infarction to be 10% in one year[6, 9] and approximately 50% in 4 to 5 years.[1, 8] In a study of 359 patients by Fields and Lemak,[8] 25% of survivors from acute internal carotid artery occlusion developed recurrent stroke in 44 months, 70% of which were ipsilateral to the occlusion. Aspirin was found to significantly reduce the risks for recurrent stroke or death only in men,[2] and no other agent is of proven efficacy in preventing recurrent strokes.

These preliminary data in our continuing follow-up study are indicative of probable beneficial value of the STA–MCA anastomosis in a group of patients with cerebral ischemia or infarction in ICA distribution in preventing recurrent cerebral infarction. Improvement in neurologic deficits could still be related to the natural course of cerebral infarction, although there was a median duration of 2 months between last ischemic episode and the STA–MCA anastomosis. These patients are continuing to be followed on a regular basis, and more definite conclusions will become available in 2 to 3 years. In spite of careful selection, there were six deaths, all related to cardiopulmonary disorders, which point out the importance of ischemic systemic risk factors for cerebrovascular disease, especially cardiac disease, in consideration of this surgical procedure and also overall management of such patients.

References

1. Acheson, J., Hutchinson, E.C. Observations on the natural history of transient cerebral ischemia. Lancet 2:871, 1964.

2. Canadian Cooperative Study Group. A randomized trial of aspirin and sulfinpyrazone in threatened stroke. N Engl J Med 299:53–59, 1978.

3. Fields, W.S., Lemak, N.A. Joint study of extracranial arterial occlusion: X. Internal carotid artery occlusion. JAMA 235:2734–2738, 1976.

4. Gratz, D., Schmiedek, P., Spetzler, R., et al. Clinical experience with extracranial arterial anastomosis in 65 cases. J Neurosurg 44:313–324, 1976.

5. Lee, M.C., Ausman, J.I., Geiger, J.D., et al. Superficial temporal to middle cerebral artery anastomosis: Clinical outcome in patients with ischemia or infarction in internal carotid artery distribution. Arch Neurol 36:1–4, 1979.

6. Pearce, J.M.S., Gubbay, S.S., Walton, J.N. Long term therapy in transient cerebral ischemic attacks. Lancet 1:6, 1965.

7. Reichman, O.H. Neurosurgical microsurgical anastomosis for cerebral ischemia: Five years' experience. In Cerebrovascular Diseases, Tenth Princeton Conference, P. Scheinberg, editor, Raven Press, New York, 1976, pp 311–330.

8. Siekert, R.G., Whisnant, J.P., Millikan, C.H. Surgical and anticoagulant therapy of occlusive cerebrovascular disease. Ann Intern Med 58:637, 1963.

9. Whisnant, J., Matsumoto, N., Elveback, L. Transient cerebral ischemic attacks in a community: Rochester, Minnesota 1955–1969. Mayo Clin Proc 48:194–198, 1973.

10. Yasargil, M. G., Yonekawa, Y. Results of microsurgical extra–intracranial arterial bypass in the treatment of cerebral ischemia. Neurosurgery 1:22–24, 1977.

Index